Special Contributors

James S. Newman, MD
Associate Professor
Internal Medicine
University of Texas Medical Branch
Galveston, Texas

Francis B. Quinn Jr., MD, FACS
Seinsheimer Professor of Otolaryngology
Professor of Pathology
University of Texas Medical Branch
Galveston, Texas

Additional Reviewers

Jack B. Anon, MD
Brian W. Blakley, MD
Deborah Carlson, PhD
Edgar L. Chiossone, MD
Keith F. Clark, MD
Gary L. Clayman, MD, DDS
Robert A. Dobie, MD
W. Jarrard Goodwin, MD
Earl H. Harley, MD

Samuel T. Kuna, MD
Samuel A. Mickelson, MD
Richard T. Miyamoto, MD
J. David Osguthorpe, MD
Samuel H. Selesnick, MD
Clough Shelton, MD
Maisie L. Shindo, MD
David M. Vernick, MD
Peak Woo, MD

Contributors

Ronald G. Amedee, MD
Professor and Chairman
Department of Otolaryngology–Head and
    Neck Surgery
Tulane University Health Sciences Center
New Orleans, Louisiana

Darryk W. Barlow, MD, FACS
Assistant Clinical Professor
Otolaryngology Clinic
Yakima, Washington;
University of Washington School of Medicine
Department of Otolaryngology–Head and
    Neck Surgery
Seattle, Washington

Donald J. Beasley, MD
St. Luke's Medical Center
Mercy Medical Center
Nampa, Idaho

Elizabeth A. Blair, MD
Walter Reed Army Medical Center
Washington, DC

Kenneth B. Briskin, MD
Assistant Clinical Professor of
    Otolaryngology
University of Pennsylvania;
Associate Clinical Professor of
    Otolaryngology
Temple University
Philadelphia, Pennsylvania

John W. Cavo Jr., MD
Clinical Assistant Professor
Department of Surgery
University of Connecticut School of Medicine and Dentistry
New Britain, Connecticut

Brian P. Driscoll, MD
The Ear, Nose, Throat and Plastic Surgery Associates
Orlando, Florida

David E. Eibling, MD, FACS
Professor of Otolaryngology–Head and Neck Surgery
Department of Otolaryngology
University of Pittsburgh;
VA Pittsburgh Healthcare System
Pittsburgh, Pennsylvania

D. Gregory Farwell, MD
Assistant Professor
Department of Otolaryngology–Head and Neck Surgery
University of Washington
Seattle, Washington

Gerard J. Gianoli, MD, FACS
Clinical Associate Professor
Tulane University School of Medicine
New Orleans, Louisiana

Lyon L. Gleich, MD
Associate Professor
Department of Otolaryngology–Head and Neck Surgery
University of Cincinnati Medical Center
Cincinnati, Ohio

David A. Godin, MD
Clinical Instructor
Department of Otolaryngology–Head and Neck Surgery
New York Eye and Ear Infirmary
New York Medical College
St. Vincent's Hospital
New York, New York

Steven M. Houser, MD, FAAOA
Assistant Professor of Otolaryngology
Case Western Reserve University College of Medicine
Cleveland, Ohio

Thomas Hummel, MD
Department of Pharmacology
University of Erlangen
Nuremberg, Germany

Mark A. Jabor, MD
Chief Resident
Tulane School of Medicine
Department of Otolaryngology
New Orleans, Louisiana

Michael Knecht, MD
Department of Otorhinolaryngology
University of Dresden Medical School
Dresden, Germany

Karen M. Kost, MD
Assistant Professor of Otolaryngology
Director, Voice Laboratory
McGill University
Montreal, Canada

J. David Kriet, MD
Assistant Professor
Director, Facial Plastic and Reconstructive Surgery
Department of Otolaryngology–Head and Neck Surgery
University of Kansas Medical Center;
Clinical Assistant Professor
Department of Surgery
University of Missouri School of Medicine at Kansas City
Kansas City, Kansas

Richard L. Mabry, MD
Professor
Department of Otolaryngology–Head and Neck Surgery
University of Texas–Southwestern Medical Center
Dallas, Texas

Eric L. Mansfield, MD
Wolmac Army Medical Center
Fayetteville, North Carolina

Peter J. Martin, MD
Director, Surgical Services
Naval Medical Center, San Diego
San Diego, California

Andrew J. Miller, MD
Edison, New Jersey

Craig S. Murakami, MD, FACS
Virginia Mason Medical Center
Clinical Associate Professor
University of Washington
Seattle, Washington

Thomas Murry, PhD
Professor of Otolaryngology
University of Pittsburgh Eye and Ear Institute
Pittsburgh, Pennsylvania

Andrew J. Nemechek, MD
Assistant Professor
Department of Otolaryngology–Head and
  Neck Surgery
Tulane University School of Medicine;
Chief, Section for Head and Neck Cancer
Tulane Cancer Center
New Orleans, Louisiana

Eric F. Pinczower, MD
Clinical Associate Professor
University of Washington
Bellevue, Washington

Karen T. Pitman, MD, FACS
Assistant Professor
Department of Otolaryngology
St. Louis University
St. Louis, Missouri

Randall L. Plant, MD
Assistant Professor
Department of Otolaryngology–Head and
  Neck Surgery
Eastern Virginia Medical School
Norfolk, Virginia

Gregory N. Postma, MD
Assistant Professor
Department of Otolaryngology
Wake Forest University School of Medicine;
Center for Voice Disorders
Wake Forest University
Winston-Salem, North Carolina

Gregory W. Randolph, MD
Director, General ENT Service and Thyroid
  Surgical Clinic
Massachusetts Eye and Ear Infirmary
Boston, Massachusetts

Clark A. Rosen, MD
Assistant Professor of Otolaryngology
University of Pittsburgh Medical Center
Pittsburgh, Pennsylvania

James D. Smith, MD
Visiting Professor of Otolaryngology
National University of Singapore
Singapore

Paul M. Spring, MD
Chandler Medical Center
Lexington, Kentucky

J. Gregory Staffel, MD, FACS
Shea Ear Clinic
Memphis, Tennessee

Thomas A. Tami, MD
Professor of Otolaryngology
Department of Otolaryngology–Head and
  Neck Surgery
University of Cincinnati College of Medicine
Cincinnati, Ohio

Luke K.S. Tan, MD
Associate Professor of Otolaryngology
Department of Otolaryngology
National University of Singapore
National University Hospital
Singapore

Jon K. Thiringer, DO
Chairman, Executive Committee of the
  Medical Staff
Vice Chair, Department of Otolaryngology–
  Head and Neck Surgery
Naval Medical Center
San Diego, California

Diana N. Traquina, MD
Director, Pediatric Otolaryngology
Robert Wood Johnson University Hospital
New Brunswick, New Jersey

Foreword

Expert Guide to Otolaryngology was prepared by the Core Otolaryngology Education Faculty of the American Academy of Otolaryngology–Head and Neck Surgery Foundation in collaboration with faculty of the American College of Physicians–American Society of Internal Medicine in an effort to provide the internist and primary care physician with a handy, user-friendly, and informative reference for the management of patients with diseases of the ear, nose, and throat.

It has been estimated that approximately one third of visits to primary care physicians are related to the diagnosis and management of conditions that affect the head and neck, particularly those of the ear, nose, and throat. *Expert Guide to Otolaryngology* has been designed to assist internists in the evaluation and administration of first-line therapy for these patients and to act as a guide for referral when tertiary intervention or surgery is required. On behalf of the Continuing Education Advisory Committee and the Board of Directors of the American Academy of Otolaryngology–Head and Neck Surgery Foundation, we are proud to present this text to you.

Jack L. Gluckman, MD
President
American Academy of Otolaryngology–Head and Neck Surgery/Foundation

Jonas T. Johnson, MD
Coordinator for Continuing Education
American Academy of Otolaryngology–Head and Neck Surgery Foundation

Preface

Because there is no medical specialty that practices independently, interdisciplinary cooperation in the management of most illnesses is the key to ensuring optimal outcomes for afflicted patients. The development of new insights into disease processes, the advances in pharmacology and technology, and changes in the strategies for diagnosis and treatment all mandate formal and informal consultation between specialists. This consultation is an integral part of all practices and becomes even more critical as the complexity of diagnosis and treatment increases.

The relationship between otolaryngologists and internists is a prime example of this interdependence and is the driving force behind this book. Most adult patients who present to an otolaryngologist also suffer from another medical illness, and the management of their primary diseases may be affected dramatically by this comorbidity. Consultation with a patient's internist is often crucial in determining the optimal treatment strategy. In a similar vein, patients often present to their internist with complaints referable to the head and neck, and consultation with an otolaryngologist may be necessary to ensure the best outcome. The American Academy of Otolaryngology–Head and Neck Surgery Foundation (AAO-HNSF) and the American College of Physicians–American Society of Internal Medicine (ACP-ASIM) have joined forces to produce *Expert Guide to Otolaryngology*, which details the strategies currently being used to manage patients who suffer from diseases of the ear, nose, and throat.

Expert Guide to Otolaryngology is designed to facilitate the treatment of these patients and to ease the communication between the specialties of internal medicine and otolaryngology–head and neck surgery. It is written not only for the internist in primary care but also for those in the medical subspecialties whose patients have diseases that involve the ears, nose, sinuses, neck, and upper aerodigestive tract. Hopefully, this text will be as valuable to the consulting internist in a tertiary care hospital as it will be to the solo primary care practitioner in a small community. The authors also hope that it will be particularly useful to internal medicine residents.

The chapters of *Expert Guide to Otolaryngology* are symptom oriented and are divided into seven major sections. There is also an introduction on the history of otolaryngology (written by an internist). Each chapter includes illustrative figures, tabular information, case studies designed to highlight key issues, and a list of suggested readings for readers who want additional information. We have also included treatment algorithms that appear on the second page of most chapters. These are designed to be helpful in the management of otolaryngologic diseases, but they are not necessarily the official recommendations or guidelines of either the authors or the American Academy of Otolaryngology–Head and Neck Surgery.

Expert Guide to Otolaryngology was written by practicing otolaryngologists and was edited by members of the Core Otolaryngology Education Faculty of the AAO-HNSF. Subspecialty committees of the Academy reviewed chapters for content.

The individual most responsible for the completion of this book is its editor, Dr. Karen Calhoun, who personally revised or contributed to every chapter. Her commitment and sacrifice resulted in a more cohesive text—one that we hope will be useful to the wide range of physicians who treat adults. Without Dr. Calhoun's contribution, this book would have been merely a series of monographs of limited practical use to the practicing internist and internal medicine resident. The AAO-HNSF and ACP-ASIM owe her a debt of gratitude.

We hope that you use this book in your practice and find it helpful in the management of your patients. As we prepare for future editions, we welcome any comments or contributions; direct these to the AAO-HNSF mailbox at ce@entnet.org.

David E. Eibling, MD
Chair, Core Otolaryngology Education Faculty
American Academy of Otolaryngology–Head and Neck Surgery Foundation

Contents

Introduction
The Unusual History of Otolaryngology 1
James S. Newman

Chapter 1
The Head and Neck Examination 13
James D. Smith and Francis B. Quinn Jr.

SECTION I: OTOLOGY

Chapter 2
Ear Pain and Drainage 31
Paul M. Spring and Ronald G. Amedee

Chapter 3
Hearing Loss. 53
Donald J. Beasley and Ronald G. Amedee

Chapter 4
Cerumen Impaction 75
Mark A. Jabor and Gerard J. Gianoli

Chapter 5
Itchy Ears 86
Eric L. Mansfield and Gerard J. Gianoli

Chapter 6
Dizziness. 102
Andrew J. Miller and Gerard J. Gianoli

Chapter 7
Tinnitus 132
David A. Godin and Gerard J. Gianoli

Section II: Sinonasal Disease

Chapter 8
Nasal Obstruction.. 145
Eric F. Pinczower

Chapter 9
Allergic Conditions of the Ear, Nose, and Throat 161
Richard L. Mabry

Chapter 10
Rhinosinusitis 179
D. Gregory Farwell and Eric F. Pinczower

Chapter 11
Epistaxis 202
Darryk W. Barlow

Chapter 12
Nasal Fractures 218
J. David Kriet and Craig S. Murakami

Section III: Upper Aerodigestive Tract

Chapter 13
Mucosal Lesions of the Oral Cavity, Tongue, and
    Oropharynx... 231
Elizabeth A. Blair and David E. Eibling

Chapter 14
Disorders of the Nasopharynx 265
John W. Cavo Jr. and Eric F. Pinczower

Chapter 15
Dysphagia 279
John W. Cavo Jr. and David E. Eibling

Chapter 16
Obstructive Sleep Apnea....................................... 304
Kenneth B. Briskin

Section IV: Laryngeal Disorders

Chapter 17
Hoarseness and Other Voice Disorders 325
Clark A. Rosen, Thomas Murry, and David E. Eibling

Chapter 18
Upper Airway Obstruction 342
Randall L. Plant

Chapter 19
Aspiration 363
David E. Eibling

Section V: The Neck

Chapter 20
Neck Masses 383
Karen M. Kost

Chapter 21
Salivary Gland Disorders 429
David E. Eibling

Chapter 22
Surgical Treatment of Thyroid and Parathyroid Gland
 Disease 450
Gregory W. Randolph, Jon K. Thiringer, and Peter J. Martin

Section VI: The Face

Chapter 23
Atypical Facial Pain and Related Entities 479
Steven M. Houser and Diana N. Traquina

Chapter 24
Facial Asymmetry 489
Brian P. Driscoll

Chapter 25
Lesions of the Face and Scalp 504
Luke K.S. Tan

Chapter 26
Facial Trauma..523
Karen T. Pitman

Chapter 27
Facial Rejuvenation......................................539
J. Gregory Staffel

SECTION VII: LOWER AERODIGESTIVE TRACT

Chapter 28
Hiccups 557
David E. Eibling

Chapter 29
Foreign Bodies 567
Gregory N. Postma

Chapter 30
Caustic Ingestion 592
Andrew J. Nemechek and Ronald G. Amedee

Chapter 31
Head and Neck Cancer: An Overview 604
Lyon L. Gleich and David E. Eibling

Chapter 32
Head and Neck Disorders in the Immunocompromised
    Patient 634
Thomas A. Tami

Chapter 33
Smell and Taste Disorders................................650
Thomas Hummel and Michael Knecht

Index 665

Special thanks to Karen T. Pitman for her development and writing of the excellent case studies for many of these chapters.

Introduction

The Unusual History of Otolaryngology

James S. Newman, MD

The history of medicine is filled with the efforts of humans to understand their corporeal and spiritual nature. The dead ends, mistaken assumptions, and bizarre therapeutic maneuvers of the past may seem quaint or unusual to modern physicians, but to the doctors of the time these were part of the fight to save lives and an attempt to comprehend the incomprehensible. In this brief chapter, I have outlined some physiologic principles, treatments, and observations from medicine and literature to set a perspective for the chapters to come.

Throughout the ages, Man has known that the upper airway is vital for respiration. In the Book of Genesis, it is noted that "The Lord God formed man from the dust of the earth. He blew into the nostrils the breath of life." In the fourth century BC, Hippocrates watched the mode of respiration closely, using its rate and temperature to help determine a patient's prognosis. He thought that the purpose of inspired air was to cool the innate heat of the heart and described that "cold breath" from the nostrils was often fatal.

"Brain Breathing"

The second-century Greek physician and physiologic experimenter Galen wrote several works describing respiration, including *De Usu Partium Corporis Humani* (*On the Usefulness of the Parts of the Body*). He distinguished three types of respiration: through the lungs, the skin, and the brain. "Brain breathing" was an accepted theory before Galen's time and survived another 1300 years after his death. Galen envisioned channels connecting the brain to the nostrils to aid in cerebral respiration. He described these "nasal channels" as being connected to "cerebral ventricles" within which "psychic pneuma" was produced. In his theory, these channels had secondary roles related to olfaction and "the evacuation of the residues" from the brain. He felt that, under stress, the brain discharged large quantities of material called "rheum" or "coryza" via these channels through the nose and out of the body. Galen thought these discharges traveled through the ethmoid bone, which also worked to moderate the temperature of air reaching the brain. Galen emphasized that the nose, rather than the mouth, was for respiration.

Galen stressed the importance of the nasopharyngeal structures in the filtration of inspired air. As the air passed along its winding path, particles were filtered out. Any particles that made their way completely through the nose were caught by the uvula. He also noted that the larynx was the primary organ of the voice, and he detailed three cartilages: the thyroid, cricoid, and arytenoid.

Galen also thought, as did many others, that toothaches were caused by worms and that a spider's web rolled into a ball and placed in a cavity would relieve the pain.

Catarrh

Of concern to our medical forebears, as well as physicians today, was the cause and treatment of nasal discharge, or catarrh. In the late 1400s, the Paduan physician Zerbi thought that these "cerebral secretions" traveled through the olfactory bulbs on their way from the brain. Andreas Vesalius (1514–1564), the great anatomist, also thought that air passed into the brain through the nose. However, he shared a doubt with the great French surgeon Ambrose Paré (1510–1590) that mucus passed from the brain through the nose. Gabriele Fallopio, who published *Observationes Anatomicae* in 1501 and was widely regarded as Vesalius' successor, believed that the sinuses acted as a reservoir for air before it entered the brain.

By the seventeenth century, dissent over these old theories was rising. Some anatomists thought that mucus was generated locally in the nose rather than in the brain. Supporting this theory was Gerolamo Cardano of Milan, who also wrote a treatise on teaching the blind to read using the sense of touch (in 1545) and a book on astrologic physiognomy based on forehead furrows. Jan Baptista van Helmont (1580–1644), a Belgian, also believed that mucus was generated in the nose rather than in the brain. However, Johann Jakob Wepfer (a Swiss) wrote in 1685 that the cerebral discharges were evacuated by the carotid arteries. By the late 1600s, the general opinion was that the catarrhal secretions could not come from the brain because the cribriform plate, sphenoid bone, and other bony structures were impenetrable. Injections of dye into the ethmoid bone did not leak out via the nose, supporting this theory. However, despite this proof, some still considered the brain to be a mucus-secreting gland; the great neuroanatomist Thomas Willis (1621–1675, of circle fame) thought those secretions perhaps traveled through hollow nerves.

Shut Your Mouth and Save Your Life

With the study of upper airway function came an interesting set of popular beliefs about the harmful effects of snoring and "mouth breathing." Even today, we know that snoring and sleep apnea can lead to adverse medical outcomes. For a classic description of this problem, one need look only to Joe the Fat Boy in Charles Dickens' *Pickwick Papers*, first published in monthly installments from 1836 to 1837: "On the box sat a fat and red-faced boy in a state of somnolency.... Joe, darn that boy, he's gone to sleep again." In 1852, a U.S. physician, Louis Dugas, tried to cure stertorism (snoring) with a tonsillectomy and uvulotomy, which is not too different than the uvulopalatopharyngoplasty currently in use. Snoring caps and other unusual devices popular at the time look odd to us today, but they are certainly no more bizarre than the CPAP (continuous positive airway pressure) mask.

In the United States, the landmark book published on mouth breathing and its dangers was George Caitlin's *Breath of Life* in 1861, which was later reissued under the catchy title, *Shut Your Mouth and Save Your Life* (Fig. 1). He

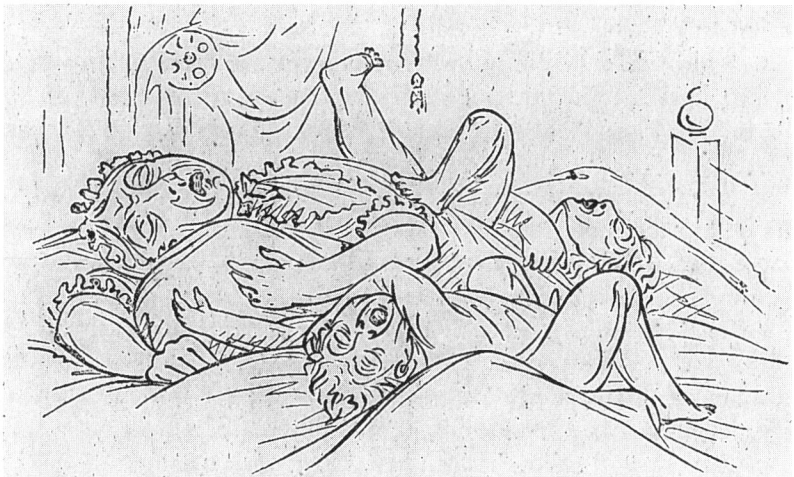

Figure 1 "Unhealthy" sleeping, i.e., breathing through the mouth while asleep. (Courtesy of the Moody Medical Library, University of Texas, Medical Branch, Galveston. Republished from Caitlin G. *The Breath of Life*. New York: Wiley; 1861.)

argued that healthy people breathe through their noses and that breathing through the mouth was harmful to health. Children were admonished to keep their mouths closed except for eating and talking and were trained to sleep with their mouths closed.

Tools of the Trade

Ancient physicians had tools for a limited inspection of the nose and ears (Fig. 2) The most simple of tools, the tongue depressor, has gone through many modifications, being fashioned from ivory, horn, or silver and ranging from straight and simple to curved and complex, with some even being spring loaded. Ironically, in today's "high-tech" world, we now use a simple wooden stick.

The otoscope was first used by Jean Itard in 1821 and was followed by a landmark atlas of otology by Adam Politzer in 1896, with detailed drawings of the tympanic membrane in health and disease. The use of the reflecting mirror aided in visualization. Although it was first held in the teeth, an easier-to-use head mirror soon followed.

No ear examination was complete without testing the mobility of the tympanic membrane. This was demonstrated using pneumotoscopy with the Toynbee otoscope and its stethoscope attachment that connected the physician's and patient's ears. The patient would perform the Valsalva maneuver and the physician would listen. This device was in use in the United States until the 1940s. In 1864, the Siegle pneumatic otoscope improved the ear examination. A tube attached to the scope's head allowed the physician to inhale and exhale air to demonstrate eardrum mobility.

It was not until the early 1800s that rhinoscopy and laryngoscopy were developed. In 1806, Phillip Bozzini described an endoscope, but it was never put to practical use. In 1848, Sir William Wilde (father of the famed playwright Oscar Wilde) suggested the use of a mirror for visualization. In 1854, Manuel Garcia, a singing instructor at the London Royal Academy, utilized two mirrors to inspect his own throat during voice production. Although his vase-shaped lamp had a short speculum and was low on candle power, he was able to describe the motion of the arytenoid cartilages and the vocal cords.

Johann Czermak used Garcia's two-mirror method in 1857 to visualize his own larynx, calling his device the "autolaryngoscope"—a large, round, perforated mirror with a second, smaller mirror to be placed in the pharynx. He suggested using a local anesthetic to aid in the procedure. His writings on and promotion of laryngoscopy brought him international fame.

Ephraim Cutter came from Boston to study under Czermak and fashioned his own laryngoscope. In 1861, he was the first to photograph his own larynx.

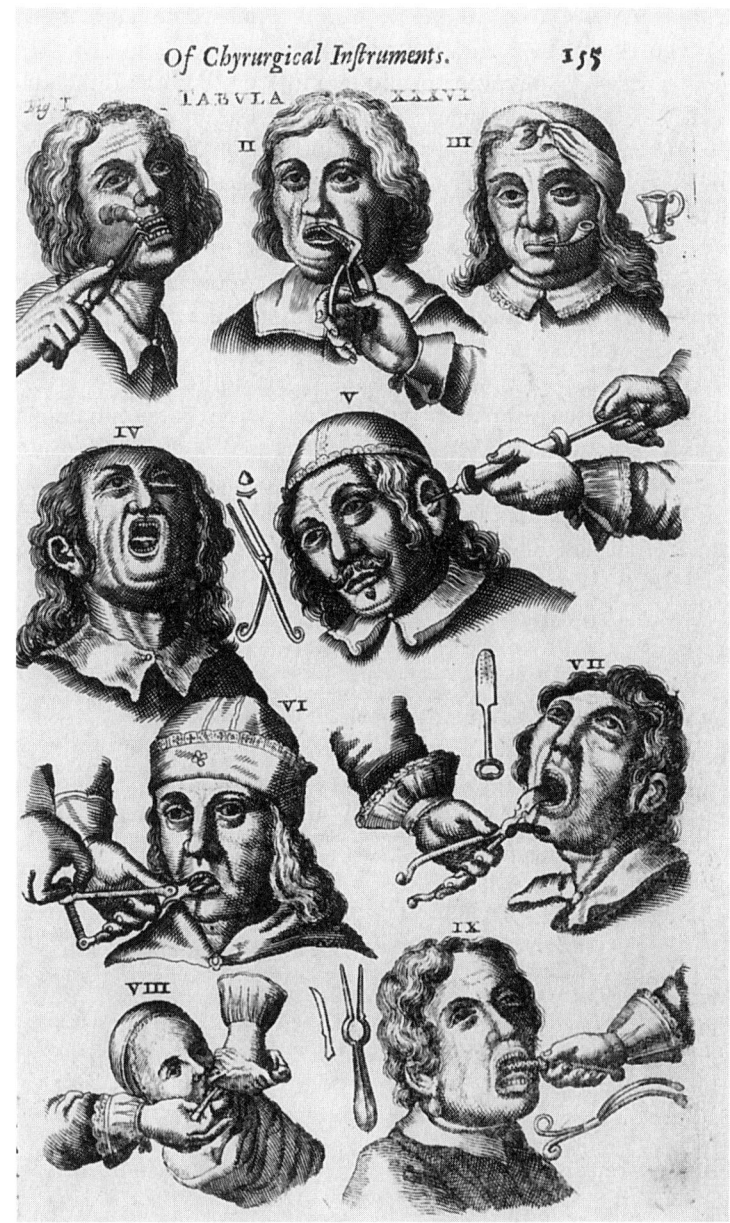

Figure 2 Various surgical instruments for use with the ears, teeth, oral cavities, and oropharyngeal structures. (Courtesy of the Moody Medical Library, University of Texas, Medical Branch, Galveston. Republished from Scultetus J. *The Chyrugeons Store-house*. London: John Starkey; 1674.)

His efforts were well received, yet his own medical school (Harvard) did not add laryngoscopy to its curriculum until 1875.

Thomas Edison's discovery of the incandescent bulb in 1880 added the powerful light source that was lacking. Another leap forward in visualization came with Heinrich Lamm's introduction of fiber optics in 1930. Light could now be transmitted through flexible bundles of glass fibers without distortion, which led to better viewing of the airways and other orifices.

Atomizers of various sorts have long been used for lubrication and the administration of medicine. Some have been simple squeeze bulbs and some are more complex (Fig. 3). Among the most toxic substances ever sprayed with an atomizer was oral mercury for the treatment of syphilis.

A final useful tool—a biological one still in sporadic use today—is the leech. Application of these creatures can remove blood from hard-to-drain places or for venous congestion. In the past, they were used occasionally to drain lesions in the nose and oropharynx (*see* section on Foreign Bodies below). George Washington suffered from a pharyngeal abscess, and his physician, Benjamin Rush, liberally phlebotomized him (as was the custom) until his death in 1799.

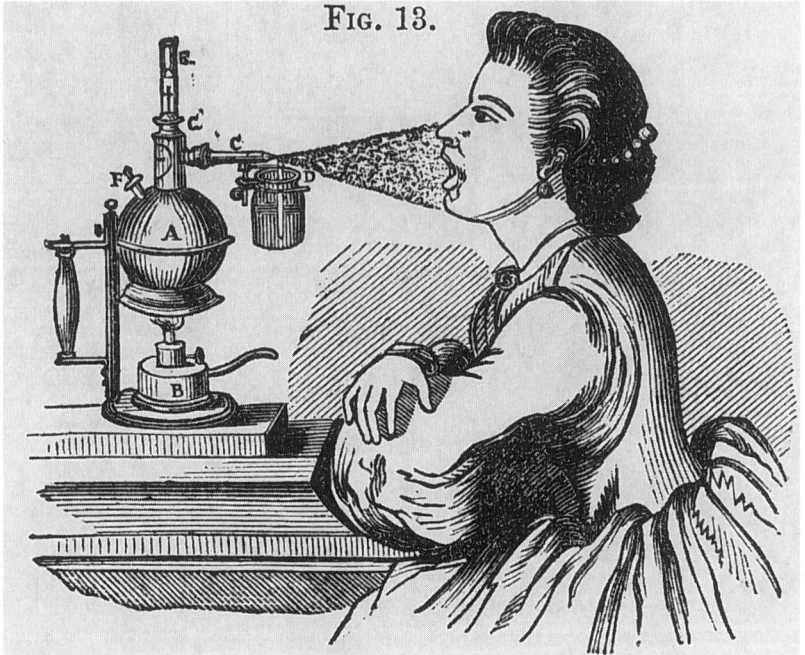

Figure 3 Siegle's apparatus (1868) for administration of nasal medication. (Courtesy of the Moody Medical Library, University of Texas, Medical Branch, Galveston.)

The Invisible Food Filter

Among the most interesting gastromedical trends of our century is that of "Fletcherization." Horace Fletcher was a self-made man, a world traveler, and a medical visionary. From humble beginnings in Massachusetts in 1849 and through dozens of careers, ranging from ink importer to the president of the New Orleans Philharmonic, he rose to international renown. However, by age 40, years of excess left Fletcher obese and ill. When he was turned down for an insurance policy, he devised a system of healthy eating. He thought that poor assimilation and an overabundance of food in general, protein in particular, led to all the ills of the world.

By Fletcher's theory, the saliva, which watered the mouth, signaled the advent of the "earned" appetite. Food was then to be chewed until no flavor remained. At that critical time, the "swallowing impulse" took over, and the food automatically slid down the gullet. Any food not ready for ingestion was blocked by the "food filter," an invisible and selective sieve. Any food that could not pass the unseen barrier was to be discreetly ejected.

An important part of Fletcher's philosophy was an optimistic outlook, and he maintained that one should eat only when hungry, never when worried, and always leave a residue of appetite as a "nest egg" for the next meal.

Fletcher's theories brought him fame, and he had many disciples. Among these was Dr. J.H. Kellogg, who coined the term "Fletcherizing" and predicted that Fletcher would go down in history with Louis Pasteur. Another follower was the author Upton Sinclair. In his landmark book, *The Jungle* (1906), a minor character embraces the masticatory mandate. This character studied the composition of foodstuffs and, by scientific chewing, tripled the value of all he ate, living on 11 cents per day.

Fletcher's greatest chewing challenge was a resistant shallot that required 722 chews before its flavor entirely disappeared. As he reported, "After the tussle, the young onion left no odor on the breath and joined the happy family in the stomach."

The Nose Knows

The proboscis, especially in its large or diseased form, has been a subject of interest in culture and medicine. Among the most notable in literature are Pinocchio's and Cyrano de Bergerac's. Shakespeare's Falstaff had a rhinophyma attributed to alcohol abuse, as did Bardolph, whose "lips blow at his nose, and it is like a coal of fire" (*Henry V*, act III, scene vi) (Fig. 4).

Among performers, the noses of Jimmy ("The Schnozz") Durante and W.C. Fields stand out. In the early 1700s, Tomas Wedders of Yorkshire made

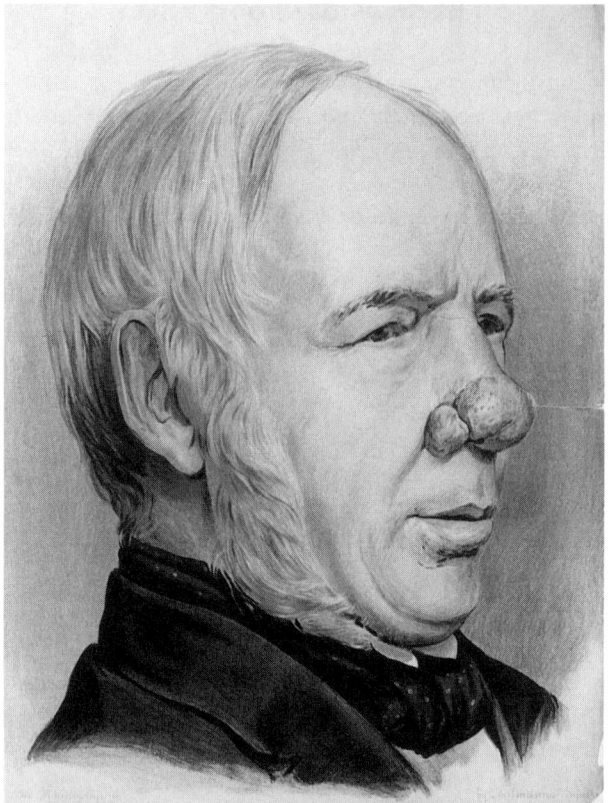

Figure 4 Rhinophyma, or the "hammer nose." (Courtesy of the Moody Medical Library, University of Texas, Medical Branch, Galveston.)

a living by displaying his enormous nose. It was said to measure 7.5 inches.

Noses have been injured in a variety of ways, from warfare to disease, and the repair of this damage has an interesting history. Approximately 1500 years ago, Hindu medicine was flourishing, and its surgeons–the most legendary one being Susruta–learned from a vigorous educational system that taught them how to "couch" for cataracts, remove bladder stones and nasal polyps, and even perform cosmetic surgery. At the time, nasal amputation was used as a punishment for adultery, and it was the lucky patient who could have his nose reconstructed using a skin graft from the forehead (a cheek flap was used for ear reconstruction). Two small tubes were placed to maintain the airway during the healing process, and the wound was smeared with honey and clarified butter, covered with cotton gauze, and dusted with clay.

Rhinoplasty fell out of favor in Western medicine; however, nose injuries continued to be a problem, especially with advancements in warfare. Ambroise Paré devised many artificial noses, some with mustaches attached (Fig. 5). In the late 1500s, Gasparo Tagliocotti used a different technique for nasal reconstruction. He attached a patient's arm to his or her head, then took a flap of skin from that arm and affixed it to the patient's nose, leaving the patient in this position for 10 days (Fig. 6A). After that, the arm and nose were separated, leaving adequate tissue behind for shaping. The nose was adjusted and supported in a sling during the healing process (Fig. 6B). Wits of the time suggested that he use gluteal tissue from another person at the donor site. The ecclesiasts of his time regarded this as meddling in God's work. After his

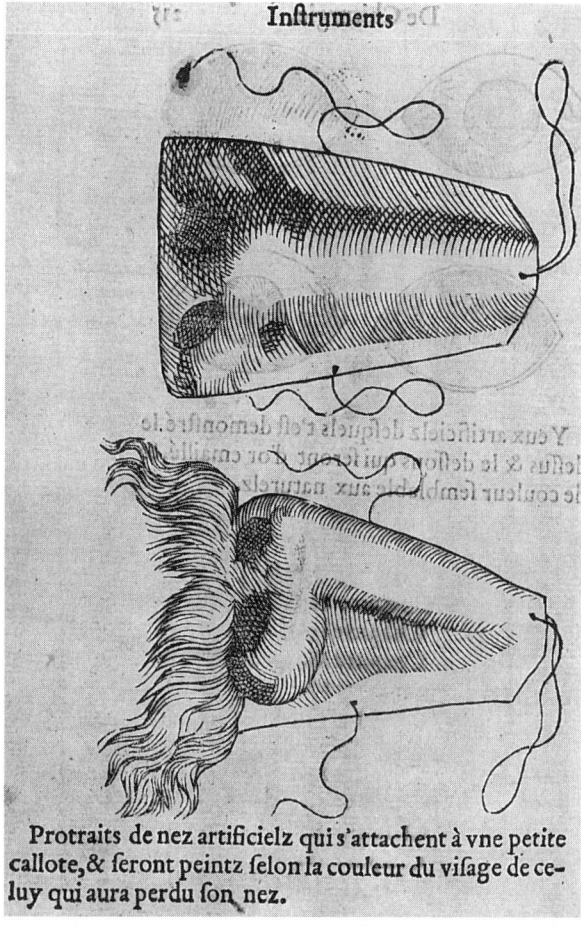

Figure 5 Artificial nose designed by Ambroise Parè in 1564. (Courtesy of the Moody Medical Library, University of Texas, Medical Branch, Galveston.)

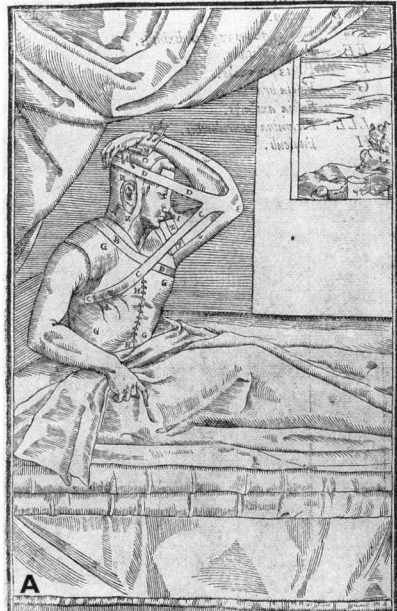 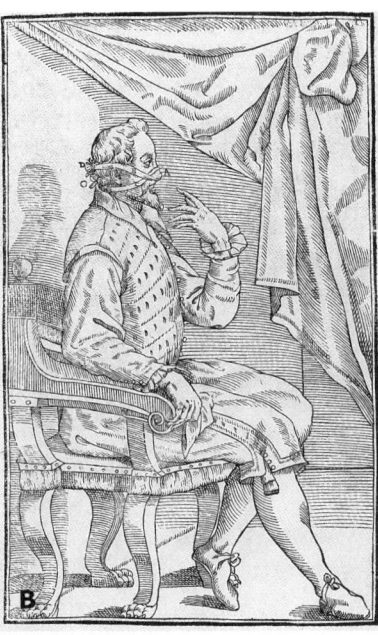

Figure 6 **A,** Gasparo Tagliacotti's patient (1597), with arm skin attached to the residual nose and an elaborate splint holding the arm to the nose while the new blood supply is established. **B,** The happy patient near the end of the nasal reconstructive procedure. (Courtesy of the Moody Medical Library, University of Texas, Medical Branch, Galveston.)

death, Tagliacotti's remains were exhumed from a convent where he had been laid to rest and reburied in unconsecrated grounds as punishment for this "meddling." In 1788, the Paris Faculty banned facial reconstruction altogether. It was not until 1829 in Germany that plastic surgery, especially of the face, was reborn through the work of Ernst Dieffenbach.

Undoubtedly the best and most graphic descriptions of rhinoplasty appear in a poem written by a fictional surgeon in Thomas Pynchon's novel *V* in the chapter titled "In Which Esther Gets a Nose Job."

"Have I told you, fellas,
She's got a sweet columella,
And a septum that sets 'em on their ass?
Each casual chondrectomy
Meant only a big fat check to me,
'Til I saved this osteoclastic lass."

Foreign Bodies

No account of the ear, nose, and throat would be complete without a brief mention of foreign objects lodged in the upper airway. Reports of insects trapped in the nose and throat are common and include maggots, centipedes, flies, and medicinal leeches. In 1893, August Weisman removed a rhinolith composed of a chalk-covered cherry pit that had been lodged for 60 years. Today, the most commonly seen foreign body is a cockroach in the tympanic canal. The advent of rhinoscopy has allowed the removal of foreign objects from the nose.

Certainly the most unusual of foreign bodies is the live fish, causing asphyxiation. In India in 1892, Norman Chevers reported five such cases in a manual of medical jurisprudence—one of a mullet that had slipped while being held between a man's teeth before baiting and another of a catfish that had made a prodigious and well-aimed leap.

Sir James Paget reported a case of a woman with blue saliva. She had a piece of aniline pencil stuck in a tooth cavity.

Sneezes

Sneezing was considered a good omen in the days of Homer, yet Aristotle wondered why the sneeze was a good omen but the cough was not. This belief also prevailed with the ancient Persians and in Africa and Mexico. Today, we automatically say "God bless you" to the sneezer, a practice that may have started around the time of Gregory the Great. During his papacy (590–604), sneezing was thought to be a sign of exposure to unwholesome vapors, and the pontiff devised a special prayer to avoid the appearance of the angel of death. The use of snuff to promote sneezing was thought to improve the health.

In 1888, Edward W. Lee reported an interesting case of a 15-year-old girl who yawned continuously for 5 weeks after a dental extraction. Belladonna was administered and thereafter the yawning turned to violent sneezing. She was given chloroform and the sneezing stopped, but on recovery the sneezes became even more vicious. Eventually she responded to ammonium and bed rest.

Hiccups

It is likely that no physical symptom has been treated with a larger variety of methods than hiccups. In Plato's *Symposium*, the physician Eryximachus recommends to Aristophanes, who had hiccuped after eating too much, to hold his breath and gargle with water. If this did not work, he should tickle his nose to induce a sneeze, which would surely halt his paroxysm. Among other approved therapies (especially for prolonged hiccups of weeks' or longer duration) are strychnine, bismuth, castor oil, camphor, hellebore, belladonna ergot, and bromides.

Summary

This chapter has highlighted many of the more interesting tidbits of the history of otolaryngology—the dead ends, bizarre practices, and false assumptions, as well as the revolutionary advances that were produced from these beginnings. As you read the chapters to come, reflect on the progress we have made but wonder what future doctors may think of our practice today.

Acknowledgements

Thanks to Sarita Oertling for help in the preparation of this chapter.

BIBLIOGRAPHY

Alasker RL. *Curing Catarrh.* New York: Grant Publishing; 1917.
Bowman IA. Historical perspective. In *Respiratory Function of the Upper Airway.* New York: Marcel Dekker; 1988.
Bynum WF, Porter R. *Medicine and the Five Senses.* Cambridge, England: Cambridge University Press; 1993.
Caitlin G. *The Breath of Life.* New York: Wiley Publishing; 1861.
Garrison FH. *An Introduction to the History of Medicine.* Philadelphia: WB Saunders; 1929.
Gould GM, Pyle WL. *Anomalies and Curiosities of Medicine.* Philadelphia: WB Saunders; 1896.
La Wall CH. *The Curious Lore of Drugs and Medicines.* Garden City, NJ: Garden City Publishing; 1929.
Paré A. *Dix Livres de la Chirugie.* Paris; 1564.
Scultetus J. *The Chyrugeons Store-House.* London: John Starkey; 1674.
Squire B. *On Rhinopyma, or "The Hammer Nose."* London: Churchill; 1889.
Tagliacotti G. *De Curtorum Chirurgia per Insitionem.* Venice; 1597.
Tobold A. *Chronic Diseases of the Larynx.* New York: William Wood; 1868.
Wilbur CK. *Antique Medical Instruments.* Atglen, PA: Shiffer Publishing; 1987.

1

The Head and Neck Examination

James D. Smith, MD
Francis B. Quinn Jr., MD

The head and neck examination is a part of every general physical examination, but it is usually abbreviated except in the patient with symptoms referable to the head and neck. Nonetheless, a wealth of clinical information can be discovered during examination of the head and neck and especially the cavities they harbor. Using a standard, consistent examination for every patient enables the clinician to recognize abnormalities when they are present.

Topographic Anatomy

Nose

The vestibule of the nose is hairy in many men and less so in women. Its most notable feature is the mucocutaneous junction denoted by a color change from yellow to reddish pink. As one looks beyond the nasal vestibule, one first encounters the anterior tip of the inferior turbinate (sometimes mistaken for a polyp), which is quite prominent, taking up most of the nasal aperture (Fig. 1.1). Immediately medial to the inferior turbinate is the cartilaginous part of the anterior nasal septum, sometimes bearing prominent blood vessels (Kiesselbach's plexus). Next, one may encounter a deviation of the nasal septum, sometimes in the shape of a plowshare (i.e., sharply angled into one nos-

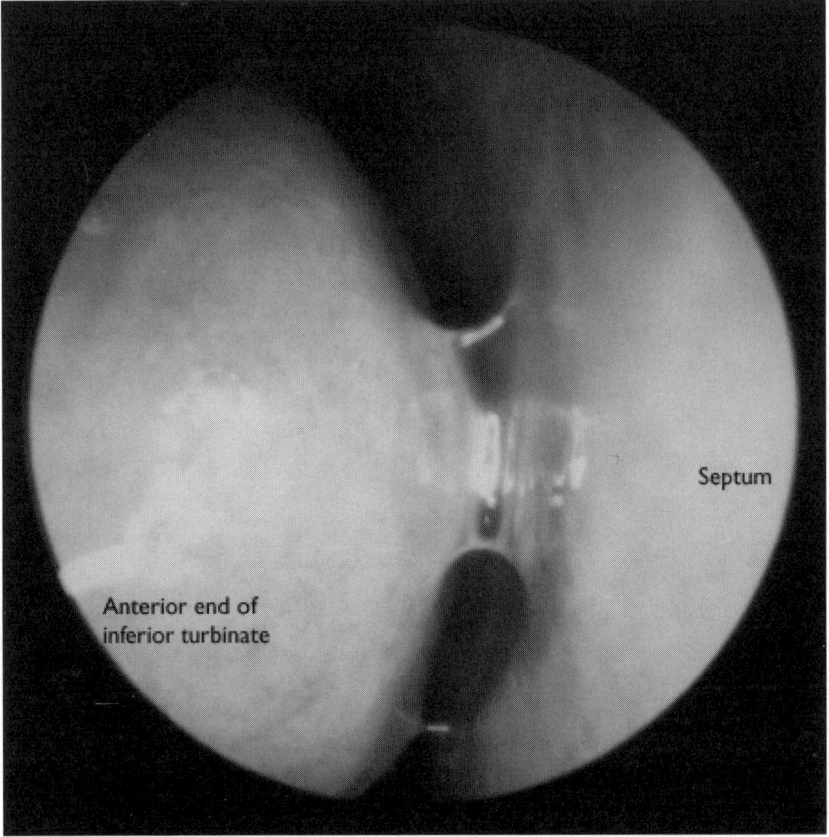

Figure 1.1 View of right nasal cavity before decongestion. The rounded object on the left (the patient's right) is the inferior turbinate. Note the minimal separation of the turbinate and the septum that will impair visualization and instrumentation (compare with Fig. 1.6). (Courtesy of Dr. James Smith.)

tril) or broadly convex, reducing the cross-sectional area of the nasal airway. Looking upward and laterally, one can often see a small lip-like structure called the *middle turbinate*. This structure is worthy of identification because it is often crucial when looking for pus or polyps that issue from the maxillary and ethmoid sinuses and drain into the middle meatus below it.

Nasopharynx

The topographic anatomy of the nasopharynx depends on whether one sees it with an examination mirror passed through the oral cavity or with a rigid or flexible endoscope passed through the nose. In a cooperative patient, the mirror displays the midline posterior edge of the nasal septum with the posterior tips of the turbinates to either side; residual adenoid at the top may be present. Rotating the mirror brings into view the donut-shaped eustachian tubes orifices (Rosenmüller's fossae). A similar view can be achieved by looking upward from below with a 90° telescope (Fig. 1.2).

After passing through the nose into the nasopharynx with the nasal endoscope (the bony choana is the posterior nasal aperture), one sees the posterior nasopharyngeal wall, which is covered with mucosa. By angling the scope right and left, the orifices of the eustachian tubes can be seen. The posterior edge of the soft palate can be seen by viewing downward.

Oropharynx

As most experienced clinicians are aware, the oropharynx is the area posterior to the anterior tonsillar pillar and superior to the vallecula. It includes the

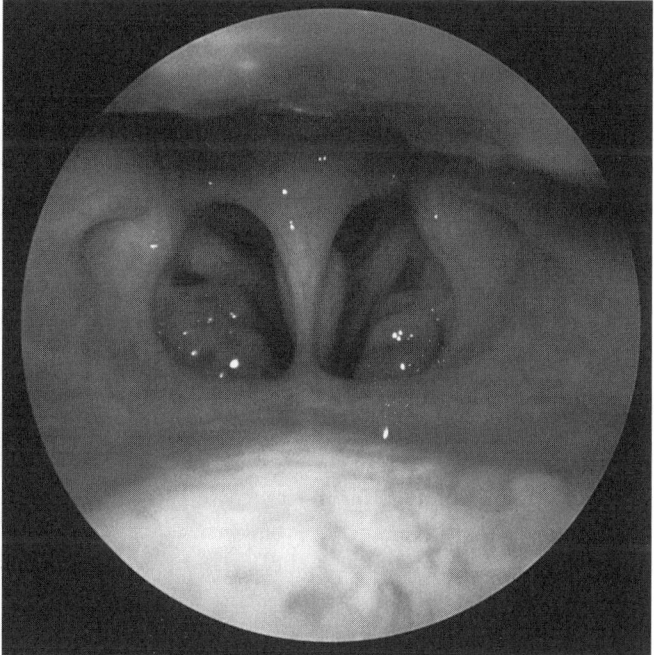

Figure 1.2 View of the nasopharynx from below using a 90° telescope passed through the oral cavity. The palate is at the bottom, and the posterior pharyngeal wall is at the top. The posterior end of the nasal septum can be seen with the inferior (larger) and middle turbinates on either side. Note the torus tubarius (eustachian tube orifices) on either side, lateral to the inferior turbinates. (Courtesy of Dr. James Smith.)

base of tongue, palatine tonsils, and soft palate. The palatine tonsils vary widely in size and appearance but are usually symmetrical.

Hypopharynx

The base of the tongue supports the giant taste buds (*circumvalate papillae*) and the lingual tonsils, an irregularly surfaced pink mass of tissue on which small fish bones and other foreign bodies can be caught. One sometimes sees the greater cornu of the hyoid bone intruding on the lateral walls of the hypopharynx. The pyriform sinuses (i.e., the entry portal to the cervical esophagus) open during phonation and can be seen posterolateral to the larynx itself.

Larynx

The first and probably most important structure that the clinician sees is the epiglottis—"first" because it sits atop the larynx, just behind the base of the tongue; "important" because acute epiglottitis is a diagnosis that can be missed all too easily and sometimes tragically. The "V" of the glottis (the space between the true vocal folds) is quickly seen and is important when orienting the viewer and assisting in the identification of adjacent structures (Fig. 1.3).

The false vocal folds are just above and parallel to the true folds. The two rounded pink arytenoids tether the posterior open end of the "V" and can be important in identifying a paralyzed vocal cord. In unilateral paralysis, one vocal cord moves freely during inspiration and phonation, whereas the other is immobile. Several tracheal rings often can be seen below the glottis, and any exudate and mucosal inflammation are noteworthy.

Neck

The topography of the neck is remarkable for the presence of the laryngeal cartilages—thyroid, cricothyroid, and hyoid. The sternocleidomastoid muscle and thyroid gland are easily palpable. Masses about which patients sometimes complain include the greater cornua of the hyoid bone, or the ptotic submandibular glands. Reassurance is the appropriate treatment. Over the past several years, the zones of the neck have been numbered (*see* Chapter 20), but the conventional terms of submandibular, anterior, posterior, and supraclavicular still apply.

Ear

Although the external ear (pinna) is topographically complex, all clinicians, from the earliest years of practicing medicine, are capable of picking out un-

The Head and Neck Examination   17

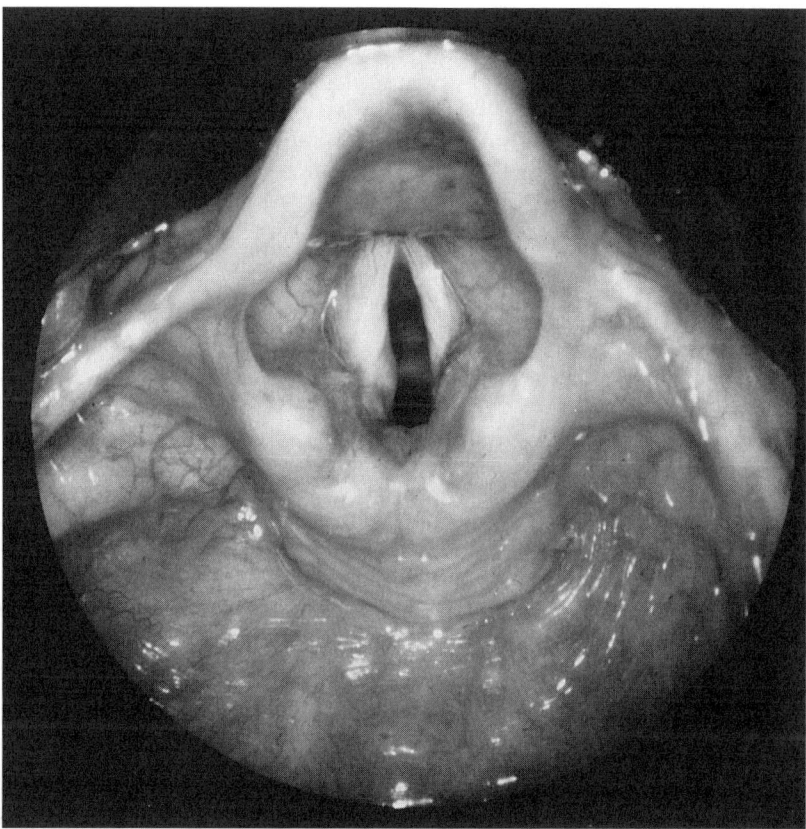

Figure 1.3 View of the larynx and hypopharynx through an operative laryngoscope. The epiglottis is at the top (anterior), and the vocal cords are seen clearly on either side of the glottic aperture. The arytenoids can be seen just posterolateral to the vocal cords, and the aryepiglottic folds connect them to the lateral aspect of the epiglottis. In this view, the laryngoscope has displaced the larynx anteriorly, opening the pyriform sinuses widely on either side and exposing the mucosa over the posterior plate of the cricoid cartilage (just inferior to the arytenoids) and the posterior hypopharyngeal wall at the top of the photograph. (Courtesy of Dr. James Smith.)

usually shaped ("abnormal") pinnae (Fig. 1.4). The ear canal is usually open and straight, but it can be difficult to examine, especially when age has allowed the external auditory meatus to collapse posteriorly to anteriorly. The anterior wall of the bony canal is often convex, reflecting the shape of the immediately adjacent temporomandibular joint and obscuring the anterior portion of the tympanic membrane. The eardrum itself is best marked by the annulus (where it joins the bony canal) and by the handle of the malleus, which can tilt inward when negative pressure exists in the middle ear, indicat-

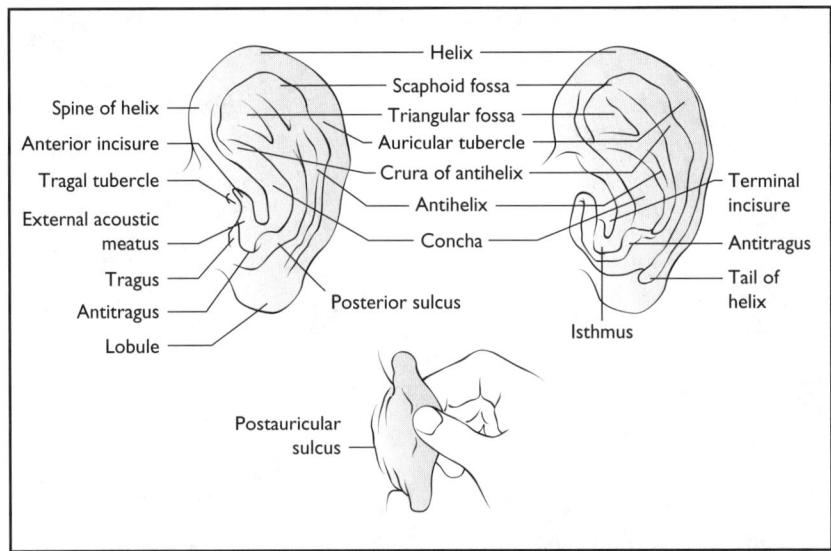

Figure 1.4 View of pinna with the cartilaginous folds labeled. (Redrawn from Bailey BJ (ed). *Head and Neck Surgery—Otolaryngology*, 1st ed. Philadelphia: JB Lippincott; 1993:1442.)

ing retraction from eustachian tube obstruction. Recall that the posteriosuperior portion of the drum is more lateral than the anteroinferior portion and that the light reflex is the only portion of the conical structure perpendicular to the line of vision (Fig. 1.5). There is a wide range of transparency encountered in normal individuals, and pneumatic otoscopy is an important aid in visualizing the three-dimensional anatomy of the eardrum.

Pearls and Pitfalls of the Head and Neck Examination

Nose

Nasal Vestibular Furunculosis
A red area on the nasal ala or on the tip of the nose in a patient complaining of pain in the same area suggests a vestibular furuncle. When this spreads along the angular vein (where the nose joins the cheek), producing a tender cord-like structure (angular vein thrombophlebitis), the patient is in danger of developing cavernous sinus thrombophlebitis. Intravenous antibiotics should be given immediately.

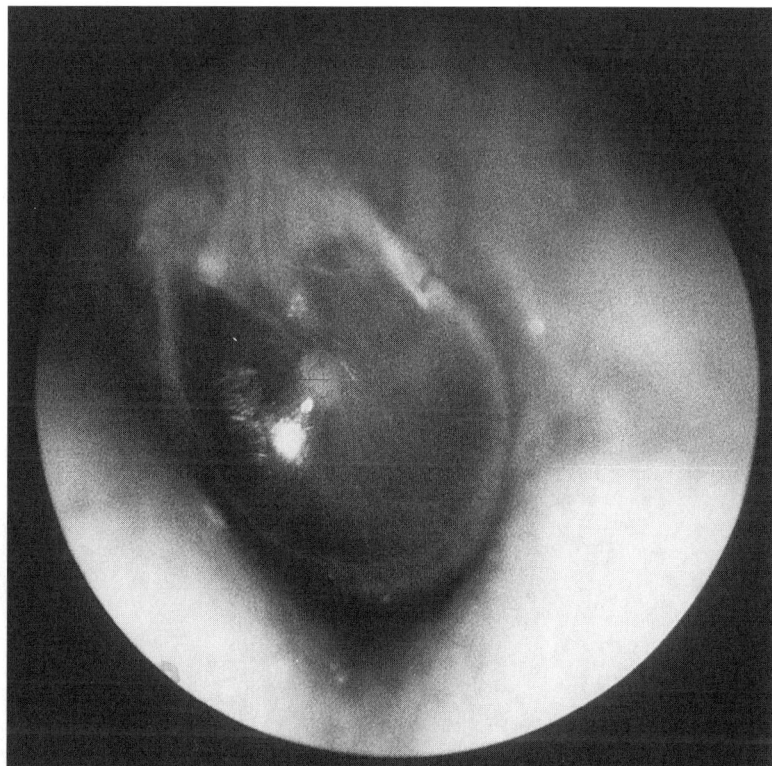

Figure 1.5 View of normal left tympanic membrane. Note that the entire annulus can be seen in this photograph, which is not usually possible in the majority of normal individuals. The light reflex is easily seen and is the only portion of the eardrum perpendicular to the light source and camera. The short process of the malleus is clearly visible, as is the umbo just posterosuperior to the light reflex. (Courtesy of Dr. James Smith.)

Nasal Septal Deviation

The caudal (anterior) edge of the nasal septum typically can be felt if one pushes the anterior columella posteriorly. The caudal edge of the cartilaginous septum sits just above the space between the medial crura of the lower lateral cartilages. One of the late effects of nasal trauma is dislocation of the anterior nasal septum, such that when the examiner lifts the tip of the nose, the edge of the septum appears in one or the other nostril.

The nasal speculum and headlight (or head mirror) permit estimation of nasal septal deviation (plowshare or convex) as well as color and engorgement of the inferior turbinate. One or two sprays of a topical decongestant (e.g., oxymetazoline, phenylephrine hydrochloride 1%, ephedrine sulfate 1%)

help one to see farther into the nose (e.g., to check the middle turbinate and middle meatus) and can indicate how much of the patient's nasal obstruction is truly skeletal and how much comes from potentially reversible mucosal edema (Fig. 1.6).

A strikingly pale nasal mucosa suggests allergic rhinitis. The failure of engorged, obstructing inferior turbinates to respond to topical decongestants indicates rhinitis medicamentosa, or nose-spray abuse. Polyps in the middle meatus raise suspicion of allergic or infectious disease of the sinuses, and pus issuing from the middle meatus confirms the existence of rhinosinusitis.

The examiner may want to mix a topical anesthetic (e.g., tetracaine [Pontocaine] 2%) with the decongestant spray to reduce discomfort when probing a

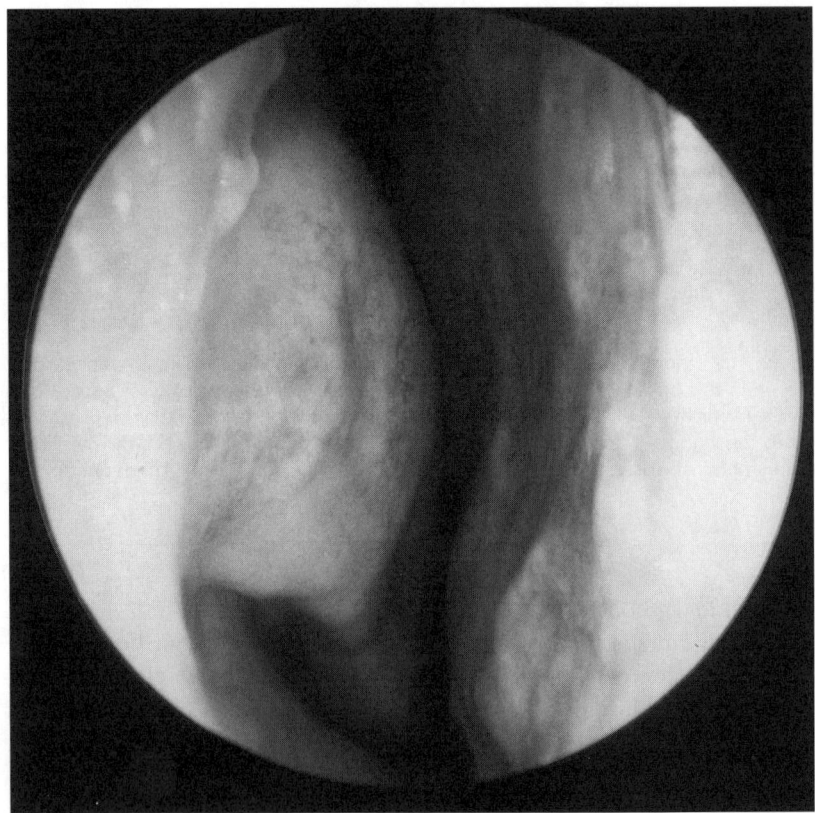

Figure 1.6 View of the interior of the right nostril after topical decongestion (compare with Fig. 1.1). The septum is on the right (the patient's left), and the inferior turbinate is on the left (the patient's right). The middle meatus is above the inferior turbinate under the middle turbinate (not shown), and the inferior meatus can be seen below and lateral to the inferior turbinate. (Courtesy of Dr. James Smith.)

polyp (polyps are soft and usually not tender on palpation; inferior turbinates are harder, and palpation may cause discomfort). Topical anesthesia combined with a decongestant greatly assists in the fiberoptic examination of the nose, nasopharynx, and upper airway. A comfortable patient is more likely to be a cooperative patient.

Nasopharynx

The traditional mirror examination of the nasopharynx is steadily being replaced by flexible fiberoptic endoscopic inspection. When meticulous and leisurely examination of the nasopharynx is necessary, a laryngeal mirror, two small urethral catheters, and a pair of hemostats assist in the viewing. After topical anesthesia of the nose and oropharynx is achieved, a catheter is inserted into each nostril, and both are brought out through the mouth where the two ends are held in each of two hemostats. Access for viewing and even for performing a biopsy is obtained in all but the most skittish of patients; however, the technique is quite uncomfortable, even with adequate topical anesthesia.

Flexible Endoscope

The flexible fiberoptic laryngoscope has multiple applications in the office environment, and its use is mastered easily (Figs. 1.7 and 1.8). However, it is costly (~$5000), requires specialized sterilization techniques, and needs frequent replacement or repair. Its primary use has been in the evaluation of vocal cord anatomy and movement. The pyriform sinuses can be examined well by asking the patient to blow against a closed mouth to increase intrapharyngeal pressure, distending the pyriform sinus area and allowing easier inspection. This examination is facilitated by having the patient turn his or her head to one side and then the other.

The inferior portion of the nasal cavity and nasopharynx also are examined easily with the flexible fiberoptic laryngoscope. It may be possible to examine the middle meatus and sphenoethmoid recesses in some patients, although most rhinologists prefer to use the rigid nasal endoscope for these regions. Assessment of pharyngeal and palatal motion also is performed easily with this scope. Recently, techniques for the evaluation of swallowing function using the flexible endoscope have been popularized (*see* Chapter 15).

The flexible laryngoscope is valuable in the evaluation of patients with sleep apnea. In addition to identifying anatomic abnormalities, the Müller maneuver can assist in determining the site of the obstruction. This maneuver is performed by inserting the scope into the nasopharynx and placing the patient in a supine position. Next, the patient is asked to breathe in with the

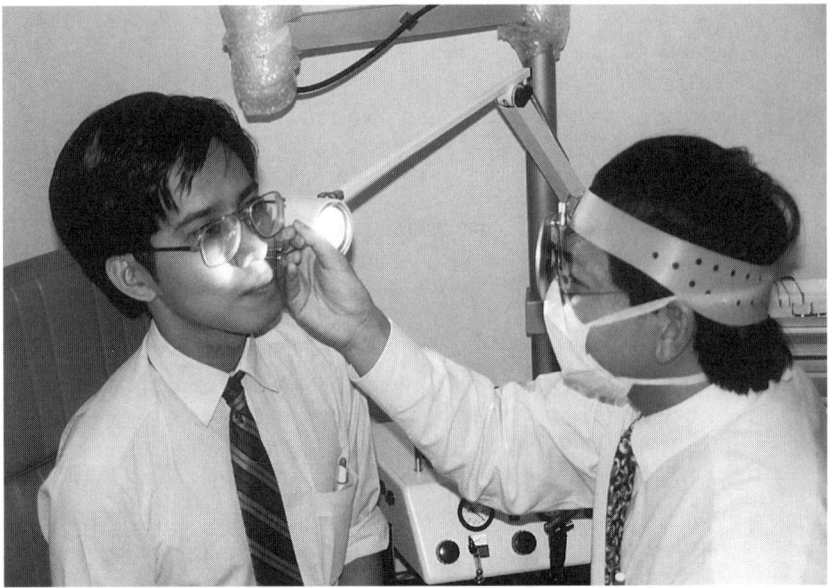

Figure 1.7 Using a head mirror and light (at the patient's left shoulder) to examine the nose. Note the bright light reflected onto the patient's face. The mirror is worn over the examiner's dominant eye, and the target object is viewed through the hole in the center of the mirror. (Courtesy of Dr. James Smith.)

mouth closed and the nose pinched shut. The examiner then notes the location of the maximal oropharyngeal and nasopharyngeal airway collapse, which may be helpful in planning treatment strategies in patients with obstructive sleep apnea.

Oral Cavity and Oropharynx

During the examination of the tonsils and posterior pharyngeal wall, it is sometimes easy to overlook the cheeks, gingiva, hard palate, floor of mouth, and tongue. Early oral cavity malignancies are encountered most frequently along the lateral inferior edge of the tongue and on the floor of the mouth and can be missed unless the area is examined specifically. Periodontitis (i.e., blunting of the interdental papillae, recession of the gingiva, and loosening of the teeth) and dental caries can indicate a need for counseling about dental hygiene or perhaps even lifestyle. Punctate red spots on the hard palate ("pipe-smoker's stomatitis") or white patches on the mucosa of the cheeks suggest tobacco consumption and provide an opportunity to discuss smoking cessation

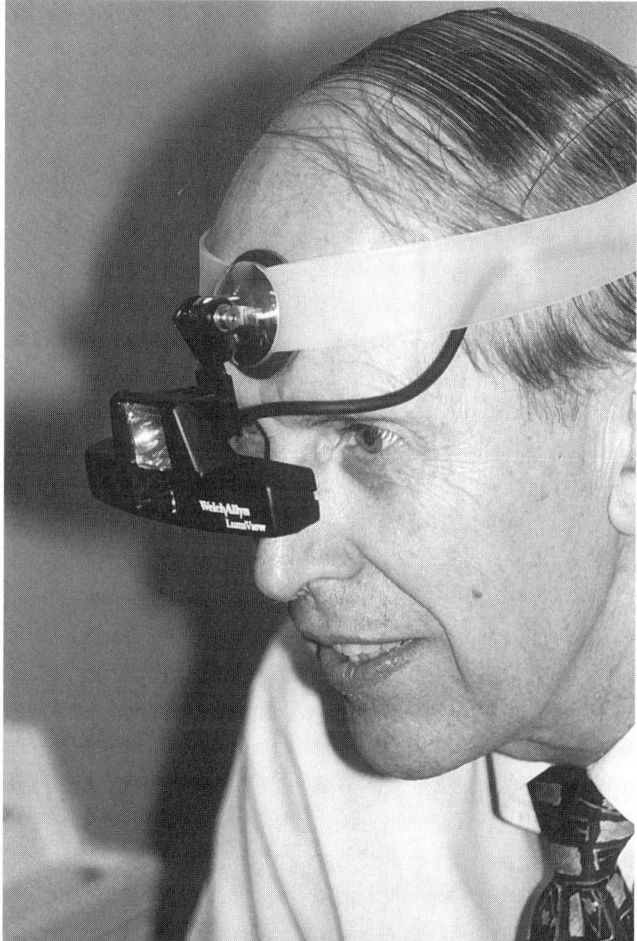

Figure 1.8 Welch Allyn LumiView, a type of headlight whose light source and magnifying loupes can be attached to a headband or eyeglass frame. (Courtesy of Dr. James Smith.)

with the patient. Protrusion of the tongue in the midline and from side to side sometimes reveals a cranial nerve lesion (e.g., of the hypoglossal nerve) or infiltration of the tongue muscle or the mouth floor by an invasive neoplasm.

Finally, holding the tip of the tongue with a gauze square and palpating the base of the tongue and tonsillar pillars with the gloved index finger of the opposite hand can ensure that no submucosal carcinoma of the tongue base escapes detection.

Larynx

Indirect Laryngoscopy

The technique of indirect laryngoscopy was invented in 1856 by a Spanish singing teacher to examine the vocal apparatus of his pupils. The required equipment is inexpensive, but the technique does require practice, hence the increasing use of alternative examination techniques.

Illumination is provided by a bright lamp, usually at the patient's right side, which is reflected by a concave mirror worn on the examiner's head (Fig. 1.9). The light source can be as simple as a gooseneck lamp with an unfrosted 100-watt incandescent bulb or a similar clip-on lamp. A headlight whose beam is nearly coaxial with the line of sight is a convenient alternative, although it is more expensive (~$250 or more) than the classic head mirror (~$35–$65). A headlight can be useful for other tasks as well and is probably a worthwhile purchase for an office-based practice (Fig. 1.10).

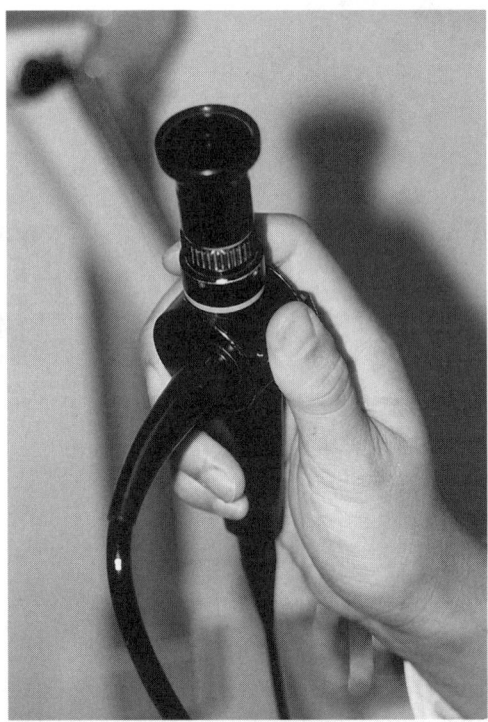

Figure 1.9 Nasopharyngoscopy technique. The nasopharyngoscope is held with the thumb on the deflection lever. The tip of the endoscope is positioned by twisting the scope and deflecting the tip in the identical manner used with a flexible bronchoscope. (Courtesy of Dr. James Smith.)

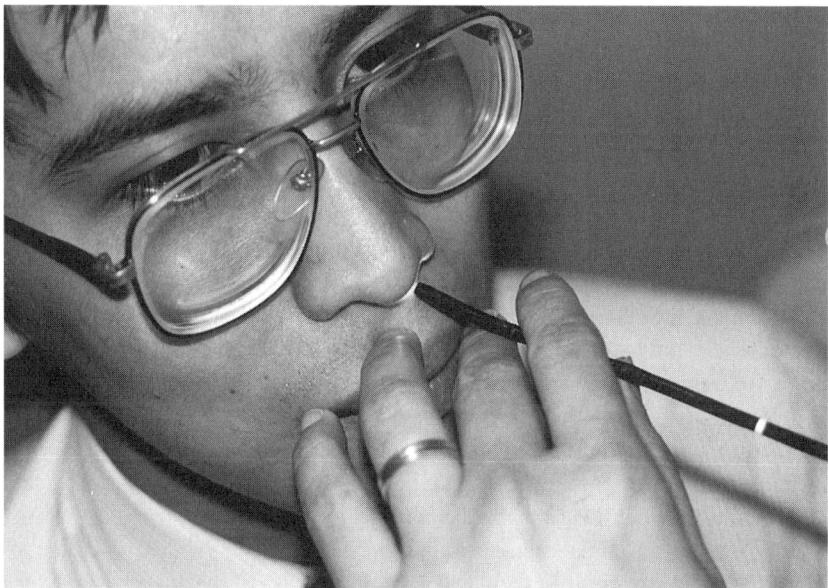

Figure 1.10 Inserting the nasopharyngoscope into the nose. The endoscope is passed under direct vision, with care being taken to avoid hitting sensitive structures, such as septal deviations. When the posterior nasal cavity is encountered, ask the patient to close his or her mouth and breathe through the nose. This will drop the palate, easing passage of the scope into the oropharynx and hypopharynx. (Courtesy of Dr. James Smith.)

A 4"-by-8" gauze square is wrapped around the protruded tongue, and the tongue is held extended by the examiner's hand, taking care not to pull the tongue too firmly onto the inferior incisors. A laryngeal mirror (#7) is dipped in defogger solution, hot water, or hot coffee (or warmed with a cigarette lighter) and then tested for temperature against the examiner's hand. The mirror is then pressed firmly upward and backward against the patient's soft palate (imagine that the soft palate is a baseball catcher's mitt and that the mirror is the catcher's fist pressed into the cupped mitt). The patient breathes only through the mouth (the patient must not breathe through the nose), and the examiner gains a clear view of the entire larynx, hypopharynx, and upper trachea in up to 80% of patients. The examination is often facilitated by a spray or two of a topical anesthetic (e.g., cetacaine, tetracaine 2%, lidocaine 4%). A rigid 90° or 70° telescope is often used for the examination in lieu of a mirror. The technique is essentially the same as that used with the mirror except that the tip of the endoscope is passed under the palate, with care taken to avoid contacting the posterior pharyngeal wall.

Some useful hints include having the patient lean extremely far forward with the hips back in the chair and the chin thrust up and out in a "sniffing" position. This posture opens the hypopharynx, allowing a better view of the anterior commissure of the vocal folds. Instructing the patient to phonate (i.e., say "EEEEEE") and then to take a sudden sharp breath, almost a gasp, reveals a recurrent laryngeal nerve paresis. The object of this procedure is to note whether each true vocal fold abducts (i.e., moves outward) to the same degree as the other. Another trick is to watch the larynx while you have the patient say "AAAAYEEEE" several times, which uncovers the vallecula–the potential space between the base of the tongue and the lingual surface of the epiglottis. If the examiner holds the mirror handle so that he or she can brace his or her ring and little finger securely against the patient's chin, he or she is able to place the mirror against the soft palate firmly and avoid "tickling" the gag reflex.

An appreciation of the normal head and neck region is gained by examining as many patients as possible, thereby building a visual database and increasing one's ability to identify any abnormalities. One soon learns to recognize the watery, floppy cord margins of polypoid corditis (with its "whiskey tenor" voice); the pinkish, faintly irregular vocal fold mucosa of the abuser (e.g., voice abuse, excessive smoking and drinking); the postintubation laryngeal granuloma; the vocal fold hemorrhages of the sports enthusiast; the ugly, granular, pinkish-white of squamous cell carcinoma; the diffuse edema and posterior laryngeal erythema of gastroesophageal reflux disease; and, most importantly, the rounded, pinkish, swollen epiglottis of acute supraglottitis.

Summary

A brief but thorough head and neck examination can expose most clinically significant pathology of the head and neck and may aid in early identification of serious diseases, such as head and neck cancer. Using a consistent, standardized technique for examining all patients enables the clinician to recognize subtle pathologies when they are present.

Additional Resources

A wealth of audiovisual materials is available to refresh examination skills. The American Academy of Otolaryngology–Head and Neck Surgery Foundation have produced a video, *The Physical Examination of the Head and Neck,* by Drs. Yanagisawa and Goodwin, which is available in most academic otolaryngology departments or may be purchased from the Academy by calling 703-836-4444 or online at www.entnet.org.

SUGGESTED READINGS

Bull TR. *A Color Atlas of ENT Diagnosis*, 2nd ed. St. Louis: Mosby Year Book; 1987.
This book is a virtual cornucopia of color pictures of a wide range of pathologic entities of the head and neck.

DeWeese DD, Saunders WH. *Textbook of Otolaryngology.* St. Louis: Mosby Year Book; 1995.
This is the standard textbook of otolaryngology and describes the examination as it has been taught to medical students for the past half-century. Although the techniques are timeless, newer endoscopic instrumentation is not covered completely.

Yanagisawa E, Goodwin G. *The Head and Neck Physical Examination.* Alexandria, VA: American Academy of Otolaryngology–Head and Neck Surgery Foundation; 1986.
This is a 30-minute video that reviews the complete head and neck examination. The images are clear, and important anatomic structures are noted. This video is available in most academic otolaryngology departments, and may be purchased from the academy (see Additional Resources).

SECTION I

Otology

2

Ear Pain and Drainage

Paul M. Spring, MD
Ronald G. Amedee, MD

History and Physical Examination

Ear pain, or otalgia, can be caused by benign or malignant conditions in the ear or elsewhere in the head and neck (called *referred otalgia*). In addition to the usual questions of pain intensity, duration, recurrences, etc., the history should elicit other ear-related symptoms such as hearing loss, tinnitus, vertigo, or pruritus. Other symptoms related to the oral cavity, larynx, pharynx, or upper esophagus are important. These symptoms include dysphagia, odynophagia, unintentional weight loss, nonhealing mucosal ulcer, neck mass, and hoarseness or other voice changes.

The head and neck examination for otalgia begins with the scalp examination. Inspection behind the ears is followed by an otoscopic evaluation of the external auditory canal (EAC) and middle ear, which often reveals an otogenic source of the pain, such as otitis media or otitis externa. (Differential diagnoses of otalgia are shown in Table 2.1.) The patency (or nonpatency) of the eustachian tube can be evaluated by asking the patient to autoinsufflate, or hold his nose and blow as though trying to pop his or her ears. Observation of the tympanic membrane (TM) during this maneuver usually shows a brief outward movement of the TM as greater-than-atmospheric pressure is introduced briefly into the middle ear via the eustachian tube. Likewise, the Toynbee maneuver—asking the patient to swallow while the mouth is closed and the nose is held closed—normally causes a brief inward movement of the

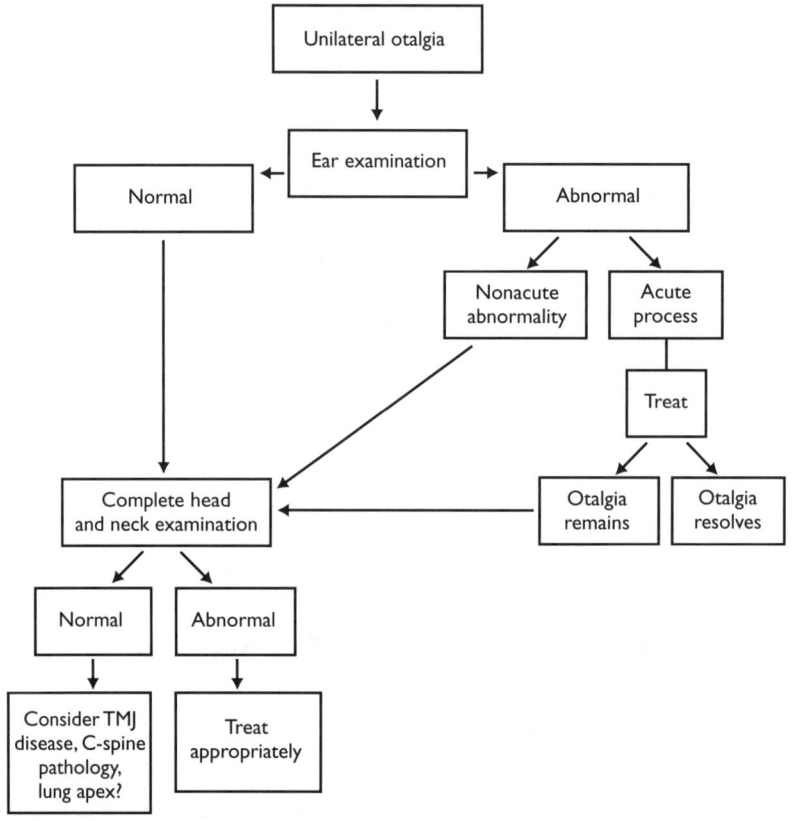

Algorithm A Management of otalgia. TMJ = temporomandibular joint.

TM as the momentary negative pressure is transmitted through the patent eustachian tube. Additionally, the physician can use the pneumatic otoscope to induce brief supra-atmospheric pressure into the EAC, causing inward TM movement (Fig. 2.1). Failure of the TM to move with any of these maneuvers suggests negative middle ear pressure.

For an evaluation of otalgia to be considered complete, the remainder of a thorough head and neck examination is required. Each of the following sections deals with specific causes of otalgia. We detail specific points for special attention in the history and physical examination in each of these sections.

Once the ears have been examined, the nose, oral cavity, oropharynx, and hypopharynx should be assessed. Significant history of smoking or alcohol use warrants a more extensive laryngeal examination. Finally, do not overlook the temporomandibular joint (TMJ). The TMJ apposes the anterior aspect of

Ear Pain and Drainage 33

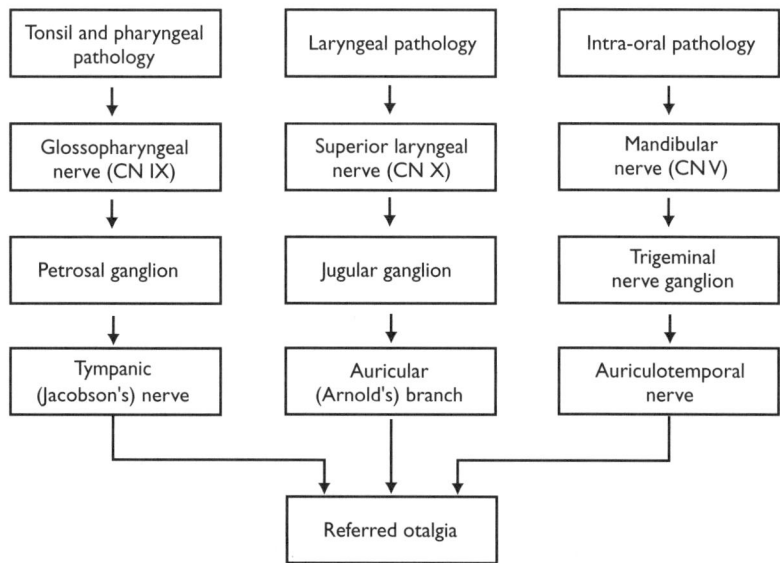

Algorithm B Causes of referred otalgia. CN = cranial nerve.

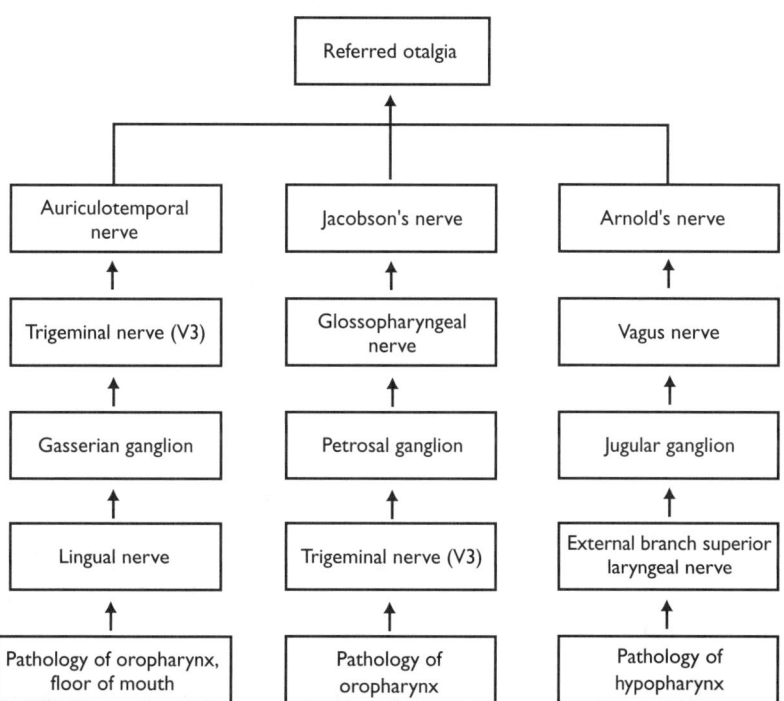

Algorithm C Neural pathways of referred otalgia.

Table 2.1 Differential Diagnoses of Otalgia and Otorrhea

Nonotogenic (Referred Pain)	Otogenic
Fifth Cranial Nerve	**External Ear**
Nose and Sinuses	Auricular trauma
Infection	Auriculitis
Neoplasm	External otitis
Septal deformity	Malignant external otitis
Nasopharynx	Cerumen
Acute infection	Foreign body
Adenoidectomy	Perichondritis
Neoplasm	Herpes zoster oticus
Teeth and Jaws	Neoplasm
Molar impaction	Otomycosis
TMJ arthritis	Perichondritis
Malocclusion	**Tympanic Membrane**
Salivary Glands	Bullous myringitis
Infection	Traumatic perforation
Stones	**Middle Ear or Mastoid**
Trigeminal neuralgia	Acute otitis media
Sphenopalatine neuralgia	Acute mastoiditis
Seventh Cranial Nerve	Barotrauma
Geniculate ganglion	Eustachian tube dysfunction
Ninth and Tenth Cranial Nerves	Chronic otitis media
Pharynx	Intracranial complications of otitis media
Tonsillectomy	Ear canal cholesteatoma
Acute tonsillitis	
Peritonsillar abscess	
Retropharyngeal abscess	
Neoplasm	
Larynx	
Neoplasm	
Granulomatous lesion	
Tongue	
Neoplasm	
Ulceration	
Esophagus	
Elongated styloid process (Eagle's syndrome)	

TMJ = temporomandibular joint.

the EAC, and any inflammation in the joint capsule may cause the perception of otalgia. Occasionally, tuning fork, audiogram, and radiologic evaluations are indicated to secure the correct diagnosis.

Algorithm A outlines the decision-making steps in the management of otalgia. The treatment of specific disorders associated with otalgia is summarized in Table 2.2.

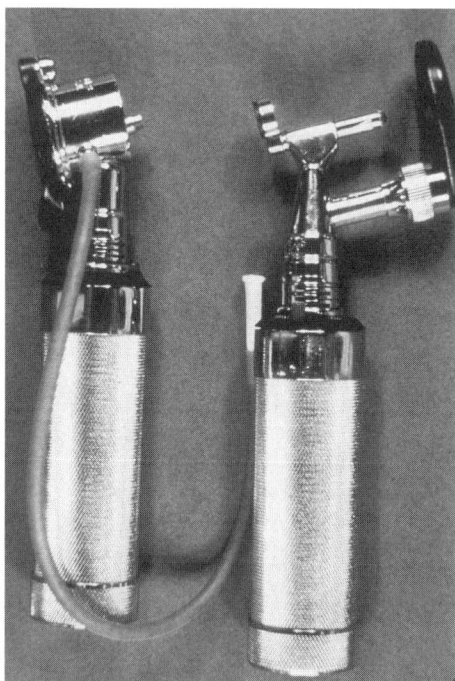

Figure 2.1 Left, The usual examining head of the otoscope can be attached to a rubber tubing and bulb that can be used to introduce pressure into the external auditory canal. **Right,** The operating head can be used when a larger access is desired for instrumentation. (Courtesy of Dr. David Eibling.)

External Ear (Auricle)

Auricular Trauma

An auricular hematoma is a sequela of trauma to the auricle. It is caused by bleeding into the space between the perichondrium and the cartilage (Fig. 2.2). Left untreated, this may deprive the underlying cartilage of its blood supply, causing its dissolution and resulting in the auricular deformity known as a cauliflower ear (Fig. 2.3).

If detected early (i.e., before firm clot formation), simple needle aspiration (under sterile conditions) may result in permanent resolution. If a firm clot has formed, incision with clot evacuation is required. After either method, reformation of the clot is prevented by placing bolsters (e.g., dental rolls, other firm sterile material) on either side of the pinna and sewing them in place with stitches of permanent, nonbraided suture through the auricle. This material is left in place for 3 to 7 days. Antibiotics are used to minimize the chance of chondritis developing (*see* Table 2.2).

Table 2.2 Treatment of Disorders of the External Ear and External Auditory Canal That Are Associated with Otalgia and Otorrhea

Disorder	Treatment
Auricular trauma	
Early diagnosis (before clot formation)	Needle aspiration followed by bolsters placed on either side of pinna; antibiotics
Later diagnosis (after clot formation)	Incision with clot evacuation followed by bolsters placed on either side of pinna; antibiotics
Auriculitis	Antibiotics
Bacterial external otitis	Topical antibiotics (e.g., Cortisporin, Coly-mycin, Vosol, gentamicin [for TM perforation])
Cerumen impaction	Aural syringing, curettage, or suction
Necrotizing external otitis	Intravenous antibiotics, local debridement, topical antimicrobials
Otomycosis	Treatment with topical antifungals
Foreign body	Removal by curette, suction, alligator forceps, irrigation (except for beans or vegetables); lidocaine or mineral oil followed by lavage for insects

TM = tympanic membrane.

Auriculitis (Auricular Chondritis)

If infection of the cartilage (auriculitis) develops, there is a greater risk for developing cauliflower ear. The auricle skin is tense and red (Fig. 2.4), and pain is often severe. The most common pathogen is *Streptococcus pyogenes*. Immediate antibiotics are required.

Diffuse Bacterial External Otitis

Bacterial external otitis arises most often in warm, humid conditions. "Swimmer's ear" describes a common presentation of this disease. Initially there is diffuse pruritus, then fullness and otalgia. The urge to scratch often leads the patient to place some object (e.g., bobby pin, pen cap) into the ear. The resultant trauma to the thin canal-wall skin further predisposes to bacterial invasion. The canal swells even more and bacterial growth continues. At this point, the EAC may be occluded, and it is difficult to visualize the TM.

As the soft tissue becomes edematous, pain worsens. Hearing decreases (conductive loss), the auricle becomes tender, and foul-smelling aural drainage may begin. Common pathogens include *Pseudomonas aeruginosa*, *Staphylococcus aureus*, and *Proteus* and *Streptococcus* species.

Ear Pain and Drainage 37

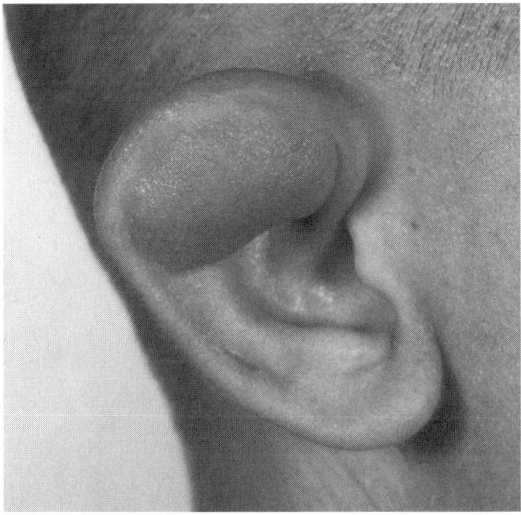

Figure 2.2 Auricle with traumatic hematoma, causing loss of definition of the fine cartilaginous landmarks. (Courtesy of Dr. Jonas T. Johnson.)

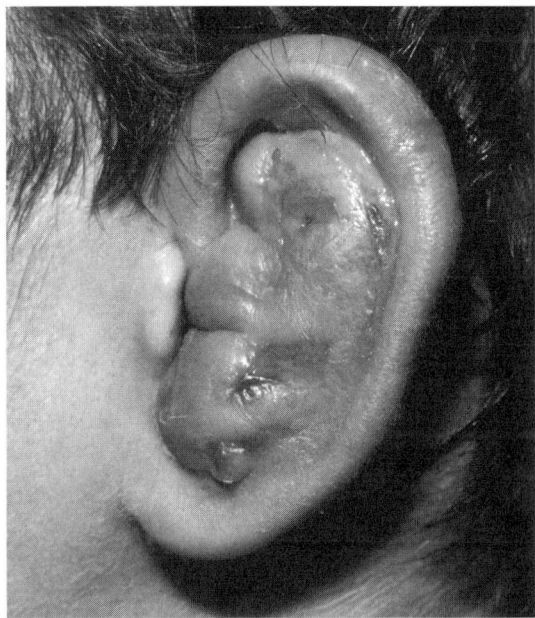

Figure 2.3 An untreated auricular hematoma eventually causes reabsorption of the underlying cartilage, with long-term deformity. (Courtesy of Dr. David Eibling.)

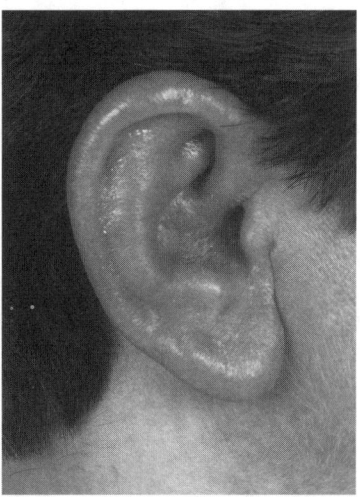

Figure 2.4 Auricular chondritis, with redness and tenderness. (Courtesy of Dr. Karen Calhoun.)

Treatment focuses on eradicating disease, restoring normal anatomy, and preventing further spread. **Topical antibiotic preparations** are the most effective medications and include polymyxin, neomycin, and an acidic solution. Some of the more familiar preparations are Cortisporin, Coly-mycin, and Vosol. Cortisporin and Coly-mycin include the anti-inflammatory hydrocortisone. Vosol-HC is acetic acid plus hydrocortisone. If a TM perforation is suspected or known to exist, nonototoxic drugs are recommended. Cipro HC and Floxin are two newer topical otic preparations that are useful in treating more severe infections. Because neomycin is effective against gram-positive bacteria, this drug is used widely in topical preparations. Ten percent to 15% of the population, however, exhibits a topical sensitivity to neomycin (Fig. 2.5). Typically, the irritation from this sensitivity will be flaking and crusting of the EAC and a streaky extrusion of fluid down the side of the face where excess drops drained. The solution should be changed to a non–neomycin-containing preparation. When redness and swelling extend beyond the pinna, pain is severe, cervical lymphadenopathy is present, or the patient is febrile. Oral antibiotics and analgesics are required.

The delivery of drops is determined by gravity and surface tension. If the canal is too swollen for drops to trickle down the entire EAC to the TM, a small **wick** (methylcellulose or cotton) is inserted gently into the canal, and the drops are applied to this. The wet wick swells (Fig. 2.6) and actively conducts drops along the entire EAC. It also exerts gentle pressure against the swollen EAC skin. The wick remains in place until the edema recedes, the acute pain lessens, and the patient is able to undergo a thorough cleaning of the canal to remove the squamous debris. Without complete cleaning to remove all pus and debris, the topical therapy cannot reach the EAC skin effectively and resolution of the infection is delayed. Generally, it is felt that if a hole in the TM exists or is suspected, nonototoxic drops should be used.

Prevention is the best defense against recurrent external otitis. Custom-fitted ear molds, acidification of the ear canal (with a commercial preparation or with a homemade mixture of one part white vinegar and one part rubbing alcohol), and avoidance of trauma to the ear canal are key preventative measures. **Neither of these solutions should be used if the TM is not intact, because they are irritating to the middle ear.**

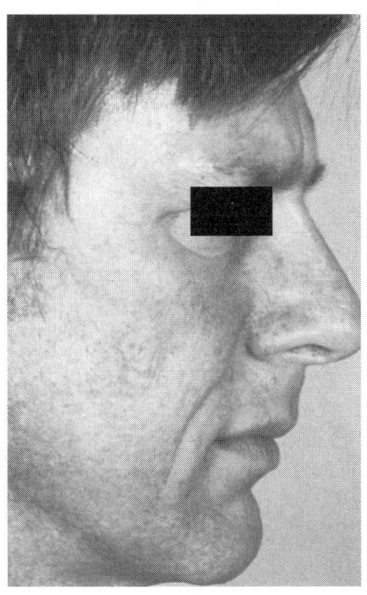

Figure 2.5 Erythema resulting from topical sensitivity to the neomycin in the ear drop. Note the typical distribution of the reaction, exactly where drops draining out of the ear would be expected to flow in an upright patient. (Courtesy of Dr. David Eibling.)

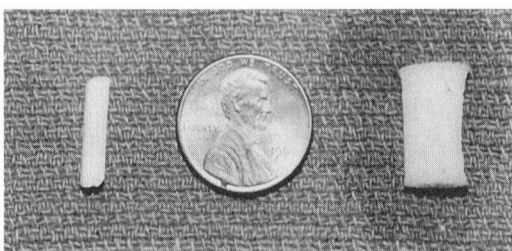

Figure 2.6 Left, The dry, unexpanded wick. **Right,** The moistened, expanded wick. (Courtesy of Dr. Karen Calhoun.)

External Auditory Canal

Cerumen (Ear Wax) Impaction

Cerumen is made of sebaceous material, a secretion of ceruminous glands and desquamated skin. The presence of cerumen is normal, yet large accumulations may cause mild to moderate discomfort to the patient. Removal is necessary, especially if the TM cannot be visualized.

Aural syringing with warm water is effective for removal. Contraindications to syringing include TM perforation either being suspected or present or in patients who are susceptible to infection when exposed to water. Curettage and suction under microscopic vision are also effective methods for removing wax (*see* Chapter 4). Improved hearing is usually immediate, but complete pain resolution may not occur for a day or two. If the skin underlying the cerumen appears very irritated or if small scratches have been caused by removal, several days of topical antibiotic may prevent a secondary otitis externa.

Necrotizing Otitis Externa

Necrotizing otitis externa, or necrotizing external otitis, is a relatively uncommon aggressive bacterial infection of the ear canal. It occurs almost exclusively in immunocompromised patients and in those with diabetes. The hallmark symptoms are a deep boring pain in the ear and granulation tissue at the bone–cartilage junction of the ear canal. In patients with AIDS, the granulation tissue may be absent. The spread of this infection causes cellulitis, chondritis, temporal bone osteitis, and intracranial complications. If the infection is not diagnosed and treated promptly, death may ensue.

Definitive diagnosis is made by computed tomography (CT) scan (Fig. 2.7). The most common pathogen is *Pseudomonas aeruginosa*. Standard care includes intravenous antibiotics and local debridement. Effective antimicrobials include ciprofloxacin, ceftazadime, and aminoglycosides with penicillins. Topical antimicrobials are considered essential. Normalizing blood glucose or otherwise improving the immunocompromised condition is also important. Hyperbaric oxygen therapy may be beneficial.

Otomycosis

Fungal infections of the external canal usually occur after prolonged use of antibacterial eardrops or in immunocompromised patients. Pain and itching are common. The most common fungi are *Candida albicans*, *Aspergillus niger*, *A. flavus*, and *A. fumigatus*. Chronic moisture in the EAC (e.g., from frequent swimming, working in the heat, use of eardrops) can predispose to fungal in-

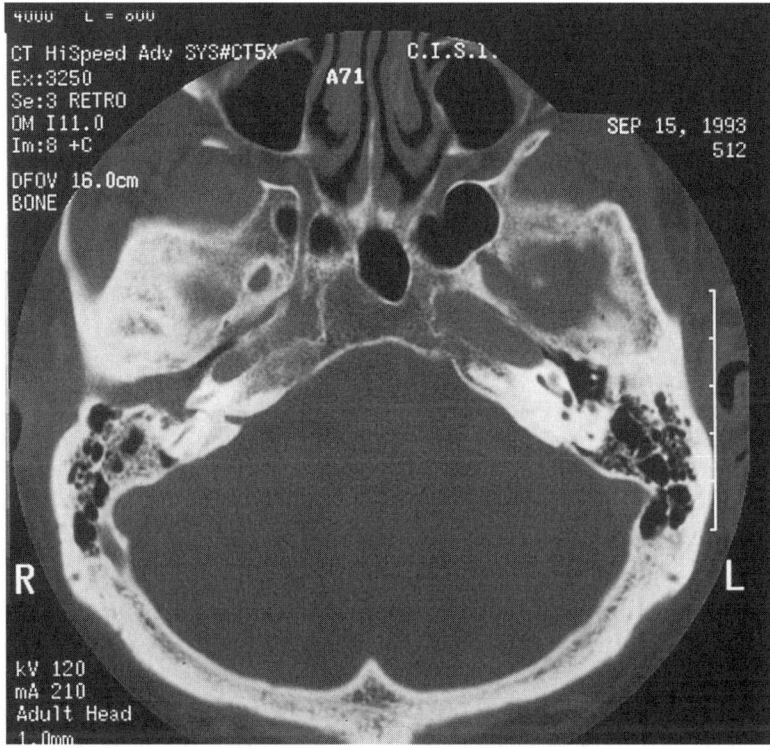

Figure 2.7 Computed tomography scan showing typical findings of malignant external otitis on the right. (Courtesy of Dr. David Eibling.)

fection. Pain is particularly severe in the early stages of the disease process. On otoscopy, the EAC may seem to contain a white fluff (sometimes mistaken for cotton strands), and mycelia are sometimes identified. *A. niger* causes a grayish-black, soft mass of conidiophores in the ear canal (Fig. 2.8). Thorough cleaning of the EAC followed by antimycotic solution (e.g., Gentian Violet, Lotrimin, Cresylate) usually results in a cure.

Furunculosis

Infection of the hair follicles causes furunculosis at the lateral aspect of the external canal. These common gram-positive (*Staphylococcus*) infections appear as localized, occasionally fluctuant swellings close to the meatus of the external canal. There is severe local pain with otoscope insertion or auricle movement.

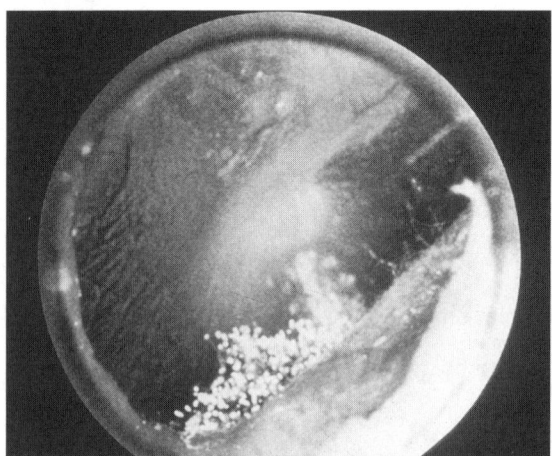

Figure 2.8 Soft mycelial elements of a fungal infection in the external auditory canal. (Courtesy of Dr. F. Kamer.)

Furuncles may be missed if the speculum of the otoscope is inserted without inspecting the superficial ear. Mastoid or mandibular-area lymphadenopathy may occur. If actual pus has developed, treatment includes incision and drainage of the abscess. Sometimes only cellulitis is present. Ear-wick insertion with Vosol solution (to acidify the canal) usually results in resolution of symptoms. If cellulitis is noted, systemic antibiotics with acceptable *Staphylococcus* coverage should be instituted (e.g., amoxicillin and clavulanate, ciprofloxacin, dicloxacillin). Pain control should include nonsteroidal anti-inflammatory drugs (or narcotics for severe pain).

Foreign Body

Beads, erasers, stones, cotton swabs, insects, and gum are among the foreign bodies that have been retrieved from EACs (Fig. 2.9). Pain varies depending on the amount of inflammation in the external canal and the presence of secondary infection.

The foreign body often can be removed in the office setting using a curette, suction, or alligator forceps. Rarely does ear washing work. Ear washing should not be used with beans or other vegetable material because it causes these to swell, making removal more difficult. Lidocaine or mineral oil may be used in the EAC for live insects, followed by lavage or removal of the insect under microscopic visualization. Less-cooperative patients must be sedated or anesthetized in the operating room for safe removal of the insect and inspection of the ear. (*See* Chapter 29 for a more detailed discussion of foreign bodies of the EAC.)

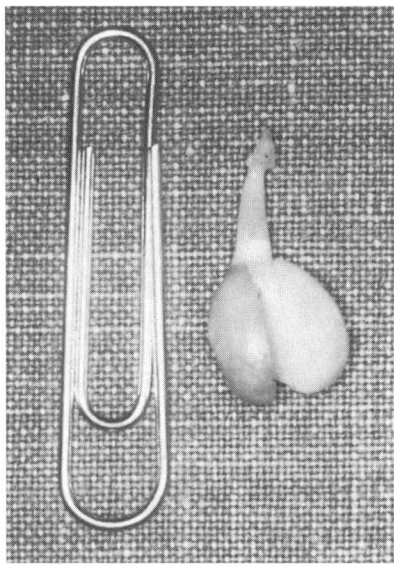

Figure 2.9 Sprouted-seed foreign body removed from the external auditory canal. (Courtesy of Dr. David Eibling.)

Tympanic Membrane (Ear Drum)

Bullous Myringitis

Bullous myringitis is characterized by blebs on the lateral TM surface (Fig. 2.10). Severe pain and aural fullness are common symptoms, but the cause is unknown (a viral infection may be involved). Occasionally, *Mycoplasma pneumoniae* has been cultured from these blebs. Pain control with Auralgen or oral treatment is necessary. Some otologists recommend rupturing the bullae, although this does not seem to decrease pain or hasten resolution. If a middle ear effusion is present, it should be treated with oral antibiotics. This disease usually is self-limited but frequently (in up to one third of patients) is associated with a reversible sensorineural hearing loss. If hearing loss is documented less than 3 weeks from onset, an audiogram should be obtained and the patient given oral steroids for 7 to 10 days.

Traumatic Perforations

Cotton swabs, bobby pins, and needles often are used by patients to "scratch the itch" in their ears. A slight miscalculation of depth and pressure or unexpected jarring of the patient's arm or head can result in TM perforations, the pain from which is sudden and frightening. These perforations are found most commonly in the posterior half of the TM, involving less than one quarter of its

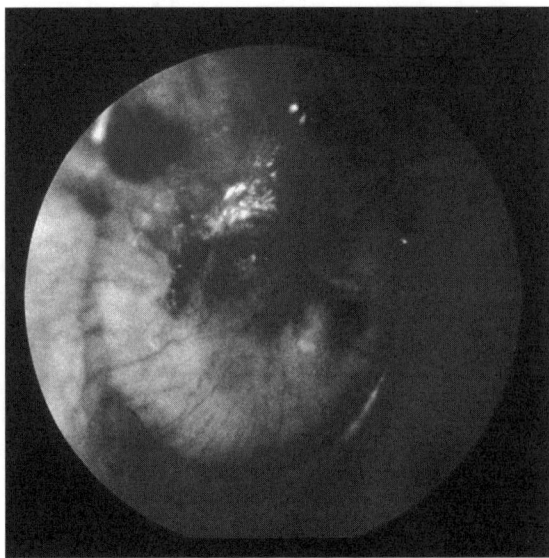

Figure 2.10 Blebs of bullous myringitis seen on the tympanic membrane. (Courtesy of Dr. Stephen Cass.)

surface area, and are seen easily with the otoscope (Fig. 2.11). A drawing documenting the size, shape, and location of the perforation is helpful for follow-up.

Performing an audiogram is recommended in all cases, and usually shows a mild conductive hearing loss that is reversible on healing or repair of the perforation. Some specialists recommend immediate "paper patching," which involves using a small instrument under microscopic vision to fold out the "pushed in" edges of the perforation. A small piece of very thin paper is moistened and placed over the TM perforation to hold these edges in place. Most practitioners, however, do not find this technique necessary, because 90% of noninfected perforations heal within 4 weeks. When the perforation does not heal, tympanoplasty may be necessary. In this procedure, a fascia graft from the temporalis is taken and placed under the native TM to make a new ear drum. Secondary infection is a concern; some physicians treat it with prophylactic topical antibiotics but, in most cases, simply keeping the EAC dry (e.g., using ear plugs while bathing or showering, avoiding swimming and diving until healed) is sufficient. If water accidentally enters the middle ear, the risk of otitis media may be lessened by several applications of topical antibiotics.

A traumatic TM perforation that is accompanied by dizziness, nausea, vomiting, and nystagmus strongly suggests a disruption of the stapes from the oval window. Such a condition requires urgent evaluation by an otologist. Although bed rest often may be all that is needed, emergent middle ear explo-

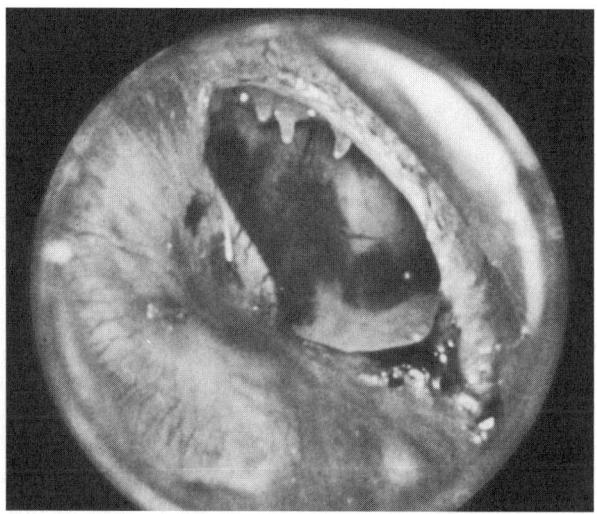

Figure 2.11 Fresh edges of a traumatic tympanic membrane perforation. (Courtesy of Dr. Jonas T. Johnson.)

ration to repair the stapes or patch the oval window may be needed to prevent further deterioration.

Middle Ear

Acute Otitis Media

The pain of acute otitis media is usually sudden in onset and variable in intensity, resulting from inflammation of the sensitive middle ear and the TM (Fig. 2.12). Tension in the middle ear space from the effusion causes exquisite pain, which may radiate to the jaw or worsen with its opening and closing.

The infection usually is caused by *Pneumococcus*, *Haemophilus influenza*, *Staphylococcus*, or *Moraxella*. The middle ear usually communicates freely with the mastoid air cells, and concomitant mastoiditis frequently develops. Pain and erythema over the mastoid tip suggest osteitis, cellulitis, or abscess.

Treatment is oral antibiotic therapy with amoxicillin, trimethoprim-sulfamethoxazole, or ampicillin as first-line therapy in adults. Second-line medications for some beta-lactamase–producing strains of *Haemophilus* or *Moraxella* species include cefaclor (Ceclor), cefuroxime (Ceftin), or amoxicillin/clavulanate (Augmentin).

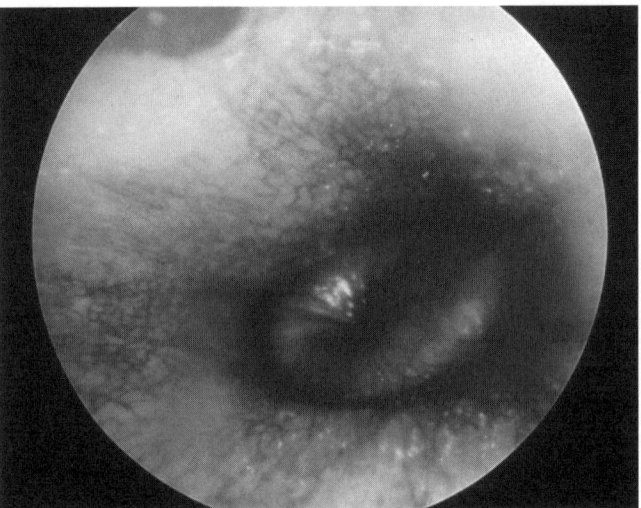

Figure 2.12 Typical appearance of the tympanic membrane in acute otitis media.

In the adult, relief of pain may be offered by a myringotomy performed under local anesthesia (usually a phenol drop on the TM) in the clinic. Decongestants and antihistamines address the usual nasopharyngeal inflammation and edema. Otic antimicrobial solutions are used if concomitant external otitis exists. Persistent pain after adequate initial therapy suggests either progressive disease or the existence of an additional cause of the pain.

Chronic Otitis Media

Chronic otitis media occurs when acute otitis media persists for longer than 3 months; it may be due to mucosal edema, poor eustachian tube function, or inadequate treatment. A chronic TM perforation often develops, and there may be a persistent painless otorrhea (Fig. 2.13). Occasionally, polypoid changes in the middle ear protrude into the external canal, causing a polyp (Fig. 2.14). Treatment of chronic otitis media is aimed at restoring middle ear and mastoid aeration, resolution of mucosal edema, and elimination of infection. Polyps must be removed so that topical medication can enter the middle ear and mastoid cavity. Typical treatment includes topical and oral antibiotics, topical steroids, and occasionally parenteral antibiotics (usually directed against *Pseudomonas* and other gram-negative organisms). Surgery also may be required (Case 2.1).

The greatest danger of progressive disease is the potential for complications. Inadequately treated otitis media can develop into acute suppurative

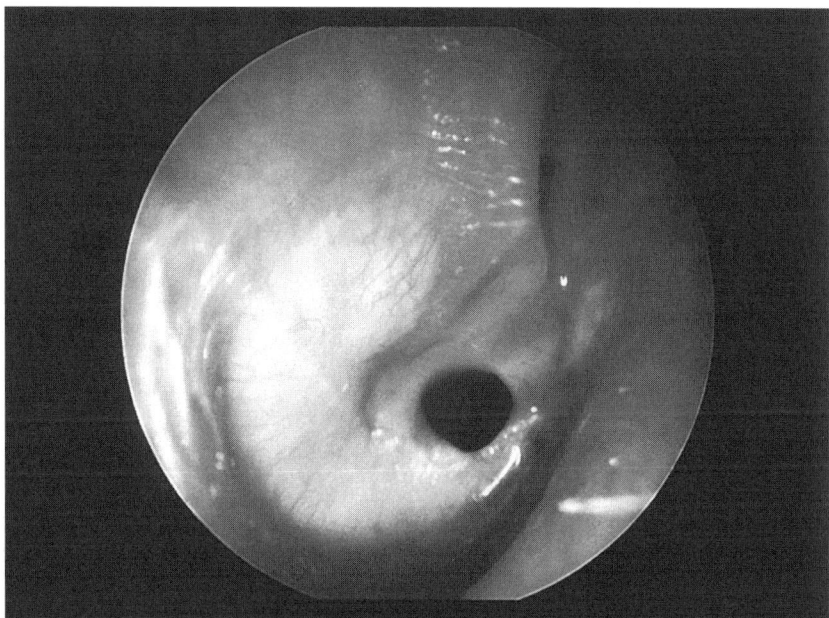

Figure 2.13 Tympanic membrane with persistent perforation of chronic otitis media. Republished with permission from (Kenna MA. *Otitis Media and Eustachian Tube Dysfunction* [*slide lecture*]. Alexandria, VA: American Academy of Otolaryngology–Head and Neck Surgery; 1998.)

mastoiditis, sometimes requiring surgery for resolution (Fig. 2.15). Chronic mastoiditis also can develop. The most serious complications are intracranial, such as an abscess, which can occur by direct extension (thrombophlebitis) or by hematogenous spread (Fig. 2.16). Intravenous antibiotics and neurosurgical drainage often are required in these cases.

In cases with persistent swelling and redness in the EAC, a biopsy of canal skin may be indicated to rule out a primary EAC tumor. Additional causes of referred otalgia include upper aerodigestive neoplasm. Endoscopic and radiographic evaluation is indicated in patients with such pain.

Otitic Barotrauma

Barotrauma to the middle ear results from failure of the eustachian tube to open and allow pressure equalization adequately during rapid pressure changes, such as when descending in an aircraft or diving under water. Normally, air passes easily from the middle ear to the nasopharynx, but passage into the middle ear is more difficult. As the middle ear pressure is maintained on ascent, air escapes easily by way of the eustachian tube into the nose with

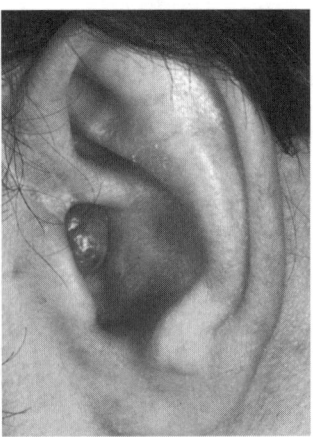

Figure 2.14 An inflammatory polyp protruding from the external auditory canal.

Case 2.1 **Young Man with Chronic Otitis Media Resulting in Tympanic Membrane Perforation**

A man 18 years of age presents with drainage and decreased hearing in his left ear. The hearing loss has developed gradually over the past 6 months. The drainage has occurred intermittantly over the past 2 to 3 months. He has a history of numerous ear infections as a child and has had pressure-equalizing tubes placed twice, most recently at 8 years of age.

Physical examination reveals that his right EAC is nearly completely blocked with an inflammatory polyp. There is scant thin pus. Audiogram shows normal sensorineural hearing, with a 30-dB CHL. His other ear is normal in appearance and hearing.

The patient is taken to the operating room, and the polyp is removed. The skin of the entire EAC appears thickened and red, and the TM is dull, retracted, and immobile, with a small anterosuperior perforation. Postoperatively, the patient's hearing is nearly back to normal. He is treated with a topical antibiotic/steroid combination and oral antibiotics. When the infection and inflammation resolve, he can taste the antibiotic drops, indicating at least minimal patency of the eustachian tubes.

Several months later, tympanoplasty (repair of the tympanic membrane perforation) is undertaken. The patient has an uneventful recovery. One year after his initial presentation, his hearing is normal, and he has no further drainage.

---

yawning. On descent, however, the middle ear air pressure is less than ambient atmospheric pressure at ground level. If the eustachian tube cannot open to allow pressure equalization, a relative negative pressure develops in the middle ear. This causes tremendous pain as the pressure pushes on the TM.

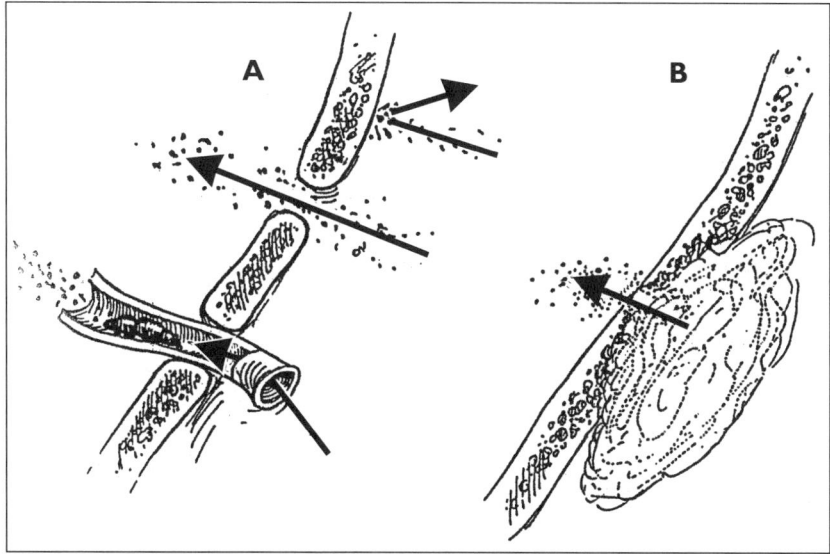

Figure 2.15 A, Acute mastoiditis can cause destruction of the fine bony septae and coalescence of the mastoid bone. **B,** Chronic mastoiditis eventually can involve surrounding bone, causing osteomyelitis. (Republished with permission from Neely JG. *SIPac on Complications of Suppurative Otitis Media.* Alexandria, VA: American Academy of Otolaryngology Head and Neck Surgery; 1978.)

Pain, hearing loss, tinnitus, and fullness may persist for several days after barotrauma. Effusions or bloody effusions (hemotympanum) also may be present. Prophylactic oral antibiotics may be used for hemotympanum. Once barotrauma has occurred, the passage of several days usually effects a cure. Occasionally, oral decongestants assist in symptom resolution.

The best treatment is prevention. When an upper respiratory infection is present, the prudent patient postpones flying or diving. If air travel is unavoidable, the use of oral and nasal topical decongestants before the flight (and antihistamines in the allergic patient) can be used before taking off and 30 to 60 minutes before landing. Active jaw opening (e.g., yawning, gum chewing) and autoinsufflation (e.g., holding one's nose, closing the glottis and popping one's ears) are also helpful.

Referred Pain

Referred otalgia occurs because numerous sensory afferents serve the external ear, external canal, TM, and middle ear. Causes of referred otalgia are listed in Table 2.1, and the pathogenesis is detailed in Algorithm B. Cranial

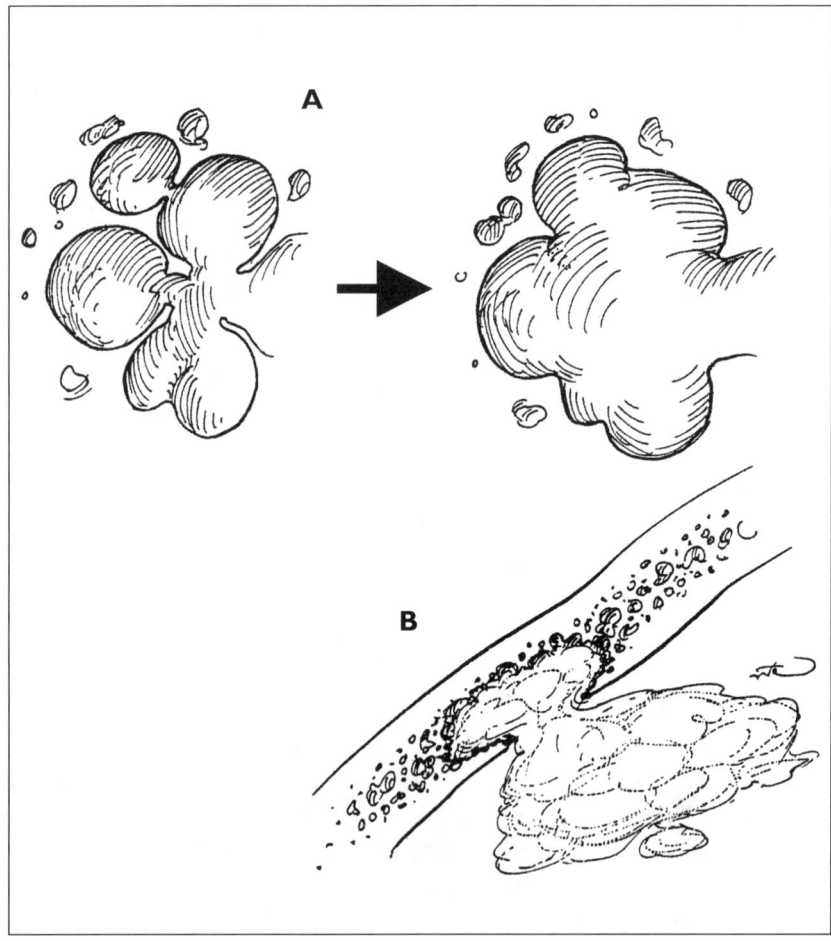

Figure 2.16 Inadequately treated middle ear infections can spread intracranially by several different routes. **A,** Direct extension can occur via extradural routes, the dural venous sinus, or subdurally. **B,** Alternately, thrombophlebitis and hematogenous spread are other routes for intracranial extension. (Republished with permission from Neely JG. *SIPac on Complications of Suppurative Otitis Media.* Alexandria, VA: American Academy of Otolaryngology Head and Neck Surgery; 1978.)

nerves V, VII, IX, X and cervical sensory innervation from C2 and C3 (great auricular nerve) are responsible for the elaborate sensory input of the ear (Algorithm C). Referred pain occurs when, for instance, stimulation of the supraglottis (the internal branch of superior laryngeal nerve) by a neoplasm causes pain via Arnold's nerve (cranial nerve X) in the EAC. Common causes of referred otalgia include pharyngitis, tonsillitis, peritonsillar abscess, cervical arthritis, and neoplasms of the entire pharynx, larynx, and upper esophagus (Case 2.2). The TMJ, which apposes the anterior wall of the EAC, frequently causes otalgia.

> **Case 2.2 Man with Referred Otalgia Caused by Neoplasm of the Pharynx**
>
> A man 57 years of age presents with persistent pain in his left ear. This began approximately 8 months ago, but he did not seek medical help until now. He is a heavy smoker and drinks an average of two six-packs of beer per day. The remainder of his history is unremarkable.
>
> Physical examination of the ear and TMJ are normal. Fiberoptic examination of his pharynx reveals a shaggy, ulcerated mass on the left lateral pharyngeal wall. Biopsy in the operating room reveals moderately differentiated squamous cell carcinoma.
>
> He undergoes surgery, followed by radiation therapy. Six months later, he has no evidence of tumor, and his ear pain has resolved completely.

Danger Signs

Patients who are immunocompromised (e.g., those who have diabetes, are taking immunosuppressives, or are on chemotherapy) or who have increasing ear pain or drainage should be referred to an otolaryngologist. Malignant otitis externa or osteomyelitis may be present. Patients with drainage or pain unresponsive to medical management may have an underlying malignancy and should be referred to an otolaryngologist.

Summary

Ear pain is a common complaint of many patients. Not all ear pain is otogenic in origin. The key to diagnosis is a good history coupled with a complete head and neck examination. Most ear pain is relatively easy to diagnose and treat. In a minority of patients with ear pain, the pain may require more involved evaluation to arrive at the correct diagnosis and treatment.

SUGGESTED READINGS

Bingham BJG, Hawke M, Kwok P. *Atlas of Clinical Otology.* St. Louis, MO: Mosby Year Book; 1992.
In-depth information about all causes of ear and hearing problems, with excellent graphics.

Bojrab DK, Bruderly T, Abdulrazzak Y. Otitis externa. *Otolaryngol Clin North Am.* 1996;29:761–82.
A detailed summary of presentations and causes of external otitis, with typical microbiology and treatment guidelines.

3

Hearing Loss

Donald J. Beasley, MD
Ronald G. Amedee, MD

Hearing loss is a symptom of a disease in the ear, ranging from a simple cerumen impaction (causing a conductive hearing loss) to middle and inner ear disorders to problems affecting the eighth cranial (or auditory) nerve (CN VIII) itself (e.g., acoustic neuroma or cerebellopontile-angle neoplasm).

The two basic types of hearing loss are *conductive* and *sensorineural*. Often the patient's complaints suggest a cause. Patients with conductive hearing loss (CHL; i.e., that which is related to ear canal or middle ear disorders) may simply complain of hearing loss or even note better hearing in noisy situations. CHL is more likely to be accompanied by ear pain (otalgia) and drainage (otorrhea) than is sensorineural hearing loss (SNHL). Patients with SNHL, however, also may experience tinnitus, dizziness, or even true vertigo. Careful questioning may reveal that the patient has a specific difficulty understanding speech. This may be apparent only in certain situations, such as when speaking on the telephone or when conversing in noisy environments or with certain individuals (e.g., children or women whose voices tend to be faint and high pitched).

Relevant Anatomy and Physiology

Understanding the detailed anatomy of the ear is key to understanding hearing loss. The "ear" should be thought of as the entire peripheral auditory system—from the auricle (pinna) to middle ear structures to the intricate cochlea and the CN VIII (Fig. 3.1). The peripheral vestibular system of the inner ear plays an important role in balance. The areas of the brain directly involved with hearing are referred to as the central auditory system.

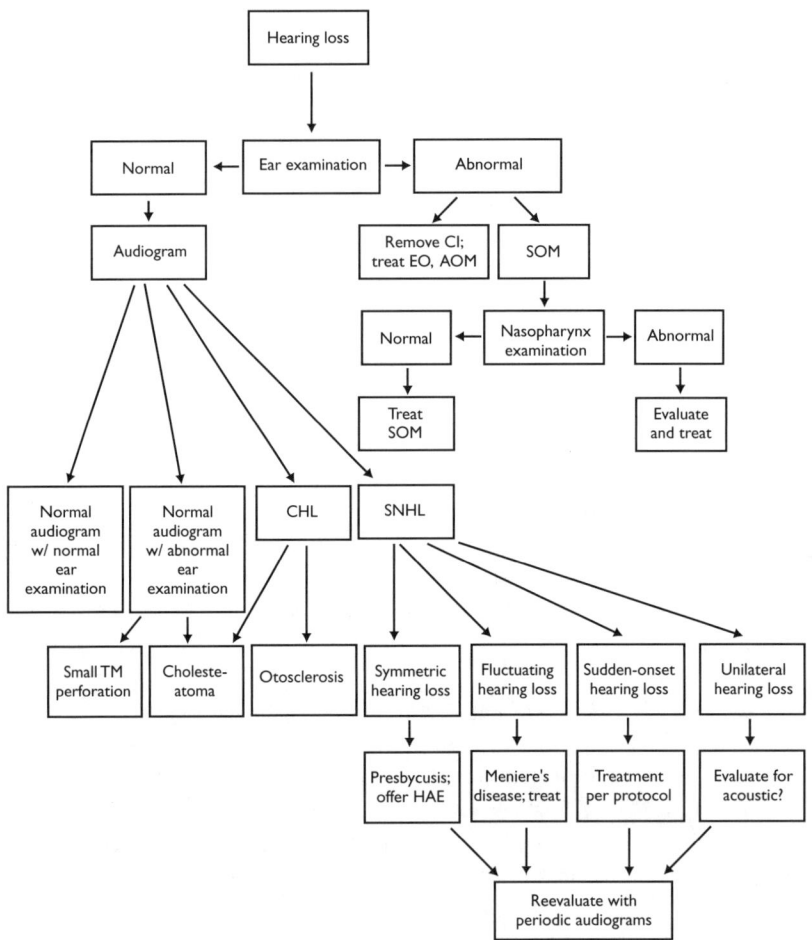

Algorithm Management of hearing loss. AOM = acute otitis media; CHL = conductive hearing loss; CI = cerumen impaction; EO = external otitis; HAE = hearing aid evaluation; SNHL = sensorineural hearing loss; SOM = serous otitis media; TM = tympanic membrane.

The auricle is the "sound collector," composed of a cartilaginous framework covered by skin (Fig. 3.2). The helix is the outermost prominent rim, running around most of the auricle. Just inside, following a similar course, is the ridge of the antihelix. The antihelix splits anteriorly and superiorly to form a depression called the fossa triangularis. The most inferior aspect of the auricle is the lobule (ear lobe). Just above the lobule is the concha, forming the mouth of the external auditory meatus. The small cartilaginous structure anterior to the external meatus is the tragus.

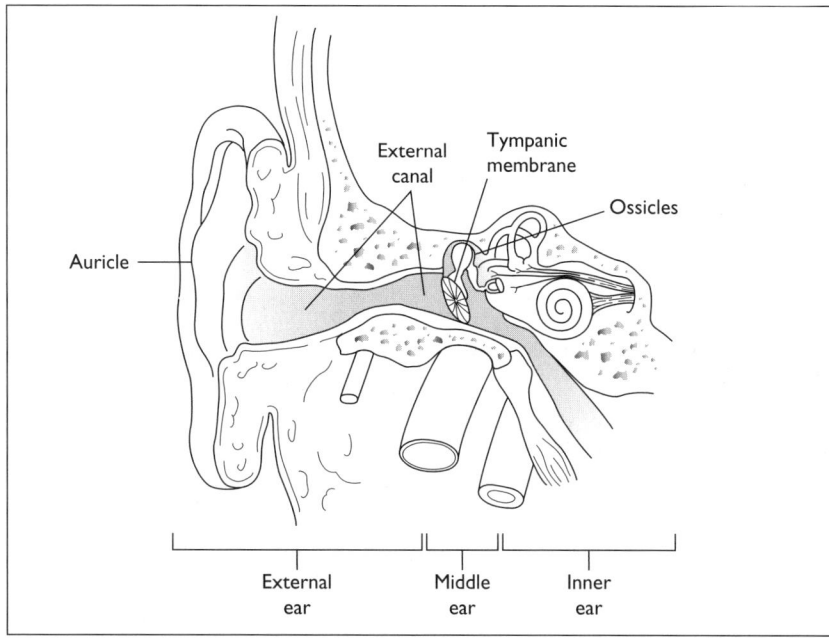

Figure 3.1 The anatomic relationships between the external auditory canal, middle ear, and inner ear.

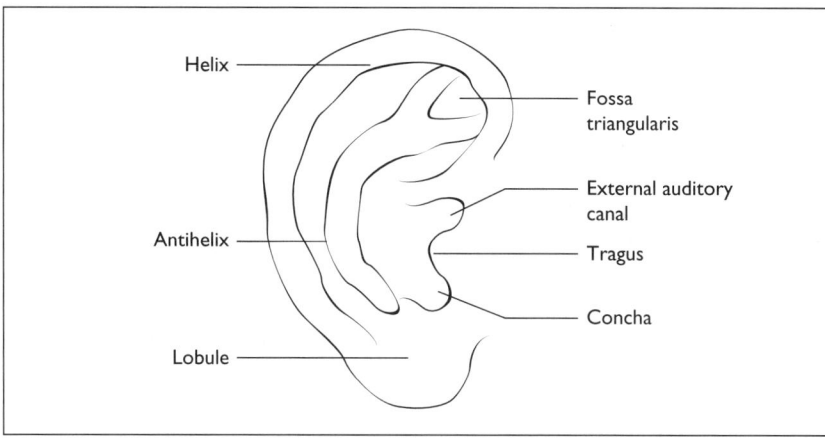

Figure 3.2 The delicate convoluted cartilage of the pinna is covered by very thin skin. The cartilage whorls form an outer rim, the helix, and an inner antihelix and fossa triangularis.

The external canal is the conduit leading medially to the tympanic membrane. The medial two thirds of the canal is a bony portion of the temporal bone lined with skin, whereas the lateral one third is skin-lined cartilage. The skin overlying the cartilaginous portion contains glands that secrete cerumen. The canal is not perfectly straight; at its midpoint there is an isthmus that bends anteriorly and slightly inferiorly—probably to protect the tympanic membrane, which is therefore best visualized by gently pulling the pinna up and back to straighten the canal. The average adult canal is approximately 9 mm in diameter and 25 mm in length.

The tympanic membrane is neither perfectly flat nor orthogonal to the external auditory canal; rather, the membrane is concave like a shallow cone pointing medially and oriented downward and forward in a sloping plane. The tympanic membrane is the most lateral aspect of the middle ear and is the first of the mechanically conducting structures encountered by sound waves. It is composed of three layers and is attached medially to the malleus bone. This attachment keeps most of the tympanic membrane under tension, so this part is named the pars tensa. Superior to the pars tensa is the pars flaccida, which is also the lateral process of the malleus.

The bony cavity of the middle ear space (Fig. 3.3) contains the three articulated ossicles and their tendons and muscles. Their primary function is to conduct sound from the external auditory canal to the fluids of the inner ear. The middle ear space extends through a small opening known as the aditus, or attic, into the mastoid air cells. Both the mastoid and the middle ear space itself may harbor infection, such as in otitis media or mastoiditis. The eustachian tube opens into the anterior middle ear cavity and connects the nasopharynx with the middle ear. When functioning properly, the eustachian tube ventilates the middle ear and equalizes middle ear pressure to the ambient pressure.

The inner ear is medial to the middle ear and deep within the temporal bone. It contains the snail-shaped cochlea (Fig. 3.4). Within the cochlea, there are two parallel chambers. The two-tiered bony labyrinth is filled with perilymph and surrounds the membranous labyrinth, which is filled with endolymph. The endolymph bathes the delicate end organs of hearing, specifically the organ of Corti, within which are tiny hair cells that connect to fibers of the CN VIII's cochlear division. Stimulated hair cells send electrical signals to the brain stem via the CN VIII for processing and then to the cerebral cortex for recognition as sound. Damage to the inner ear or the CN VIII can produce sensorineural hearing deficits.

Sound is the compression and rarefaction of air in a regular pattern. This vibration stimulates the tympanic membrane, which transmits the vibration to the ossicles of the middle ear. As the ossicles vibrate, a pressure wave of perilymph is created in the cochlea, which in turn causes hair cell movement that ultimately transduces sound into neural impulses. These impulses travel along the auditory nerve to various brainstem nuclei until they are received in the cerebral cortex of the brain and perceived as meaningful.

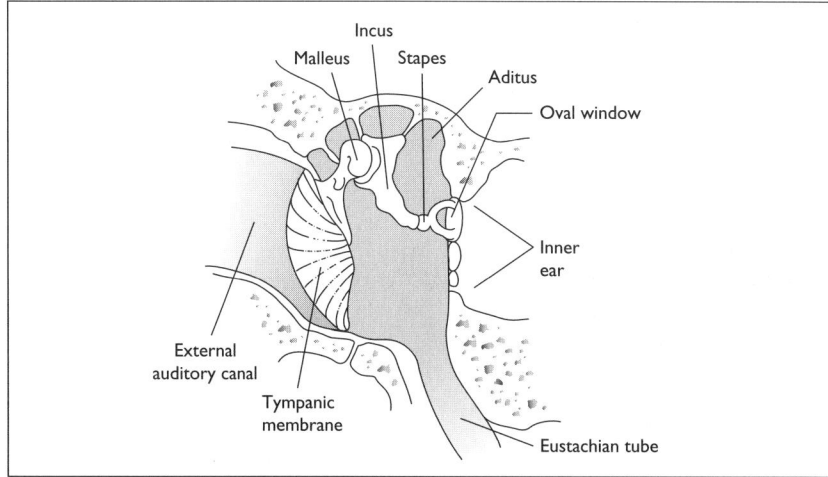

Figure 3.3 The malleus, incus, and stapes form a sound-transmitting bridge between the tympanic membranes and the oval window of the inner ear.

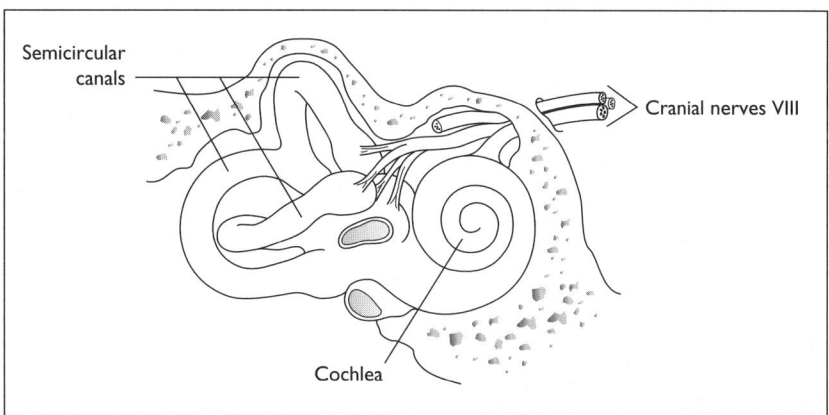

Figure 3.4 The hair cell–containing cochlea is coiled like a snail, and the three semicircular canals are oriented at right angles to each other.

History

Assessing whether one or both ears are affected with hearing loss is important. Appropriate questions in this assessment include the following:
- When did the hearing loss start?
- Is it getting better, worse, or staying the same?
- Does it remain constant or does it fluctuate?
- How much does it bother or handicap the patient?

A related otologic review of systems should assess for the presence of the following:
- Tinnitus
- Aural fullness or pressure
- Vertigo, dizziness, lightheadedness, or disequilibrium
- Drainage, discharge, or pain
- History of head trauma
- History of noise exposure
- Ototoxic medications (now or in the past)
- Family history of hearing loss

Physical Examination

The pinna is inspected for **congenital malformations**, including pre-auricular skin tags and pits (Fig. 3.5). External auditory canal patency is assessed, along with the presence of skin abnormalities (e.g., erythema, edema, scale) and drainage. The removal of cerumen can be difficult, but it is imperative for a complete physical examination to be performed. If the tympanic membrane can be seen adequately and is intact, then attempting irrigation is safe. **However, irrigation should not be used if a history of ear surgery or a possibility of perforation exists, if otalgia is present, or if the patient is diabetic.** At times, a cerumen softener (e.g., Colace) should be used for several days. When available, an operating microscope, specialized suction, and curettage and grasping instruments enable the removal of almost all cerumen impactions.

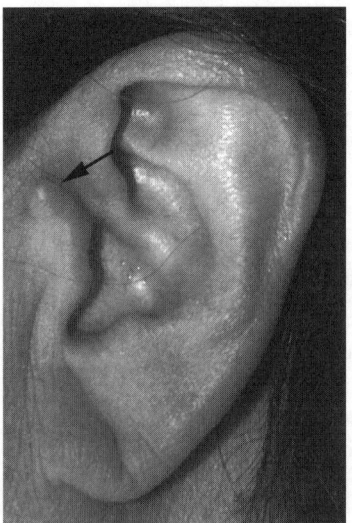

Figure 3.5 Small skin tag on the tragus (*arrow*), with no associated hearing deficits. (Courtesy of Dr. Karen H. Calhoun.)

Inspection of the tympanic membrane for normal landmarks and pathology should be performed. The clinician should determine if there are any perforations or retraction pockets. Is the appearance of the tympanic membrane a normal translucent, shiny gray? Are there areas of thickening, discoloration, or perforations?

When the tympanic membrane has its normal translucency, fluid in the middle ear can be seen clearly. The character of this fluid and the presence of air bubbles or a meniscus should be noted. Indirect assessment of middle ear pressure can be made with the pneumatic bulb by instilling air gently into the external auditory canal while assessing the tympanic membrane for movement.

Tuning fork tests are an important part of the physical examination in a patient with hearing loss. These forks can help to distinguish normal from abnormal hearing and to differentiate between CHL and SNHL. Tuning forks provide a screening evaluation of the hearing, but they are not a substitute for an audiologic evaluation.

The **Weber** and **Rinne** tests are performed with **512- and 1024-Hz tuning forks**. For the Weber test, the tuning fork is gently struck and then placed in the center of the patient's forehead. The patient is asked if the sound is louder on either side or if they are equal. If the patient cannot hear the sound, the clinician may try to place the fork on the bridge of the nose or upper central incisors. In a person with normal hearing, the sound will be equal in both ears. With CHL, the sound lateralizes to (i.e., is louder in) the impaired ear. This may seem counterintuitive, but it is important to remember that the tuning fork is measuring sound transmission through bone, which does not attenuate sound transmission effectively. If both nerves receive the sound equally (i.e., there is no difference in SNHL), then the ambient noise in the ear that is hearing normally will partially mask the sound, whereas the ear with CHL will provide no such masking. With SNHL, the sound lateralizes away from (i.e., is softer in) the impaired ear.

The Rinne test is performed by gently striking the tuning fork and placing it on the patient's bony mastoid tip (Fig. 3.6); he or she usually hears the sound well. When the patient signals that the sound is no longer heard, the fork is moved away from the skull and held in front of the external auditory meatus. The residual vibrations should now be heard. Failure to hear this second sound is termed a "reversal" of the Rinne test or a "negative" Rinne test, indicating that bone conduction is better than air conduction. Because air conduction is normally more acute than bone conduction, this is an abnormal finding consistent with CHL.

Differential Diagnosis

Conductive hearing loss results from problems in the external ear, tympanic membrane, or the middle ear space or its contents. CHL impedes amplification and transmission of sound to the cochlea, whereas SNHL results from malfunction of the cochlea or the acoustic nerve and can be worsened functionally by concomitant malfunction of the central auditory pathways. The differential diagnoses of these two basic types of hearing loss are detailed in Table 3.1.

Additional Diagnostic Evaluation

Laboratory Testing

Laboratory testing for hearing loss usually is reserved for patients who present with new-onset SNHL. In these cases, a **fluorescent treponemal antibody absorbed (FTA-Abs) test** may detect late secondary or tertiary

Table 3.1 Differential Diagnosis of Conductive and Sensorineural Hearing Loss

Conductive Hearing Loss	Sensorineural Hearing Loss
Impacted cerumen	Presbycusis
Foreign body	Noise-induced hearing loss
Otitis externa	Meniere's disease
Middle ear effusion	Congenital hearing loss
Otitis media	Ototoxicity
Cholesteatoma	Sudden hearing loss
Otosclerosis	Acoustic neuroma
Middle ear neoplasm	

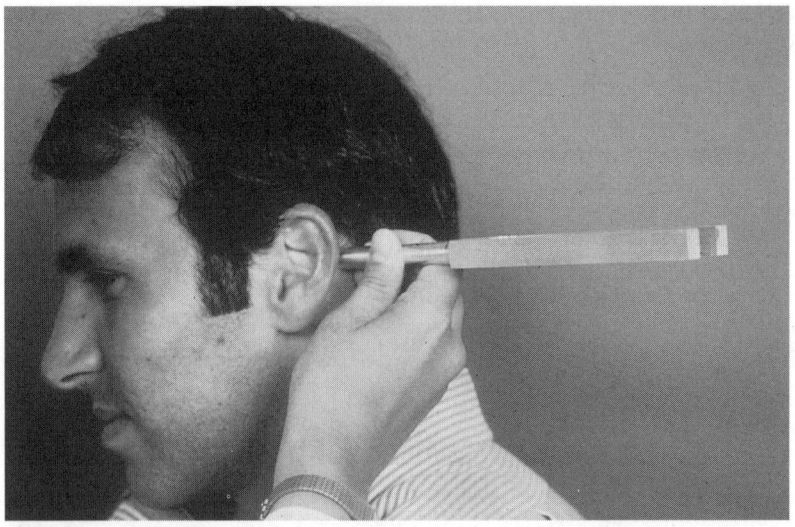

Figure 3.6 Physician performing the Rinne test, holding the 512-Hz tuning fork directly on the mastoid tip to assess bone conduction. (Courtesy of Dr. Jonas T. Johnson).

syphilis. A **complete blood count (CBC)** may provide evidence of an inflammatory process or an occult hematologic malignancy. Obtaining an **erythrocyte sedimentation rate (ESR)** may reveal the presence of an inflammatory or autoimmune process. Because hyperlipidemia, hypothyroidism, and the small-vessel disease that occurs with diabetes can be associated with SNHL, one may want to obtain a fasting blood sugar level and lipid profiles and to perform a 2-hour postprandial glucose tolerance test and thyroid function tests. Other conditions associated with hearing loss include Lyme disease and HIV, so the physician may wish to obtain Lyme titers (if in an endemic area) and HIV serology in selected cases.

Imaging Studies

Computed tomography (CT) and magnetic resonance imaging (MRI) are the most useful imaging studies for elucidating hearing loss. CT gives the best bony definition of the temporal bone; the assessment of congenital abnormalities and bone destruction by tumor are best shown by this type of study (Case 3.1) (Fig. 3.7). MRI with gadolinium offers excellent soft tissue definition of structures in and around the temporal bone (Fig. 3.8), and inflammatory lesions and tumors also are well defined.

Case 3.1   Woman with Acoustic Neuroma

A righthanded woman 45 years of age complains of a gradual onset of leftsided hearing loss. She denies trauma, noise exposure, ear pain, and drainage. She denies dizziness, headache, and any other neurological symptom. Past medical history is insignificant.

Physical examination is completely normal, with the exception of the Weber tuning fork test, which lateralizes to the right ear. An audiogram reveals an asymmetric hearing loss, with normal hearing on the right and a 45-dB high-frequency loss on the left. Speech discrimination scores are 100% on the right, and 32% on the left. Acoustic-reflex testing reveals absent reflexes on the left. An auditory brainstem response test is performed and reveals poor waveforms on the left, with normal waves on the right. An MRI scan with gadolinium reveals a 2-cm acoustic neuroma in the left cerebropontile angle, with widening of the internal auditory canal. A translabyrinthine resection of the tumor is performed, with no attempt to preserve hearing. Her recovery is uneventful, with the exception of several weeks of mild vestibulopathy (dizziness) that responds well to rehabilitation exercises.

Discussion
Acoustic neuroma is an important cause of asymmetric hearing loss, and its presence should be ruled out, particularly in younger patients. The definitive test is the MRI scan with gadolinium, although audiologic testing and the auditory brainstem response test may provide significant clues to its presence.

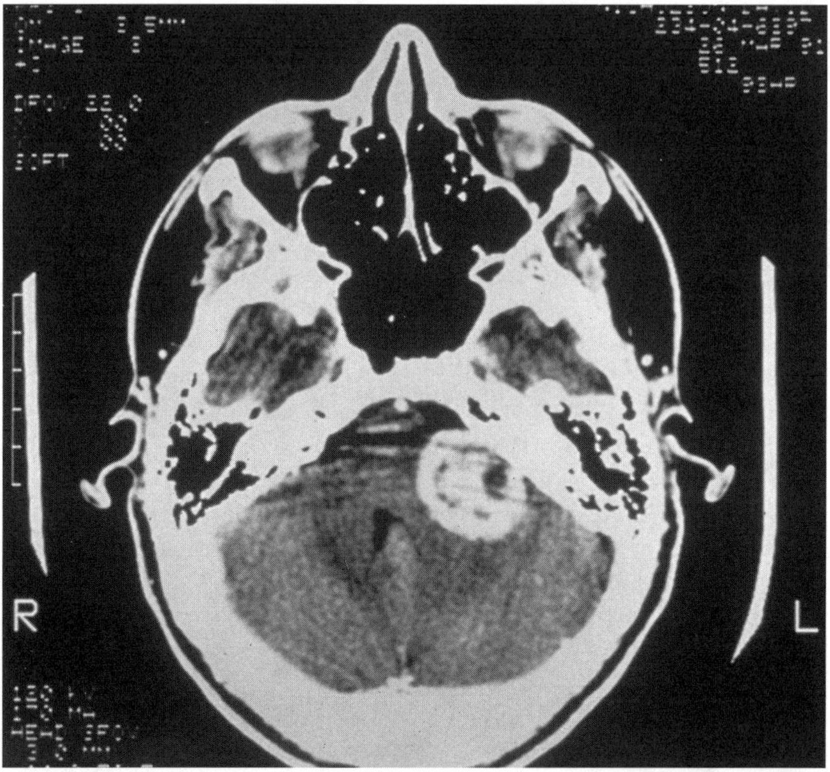

Figure 3.7 Computed tomography scan of temporal bone showing a large acoustic neuroma in the left cerebellopontile angle. (Courtesy of Dr. Stephen Cass.)

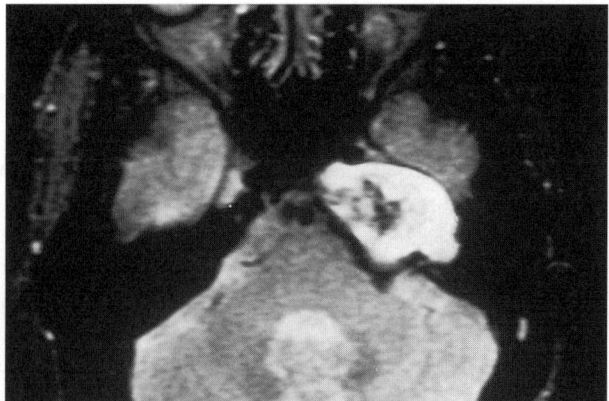

Figure 3.8 Magnetic resonance imaging scan of a temporal bone showing a large cholesterol granuloma of the petrous bone. (Courtesy of Dr. David Eibling.)

Audiograms

The basic instrument used to assess hearing quantitatively is the pure-tone-and-speech audiometer, which produces pure tones and speech of varying frequency and intensity. Plotting the frequency against the intensity provides an audiogram (Fig. 3.9). The **air conduction** of sound is the transmission of sound through to the external, middle, and inner ear. **Bone conduction** represents the transmission of sound directly through the inner ear and reflects on the health of the inner ear and the neural transmission of sound. Six threshold levels are tested at octave frequencies from 250 to 8000 Hz. Both air- and bone-conduction measurements are recorded at the hearing threshold level (HTL) to detect the presence of CHL and SNHL. The human ear can detect sounds from 20 to 20,000 Hz, but the most important range of hearing for conversational speech is 300 to 3000 Hz.

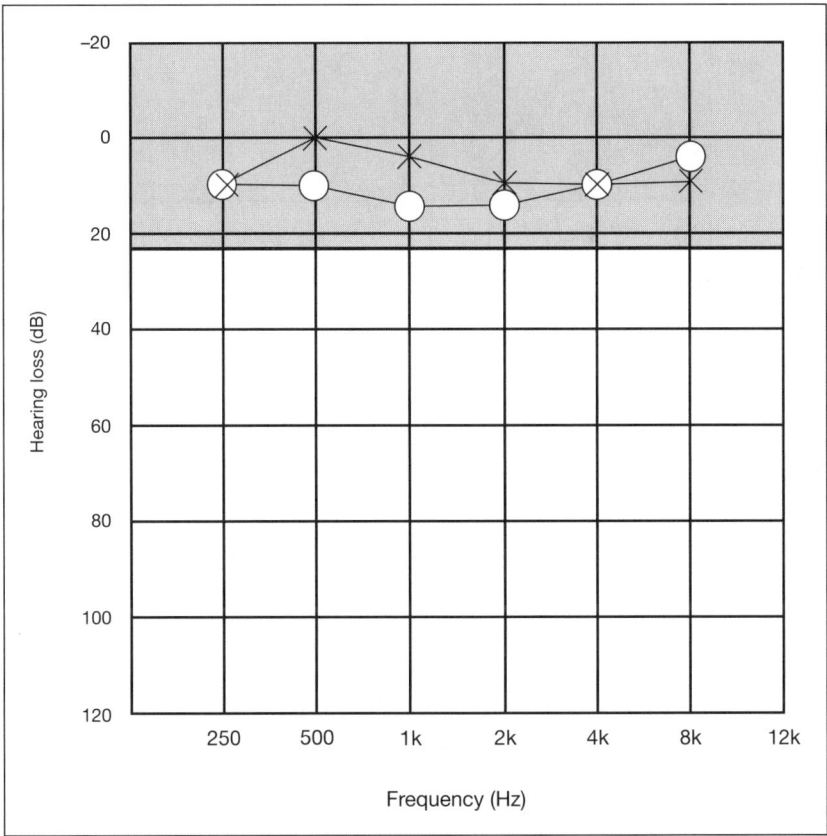

Figure 3.9 This audiogram shows normal air-conduction hearing in both ears. The left ear is represented by "×" and the right ear by "○."

The normal hearing range for adults is 0 to 20 dB, as seen in Figure 3.9. Pure-tone testing that reveals impaired hearing on air conduction but normal hearing on bone conduction is indicative of **CHL**–pathology in the part of the hearing mechanism that conducts sounds waves or vibrations to the cochlea (i.e., external auditory canal, eardrum, and ossicles) (Fig. 3.10). This **"air–bone gap"** characterizes the conductive loss. If both air- and bone-conduction measurements are depressed to the same level (i.e., an air–bone gap of <10 dB), then **SNHL** is present (Fig. 3.11). Figure 3.12 is an example of a patient with a noise-induced SNHL; there is a characteristic shape with a 4000-Hz "notch."

Ambient noise can diminish the accuracy of an audiogram markedly. The most accurate audiograms are those obtained in a soundproof booth in which the tester communicates with the patient being tested via a microphone (Fig. 3.13).

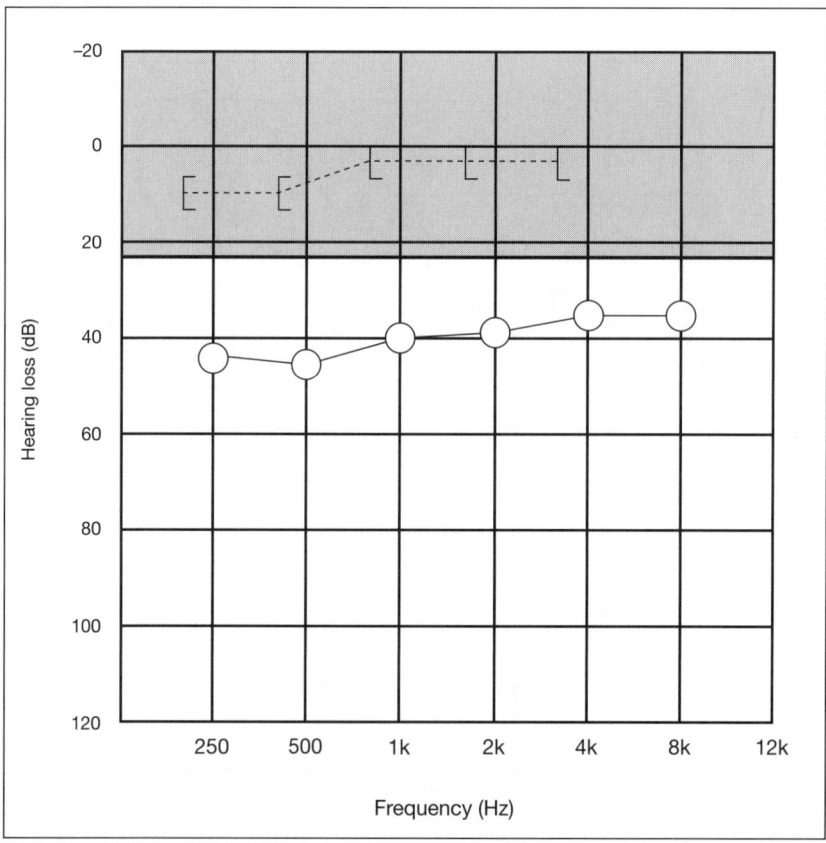

Figure 3.10 This audiogram shows a conductive hearing loss in the right ear. The line with brackets shows the hearing level when bone conduction is assessed (sensorineural hearing level), and the line with circles shows the impaired air-conduction hearing in the right ear.

Auditory Brainstem Response

The auditory brainstem response (ABR)—also called the brainstem auditory evoked response (BAER) or the brainstem evoked response (BSER)—is a sensitive, noninvasive, and inexpensive measure of cochlear, CN VIII, and central auditory function that is available in most hospitals and other medical facilities (Fig. 3.14). ABR is not affected by a patient's state of arousal; therefore, if necessary, sedation may be used for testing. An ABR uses clicks or tone bursts administered via headphones. The resultant electrophysiologic responses are recorded from the surface of the patient's scalp and ears. A signal-averaging computer compiles the results as a waveform. Each component originates from a location along the central auditory system. These components are labeled with Roman numerals (I–VI) and are described by their latency (in milliseconds [ms]) and amplitude from one peak to the following trough (in microvolts

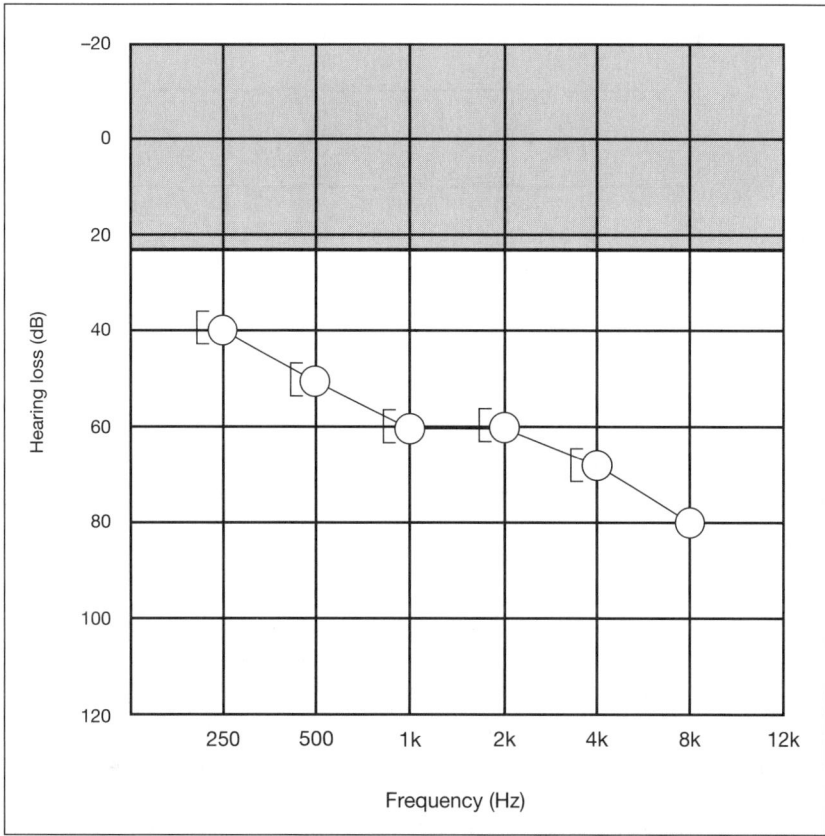

Figure 3.11 This audiogram shows the air- and bone-conduction lines superimposed but depressed, indicating a sensorineural hearing loss.

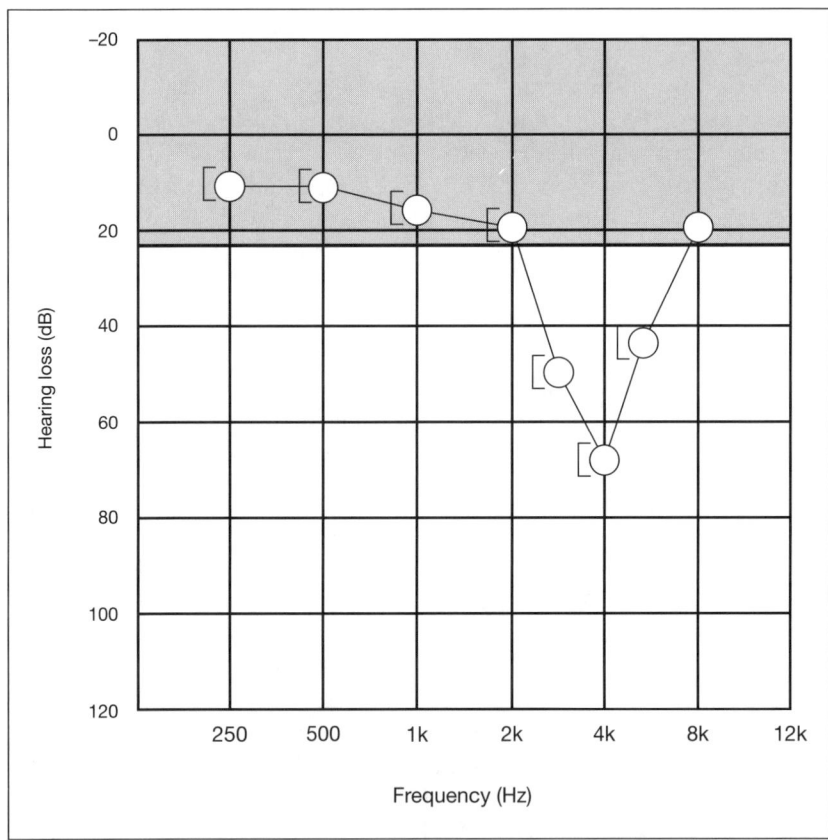

Figure 3.12 This audiogram shows a superimposed air- and bone-conduction level, both of which "dip" at 4000 Hz. This configuration is typical of noise-induced hearing loss.

[μV]). Analysis of the wave components provides neurodiagnostic information of cochlear, auditory nerve, and brainstem auditory function.

Management and Follow-Up

Management depends on the cause of the hearing loss (*see* Algorithm). **CHL** caused by cerumen impaction or a foreign body is treated by removing the offending mass, whereas middle ear infections are treated with antibiotics. Other causes of CHL, such as persistent effusion or otosclerosis, often are correctable with surgery. A **cholesteatoma** is a slow-growing epithelial cyst that can destroy the ossicles and erode into the inner ear; thus, surgical removal is nearly always indicated.

Hearing Loss 67

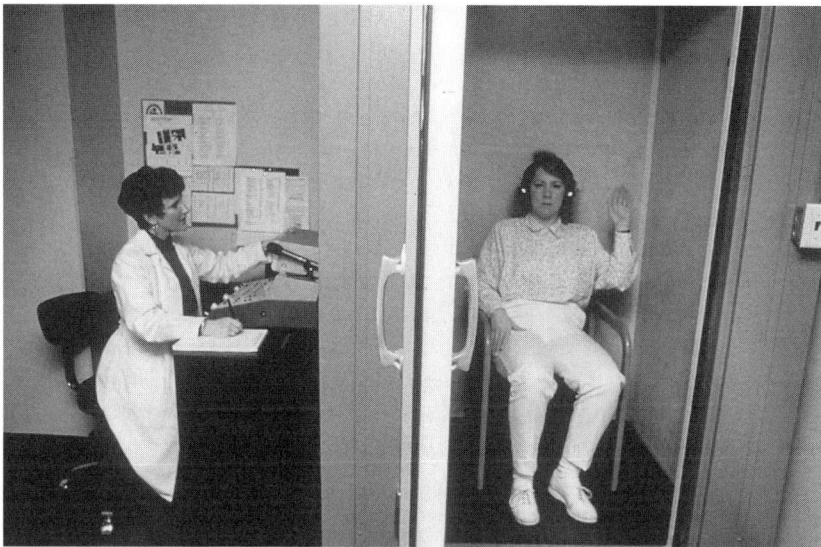

Figure 3.13 Photo of a soundproof audiologic testing booth with the door open. The examinee indicates that she has heard the sound in her left ear by raising her left hand. In actual testing, the door would be closed. Without a soundproof booth, audiometric testing is only an approximation. (Courtesy of Dr. David Eibling.)

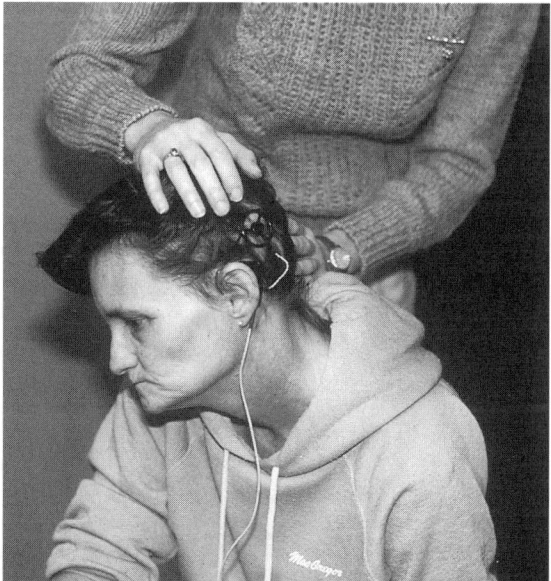

Figure 3.14 The auditory brainstem response test. Sound is presented to the external auditory canal, and evoked potentials are measured transcranially. Wave presence and morphology provide objective evidence of hearing function. This test has significant benefit in site-of-lesion testing and in identifying malingerers. (Courtesy of Dr. Barry Hirsch.)

Many patients with significant **SNHL** may benefit from hearing aids, but patients first must be evaluated appropriately. **Ototoxicity** may be caused by the administration of life-saving medications and, in some cases, may be reversible if the offending agent can be discontinued. Acoustic neuromas and other cerebellopontine-angle neoplasms may present with SNHL and generally require surgical removal. Progressive **Meniere's disease** signifies endolymphatic hydrops and sometimes can be slowed by medical treatment (*see* Chapter 6). At present, the main causes of SNHL (e.g., **presbycusis**, noise-induced, congenital) have no effective medical or surgical treatment; SNHL patients should be encouraged to use hearing aids (Case 3.2).

Sudden hearing loss represents an enigma, and numerous therapeutic strategies exist (Case 3.3). For example, one theory is that sudden hearing loss is a manifestation of an autoimmune disorder. Other theories include viral inflammation and vascular insufficiency of the cochlea. Management options include

---

Case 3.2 Elderly Man with Sensorineural Hearing Loss Caused by Aging and Noise Exposure

A man 75 years of age and a veteran of World War II worked in a metal-fabrication plant for 35 years. He has noted hearing loss that interferes with his interpersonal relationships. His hearing loss tends to be more problematic when he is in groups or when his wife is speaking to him in a noisy environment, such as when the grandchildren are visiting. He denies ear pain and drainage but does admit to constant, high-pitched tinnitus that seems to be worse in the left ear. He does not smoke, takes only an antihypertensive agent, and has no other significant medical history.

Physical examination reveals normal ear canals and tympanic membranes, and the rest of the physical examination is normal. There is no objective tinnitus. An audiogram was performed and showed binaural, high-frequency SNHL, with thresholds dropping to 70 and 80 dB at 6000 Hz. Speech-reception thresholds were 35 and 45 dB in the right and left ears, respectively. Discrimination scores were 76% and 74%, respectively.

The patient is counseled about amplification. He and his wife are counseled about lifestyle changes to improve their ability to communicate.

Discussion
This patient presented with the classic high-frequency SNHL that is associated with aging and noise exposure. Like most patients, he complained chiefly about the inability to understand speech due to the loss in discrimination that occurs with high-frequency hearing loss. Newer programmable hearing aids as well as other advances in auditory rehabilitation can provide significant enhancement of day-to-day communication for individuals who have similar deficiencies. Hearing-conservation programs have the potential to reduce or eliminate many of the hearing disabilities that affect today's older population.

watchful waiting and treatment with steroids, intravenous histamine, and antiviral agents. Because the cause is usually unknown, steroids are used in an attempt to decrease any inflammatory component. Unfortunately, a significant number of patients are helped only by a hearing aid. Many patients with sudden hearing loss will experience a return of their hearing, although it is not clear whether this return is facilitated by any administered therapy. Nevertheless, most patients elect to be treated because the potential benefits outweigh the risks.

Used to ameliorate hearing loss, hearing aids are miniaturized sound-amplifying devices that contain a microphone to receive sound, an electronic processor (amplifier) that manipulates the qualities of the sound to make it more usable to the listener, a speaker (receiver) directed toward the ear, and a power source (Fig. 3.15). Patients may express concerns about the cosmetic appearance of wearing a hearing aid; however, more than 80% of the hearing aids dispensed in the United States are small enough to fit within the ear canal, and the latest generation of hearing aids can be worn deep inside the ear canal, within millimeters of the tympanic membrane. Many sophisticated variations are available (Figs. 3.16–3.19). Proper selection of hearing aids requires evaluating the hearing loss precisely, choosing a device that is appropriate for the hearing loss, fitting the aid to the ear, and training the patient in proper use of the device. Some patients with CHL also may benefit from amplification. Less sophisticated, often overlooked, but extremely useful to hearing-impaired individuals are **assisted-listening devices**, such as amplified

---

Case 3.3   Woman with Sudden Sensorineural Hearing Loss

A woman 45 years of age awakened with a sudden leftsided tinnitus and complete hearing loss. She had had no history of ear drainage, URI, or pain. Her past medical history is unremarkable, and she takes no medications.

Physical examination reveals normal tympanic membranes and ear canals, and the remainder of her head and neck examination is normal as well. An audiogram reveals an ipsilateral, flat SNHL, with a speech-reception threshold of 60 dB. Speech discrimination is 82%, with a sensation level of 100 dB. MRI scan with gadolinium is normal.

The patient is diagnosed with sudden SNHL. She is treated with prednisone (60 mg/d for 3 weeks). She returns 3 weeks later with persistent symptoms, and a repeat audiogram reveals no change.

Discussion
Numerous therapeutic strategies are considered for sudden hearing loss. Because one theory is that sudden hearing loss is a manifestation of an autoimmune disorder, it was decided that this patient should be treated with steroids.

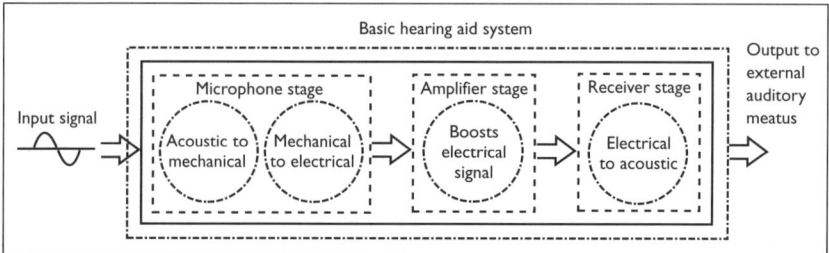

Figure 3.15 The basic components of a hearing aid system. (Reprinted with permission from Bailey BJ. *Head and Neck Surgery–Otolaryngology*. Philadelphia: JB Lippincott; 1993:1860.)

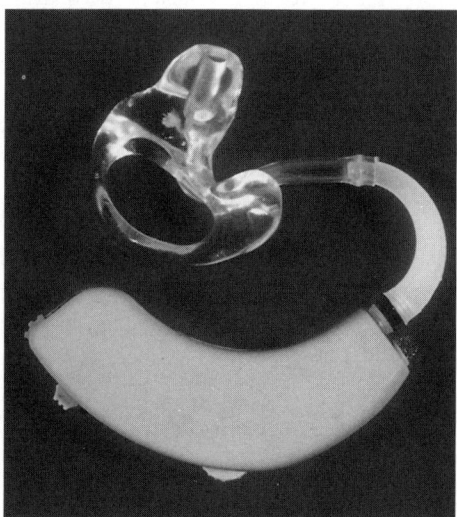

Figure 3.16 Behind-the-ear hearing aid. A behind-the-ear aid tends to be of lower cost than in-the-ear or in-the-canal aids, and they also are more powerful. The separation of the microphone from the speaker reduces problematic feedback. (Courtesy of Dr. Deb Carlson.)

telephone receivers and various forms of direct sound transmission from the source to individual receivers in auditoriums, classrooms, and personal television-viewing areas (Fig. 3.20).

Some **implantable hearing aids** also are currently available. The **cochlear implant**, which is the most sophisticated of these devices, can provide useful hearing to certain totally deaf patients (Fig. 3.21).

Danger Signs

Signs or symptoms that require urgent evaluation and treatment include severe otalgia, aural discharge with or without a tympanic membrane perfora-

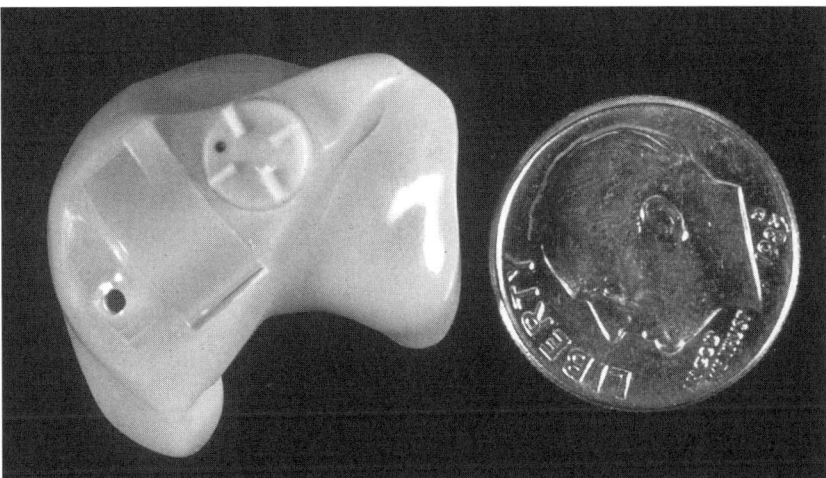

Figure 3.17 In-the-ear hearing aid. The small knob is the volume control. These smaller aids are limited in amplification because of feedback. (Courtesy of Dr. Deb Carlson.)

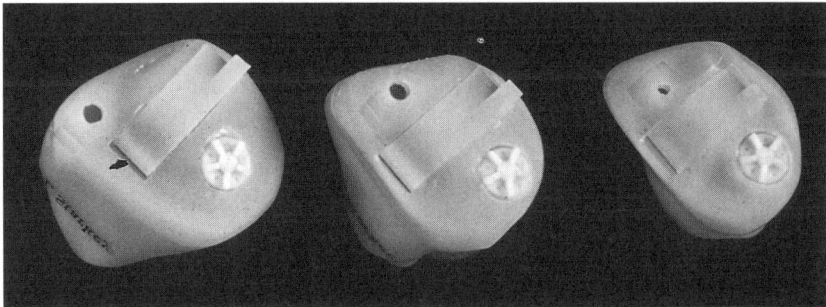

Figure 3.18 In-the-canal hearing aid. Completely in-the-canal aids are nearly invisible but more difficult to fit because they must conform perfectly to the ear canal. (Courtesy of Dr. Deb Carlson.)

tion, headaches, mental status changes, or cranial-nerve deficits associated with aural discharge or hearing loss. Patients with sudden hearing loss, even in the absence of pain or other symptoms, should be examined immediately for cerumen impaction. If earwax is not present, they should undergo an audiologic evaluation and, if indicated, additional specialized testing.

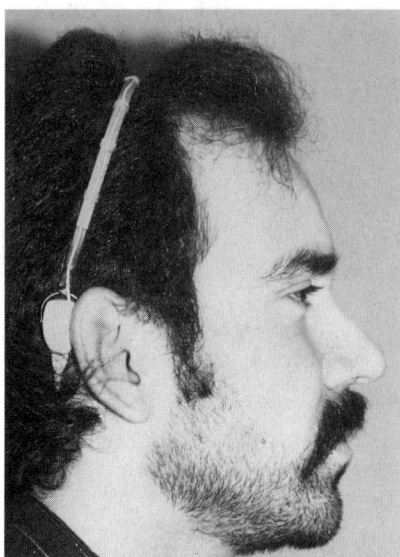

Figure 3.19A Bone-conducting hearing aid. A bone-conducting aid transmits sound directly through the scalp to the bone of the skull in patients suffering from otherwise uncorrectable hearing loss. (Courtesy of Dr. Deb Carlson.)

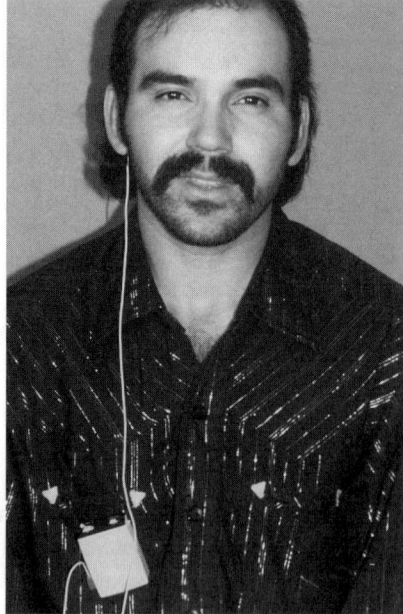

Figure 3.19B Patient with body hearing aid in place. Maximal amplification without feedback is facilitated by the placement of the microphone away from the ear piece and by the larger "box." (Courtesy of Dr. Deb Carlson.)

Hearing Loss 73

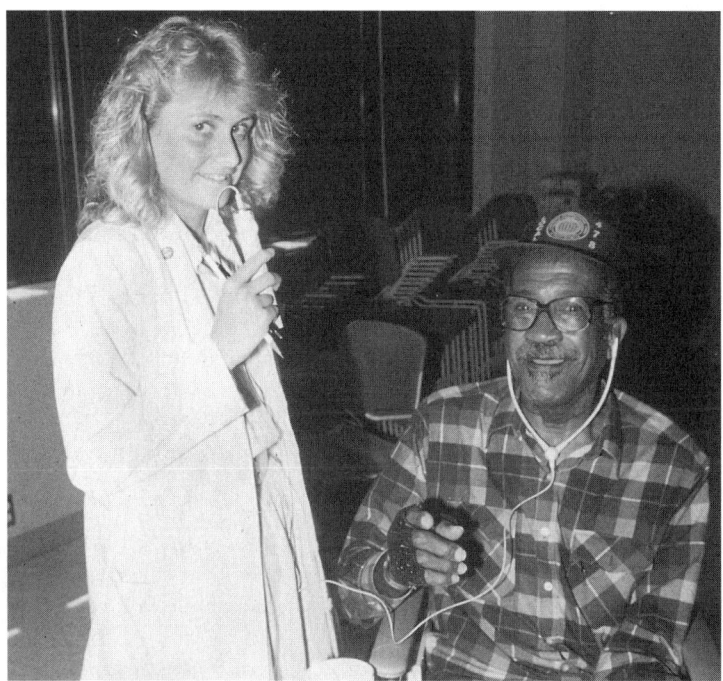

Figure 3.20 An assisted-listening device. High-powered amplification can be provided at relatively low cost via assisted listening devices such as the one pictured here. Particularly valuable for hospitalized or institutionalized patients, these devices should be widely available, especially in intensive-care settings. (Courtesy of Dr. Deb Carlson.)

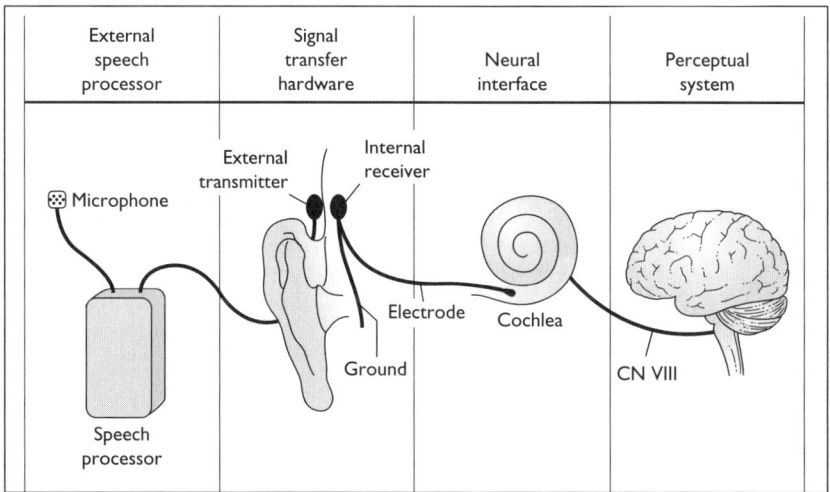

Figure 3.21 The basic cochlear implant system. CN VIII = eighth cranial nerve. (Republished with permission from Kartush JM, Cass SP, Leder SB, Koch DB. *The SIPac Cochlear Implantation*. Alexandria, VA: American Academy of Otolaryngology–Head and Neck Surgery; 1998.)

SUGGESTED READINGS

Arlinger S. Recent developments in air-conduction hearing aids. *Ear Nose Throat J.* 1997;76:310–5.
Updates the reader on the newest developments in hearing aids.

Gates GA, Rees TS. Hear ye? Hear ye: successful auditory aging. *West J Med.* 1997;167: 247–52.
Describes age-related hearing-loss mechanisms, accurate diagnostic methods, and treatments that are available for the more common causes of hearing loss.

Hetu R. The stigma attached to hearing impairment. *Scand Audiol Suppl.* 1996;43:12–24.
Discusses the negative consequences of being hearing impaired, and explores issues relating to positive rehabilitation of social image as well as actual hearing in the hearing-impaired patient.

Malchaire J, Piette A. A comprehensive strategy for the assessment of noise exposure and the risk of hearing impairment. *Ann Occup Hyg.* 1997;41:467–84.
Explains the technical details of evaluating occupational noise exposure and risk of hearing impairment.

Ruth RA. Evaluation of sensorineural hearing loss. *Compr Ther.* 1997;23:742–9.
Details the precise evaluation of SNHL, with review of methods of differentiating inner ear disorders from retrocochlear disorders. Also reviews various assisted-listening devices and hearing aids.

Sha SH, Schacht J. Prevention of aminoglycoside-induced hearing loss. *Keio J Med.* 1997;46:115–9.
Explains a potential method for ameliorating some of the crippling ototoxicity currently associated with worldwide aminoglycoside use and the coadministration of iron chelators.

4

Cerumen Impaction

Mark A. Jabor, MD
Gerard J. Gianoli, MD

Cerumen impaction (CI) is a common otologic problem. Cerumen (ear wax) provides a protective coating for the delicate skin of the external auditory canal (EAC). However, when cerumen accumulates in excess, it can block the EAC completely (causing discomfort and conductive hearing loss) and can impede inspection of the tympanic membrane (TM). Removing an impaction can be painful for the patient and frustrating for the physician. This chapter details a stepwise approach to this simple but challenging problem.

Relevant Anatomy and Physiology

The S-shaped EAC has a lateral cartilaginous portion and a medial bony portion. The skin over the bony portion is thin, without hair or other skin appendages, whereas the cartilaginous portion's skin is thick, adherent, and contains hair follicles and numerous glands.

Cerumen Composition

Cerumen is a mixture of sebum from the sebaceous glands and secretory products of the ceruminous glands (modified apocrine sweat glands). There are no eccrine sweat glands in the EAC. Desquamated epithelial cells, shed hairs, and foreign bodies also are mixed into the cerumen.

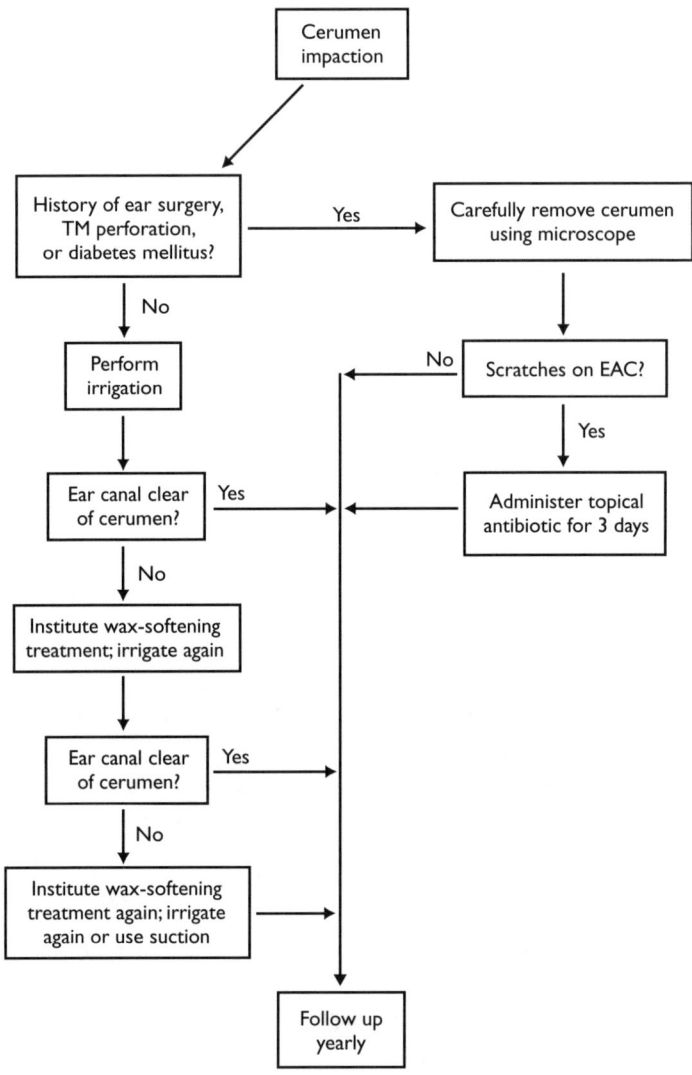

Algorithm Management of cerumen impaction. EAC = external auditory canal; TM = tympanic membrane.

Cerumen is hydrophobic, contains immunoglobulins and lysozyme, maintains an acidic pH (6.15), and is probably bacteriostatic. With respect to age or sex, no differences in chemical composition of cerumen have been noted among patients. There are two distinct types of cerumen: 1) a wet type found predominantly in white and black populations, and 2) a dry, scaly type found mostly in Asians. Wax phenotype is determined by a single gene pair, with the "wet" allele being dominant.

Epithelial Migration

Under normal conditions, the EAC is self-cleaning. Migration of the squamous epithelium occurs in a centrifugal pattern away from the umbo (the attachment of the malleus handle at the center of the TM) and proceeding from the tympanic annulus toward the lateral end of the EAC (from medial to lateral). The mean rate of this migration is 0.07 mm/d.

Etiology

Cerumen impaction afflicts 2% to 6% of the normal adult population and 25% to 34% of the geriatric nursing-home and institutionalized, mentally retarded patients. The reason for these differences is not known. In normal adults, some known causes of CI include abnormal EAC anatomy (e.g., stenosis of the external meatus, osteoma, presence of a mastoid cavity, occlusion of the EAC by a hearing-aid mold), associated dermatosis, and inappropriate attempts at removing wax (e.g., with a cotton swab, which pushes wax farther into the EAC and impacts it against the TM). Nevertheless, these represent a small number of patients who require regular disimpaction of cerumen. The primary problem may be a disorder of keratinocyte separation in the superficial EAC during the desquamation phase of migration.

History and Physical Examination

Cerumen impaction often is found incidentally while examining the ear for other reasons. Patients complain of otalgia, hearing loss, or both. The degree of hearing loss is proportional to the amount of occlusion; however, the patient may not perceive any diminution in hearing until complete occlusion occurs. An 80% occlusion may cause only mild conductive hearing loss, whereas complete occlusion causes moderate hearing losses (from 40–45 dB). Patients may notice a sudden change in hearing after irrigating their ears with water to clean them out or after swimming, bathing, or showering. Water can convert a partial obstruction to a complete one. Otoscopic examination usually reveals a light or dark brown mass (either sticky or dry and flaky) that partially or completely occludes the EAC.

Management and Follow-Up

There are three basic treatments for CI: direct removal, irrigation, and the use of cerumenolytics. In most situations, direct removal or irrigation is effective for the removal of CI (Case 4.1). However, when a solid, complete CI exists, using cerumenolytics with one of the first two methods usually works best.

For a patient with a low pain threshold, filling the EAC with a eutectic mixture of local anesthetics (EMLA) approximately 1 to 2 hours before instrumentation markedly increases patient comfort and cooperation. The EMLA cream is squeezed from its container into a 1-cm^3 tuberculosis-type syringe, and an 18-g Angiocath is used to introduce the EMLA into the EAC.

Complete removal of a large, "stubborn" CI may take more than one office visit. The Algorithm outlines the decision-making steps involved in the management of CI.

Direct Removal

Direct cerumen removal is an especially effective method that is accomplished with suction or a cerumen curette under direct vision via an otomicroscope or a hand-held otoscope equipped with a surgical head (Fig. 4.1). We prefer the microscope (when available), because it allows the use of both hands for removing the CI (Fig. 4.2). Using the regular (pneumatic) head of the otoscope with the sliding door partially opened provides suboptimal viewing and increases the difficulty of CI removal. Curettes come in a variety of shapes and forms (Fig. 4.3). Plastic curettes probably are the safest but may be ineffective with hard, dry cerumen. Our preference is a wire-loop curette, using the largest speculum that can be placed comfortably in the EAC to maximize vision. **Cerumen should never be scraped directly off the TM because this is extremely painful and may cause a TM perforation.**

Suction is also an effective way to remove a CI and often complements removal by curette. A #5 or #7 Frasier-tip suction works best for most patients' ears. However, patients should be warned that the suctioning sounds very loud. If the suction tip becomes clogged, it can be cleared with a stylet. Periodic suctioning 1 to 2 oz of water clears debris from the catheter, minimizing

---

Case 4.1 **Young Man with Sudden Hearing Loss in One Ear**

A man 25 years of age presents complaining of a sudden hearing loss in his right ear. Examination of the ear reveals total occlusion of the external auditory canal by soft cerumen. After irrigation of the cerumen from the ear canal, the patient reports that his hearing is restored immediately.

frustrating episodes of suction-tip blockage (Fig 4.4). Cerumen adjacent to the TM usually can be removed by this method, but suctioning directly on the TM causes much discomfort and can damage the TM.

A suction or curette should never be used "blindly" (i.e., without being able to see exactly where the tip of the instrument is in the EAC) because this nearly always results in trauma to the EAC, TM, or both. A delicate touch with the instrument is helpful because the thin EAC skin is very susceptible to trauma. Blunt trauma to the canal-wall skin may cause a hematoma that can obscure the view of the EAC completely, causing postponement of CI removal. Advantages of these direct-removal methods include excellent visualization, and they may be used in nearly every situation. Disadvantages include high cost and the need for additional space for the equipment.

In patients who have had previous ear surgery, are diabetic, or are otherwise immunocompromised, any ear canal instrumentation should be performed cautiously, if at all.

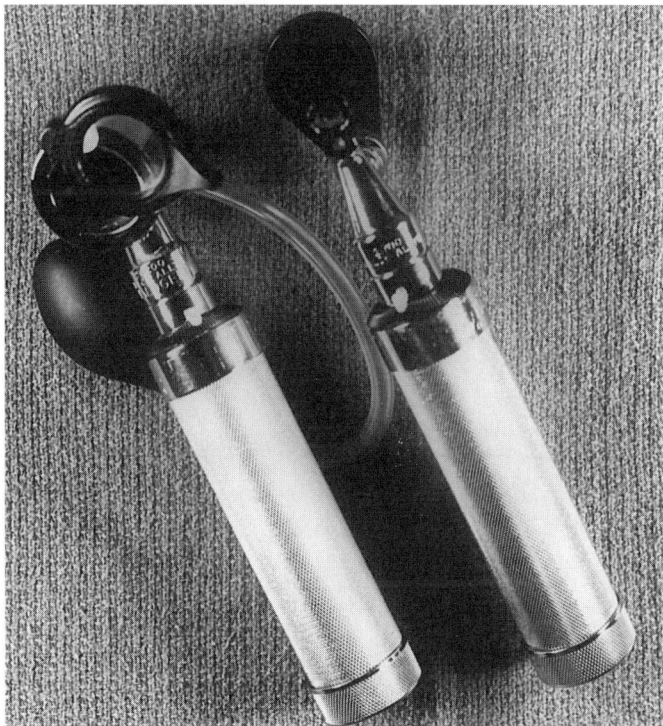

Figure 4.1 A pneumatic (*left*) and surgical otoscope (*right*). Note the door is partially slid over on the pneumatic scope, which makes it very difficult to view the external auditory canal (EAC) through magnification and to insert instruments simultaneously. Contrast this with the surgical head that allows easy placement and maneuvering of instruments and that should always be used when examining the EAC.

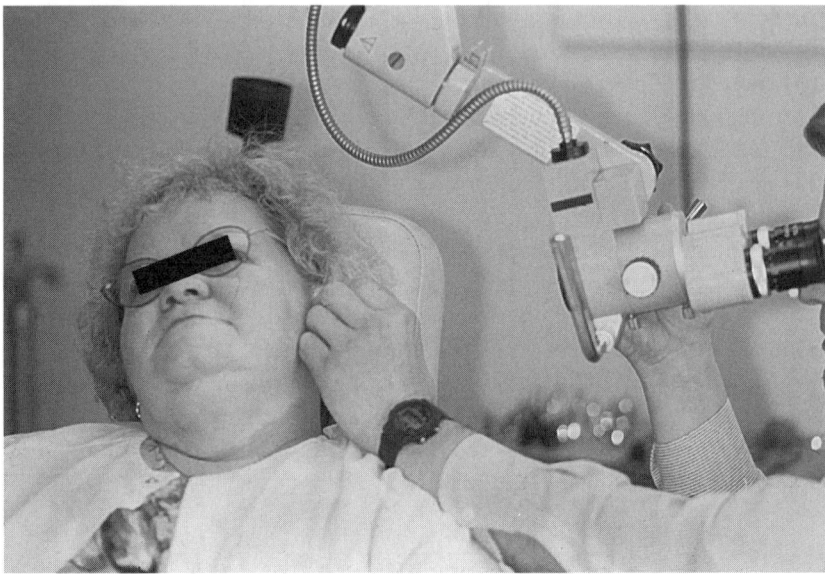

Figure 4.2 Removal of the cerumen via the operating microscope.

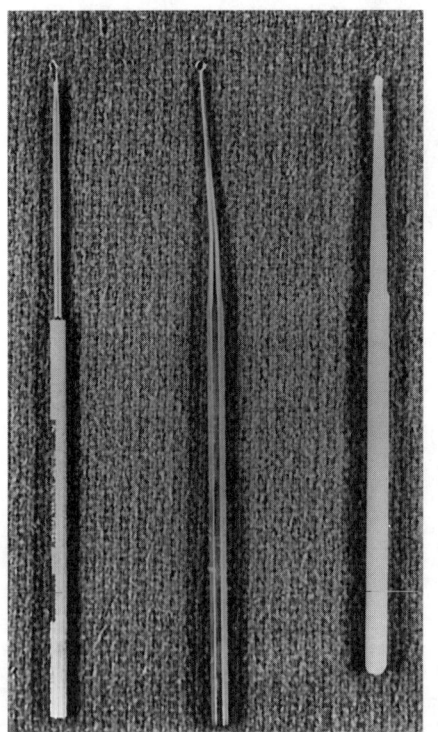

Figure 4.3 Cerumen curettes.

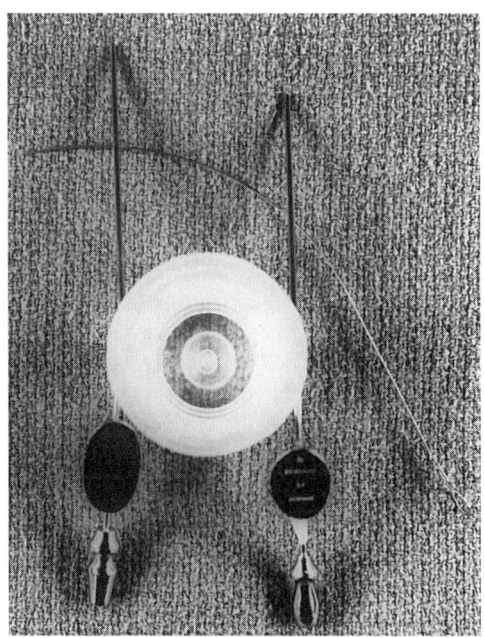

Figure 4.4 Frazier suction tips (#5 and #7), small medicine cup of water, and suction-tip stylet should be available for removal of a cerumen impaction via the suction technique.

Irrigation

There are many effective irrigation systems, some available commercially and others "home made" (Fig. 4.5). All are equal in effectiveness; however, ease of use may vary. **The syringe or catheter tip should never be placed directly on the EAC skin or on the TM, and irrigation is not used if a TM perforation exists or is suspected.** The tip is inserted no farther than 1 cm into the external meatus and is aimed away from the TM, toward the EAC (Fig. 4.6). During irrigation, periodically changing the direction of the tip is helpful. Studies have shown that syringe irrigation is safe in most situations because the pressures developed in the EAC are insufficient to rupture the TM, even when the EAC is wide, a metal syringe is used, or the patient is elderly. However, irrigation can cause TM rupture if the TM is atrophic or, rarely, by direct trauma of the syringe tip.

Warm (i.e., body temperature) water is used to avoid thermal stimulation of the semicircular canals that can result from the use of hot water. Such thermal stimulation can cause nystagmus, dizziness, nausea, and vomiting. However, even with warm water, low-pressure irrigation, and an intact TM, some patients still experience mild dizziness that subsides in a few minutes.

If performing irrigation with an **oral jet irrigator**, adjust it to the lowest possible setting and use a modified tip to direct the stream away form the

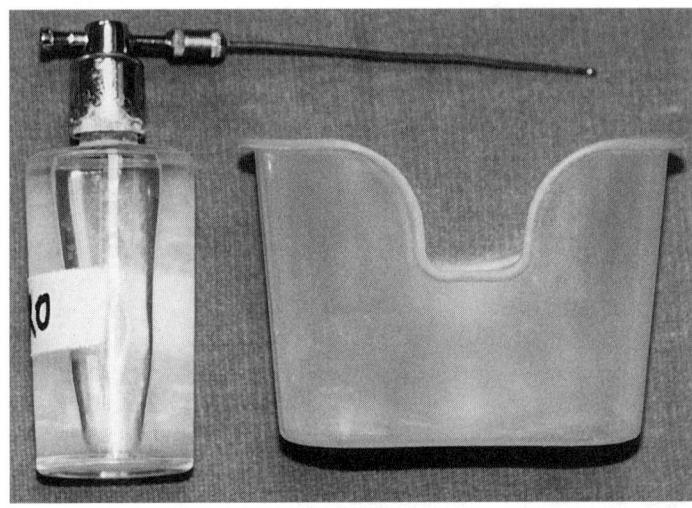

Figure 4.5 One common irrigation apparatus. The glass jar holds warm irrigating solution. A pressure source is attached to the top and, when a finger occludes the air-escape hole, a gentle stream of solution is delivered from the tip. Pressure can be modulated by varying the degree of finger occlusion. The oddly shaped container is made so that one side fits snugly around the patient's ear and irrigation can be performed via the other side. This protects the patient and his or her clothing from being spattered.

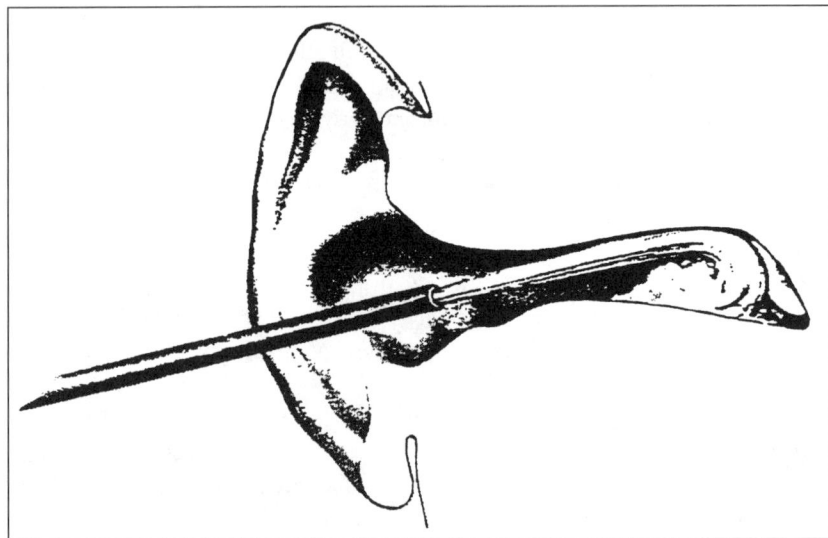

Figure 4.6 Correct placement of an irrigating device into the external auditory canal. Note that the direction of the water column is against the external ear canal, not the tympanic membrane.

TM; **at high settings, it is possible for this irrigator to exceed the mean TM rupture pressure.** Advantages of irrigation are low cost, high effectiveness, and relative safety. The disadvantages are that 1) it is contraindicated with a TM perforation; 2) it is impossible to visualize the TM, allowing debris to be flushed into the middle ear space through an undiagnosed TM perforation; 3) there is an increased susceptibility to external otitis, especially in patients with diabetes, possibly leading to necrotizing otitis externa; and 4) irrigation alone is not effective in removing complete, solid CIs. Rare complications include ossicular disarticulation, perilymph fistula, and complete sensorineural hearing loss.

Cerumenolytics

Cerumenolytics are used to soften hard wax plugs before irrigation or direct removal. Numerous cerumenolytic agents are available, but many are used without any scientific proof of their effectiveness. The only effective cerumenolytics are aqueous based (Table 4.1), and the best of these are docusate sodium (a stool softener) and a 10% solution of sodium bicarbonate. The success of sodium bicarbonate and docusate sodium may be due to their water bases. Additionally, distilled water is an effective cerumenolytic; however, because there is a well-established association between water exposure and otitis externa, prolonged placement of distilled water alone into the EAC is not recommended.

Docusate sodium has been used clinically for several years without adverse effects. It is available as a 1% solution in a 30-mL dropper but does not have specific indications as a cerumenolytic. Before use, it should be warmed to near body temperature. Eight to 10 drops are placed in the EAC for 10 minutes, which softens the mass, making removal with instrumenta-

Table 4.1 Cerumenolytic Agents*

Organic-Based Preparations	Aqueous-Based Preparations
Glycerin	Docusate sodium
Olive oil	Distilled water
Propylene glycol	Sodium bicarbonate
Turpentine spirit	Hydrogen peroxide
Formaldehyde (10%)	Sialic acid
Alcohol (95%)	Buro-Sol
Liquid paraffin	
Cerumenex	
Cerumol	
Auralgan	

* All aqueous-based preparations act as effective cerumenolytics, whereas organic-based preparations show minimal cerumenolytic properties.

tion or irrigation easier. This method may obviate the need for a second office visit.

Prevention

For patients with repeated CIs, the docusate sodium solution used in cerumenolytics may be used monthly to prevent accumulation of impacted cerumen. After an infusion of the docusate sodium solution in the EAC for 10 minutes, the ear is lavaged with lukewarm water with a syringe. The small amount of cerumen accumulated each month is easily removed, preventing impaction. The ear canal may be dried using a hair dryer set at body temperature. This procedure may be performed either by the patient or by a health care provider.

Alternative Health Methods

Ear candles have become a popular CI treatment. A hollow candle is burned with the unlit end in the EAC with the intent of creating negative pressure and drawing cerumen from the EAC. Clinical evaluation of this method has determined that ear candles produce no such negative pressure; thus, they do not remove cerumen. In fact, **ear candles can actually drip candle wax into the EAC and cause EAC skin burns and other ear injuries.** They have no clinical benefit, and their use is discouraged.

Otitis Externa and the Traumatized External Auditory Canal

If external otitis or trauma to the EAC (either self-inflicted or iatrogenic) is present in addition to CI, a topical antibiotic/steroid preparation is initiated. With proper instillation of drops and careful cleansing of debris and exudate of the EAC, the inflammation will subside. Cerumen can then be removed with minimal discomfort to the patient. The eardrops liquefy the cerumen, simplifying its removal. Once cerumen is removed, the topical antibiotic drops are more effective in treating residual inflammation of the EAC. Case 4.2 illustrates the use of antibiotic drops in the treatment of EAC irritation after curettage and suction.

Danger Signs

The most significant danger sign associated with CI is persistent otitis externa despite appropriate treatment, especially in patients with diabetes. In such cases, perform diligent cleaning with suction, avoid irrigation, and be highly suspicious of malignant external otitis.

Case 4.2 Use of Topical Antibiotic Drops After Curettage and Suction

A woman 72 years of age complains of excessive wax accumulation in her ear canals. Examination shows both external auditory canals nearly occluded by hard, dry cerumen. Irrigation does not remove much of the cerumen. Using the operating microscope and a combination of curetting and suction, you painstakingly remove all the cerumen. You note that there are some small areas of irritation on the EAC skin afterwards, and prescribe topical antibiotic drops for 3 days. On 2-week follow-up, both ear canals are clear, the TMs look normal, and the patient is satisfied.

SUGGESTED READINGS

Andaz C, Whittet HB. An *in vitro* study to determine efficacy of different ear-dispersing agents. *J Otorhinolaryngol.* 1993;55:97–9.

This article compares in vitro use of various solutions used for treatment of cerumen impaction. Water, which the researchers originally used as a control, turned out to be the most effective treatment, whereas the commonly recommended olive oil was ineffective.

Grossan M. Cerumen removal: current challenges. *Ear Nose Throat J.* 1998;77:541–6.

This article details the techniques of removing cerumen, the potential complications, and methods for preventing complications.

Wilson PL, Roeser RJ. Cerumen management: professional issues and techniques. *J Am Acad Audiol.* 1997;8:421–30.

Although intended for audiologists, this article nevertheless offers a good review of techniques for cerumen removal.

5

Itchy Ears

Eric L. Mansfield, MD
Gerard J. Gianoli, MD

There are many causes of itchy ears, ranging from simple skin dryness of the external auditory canal (EAC) to squamous cell carcinoma. Allergic reactions and superficial infections are the most common causes; however, because the ear canal is essential for normal hearing, many of the diseases that cause pruritus affect hearing. This not only complicates the issue but also makes the patient more uncomfortable. Symptoms are magnified because of the structure of the EAC, and the inability to alleviate the itch by scratching leads to the insertion of foreign objects into the EAC, which in turn may cause an infection that overshadows the underlying problem. Thus, pruritus is a symptom that should not be ignored.

Anatomy and Physiology

The EAC is the only squamous epithelium–lined *cul de sac* in the body. In the medial two thirds, the skin is very thin and lies directly on the underlying bone, with no intervening connective tissue. Other than the nail beds, this squamous epithelium is the only epithelium in the body that migrates. With the production of cerumen, the EAC becomes self-cleaning, removing debris and tiny foreign bodies in the cerumen as the epithelium migrates to the edge of the EAC.

Itchy Ears 87

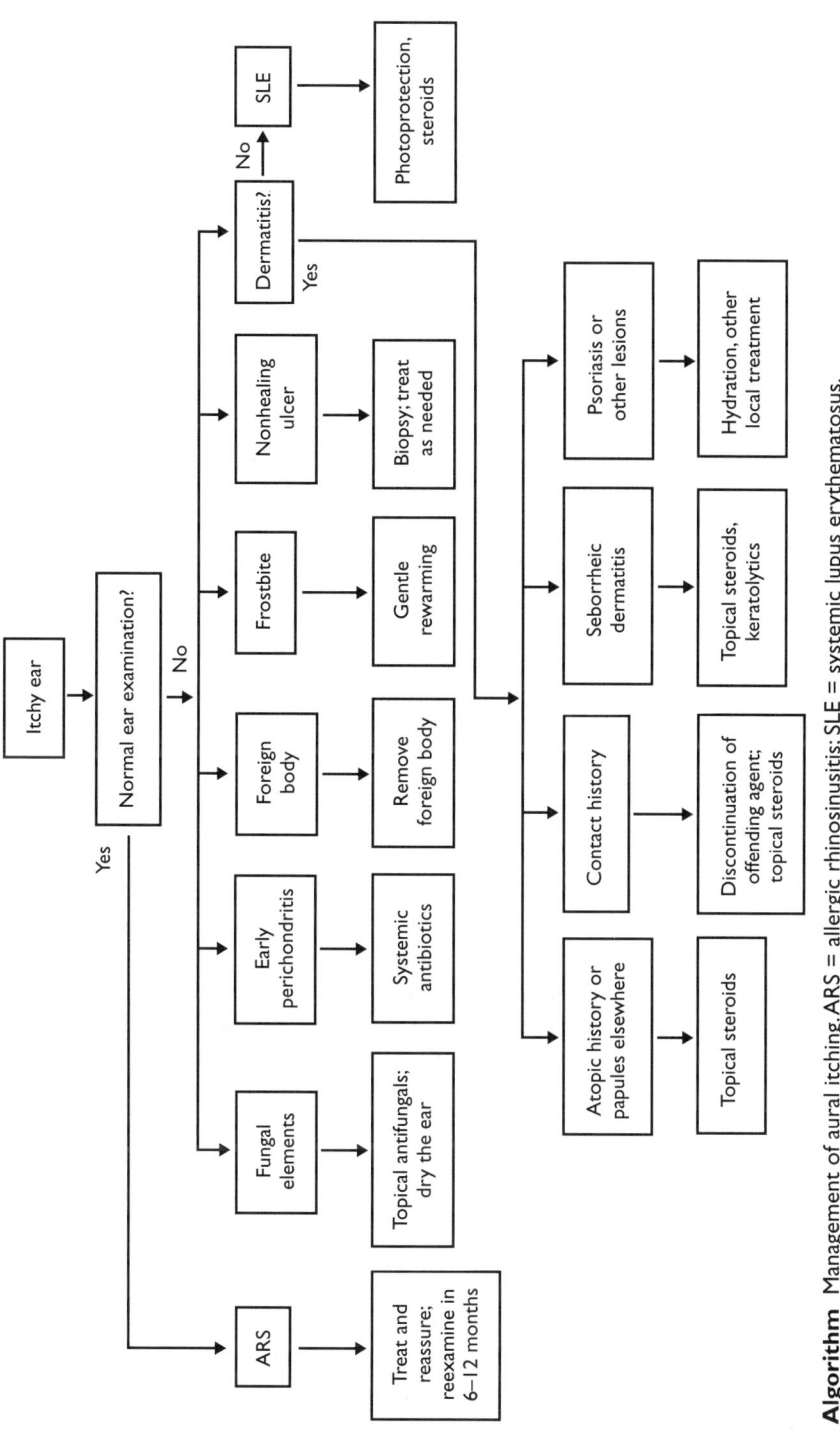

Algorithm Management of aural itching. ARS = allergic rhinosinusitis; SLE = systemic lupus erythematosus.

History

Specific points to be covered in the history during an evaluation of itchy ears include the following:
- History of ear infections or other problems
- Ear-related symptoms (e.g., otorrhea, otalgia, tinnitus, vertigo, hearing loss)
- Allergic rhinosinusitis history
- Whether an instrument (e.g., cotton swab, bobby pin) was inserted in the ear in an attempt to relieve the itching
- Systemic dermatologic problems
- Swimming and bathing habits (e.g., if the patient is an enthusiastic scuba diver, the resulting water in the ear canals may make a perfect medium for infection, and the itching may represent an early otitis media)
- Exposure to cold (frostbite) and the use of hair dyes, sprays, perfumes, etc. (contact dermatitis)

Physical Examination

Examination of the patient with itchy ears begins with inspection of the pinna. One looks at skin quality on both the medial and lateral surfaces of the pinna and for signs of irritation in the postauricular sulcus. Any signs of extreme dryness, scaliness, edema, erythema, or discrete masses or lesions are noted. It is important to inspect the entire meatus, just as the concha becomes the opening of the EAC. The otoscope light can be shined in this area before inserting the speculum into the ear canal. Fissures and furuncles are common findings in this area. In the external canal, one notes skin quality, dryness, and signs of trauma (e.g., scratches that might indicate instrumentation). Foreign bodies, mycelial elements (indicating a fungal infection), pus, and cerumen location (e.g., a thin sheet of cerumen pushed against the tympanic membrane may be a sign of chronic cotton swab use) should be noted.

Diagnosis and Management

Local Causes

The Algorithm outlines the diagnosis and treatment of the causes of aural itching.

Chronic Otitis Externa

An early or chronic low-grade infection of the EAC is a common cause of itchy ears (Case 5.1). Bony exostoses may partially occlude the EAC. They may trap water between them and the tympanic membrane, also leading to maceration of the external canal skin and an infection of the external canal (Fig. 5.1). Early in the course of an infection, the patient often becomes aware of itching that progresses to pain as the infection develops (Fig. 5.2). Similarly, in a chronic infection, the inflamed skin of the EAC becomes thickened, reac-

---

Case 5.1 Man with Chronic Otitis Externa Exacerbated by Use of Cotton Swabs

A male veteran 59 years of age complains of chronic itching ears. He admits to scratching his ear frequently and recently has noted increased drainage and pain from the right ear. He reports that the chronic itching began while he was stationed in Southeast Asia in 1967 and that it has been present in varying degrees since then. He has no history of diabetes, hypertension, or known cardiac or pulmonary disease. The rest of the history is negative.

Physical examination reveals bilateral erythematous ear canals, with edema and exudate. There is crusting around the meatus but no evidence of perichondritis. The right ear canal is partially obscured with pus. After suction, the medial portion of the canal is found to be filled with impacted cotton. This is removed to reveal an intact but thickened tympanic membrane. Examination of the nasal passages, oral cavity, oropharynx, larynx, and hypopharynx is unremarkable, and there are no neck masses.

The patient is instructed to avoid using cotton swabs (e.g., Q-Tips) and is placed on antibiotic steroid drops for 2 weeks. When seen in follow-up, he complains of persistent itching, but the ear canals appear much improved. The drops are discontinued, and he is placed on a steroid cream that is to be applied daily. Six months later when seen in routine follow-up, he has evidence of cotton fibers imbedded in the dry cerumen.

Discussion
This is a common presentation of chronic otitis externa perpetuated by continued cotton-swab use. The physician performs a complete head and neck examination to rule out another disease (e.g., head and neck cancer) that could cause referred otalgia. A possible triggering factor might have been gastroesophageal reflux with referred ear discomfort, and, if there were suggestive symptoms, the physician might have elected to treat the suspected reflux empirically. Possibly the ear discomfort was caused by chronic fungal otitis, even in the absence of visible fungal elements, and empirical antifungal topical therapy also might be tried. The patient should be reminded at each visit to avoid cotton swabs because continued use will exacerbate and perpetuate the condition.

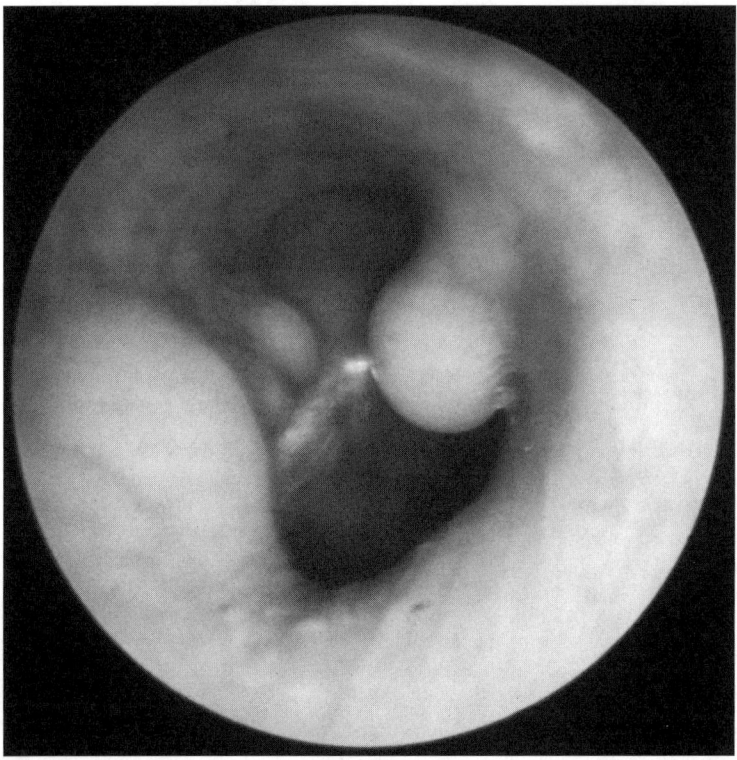

Figure 5.1 Bony exostoses such as these can partially or completely block the external auditory canal, predisposing the patient to external otitis. If necessary, they can be surgically removed. (Courtesy of Dr. David Eibling.)

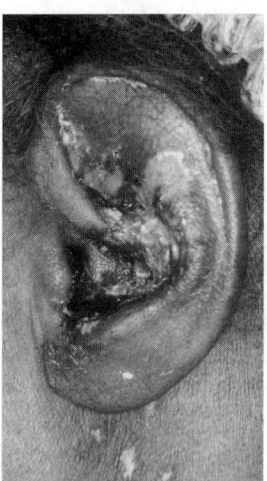

Figure 5.2 Even severe infections such as herpes zoster oticus (Ramsey-Hunt) syndrome can present with itching early in their course. (Courtesy of Dr. Jonas Johnson.)

tive, and itchy (Fig. 5.3). If the infection is bacterial, use of a topical antibiotic ointment that also contains a steroid is particularly efficacious. However, chronic otitis externa often represents an otomycosis, a fungal infection of the EAC (Case 5.2). Otomycosis can be treated effectively with thorough cleaning of the EAC, followed by the use of an antimycotic solution such as Gentia violet, Lotrimin, or Cresylate.

Nonspecific Dermatitis
Some patients, especially elderly ones, present with distressingly persistent itching of the ear canals. Often, the itching precedes and announces an impending acute diffuse otitis externa. The opening of the canal is red, scaly, and dry, and one may see a tiny fissure at the 12 o'clock position at the meatus. The remainder of the canal is free of wax (or has only small amounts of dry, crumbly cerumen), with little evidence of inflammation. The ear does not discharge, but the erythema and scaling sometimes can extend into the cavum conchalis. There is little pain, but the appearance of excoriation

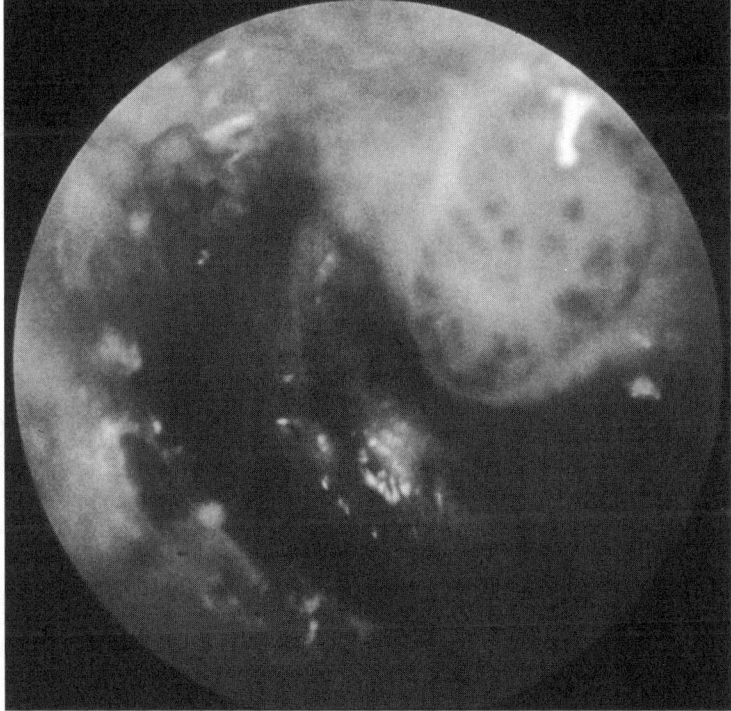

Figure 5.3 Typical chronic external otitis. Granulation tissue has formed near the tympanic membrane. (Courtesy of Dr. Steven Cass.)

about the meatus attests to the intensity of the itching. It is sometimes difficult to distinguish this condition from psoriatic or seborrheic disease (*see* sections on these conditions below), except that eczematoid external otitis exists without concomitant lesions elsewhere. Initial treatment with hydrocortisone cream and then prophylaxis with Furstenburg's ointment is almost always effective. (Dr. Furstenburg's Supplementary Salve for Sufferers of Scanty Ceruminous Secretions: 3% each of phenol, salicylic acid, and sulfur precipitate in a petrolatum base; dispense 60 g.) One instructs the patient to apply the ointment with the finger, massaging the tragus gently afterward to distribute the medication. It is applied at least twice a day and more often if needed for itching.

Case 5.2   Elderly Man with Fungal Otitis Externa

A man 68 years of age with insulin-dependent diabetes mellitus complains of chronic itching in his right ear. He has significant hearing loss and wears an in-the-ear hearing aid in his right ear. He does not have an aid for his left ear because he says it is "too expensive." He lives alone and often sleeps with his hearing aid in place so that he can hear sounds in the house at night. He denies significant otalgia, pharyngeal discomfort, dysphagia, and voice change.

Physical examination reveals dried cerumen in the left ear canal and moist debris in the right ear, with obvious fungal fruiting bodies in the right ear. Both canals are debrided with microscopic control; care is taken to avoid trauma to the ear canal or contamination of the left canal with debris from the right. The hearing aid also is cleaned, during which moist debris is suctioned from the speaker channel. The right ear canal is painted with Gentian violet, and the patient is begun on Lotrimin (metronidazole) "spelling" drops. He is instructed to leave his aid out and to return for recleaning in 1 week. When reexamined, his ear canal is clean and is repainted. He is instructed to continue the antifungal topical drops and to leave his hearing aid out at night.

Discussion

Fungal otitis externa is a common problem in elderly diabetic patients, especially for those who require the use of a hearing aid. Unfortunately, this patient had only one aid, so he could not alternate aids ear to ear. Furthermore, if he had had a behind-the-ear aid, an open mold (or two; one for each ear) could be used, which would permit better aeration of his canal. Careful cleaning of the canal is critical to clean out fungal debris and to avoid trauma, which could precipitate a more serious bacterial infection. Antifungal agents are important, but canal debridement is the most critical component of therapy. Use of the hearing aid is critical to patients such as this because of the inability to hear doorbells, alarms, the phone, etc. The physician must carefully consider the implications of withholding amplification, even for a brief time, from a patient who has become accustomed to its use.

Contact Dermatitis

Contact dermatitis is common on the pinnae. When the conchae and periauricular skin are primarily affected, allergy to grooming products (e.g., shampoos, hair dyes) is suspected. The most common offending ingredients are fragrances, preservatives, and paraphenylenediamine, a common hair dye ingredient. Dermatitis restricted to the EAC may result from contact with hearing-aid components, including vinyl plastic, methylmethacrylate, and rubber. Silicone hearing aids are rarely irritating. The pinna can become excoriated by coming in contact with nickel (e.g., in earrings, glasses, ear pieces) and by any subsequent dermatitis. Stroking or scratching the ear with nickel-containing objects such as bobby pins or writing pens can induce the same reaction.

A more common offender in contact dermatitis is neomycin, which is contained in numerous otologic drops, including Coly-Mycin, Cortisporin, Otobione, Otocidin, and Otocort. Approximately 15% of patients treated for external otitis have or develop neomycin sensitivity. Many topical agents available over the counter also cause contact dermatitis, including benzocaines, para-aminobenzoic acid (PABA) in sunscreens, propylene glycol (in Cerumenex), hygroscopic alcohol in otic preparations, and others.

Treatment consists of the identification and discontinuation of the offending agent. Topical steroids speed symptom resolution. Burow's aluminum solution (Domeboro) dries weeping lesions, removes crusts, and re-acidifies the skin. It is helpful for exudative lesions. Occasionally, systemic steroid therapy is indicated.

Allergic Rhinosinusitis

Patients with known inhalant allergy problems may complain of intensely itchy ears. Sometimes they have attempted to scratch the canals with assorted instruments (e.g., cotton swabs, bobby pins, parts of pens), causing excoriations that develop into bacterial external otitis. Other times, the physical examination of the ears is completely normal. Many of these patients also complain of itching of the palate. Aggressive treatment of the allergic problems, particularly with systemic antihistamine therapy, improves the itching.

Foreign Bodies

Itchy ears can be caused by foreign bodies in the EAC, either animate (e.g., cockroaches, flies, other insects) or inanimate (e.g., beads, erasers) (Fig. 5.4). History usually reveals the diagnosis. Physical examination confirms the diagnosis. A living EAC foreign body can be distressing because its movements on the tympanic membrane can sound as loud as an earthquake. Sometimes shining a bright light onto the ear encourages the bug to leave the ear canal. If this is not successful, the next treatment is to still the bug's movements, im-

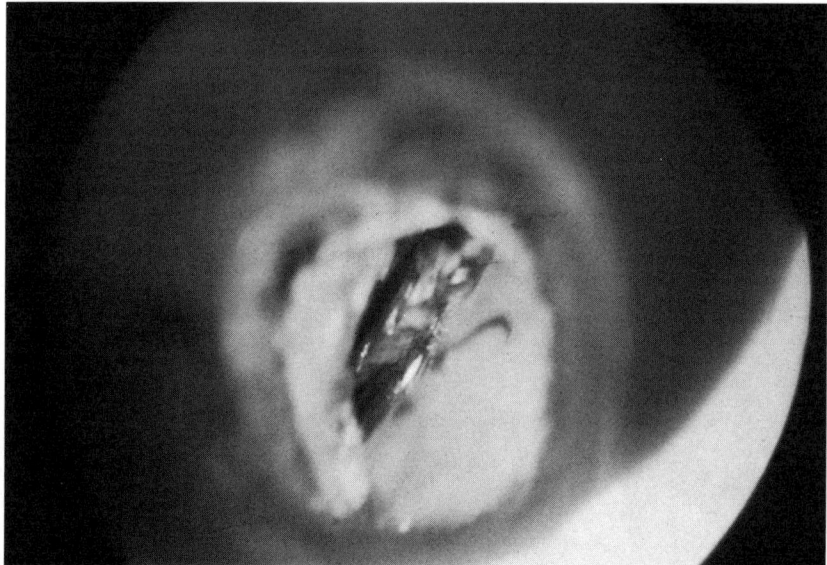

Figure 5.4 A bug can be seen in the external auditory canal. (Courtesy of Dr. Jonas Johnson.)

mobilizing or drowning it by administering 1% plain lidocaine or isopropyl alcohol in the EAC. These are not used if a tympanic membrane perforation exists or is suspected, and they are very irritating to the middle ear. Once the insect is still, traditional removal methods can be used (Case 5.3).

Another common foreign body is cotton, either from a plug of cotton that the patient placed in the meatus and then was unable to retrieve or that which has come off a cotton swab. This may cause an itchy sensation in the EAC. If the patient seeks medical care promptly, removal with a small forceps under microscopic visualization is simple. Sometimes, however, the patient either does not realize that the retained cotton is in the ear canal or is embarrassed to seek treatment. In such cases, external otitis often ensues, and the infection may need to be treated before the presence of the foreign body is evident. (*See* Chapter 29 for a more detailed discussion of foreign bodies in the EAC.)

Perichondritis

Early perichondritis can cause itchy ears and usually originates with simple trauma or an otitis externa (Fig. 5.5). Because the skin of the external ear and EAC is so thin, the perichondrium is particularly susceptible to infection. The early itching soon becomes edema and erythema, and exquisite

> **Case 5.3** **Young Man with a Foreign Body (a Spider) in the Ear**
>
> An upset man 23 years of age presents to the otolaryngology clinic (at a military base in California) at 7 AM, holding his hand over his ear and asking that the doctor be called to "take the spider out." The patient states that he was awakened by an uncomfortable sensation of motion in his ear canal and that his roommate had looked in his ear and had seen a spider. The clinic technician examines the ear, notes a gray fuzzy object filling the canal, and calls the physician.
>
> Treatment begins with filling the ear canal with 4% xylocaine. The spider immediately crawls out of the ear canal, and the patient brushes it to the floor, effectively dispatching it with the heel of his boot.
>
> ### Discussion
> This case is typical of cases in which an insect (or in this case, an arachnid) becomes lodged in the ear canal because the patient knew that the object was alive; however, it was atypical because the patient knew that it was a spider. The technician correctly did not attempt to remove it, because grasping an insect or spider in the ear canal can lead to it struggling, scratching, and biting and, subsequently, severe pain for the patient. Once the insect has been immobilized, it can be removed easily by forceps. Care must be taken to avoid trauma to the ear canal and to assure that all insect parts are removed. (Case contributed by Dr. David Eibling.)

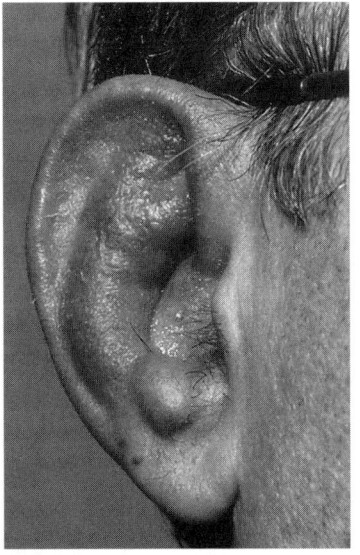

Figure 5.5 With perichondritis, the ear is thickened and tender, with edema and erythema of the overlying skin. (Courtesy of Dr. Steven Cass.)

tenderness follows. Gram-negative organisms are the most common cause, and treatment with intravenous antibiotics is usually required. If the infection is pure *Pseudomonas aeruginosa*, ciprofloxacin is a good antibiotic choice. For a mixed gram-positive/gram-negative organism infection, quinolones are good choices.

Other Local Causes

Mild thermal injury (e.g., frostbite) can cause an itchy sensation early in its course. There is always a history of exposure to cold temperatures. Gentle rewarming is achieved with cotton pledgets of approximately 38° to 42°C.

Carcinomas of the EAC are rare (1–2 per 100,000 population per year) (Fig. 5.6). However, any nonhealing ulcer on the pinna or in the EAC, itchy or not, deserves biopsy to rule out malignancy.

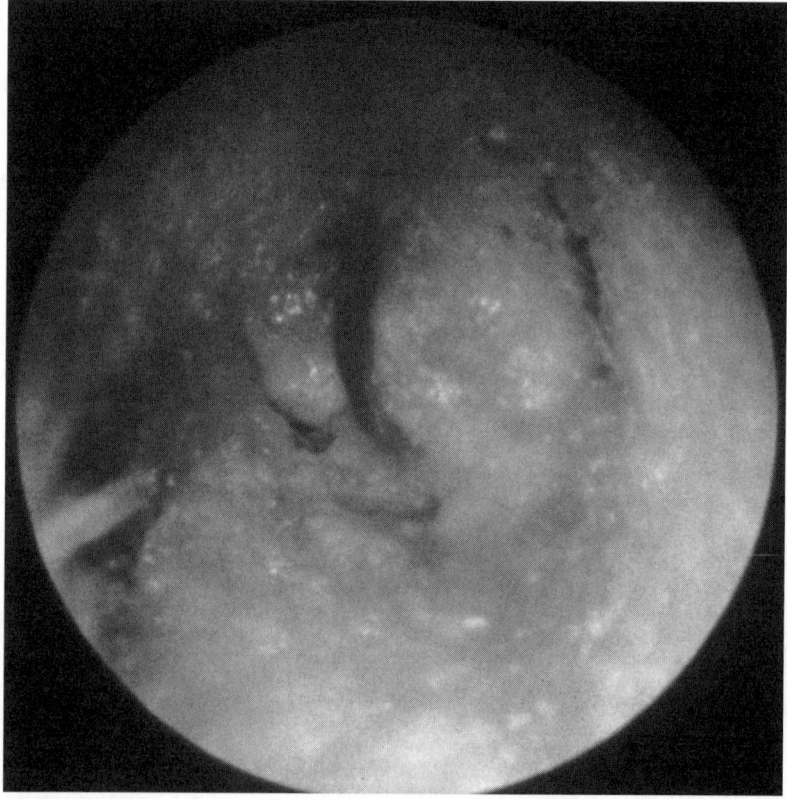

Figure 5.6 Ulcerating squamous cell carcinoma in the external auditory canal. (Courtesy of Dr. David Eibling.)

Systemic Dermatologic Diseases

Atopic Dermatitis

Any skin diseases that occur elsewhere in the body also can occur in the EAC. Atopic dermatitis is an acute exudative inflammation usually associated with atopic eczema. When it occurs on the pinna, other parts of the neck, face, or body usually are involved. Atopic dermatitis of the pinna or EAC, for which there may be a strong family history, often is accompanied by allergic rhinitis, conjunctivitis, or asthma.

This disease often begins in early childhood and has an unpredictable course. It may abate during puberty, or it may wax and wane during an entire lifetime. It tends to be exacerbated by stress, contact irritants, trauma, temperature changes, foods, and pollen exposures.

On the pinna and elsewhere, there is poorly circumscribed erythema with small, slightly elevated papules. There is usually intense pruritus, with excoriations that sometimes obscure the EAC lesions or even cause an overlying external otitis. Chronic rubbing can cause lichenification, in which the normal skin markings are broadened and coarsened, often with hyperpigmentation.

Diagnosis is based on morphology, age of onset, chronicity, and positive family history. The differential diagnosis includes contact dermatitis and seborrheic dermatitis. Contact dermatitis usually has an isolated focus and a history of contact, such as with a hat, earband, earplug, or earring. Atopic dermatitis, on the other hand, is usually more generalized, and the patient often has a family history of atopic dermatitis.

Treatment of acute exacerbations is with a topical steroid, which, in the EAC, can be applied as either a suspension or a cream. Systemic antihistamines may help for intense pruritus, but systemic steroids may be necessary for generalized flare-ups.

Atopic dermatitis can become infected secondarily, most often with *Staphylococcus aureus*. A topical antibiotic solution works well for this, especially combined with a steroid cream to combat the pruritus and inflammation.

Psoriasis

Patients with psoriasis often have ear involvement. This idiopathic, chronic, inflammatory, and proliferative skin disease presents with raised, scaly primary lesions (Fig. 5.7). The peak onset incidence is in the second decade, but it can begin at any time of life. As with atopic dermatitis, psoriasis is multifactorial with a genetic component and can be exacerbated by infections, mental or emotional stress, and medications (e.g., beta-blockers, lithium, nonsteroidal anti-inflammatory drugs).

The primary lesion of psoriasis is a sharply circumscribed, bright-red papule with a surface scale that is thick, broad-based, and silvery white. Psori-

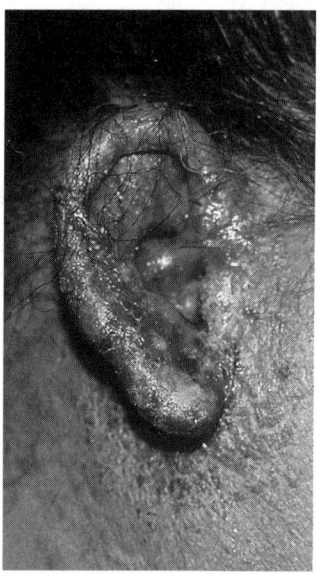

Figure 5.7 Infected psoriasis of the auricle. (Courtesy of Dr. David Eibling.)

asis of the EAC usually has a dense, thick, adherent, psoriatic scale. Lifting away this scale exposes pinpoint bleeding (Auspitz's sign). Examining other areas, including the scalp, fingernails, elbows, and knees, helps with the diagnosis. All psoriasis causes itching, especially in the EAC. Psoriasis of the skin can clinically resemble other inflammatory scaly dermatoses. The main differential diagnosis is seborrheic dermatitis, which exhibits scruffy, diffuse scales with much less erythema than psoriasis.

Treatment of psoriasis of the EAC is similar to treatment of other areas, modified only to accommodate the thin skin. Simple warm-water soaks (applied by placing saturated gauze against the affected pinna) hydrate the skin, gently debride it, and help topical preparations penetrate the skin. Petroleum-based or other occlusive moisturizers are helpful when carefully applied.

Even mild trauma can induce localized lesions, so the wearing of earrings, tight hats, etc. should be avoided. Low-potency topical steroids are the first line of therapy but are limited by potential side effects of atrophy, telangiectasia, and acneform eruptions. Topical calcipotriene, a topical form of activated vitamin D, recently has been approved for treatment in the United States. Systemic therapy (e.g., azulfidine, methotrexate, hydroxyurea, cyclosporine, etretinate) is rarely used.

Seborrheic Dermatitis

Seborrheic dermatitis is a common disease, with peaks in infancy and old age. It is a commonly acquired inflammatory disorder affecting the oil-rich, high-sebum regions of the skin. Severe disease is often associated with Parkinson's disease, Down's syndrome, and other neurological conditions, perhaps secondary to an increase in sebum in this population. It is found in nearly 85% of patients with AIDS.

Clinical features of seborrheic dermatitis are varied. The lesions are neither circumscribed nor elevated, as is seen with psoriasis. The scalp, face, trunk, and ears are involved, displaying a powdery or greasy scale (as opposed to the thick scale of psoriasis). Histologically, there is focal hyperkeratosis, with a superficial perifollicular lymphocytic dermal infiltrate. The lipophilic yeast *Malassezia furfur* is thought to be involved in the pathogenesis.

As with psoriasis, definitive diagnosis is based on an examination of the whole body. Generally, dry, scaly dandruff is seen around the EAC and pinna (concha and scapha). On the face, there is a predilection for the T-zone, eyebrows, and nasal alae.

Treatment involves mild topical corticosteroids and keratolytics. Patients with ear involvement usually have scalp involvement as well. A shampoo containing selenium sulfide (e.g., Selsun Blue, Desenex), zinc pyrithione (e.g., Head and Shoulders), or coal tar (e.g., Neutrogena T-gel) decreases the dermatitis. Antifungal creams and shampoos directed at *Malassezia furfur* are also effective. Shampoo can be used daily at first, then less often as needed to maintain control.

Lupus Erythematosus
Systemic lupus erythematosus (SLE) is a multisystem autoimmune disease, and approximately one quarter of patients with SLE develop discoid skin lesions, which may be the first sign of the disease. The skin manifestations range from local (discoid) lupus to subacute cutaneous lupus to true SLE.

Discoid lupus lesions manifest as epidermal atrophy with erythema and scaling. Hypopigmentation is common and becomes more noticeable and disfiguring with the darker the patient's natural skin color. Treatment involves stringent photoprotection and topical or intralesional steroids. Occasionally, systemic steroids or antimalarial agents are needed.

Danger Signs

Some EAC diseases present with relatively mild itching and other symptoms that can become hearing- or life-threatening. These include the following:
- **A beefy or ulcerative EAC lesion that is refractory to medical treatment:** may be an early carcinoma (Fig. 5.8); biopsy is indicated

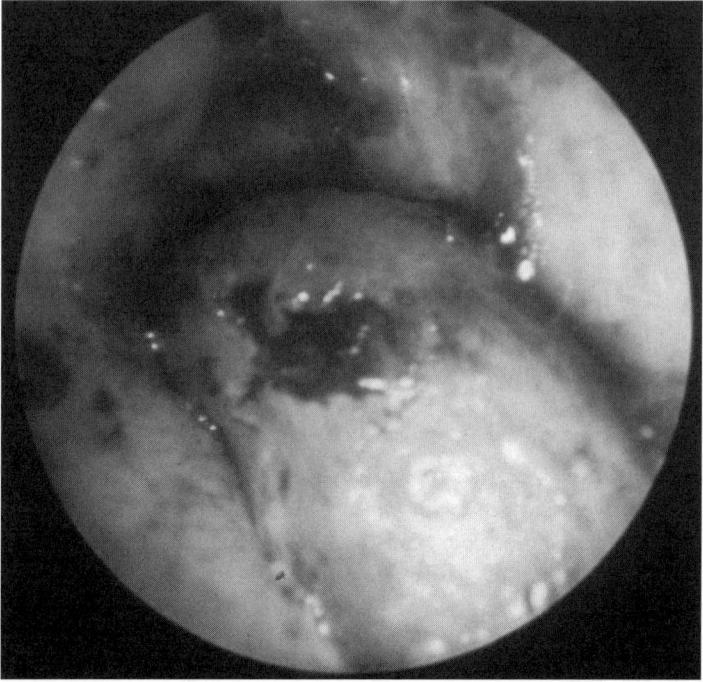

Figure 5.8 Adenoid cystic carcinoma of the external auditory canal. (Courtesy of Dr. David Eibling.)

- **A generalized peri-auricular edema:** may be an early perichondritis or chondritis
- **Otorrhea with the EAC closed by edema, with or without mastoid tenderness:** can indicate middle ear or mastoid disease
- **Any aural polyp:** may be the sign of a serious underlying disease such as a cholesteatoma, especially one that protrudes through the tympanic membrane
- **A tympanic membrane perforation, with or without otorrhea**
- **Continued complaints of an itchy ear with a normal examination:** the same detailed head and neck examination used for unexplained otalgia should be preformed; an occult pharyngeal malignancy must be ruled out

Summary

Diseases of the EAC are varied. Dermatologic diseases contribute to a large part of the pathology in this region. Careful diagnosis and accurate treatment, with special attention to the danger signs, should soothe the "itchy ears" and the patient.

SUGGESTED READINGS

Roland MS, Marple PE. Disorders of the external auditory canal. *J Am Acad Audiol.* 1997;8:367–8.

This article reviews normal anatomy and physiology of the EAC and describes in detail all common disorders. It also includes a good review of diagnosis and treatment of malignant external otitis.

Roeser RJ, Ballachanda BB. Physiology, pathophysiology, and anthropology/epidemiology of human ear canal secretions. *J Am Acad Audiol.* 1997;8:391–400.

This fascinating article discusses the components of the EAC secretions, the sequelae of excessive or impacted secretions, and the anthropologic and epidemiologic importance of these secretions.

Shea CR. Dermatologic diseases of the external auditory canal. *Otolaryngol Clin North Am.* 1996;29:783–94.

This article discusses both EAC manifestations of systemic dermatologic diseases and local reactive or irritative conditions of the EAC.

Tran LP, Grundfast KM, Selesnick SH. Benign lesions of the external auditory canal. *Otolaryngol Clin North Am.* 1996;29:807–25.

This article details the common mass lesions of the EAC, some of which present with itching.

6

Dizziness

Andrew J. Miller, MD
Gerard J. Gianoli, MD

Dizziness is a word patients use to describe unsteadiness, lightheadedness, whirling and floating sensations, headache, and imbalance. The three primary systems that control balance are the vestibular, visual, and proprioceptive systems—all of which are components of the central nervous system (CNS). Dysfunction of the vestibular system usually causes "true" vertigo, a sensation of spinning or an illusion of spinning motion, which must be distinguished from unsteadiness, lightheadedness, or a change in the awareness of the environment.

Anatomy

The vestibular labyrinth—the end organ of the peripheral vestibular system—and the cochlea comprise the inner ear, which is found in the petrous portion of the temporal bone. Each labyrinth is composed of a superior, posterior, and horizontal semicircular canal (SCC), a utricle, and a saccule (Fig. 6.1). The SCCs are orthogonal to each other and respond to angular acceleration. Each canal is composed of a dense bony capsule containing a membranous structure supported by a fluid that is high in sodium and low in potassium (perilymph). Inside the membranous labyrinth, the fluid is high in potassium and low in sodium (endolymph). Near the entrance of each canal into the vestibule, there is a dilation called the ampulla. An elevation inside each ampulla (the crista) contains hair cells that project into a

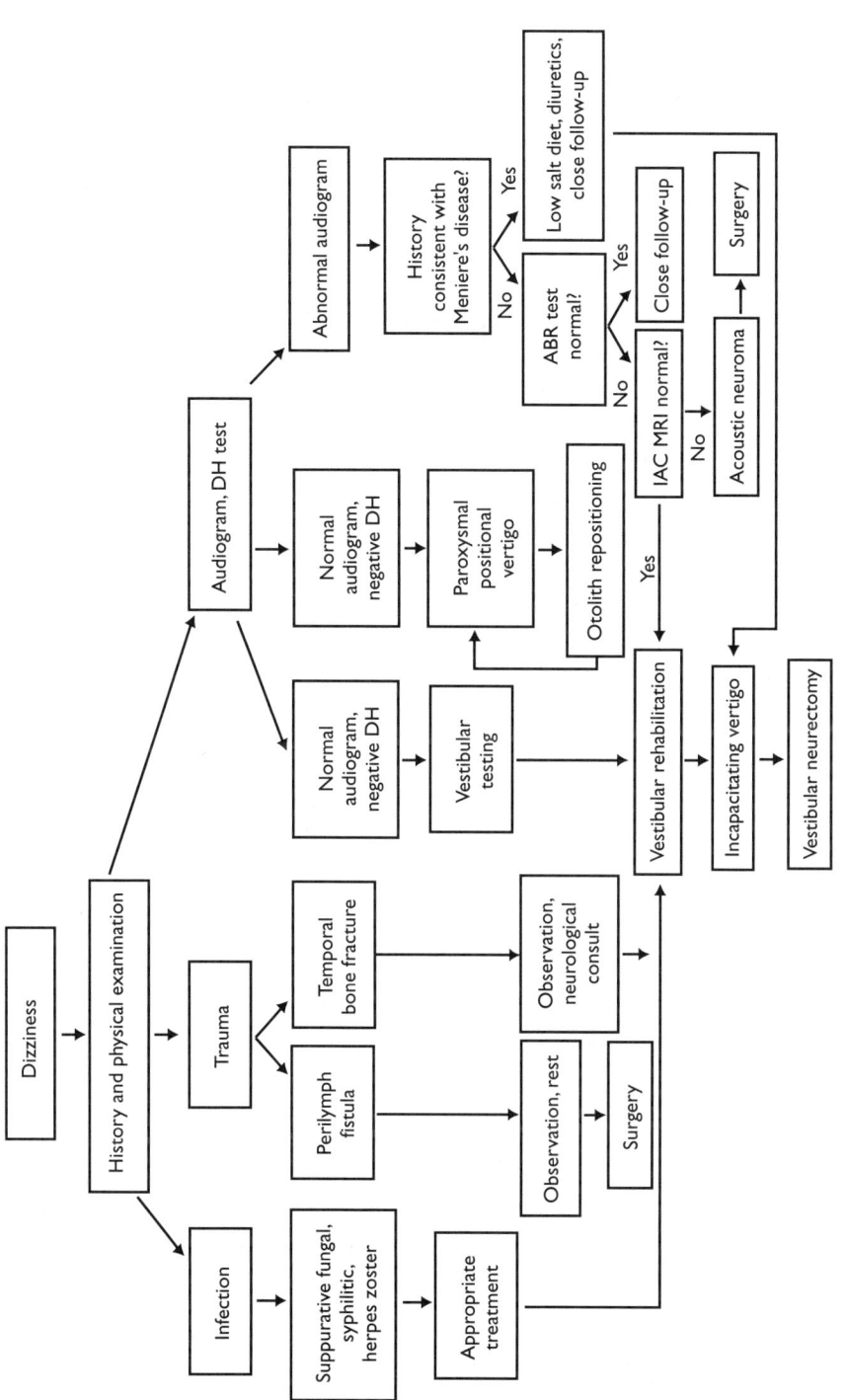

Algorithm Management of dizziness. ABR test = auditory brainstem response test; DH test = Dix–Hallpike test; IAC = image-analysis cytometry; MRI = magnetic-resonance imaging.

gelatinous material (the cupula) (*see* Fig. 6.1). The cupula responds to fluid motion in the canal, stimulating the hair cells. The utricle and saccule both contain an area of sensory epithelium (macula) that also have projecting hair cells; however, these hair cells project into a membrane (otoconia) upon which are many granules of calcium carbonate (1). These granules move in response to linear and gravitational acceleration, activating the hair cells. The utricle is excited by horizontal acceleration, whereas the saccule is sensitive to vertical acceleration.

Physiology

The right and left vestibular systems each emit baseline signals that the brain interprets as equal. When the activity on one side changes with respect to ac-

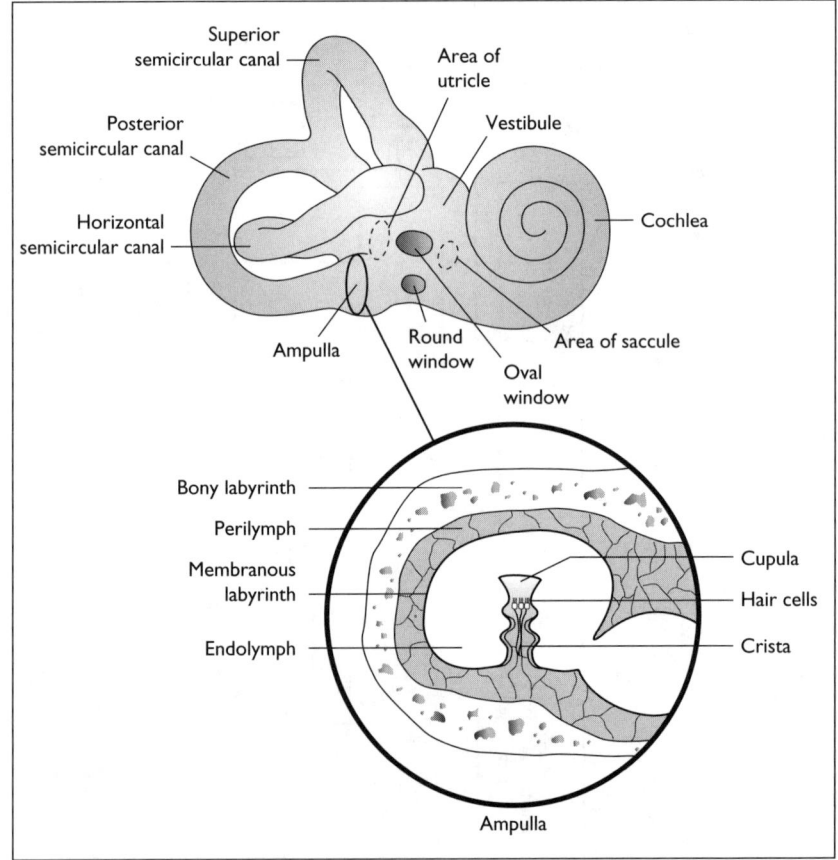

Figure 6.1 Structures of the bony labyrinth, with expanded view of the internal structures of an ampulla.

tivity on the other, complex responses are evoked (Fig. 6.2). One of these, the vestibulo-ocular reflex, keeps the eyes focused on an object while the head is in motion. Rotating the head activates the hair cells and sends a signal to the vestibular nucleus. The impulse travels to the contralateral sixth cranial nucleus, ascends the medial longitudinal fasciculus, and crosses to the third and fourth ipsilateral cranial nerve nuclei (*see* Fig. 6.2), resulting in the slow phase of eye movement in the opposite direction of the head turn. When one vestibular labyrinth is hypofunctional, the brain perceives the constant unequal signals between the two sides as persistent stimulation. Because the eyes cannot move indefinitely in one direction, the slow phase of eye movement is followed by a cortically generated, rapid, compensatory movement in the opposite direction (2). This rhythmic alternation between slow and fast eye motions is called nystagmus. By convention, the direction of the nystagmus is named for the direction of the fast component (i.e., "left-beating nystagmus" indicates fast movement in the left direction).

The vestibulospinal reflex results from activation of the vestibular system. The signal causes muscle contraction on the ipsilateral side and relaxation on the opposite side, resulting in a falling toward the side of hypoactivity.

The flocculonodular lobe of the cerebellum receives input from both the labyrinth and the vestibular nucleus, and its output possibly helps suppress vestibular hyperactivity (*see* Fig. 6.2). The vermis of the cerebellum receives input from the dorsal spinal cerebellar tract, which provides information on muscle position and tension. Multiple connections through the reticular system provide pathways to the phrenic nucleus, salivatory nuclei, and nucleus ambiguous and account for the vomiting, salivation, and regurgitation seen with some disorders. Connections between the reticular and sympathetic systems mediate pallor and sweating. Discrete tracts between the vestibular nucleus and the dorsal efferent nucleus of the vagus nerve contribute to nausea and vomiting during labyrinthine disturbance.

Over time, the CNS can become accustomed to prolonged vestibular inequalities. The visual and proprioceptive systems also assist in compensating for vestibular disorder (3).

History

One begins the history interview by attempting to understand the patient's use of the word *dizziness*, distinguishing between true vertigo (a sense of motion) and disequilibrium, lightheadedness, or imbalance. Note frequency, duration, time of onset, and cessation. Record the existence of the following symptoms:
- Hearing loss
- Tinnitus

- Nausea and vomiting
- Fever and chills
- Upper respiratory infection
- Headache
- Visual changes
- Otalgia
- Aural fullness
- Motion sickness
- Weakness
- Ataxia or falling to one side
- Facial numbness
- Chest pain
- Palpitations
- Sweating

Look for precipitating events such as a recent upper respiratory infection, head turning, change in position (e.g., going from sitting to standing), straining, history of head trauma, loud noises, chemical exposure, and menstruation. A positive history of any of the following conditions can influence symptoms and treatment:
- Birth defects
- Diabetes mellitus
- Thyroid disease
- Coronary artery disease
- Peripheral vascular disease
- Collagen vascular disease
- Autoimmunity
- Hypertension
- Allergic rhinitis
- Ear infections
- Endocrinologic, CNS, or ocular disorders
- Current medications
- Caffeine, alcohol, and salt consumption

A history of previous ear surgery is vital to diagnosis. Family and occupational histories may have implications for diagnosis and treatment.

Physical Examination

Vital signs may reveal **tachycardia**, **irregular pulse**, or hyper- or hypotension. Check **orthostatic hypotension** by recording the blood pressure with the patient in the supine position, and then again immediately on standing up. A difference of 20 mm Hg in these two systolic blood-pressure measurements

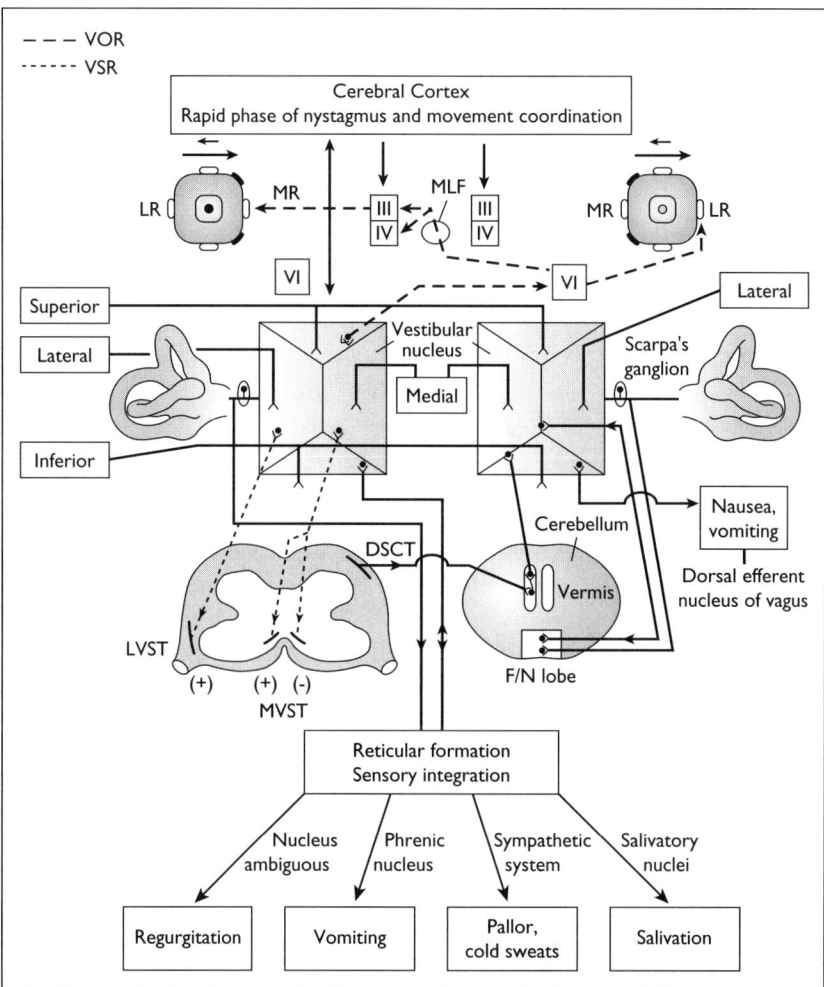

Figure 6.2 Pathways of the vestibular system. DSCT = dorsal spinal cerebellar tract; F/N lobe = flocculonodular lobe; LR = lateral rectus; LVST = lateral vestibular spinal tract; MLF = medial longitudinal fasciculus; MR = medial rectus; MVST = medial vestibular spinal tract; VOR = vestibulo-ocular reflex; VSR = vestibulospinal reflex.

(in a patient with a blood pressure in the normal range) is generally significant. The quality of the sensation felt by the patient usually is clearly light-headedness or presyncope, not true vertigo.

Check the ears for **otorrhea**, perforated eardrum, and diminished hearing. Examine the eyes for **pupillary reaction**, nystagmus, retinal disease, and papilledema. Auscultate the neck for **carotid bruits**, then palpate for lymphadenopathy or thyromegaly. Follow this with testing of the cranial nerves.

Check **cerebellar function** with rapid, alternating hand motions. **Gait** is evaluated; a broad-based unsteady gait suggests cerebellar dysfunction. Perform the **sharpened Romberg test** by having the patient stand with his or her feet close together, arms folded, and eyes closed; watch for any swaying or unsteadiness. The **tandem walk** involves the patient standing with his or her arms folded, then walking a straight line, positioning his or her feet heel to toe; record estimates of proprioception, peripheral sensation, and strength. The Fukuda test, in which the patient marches in place with his or her eyes closed for 45 seconds, is useful because turning the body while marching in this manner indicates hypofunction of the vestibular system on the same side.

Nystagmus, if present, is an important indicator of vestibular dysfunction but difficult to detect during the usual physical examination. If the patient fixes his or her vision on any object, nystagmus will be suppressed. Furthermore, if the patient closes his or her eyes to avoid any visual fixation, nystagmus cannot be assessed. This dilemma is solved by using **Frenzel (+20 diopter) lenses**, which are so strong that looking through them makes everything blurry; hence, no visual fixation is possible. A tiny light in the Frenzel frame permits the examiner to see a patient's nystagmus in any gaze field (Fig. 6.3). The patient is asked to report the quality and time course of any dizziness experienced. Some vestibular testing laboratories have video-Frenzel equipment that projects the patient's eye movements onto a video screen and records them (Fig. 6.4).

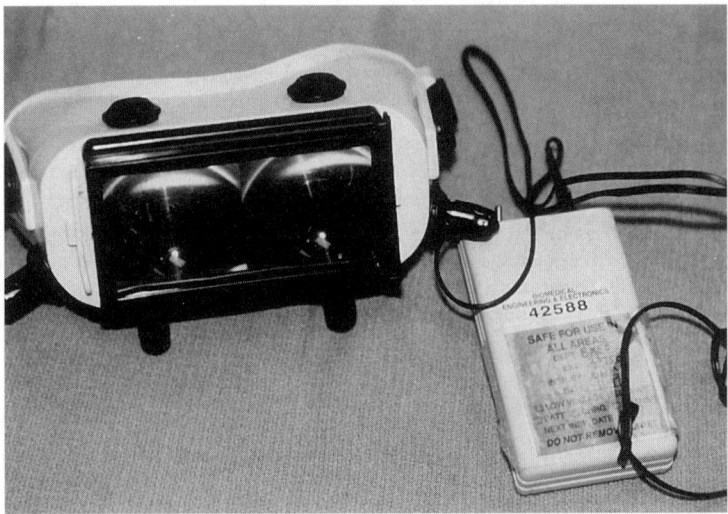

Figure 6.3 These reasonably priced Frenzel lenses are battery powered and contain a small light within the frame to allow the physician to observe the patient's eye movements.

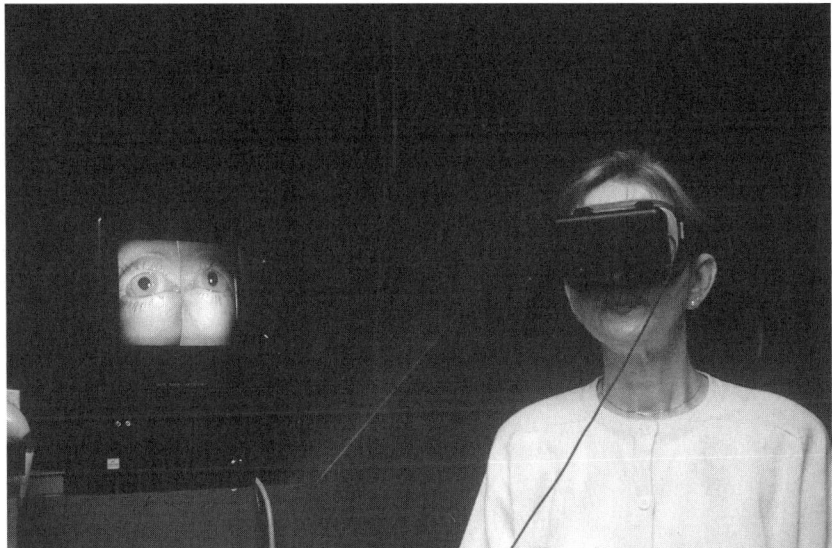

Figure 6.4 These video-Frenzel lenses have a small camera within the frame, allowing projection of the eye movement onto a video screen and recording it for later serial comparisons.

In the positioning test (**Dix–Hallpike maneuver**) (Fig. 6.5), the patient (in whom there has been no cervical movement restrictions or previous cervical spine surgery) sits up and, with his or her head turned to one side, quickly reclines (with help from the physician) until supine, with the head hanging over the edge of the table at 30° below the horizontal and still turned to the side. Watch the eyes for at least 20 seconds with Frenzel lenses in place and look for nystagmus; question the patient about any symptoms. Note the latency, duration, direction, and fatigability of any nystagmus. Then raise the patient back to a sitting position and again watch the eyes, noting any change in nystagmus or symptoms. The same maneuver is then repeated with the head turned in the opposite direction.

Caloric testing of the labyrinth can be done in the office. When the patient reclines 60° from the sitting position, the horizontal SCC is positioned vertically. With Frenzel lenses in place, the physician irrigates one ear with cool (30°C) water for 30 seconds. This causes the endolymph to move by convection in a direction that causes the vestibular output to be hypoactive with respect to the opposite side. Normally this is followed by nystagmus, with the slow phase toward the irrigated ear and the rapid phase toward the opposite direction (Table 6.1). After noting the nystagmus, the lenses are removed, and the patient fixates on a point to determine if the nystagmus is suppressed with fixation, as is normal. The opposite ear is then irrigated with cool water, and

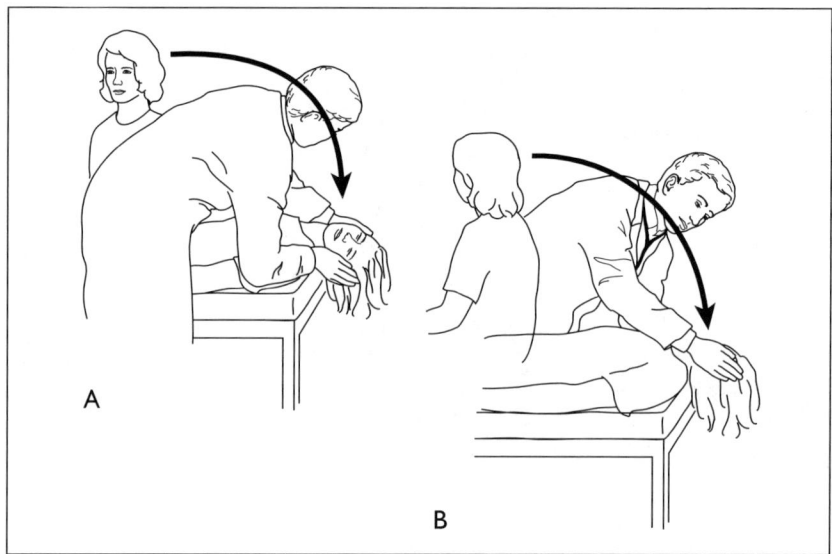

Figure 6.5 The Dix–Hallpike maneuver. **A,** The patient starts with the head turned to the left. The physician reclines the patient to the supine position, with the head hanging 30° off the edge of the table. After viewing any nystagmus, the patient is brought back to the sitting position, and the physician observes the eyes again. **B,** The maneuver is repeated, with the patient's head turned the other way.

Table 6.1 Results of Caloric Testing

Water Temperature	Ear	Eye (Slow Phase)	Eye (Fast Phase)
Cold	Right	Right	Left
Cold	Left	Left	Right
Warm	Right	Left	Right
Warm	Left	Right	Left

the physician observes the nystagmus, comparing the result to the first side. Next, the entire sequence is repeated with warm (44°C) water. This time, the nystagmus occurs in the opposite direction to that produced by the cool-water irrigation. Furthermore, the slow phase now is directed away from the irrigated ear, and the rapid phase is toward the irrigated side. If an irrigation system is not available, water may be injected into the external auditory canal using a 60-cm^3 syringe with an intravenous catheter tip.

Additional Diagnostic Evaluation

Because an underlying disorder can affect both hearing and balance systems, **audiometric testing** is routine. Testing for air- and bone-conduction thresholds, speech discrimination, acoustic reflexes, and tympanometry is standard. The **auditory brainstem response test** can be useful when patient compliance is inadequate, and it can help locate the responsible lesion.

Many aspects of the specific vestibular testing performed during the physical examination may be evaluated with **electronystagmography (ENG)** (4), a quantitative examination of vestibular function that can enhance or even replace office caloric testing. ENG measures eye movement and is based on the difference in voltage between the cornea (positive) and the retina (negative). The patient must abstain from drinking alcohol and taking anticholinergics, antihistamines, barbiturates, and other CNS depressants for 1 week before testing. Electrodes are applied to the patient's face above, below, and lateral to the eyes to record the corneoretinal potential (Fig. 6.6). Next, a series of evaluations amounting to an extension of the caloric examination (described earlier in this chapter) is performed in a dark room, and the results are recorded automatically on chart paper. The details of the ENG examination are beyond the scope of this chapter, but interested readers can consult the references provided (5).

Advanced tests of vestibular function are available in specialized centers (6). **Sinusoidal harmonic acceleration** uses a spinning chair to increase diagnostic sensitivity (Fig. 6.7). Some practitioners obtain useful information from **vestibular autorotation testing**, during which the patient moves his or her own head in both the horizontal and vertical planes. These tests may be

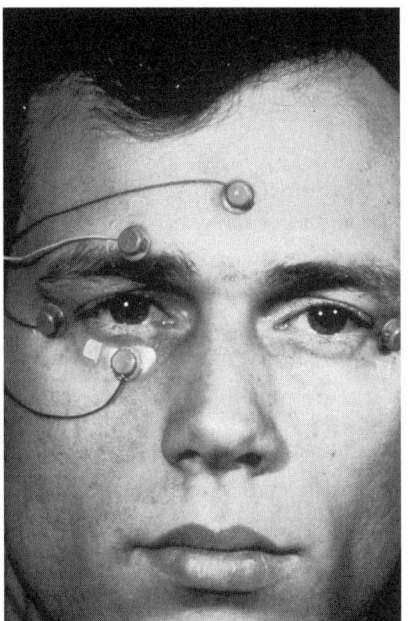

Figure 6.6 The placement of the electrodes around the patient's eyes during ENG testing.

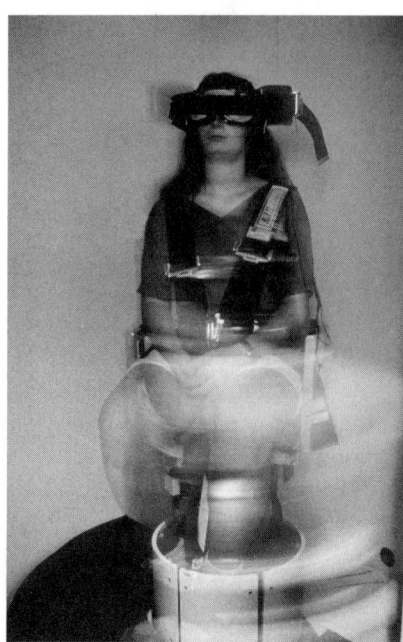

Figure 6.7 Rotation chair testing, used with the video-Frenzel lenses.

able to identify early vestibular dysfunction and can assist in vestibular rehabilitation. **Dynamic posturography** helps localize the disorder to the vestibular, visual, or proprioceptive systems by using the various combinations of open or covered eyes, a stable or moving horizon, and a stable or moving platform (Fig. 6.8).

Laboratory testing can be used when the history suggests a systemic cause of the dizziness, such as coronary artery disease, cardiac arrhythmias, peripheral vascular disease, diabetes mellitus, hypertension, hypothyroidism, and collagen vascular disease. Tests that may prove helpful include antinuclear antibody level, erythrocyte sedimentation rate, rheumatoid factor, fluorescent treponemal antibody absorbance (FTA-Abs), complete blood count, and PT/PTT (looking for hypercoagulable states). Cervical spine radiography can confirm cervical arthritis or calcified vessels.

High-resolution axial and coronal temporal bone CT (computed tomography) scans show bony structures, congenital malformations, temporal bone fractures, or infectious processes in the ear. A magnetic resonance imaging (MRI) scan, including T_1- and T_2-weighted images and T_1 with gadolinium, is useful for evaluating possible cerebellopontile-angle masses.

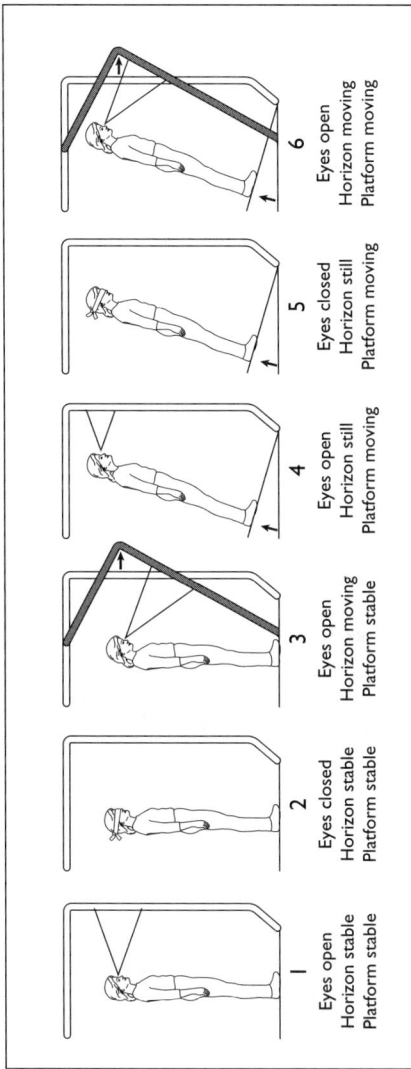

Figure 6.8 The six positions used in posturography.

Differential Diagnosis

Although the differential diagnoses for dizziness are numerous (Table 6.2), a comprehensive history (Table 6.3) and physical examination with directed evaluation can limit the options considerably. Some causes affect only the peripheral vestibular system (including the labyrinth, vestibular nerve, and vestibular nucleus), whereas other types of pathology affect the CNS; some

Table 6.2 Differential Diagnosis of Dizzines

Idiopathic Disorders	Cardiovascular Disorders
Meniere's disease	**Vascular Disorders**
Infection	Hypertension
Vestibular neuronitis	Vertebrobasilar insufficiency
Herpes zoster oticus	Transient ischemic attack
Suppurative labyrinthitis	Stroke
Serous labyrinthitis	Wallenberg's syndrome
Otitis media/externa	Subclavian steal
Syphilis	Vascular-loop compression syndrome
Fungal infection	Carotid sinus syndrome
CNS infection	Postural hypotension
Trauma	Migraine headache or equivalent
Benign paroxysmal positional vertigo	Blood components
Temporal bone fracture	Hyperviscosity
Perilymph fistula	Anemia
Labyrinthine concussion	Decreased oxygen capacity
CNS trauma (subdural hematoma)	**Cardiac Disorders**
Cerebellopontine-angle masses	Arrhythmia
Neoplasm (acoustic neuroma, meningioma)	Cardiac failure
Cholesteatoma	Hypoxia
Cholesterol granuloma	**Pediatric Disorders**
Aneurysm	Congenital anomalies
Allergic and Immunologic Disorders	Hereditary syndromes
Autoimmune inner ear disease	Arnold–Chiari syndrome
Allergic reaction	Large vestibular aqueducts
Cogan's syndrome	Perilymph fistula
Relapsing perichondritis	Benign paroxysmal vertigo (in children)
Endocrine/Metabolic Disorders	**Other Disorders**
Diabetes mellitus	Toxic agents
Hypothyroidism	Ocular disorders
Addison's disease	Proprioceptive disorders
Central Nervous System Disorders	External and middle ear disorders
Epilepsy	Motion sickness
Multiple sclerosis	Aging
Cerebellar disorders	Psychogenic disorders

CNS = central nervous system.

processes affect both systems. The general diagnosis and management Algorithm may assist in arriving at the correct diagnosis and starting treatment. However, it is important to remember that symptom complexes of many processes can overlap, so a complete understanding of the specific causes of dizziness is desirable.

Table 6.3 Key Points of History

Patient's definition of dizziness (vertigo vs. unsteadiness or lightheadedness)	Past medical history
	Past surgical history
Time course and pattern	Factors that improve or worsen dizziness
Presence of hearing loss, tinnitus, or aural fullness	Drug, cigarette, caffeine, or alcohol use
	Family history
Associated symptoms	Occupational history
Precipitating factors	

Diagnosis and Management of Specific Disorders

The Algorithm outlines the decision-making steps in the management of dizziness.

Meniere's Disease

Meniere's disease is a vestibular disorder usually presenting in adults 30 to 50 years of age. The classic symptoms are episodic vertigo; low-pitched tinnitus; fluctuating, low-frequency sensorineural hearing loss (SNHL); and a feeling of fullness in the affected ear. The vertigo is intense for 1 to 2 hours, followed by unsteadiness for a few days. The hearing loss and tinnitus usually resolve after an attack but may increase with each episode, and the vertigo may persist. Drop attacks (**"crisis of Tumarkin"**), during which the patient loses extensor tension and falls to the ground fully conscious, may occur late in the disease. The cause of Meniere's disease is unknown, but autoimmunity, endocrine disorder, and disturbed labyrinthine electrolyte balance are suspected. The diagnosis is made by the history because the physical examination is normal except during an attack. Audiometry shows low-frequency SNHL, and ENG shows hypoactivity on the affected side (7).

The treatment begins with eating a low-salt diet, avoiding tobacco and caffeine, and taking a diuretic (hydrochlorothiazide). **Vestibular suppressants** are needed only during an acute attack. If medical treatment fails, surgery (e.g., endolymphatic shunt, vestibular nerve section, labyrinthectomy) may help. Chemical destruction of the vestibular system with transtympanic aminoglycosides has succeeded in controlling vertigo in some patients (8). Case 6.1 provides an example of a patient with Meniere's disease who initially did well with medical therapy but who eventually required surgical intervention.

Infections

Vestibular neuronitis typically follows a nonspecific viral illness. It begins with an episode of severe vertigo that lasts weeks to months and is accompanied by

Case 6.1 — Man with Meniere's Disease

A man 47 years of age presented with a history of sudden-onset vertigo 3 days before his current visit. The vertigo began in the mid-morning while he was at work and increased in intensity over an hour to the point he was nauseated and vomiting. Unable to work, he took a meclizine tablet and was driven home by a coworker. Later that afternoon, he felt much improved but "drained." He had noted a sense of fullness and buzzing in his right ear on awakening that morning, and the sensation has persisted up to now.

His past medical history is pertinent because he had experienced a similar, less-severe episode 4 years ago that lasted only 3 hours. An audiogram done at that time demonstrated a right SNHL, and he was diagnosed with presumptive Meniere's disease. He had been symptom free between the attacks. He denies having any other neurological symptoms, headache, cardiac disease, and hypertension. He is taking no medication except for the meclizine he had begun at the time of his first vertigo event.

Physical examination is normal, with normal ears and no evidence of any cardiac or neurological abnormality. An audiogram is preformed and reveals a right-sided SNHL of 40 dB, a 15-db increase since his first audiogram. Speech discrimination scores were normal. An MRI scan is obtained and reveals no evidence of acoustic neuroma or other abnormality.

The patient is counseled about the natural history of Meniere's disease and is begun on a thiazide diuretic. He does well initially, but within 2 years is experiencing several attacks each month, many of which require that he leave work. He is asked whether further treatment might be possible, particularly due to the effect on his employment and his ability to safely operate an automobile. After consultation with a neurotologist, the decision to proceed with vestibular nerve section is made. Several other treatment options are discussed, including endolymphatic shunt and vestibular ablation with intratympanic gentamicin, but he and his surgeon decide on retromastoid craniotomy and nerve section. The procedure is performed uneventfully, and he is discharged on the second postoperative day with minimal residual vertigo. However, he experiences significant postoperative disequilibrium and begins outpatient vestibular adaptive exercises 1 week after surgery. He is able to return to work within 3 weeks and notes progressive improvement over the next 3 months. He has no further attacks of vertigo but has minimal residual disequilibrium with rapid head movement, to which he has accommodated easily.

Discussion

Meniere's disease is a life-long chronic disease that is managed by progressive levels of intervention. Some patients experience only minimal, infrequent symptoms and require no treatment. Others who are more symptomatic respond to diuretics, and a few may require surgical management. In older individuals for whom surgical management is not an option, vestibular ablation with intratympanic gentamicin is often effective. Treatment decisions are best made in consultation with a neurotologist—a subspecialist who treats diseases of the ear and cerebellopontile angle. Patients often request disability for Meniere's disease but should be advised that treatment is available for the symptoms of the disease and that the assumption of a sedentary lifestyle or disability is not the optimal strategy.

nausea and vomiting. Hearing usually is not affected (9). There is spontaneous nystagmus toward the unaffected ear and hypoactivity of the involved side on ENG. Treatment consists of rehydration, vestibular suppressants, and rehabilitative vestibular exercises. Case 6.2 illustrates a typical case of vestibular neuronitis.

Case 6.2 Man with Vestibular Neuronitis

A man 35 years of age awakens with profound vertigo, nystagmus, and nausea and is unable to walk without assistance. He is taken to the emergency department of the community hospital for evaluation. He has had no previous episodes and has no significant past medical history.

Review of symptoms is unremarkable, with the exception of an upper respiratory infection the previous week. His vital signs are normal, with the exception of mild tachycardia. He has a brisk left-beating nystagmus that did not alter with changes in position. He is profoundly nauseated and has vomited several times. Neurological examination fails to reveal any specific muscle weakness or sensory changes, and cranial nerve testing is normal. He states that his hearing seems to be normal and does not note any headache or nuchal rigidity.

An electrocardiogram and an urgent head CT scan with contrast are normal.

He is diagnosed with probable vestibular neuronitis and admitted for intravenous fluids and vestibular sedation with parenteral benzodiazepam. He improves significantly after therapy and was able to resume eating within 24 hours. An audiogram is normal, and the diagnosis of vestibular neuronitis is confirmed. After discharge, he continues to improve and, several weeks later, has only minimal disorientation with sudden head movement. These symptoms abate slowly, but he notes persistent minor disequilibrium for months.

Discussion

This case illustrates typical vestibular neuronitis, i.e., an isolated episode of severe vertigo with associated nausea but without hearing loss. The diagnosis is one of exclusion, because other injury to the vestibular portion of the eighth cranial nerve or vestibular nuclei (secondary to infarct or brainstem neoplasm) may mimic this diagnosis. The presentation at a young age and the history of a recent viral upper respiratory infection suggest the diagnosis. Imaging usually is not required, especially in the absence of focal neurological signs, unilateral hearing loss, or recurrent or persistent symptoms.

The persistent disequilibrium that often follows acute vestibular disorders is due to permanent residual dysfunction and can be troublesome for patients. If this patient had been employed as a roofer, steel erector, or other similar occupation, he would have to quit his job. Younger patients typically accommodate rapidly, but older patients can become essentially disabled. Accommodation can be enhanced by activity, avoidance of vestibular suppressants, and formal vestibular exercises taught by a physical therapist versed in vestibular rehabilitation. Classic BPPV may occur later in these patients and may respond to otolith repositioning.

Herpes zoster oticus (Ramsey–Hunt syndrome) presents with facial pain and vesicles on the skin of the external ear; it can be accompanied by hearing loss, tinnitus, vertigo, and facial paralysis. Treatment includes oral acyclovir 800 mg five times daily for 7 to 10 days, corticosteroids, rehydration, and evaluation by an otologist if facial palsy occurs.

Suppurative labyrinthitis, a bacterial infection of the inner ear, is a medical and surgical emergency that arises from a middle ear infection. It also can result from bacterial meningitis spreading to the inner ear through the internal auditory canal or cochlear aqueduct. Chronic otitis media may erode the horizontal SCC wall, allowing bacterial invasion of the inner ear. Symptoms include fever, chills, nausea, vomiting, severe vertigo, profound and permanent SNHL, and nystagmus. ENG shows hypoactivity of the affected ear. The patient requires immediate hospitalization, intravenous fluids, antiemetics, vestibular suppressants, and treatment of the initiating pathology. Steroids given concomitantly with the antibiotics may prevent hearing from deteriorating further. The severe vertigo peaks in 24 hours and resolves in a few days, but persistent disequilibrium may require rehabilitative vestibular exercises. Although most patients respond to medical therapy, there are those whose symptoms worsen or remain the same. Others may develop intracranial complications, requiring surgical intervention.

Syphilis must be considered in the diagnosis of vertigo and progressive or fluctuating SNHL. Congenital syphilis can occur as a severe early infection or as a more insidious latent form. Secondary syphilis may present with luetic labyrinthitis caused by meningoencephalitis. Tertiary syphilis causes inflammation and fibrosis in the inner ear. Hennebert's sign (vertigo and nystagmus on pneumatic otoscopy) and Tullio's phenomenon (vertigo and nystagmus in response to intense sound) may be seen. Laboratory tests (e.g., rapid plasma reagin test, Venereal Disease Research Laboratory test for syphilis) confirm active infection, whereas the FTA-Abs test establishes previous infection. Treatment is penicillin for 3 months. Corticosteroids may improve auditory function.

Fungal infection of the labyrinth is seen mainly in the immunocompromised patient. Common infections are candidiasis, aspergillosis, mucormycosis, cryptococcosis, and blastomycosis. Systemic antifungal agents with aggressive surgical debridement may avoid the usual poor outcome.

Serous Labyrinthitis

Serous labyrinthitis, a severe noninfectious inflammatory process of the inner ear, results from the introduction of toxic substances into the labyrinth (e.g., chemicals, products of otitis media, allergens), with no evidence of bacterial invasion. Vertigo is less severe, and hearing loss is usually minimal. As with otitis media, aggressive antimicrobial treatment is warranted to prevent suppurative labyrinthitis. A pressure-equalizing tube inserted through the tympanic membrane also can help alleviate symptoms. Vertigo and hearing loss usually subside gradually.

Trauma

Head trauma can cause symptoms of vertigo (due to vestibular injury) and disequilibrium and lightheadedness (secondary to CNS injury [e.g., stroke]).

Benign paroxysmal positional vertigo (BPPV) can be caused by trauma, infection, surgery, or aging (10). In BPPV, a few otoconia are dislodged from the macula and find their way into the posterior or horizontal SCCs. These otoconia may roam free in the canal (**canalithiasis**) or adhere to the cupula (**cupulolithiasis**). With head motion (e.g., rolling over in bed), the resulting otoconia movement stimulates the hair cells, inducing vertigo. This can be reproduced by the Dix–Hallpike maneuver (*see* Fig. 6.5). Patients may complain of a constant vague dizziness secondary to cupulolithiasis, which is thought to transform the SCC from an angular-acceleration detector to a linear-acceleration or gravity detector. With posterior SCC BPPV, nystagmus appears after a short latency and is rotary in the direction of the ear that is turned down. In horizontal SCC BPPV, nystagmus is immediate and horizontal toward the turned-down ear. Vestibular exercises and canalith repositioning are the initial treatment (Case 6.3) (11,12).

Canalith repositioning is based on the theory that the otoconia can be rotated from the SCC into the vestibule (Fig. 6.9). For posterior SCC BPPV, the patient lies supine with the affected ear down. At 30-second intervals, the physician gradually turns the patient's head to the opposite side while turning his or her entire body to the opposite side as well, finally bringing the patient back to the sitting position. A mastoid vibrator helps facilitate otoconia movement.

For horizontal SCC BPPV, the patient begins in the supine position with the affected ear down. At 30-second intervals the patient's head and body are turned a complete 360° (*see* Fig. 6.9) (11). After the procedure, the patient keeps his or her head elevated and avoids rapid turning or bending for 3 days. If these measures fail, surgical interventions (e.g., **posterior SCC occlusion, singular neurectomy**) are available.

Most **temporal bone fractures** are a combination of the two types, transverse and longitudinal. A transverse temporal bone fracture results from a severe blow to the frontal or occipital areas and carries a high incidence of severe vertigo and SNHL secondary to disruption of the labyrinth. The tympanic membrane is intact, and nystagmus is seen to the side contralateral to the injury, with facial paralysis in 50% of the patients. Severe vertigo can be controlled with vestibular suppressants until it subsides in approximately 1

> ### Case 6.3 — Woman with Benign Paroxysmal Positional Vertigo
>
> A woman 52 years of age presents with a complaint of awakening with the room spinning. After nearly a minute, the dizziness seems to clear. However, when she tries to get out of bed, the vertigo recurs, lasting 15 to 30 seconds. As the day goes on, she has gradual improvement, but many times during the day notes several seconds of vertigo. She does not experience nausea, denies tinnitus and hearing loss, and has no history of ear disease.
>
> Physical examination reveals normal vital signs, no nystagmus, and normal neurological examination. Tympanic membranes and gait are normal. Tuning fork and cerebellar tests are all normal. A Dix–Hallpike test reveals brisk, downbeating, rotatory nystagmus with the right ear down. Vertigo appears 6 seconds after being placed in the precipitating position, increases for 15 seconds, then resolves by the end of 1 minute, duplicating her complaint. Repeating the test several minutes later demonstrates reduced nystagmus and symptoms of vertigo.
>
> An audiogram is normal, and she is diagnosed with BPPV. An otolith-repositioning procedure was performed, and she was instructed to maintain her head in the upright position for 24 hours. When contacted by the office nurse 2 days later, the patient has no recurrence of her symptoms.
>
> Nine months later, she represents with similar symptoms of a somewhat lesser degree. A second Dix–Hallpike test was positive, and an otolith repositioning maneuver was performed again with excellent response.
>
> #### Discussion
>
> This patient presented with the classic symptoms of BPPV. Her initial attack probably occurred when she rolled over in bed as she was awakening. The nystagmus began after a short latency and was fatigable, classic for BPPV. The clinical response to repositioning is often dramatic and can be repeated if the symptoms recur, which they typically do. This diagnosis is important to rule out, because it often is treated easily. Using meclizine is discouraged because vestibular suppressants are unlikely to improve the symptoms.

week; residual unsteadiness may last for 3 to 6 months. Prompt referral to the specialist is important if there is facial nerve paralysis; surgical decompression of the bony canal may be necessary.

Longitudinal temporal bone fractures are more common than transverse fractures and usually result from a blow to the side of the head. The external auditory canal and tympanic membrane may be lacerated and, with ossicular discontinuity, can cause conductive hearing loss. Facial nerve paralysis is observed in only 20% of patients, and SNHL is much less common. Vertigo is usually mild, presenting with changes in head po-

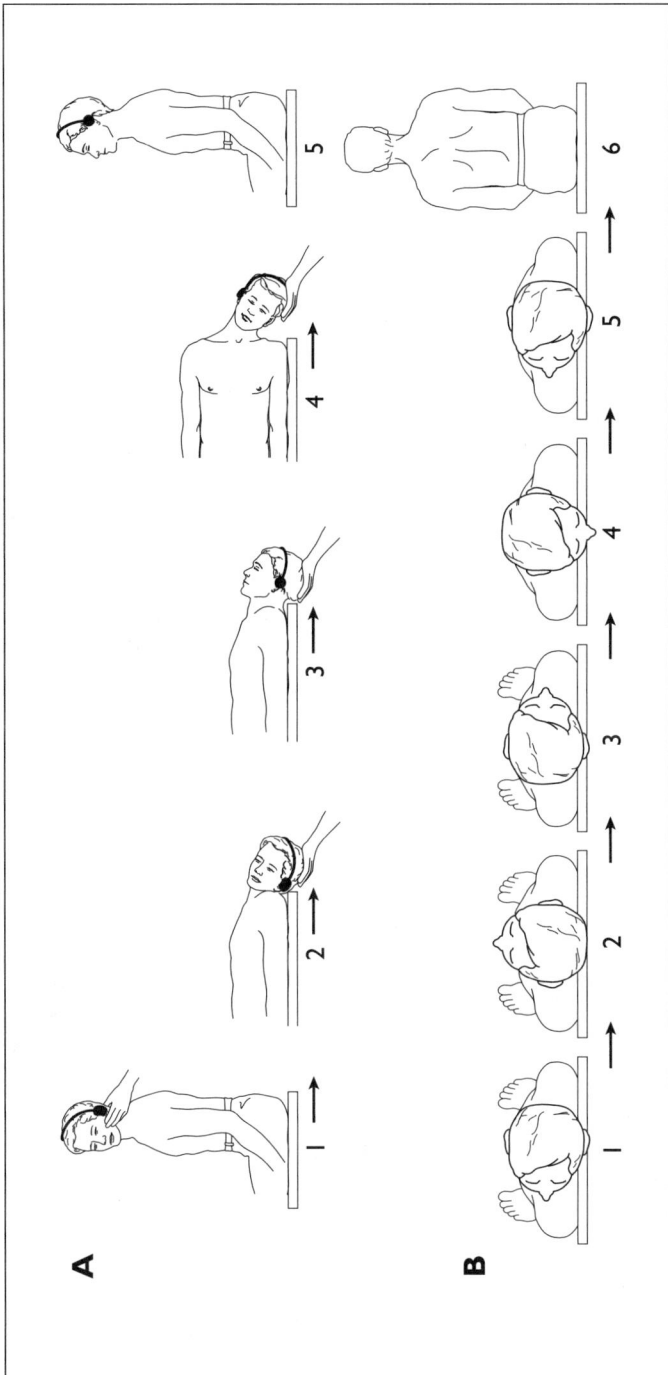

Figure 6.9 Canalith repositioning procedure (CRP). **A,** CRP for posterior semicircular canal (SCC) benign paroxysmal positional vertigo (BPPV) starts with the patient in a seated position and his or her head turned to the affected ear. With the mastoid vibrator in place, the patient then is moved through each position in 30-second intervals, arriving back in the sitting position. **B,** CRP for horizontal SCC BPPV starts with the patient in the supine position with his or her head turned to the affected ear. The patient then is moved through each position in 30-second intervals, with the mastoid vibrator in place, arriving back in the sitting position.

sition and often resolving after rehabilitative vestibular exercise (*see* section on Management below).

Controversy surrounds the cause of perilymph fistula (PLF), the leakage of perilymph from the oval or round windows. It may result from trauma, infection, strenuous physical activity, scuba diving, or airplane travel or may simply occur spontaneously (13). The patient presents with vertigo, fluctuating or sudden SNHL, tinnitus, and aural fullness much like Meniere's disease, and symptoms may be increased by straining. The physical examination is not much help, but some patients may have vertigo and nystagmus on pneumatic otoscopy (positive fistula test) (14). With a large PLF, cerebrospinal fluid otorrhea may be encountered, as shown by the presence of β_2-transferrin. High-resolution CT scan usually does not reveal the presumptive fistula except in children with a malformation of the temporal bone.

Treatment is bedrest, head elevation, antitussives, stool softeners, and reduced physical activity. If the symptoms appear after a head trauma, the fistula may be the result of a dislocated stapes, and surgical repair may be necessary. Some surgeons explore the middle ear in PLF patients who do not respond to medical treatment. In such cases, surgery involves patching the oval and round windows with soft tissue. This procedure often helps vertigo but rarely restores hearing. Vertigo in patients with a history of otologic surgery, especially stapedectomy, deserves prompt referral to an otologist with a presumptive diagnosis of PLF.

A **labyrinthine concussion** may cause vertigo and SNHL. Although SNHL may not improve, vertigo and disequilibrium usually respond to vestibular exercises. One must not confuse this with subdural hematoma, which also can cause unsteadiness after head injury.

Cerebellopontile-Angle Masses

Cerebellopontile-angle masses include neoplasms, cholesterol granuloma, cholesteatoma, and aneurysms (Case 6.4), but the most common mass by far is acoustic neuroma. (Meningiomas, glomus tumors, CNS tumors, and other neuromas make up a smaller percentage.) Acoustic neuromas are benign, grow slowly, and originate from Schwann's cells of the vestibular nerve. Patients with an acoustic neuroma are more likely to present with unsteadiness than with vertigo. The mass encroaches on the cochlear nerve, with progressive asymmetrical SNHL marked by loss of speech discrimination. ENG may be hypoactive. Cranial nerve V (and, later, cranial nerves VII, IX, X, and XI) may be affected. Approximately 15% of patients with an acoustic neuroma present with acute vertigo and a sudden, asymmetrical SNHL, suggesting cochleovestibular cerebrovascular accident. MRI with gadolinium of the internal auditory canals demonstrates

Case 6.4 Man with Vertigo Caused by a Cholesteatoma

A man 58 years of age presents to the emergency department with an acute attack of vertigo and associated nausea and vomiting. The patient is unemployed and uninsured and has not sought treatment for any aliment for many years. He has a long history of drainage from his left ear and has not been able to hear from that ear since childhood.

Physical examination reveals a thin, unkempt man with a strong odor of alcohol and a brisk right-beating nystagmus. He is unable to walk and cannot stand without assistance. The nystagmus does not change with positional changes, nor does it fatigue with time. Facial nerve function and the remainder of the neurological examination are normal. Otologic examination reveals foul drainage in the left ear canal. After suctioning the canal, microscopic examination reveals a large cholesteatoma with erosion of the ear canal and granulation tissue obscuring the margin of the erosion.

The patient is admitted and intravenous benzodiazepam is administered, markedly decreasing his symptoms. An urgent head CT scan with contrast and 1-mm cuts through the temporal bone reveal a large lucency in the left mastoid cavity, with erosion of the lateral semicircular canal. There is no evidence of intracranial fluid collection or enhancement of the dura to suggest intracranial extension. An audiogram demonstrates profound hearing loss in the affected ear; however, because of the normal hearing of the contralateral ear, adequate masking could not be performed to determine accurately the degree of conductive loss.

The patient is placed on intravenous antibiotics and local ear care. Several days later he undergoes modified radical mastoidectomy and removal of the cholesteatoma and fascial grafting over the fenestration in the horizontal semicircular canal. His vertigo gradually improves, although he is left with significant permanent disequilibrium for which he is prescribed vestibular rehabilitation as an outpatient. His hearing does not return, and he becomes lost to follow-up after his third postoperative visit.

Discussion

Vertigo can be the initial manifestation of inflammatory ear disease; however, other symptoms (e.g., pain, hearing loss) typically occur first. Most patients encountered in a physician's office have been evaluated previously; hence, large infected cholesteatomas are rare. However, in underserved areas where routine health care is not readily sought or available, cases such as this are still encountered.

---

the tumor. Treatment usually involves surgical excision, with stereotactic radiation reserved for patients unsuited for general anesthetic or unwilling to undergo operation. In reviewing reported results of treatment, one must differentiate between simply preserving a patient's hearing and preserving his or her *useful* hearing.

Allergic and Immunologic Diseases

Autoimmune inner ear disease may present with vertigo or disequilibrium and a rapidly progressive or fluctuating SNHL that may be asymmetric. Symptoms may be associated with rheumatoid arthritis, scleroderma, or systemic lupus erythematosis. Tests for antinuclear antibody, rheumatoid factor, erythrocyte sedimentation rate, and antibodies to inner ear antigens (with the lymphocyte transformation test or a Western blot assay looking for antibodies to the 68-kD inner ear protein) may assist in establishing a diagnosis (15). These tests have shown moderate sensitivity and high specificity to autoimmune diseases of the inner ear.

Treatment consists of high-dose steroids for 4 weeks, tapering off as symptoms allow. If no benefit is seen, a cytotoxic agent (e.g., cyclophosphamide) or plasmapheresis may be appropriate.

Cogan's syndrome (autoimmune interstitial keratitis, episodic severe vertigo, progressive SNHL, and tinnitus) can be seen with systemic disorders or vasculitides such as rheumatoid arthritis, polyarteritis nodosa, or inflammatory bowel disease (16). The interstitial keratitis of Cogan's syndrome produces rapid visual loss with inflammatory symptoms, whereas the interstitial keratitis of syphilis is insidious and without acute inflammation. Treatment is with steroids; if there is no response, cytotoxic agents are added.

Allergic reaction to various substances may cause symptoms of vertigo, hearing loss, and tinnitus usually through a non–IgE-mediated process that causes edema of the labyrinth. The symptoms usually resolve once the allergen is removed. Allergy testing and immunotherapy may prevent future episodes.

Endocrine and Metabolic Diseases

Diabetes mellitus may induce dizziness by a variety of mechanisms (17). Hypo- or hyperglycemia may evoke lightheadedness. Damage to small vessels due to diabetes mellitus may cause labyrinthine ischemia. Diabetes mellitus also can cause a primary neuropathy of the vestibular nerve. **Hypothyroidism** may present with dizziness, SNHL, tinnitus, aural fullness, and other symptoms of hypothyroidism, such as weight gain, dry skin, and constipation. The symptoms improve with thyroid replacement therapy. **Addison's disease** (adrenocortical insufficiency) may cause lightheadedness and postural hypotension.

Cardiovascular Diseases

Cardiovascular diseases can produce varying degrees of cerebral anoxia, resulting in complaints of imbalance, unsteadiness, or lightheadedness that are often presyncope (Case 6.5). If the disorder affects the blood supply to the labyrinth or to the vestibular nucleus, the patient may present with true vertigo. The internal auditory artery supplies blood to the labyrinth and is a branch of the anterior inferior cerebellar artery, which derives from the vertebrobasilar artery system. Because the internal auditory artery is an end artery, any disease affecting it or its feeding vessels may result in ischemia to the labyrinth, causing vertigo and hearing loss (18).

Many patients believe that **hypertension** causes dizziness; however, more often dizziness is a side effect of the medications used to treat hypertension. **Atherosclerosis**, when present in the vertebrobasilar artery system, can result in vertebrobasilar insufficiency, causing dizziness, vertigo, syncope, ataxia,

---

Case 6.5   **Man with Syncope Caused by a Cardiovascular Disorder**

A man 42 years of age with no history of significant medical problems presents to his physician complaining of "dizzy spells." He has experienced six or seven episodes of dizziness in which he felt like he was "floating" and was about to "pass out." He denies a sense of spinning or illusion of motion but notes that his vision becomes gray at the time of the spells. Each of these lasted only several seconds, and, although he occasionally had to hold onto objects to keep from falling, he had not fallen nor suffered syncope. Friends who witnessed the episodes stated that he looked pale and had him sit to "get his balance."

His past medical history is completely benign, with no history of hearing loss, true vertigo, other neurological symptoms, chest pain, or cardiac symptoms. His physical examination and an electrocardiogram are normal. He is thought to be suffering from "near" syncope and is evaluated for a possible cardiac or neurological cause. A Holter monitor is placed, and a review of the strip reveals a period of arrhythmia with aberrant conduction and 4 seconds of asystole. After further investigation, he undergoes insertion of a cardiac pacemaker and has no further episodes of dizziness.

Discussion

This case illustrates that symptoms that the patient describes as dizziness may not be vestibular in nature but rather some other process (e.g., "near" syncope). Differentiation while taking a history may be challenging and is time consuming. The difficulty is increased further because patients with true vertigo often state that they thought that they were about to "pass out" and may report that they became quite agitated and diaphoretic (due to fear). The astute physician in this case recognized that the history did not include symptoms of an illusion of motion and therefore evaluated the patient for near syncope, probably saving his life.

dysarthria, weakness, and visual changes. Emboli in the carotid or vertebrobasilar systems may result in **transient ischemic attacks**, causing these same symptoms. If an embolus occludes the internal auditory artery, a condition called **labyrinthine apoplexy** results, causing acute vertigo, nausea, vomiting, SNHL, and tinnitus. If atherosclerosis is suspected, evaluation includes carotid imaging studies. Depending on the results of the evaluation, endarterectomy may be indicated. Although the patient's strength may return gradually during the recovery from a stroke, the unsteadiness (caused not only by damage of the labyrinth and CNS but also by decreased proprioception and vision) may be permanent.

Occlusion of the subclavian artery proximal to the branching of the vertebral artery may cause a **subclavian steal** that causes episodic dizziness, headache, vision changes, dysarthria, audible bruit, and a 20–mm Hg difference in blood pressure between both arms and a weakened radial pulse on the steal side. Bypass of the occluded segment may resolve the symptoms. **Wallenberg's syndrome** results from ischemia of the lateral medulla from an occlusion of the posterior inferior cerebellar artery. Vertigo, nausea, vomiting, nystagmus, dysphagia, Horner's syndrome, and ipsilateral vocal cord paralysis are seen with the loss of pain and temperature sensation on the ipsilateral face and the contralateral trunk. A **basilar artery aneurysm** can decrease blood flow to the labyrinth or allow the development of thrombus.

A **vascular loop** is a vascular structure compressing the eighth cranial nerve that can be seen on MRI. This is a diagnosis usually made at surgical exploration (19). Mild compression may produce dizziness and tinnitus, but it is difficult to prove. Surgery during which a synthetic material is placed between the vessel and the eighth cranial nerve sometimes will eliminate the symptoms. Surgical intervention usually includes vestibular nerve section.

Polycythemia, sickle cell anemia, and macroglobulinemia may cause a **hyperviscosity syndrome** that affects the small vessels of the vestibular system. Symptoms include vertigo, hearing loss, and visual disturbance. **Hypoxia** of the labyrinth or CNS may occur with carbon monoxide poisoning, leukemia, lung disease, and severe anemia, resulting in vertigo. **Cardiac arrhythmias** usually cause lightheadedness or presyncope but not true vertigo.

Central Nervous System Diseases

Disorders of the CNS (e.g., **tumors, meningitis, abscess**) often evoke dizziness or unsteadiness, usually without true vertigo. A neurological examination forms an important part of the work-up for dizziness. If a CNS disorder is suspected, then CT or MRI should be considered.

Epilepsy may be associated with dizziness or vertigo either in the form of an aura preceding a general seizure or as a symptom of temporal lobe epilepsy. The vertigo ranges in severity and usually is not accompanied by hearing loss; however, the patient may lose consciousness or suffer auditory or visual hallucinations. Management aimed at seizure control usually eliminates episodes of dizziness.

Multiple sclerosis presents with vertigo in 5% to 10% of patients diagnosed and is eventually present in 30% to 40% of all those with the disease (20). Demyelinization can cause dysfunction of the medial longitudinal fasciculus, resulting in internuclear ophthalmoplegia, which is the inability of the medial rectus muscle to return the eye medially after looking laterally. Nystagmus is often present on lateral gaze. Multiple sclerosis also may cause visual disturbances and can injure the long nerve tracts of the spinal cord, causing a loss of proprioception. Because proprioception and visual function contribute to the patient's balance, disturbance of these functions compounds any vestibular problem already present and increases the difficulty of rehabilitation.

Cerebellar disorders may be seen with infection, tumor, vascular disease, toxic ingestion, or aging. Degradation of the connections between the cerebellum and the vestibular system that mediates inhibitory impulses may impair inhibition, resulting in vertigo or dizziness.

Miscellaneous Disorders

Ocular disorders (e.g., decreased acuity, muscle movement, and intraocular pressure) may produce dizziness. Because the visual system is important to spatial orientation, visual disorders intensify symptoms of vestibular disease.

Proprioceptive disorders of the peripheral nervous system caused by alcohol abuse, diabetes mellitus, tabes dorsalis, pernicious anemia, or pellagra may cause imbalance, compounding symptoms of vestibular disease. Posturography may identify a proprioceptive component of the disequilibrium (*see* Fig. 6.8).

Toxic agents that cause vertigo include the same medications that cause hearing loss secondary to hair cell destruction. These medications include aminoglycosides, aspirin, quinine, chemotherapy, and diuretics (21). Audiogram and ENG may be normal early in toxic exposure, but subtle vestibular-system deficits may be detected on sinusoidal harmonic acceleration and the vestibulo-autorotation test. If vestibular function is present on testing, then vestibular exercises help the CNS to compensate. If the drug destroys both vestibular systems, then oscillopsia (i.e., the inability to maintain a stable horizontal visual reference while walking) may occur. This situation presents a difficult problem because the brain is receiving no input with which to generate compensation. ENG shows bilateral hypoactivity on caloric testing. However, if some vestibular activity persists, then rehabilitative vestibular exercises may help (*see* section on Management below).

Cerumen or a foreign body in the external auditory canal may create pressure on the tympanic membrane, causing vertigo. **Eustachian tube dysfunction** caused by allergic rhinitis or upper respiratory infection also may cause dizziness.

Otosclerosis, either of the stapes or the labyrinth, may cause vertigo. It is diagnosed by history, tuning fork tests, and audiometry. When the stapes is involved, a stapedectomy may be performed if the patient does not have active Meniere's disease. If the otosclerosis involves the labyrinth, oral sodium fluoride may halt the progression of disease.

Motion sickness is due to unaccustomed periodic movements and causes dizziness, nausea, and vomiting. The absence of compensation by vision or proprioception worsens the symptoms. An example is a ship passenger whose *mal de mer* becomes worse when he goes below deck and loses a visual reference (e.g., the horizon, the surface of the sea). Occasionally, after a prolonged voyage, the patient may experience recurrent sensations of imbalance on solid land for a period of months to years, a condition called ***mal de debarquement*** syndrome (22). Motion sickness is treated with antihistamines, diazepam, scopolamine, and other vestibular suppressants.

The natural process of **aging** can be accompanied by dizziness and impairment of balance (23). The connections between the different areas of the vestibular system weaken with age, and the hair cells slowly atrophy. The receptors within the vasculature may decrease in sensitivity, causing postural hypotension on rapid position change. The patient learns to change positions more slowly. Additionally, the proprioceptive and visual systems decrease in efficiency over the years.

Psychogenic vertigo is a diagnosis of exclusion. These patients present with an atypical or bizarre story, hyperventilation, an impending lawsuit, or symptoms of other psychiatric disorders. The most useful test for distinguishing these patients is posturography.

Management

The treatment of vertigo begins only after an appropriate history interview, physical examination, and directed evaluation. Most conditions that produce dizziness are not emergencies, usually resolve spontaneously, and can be evaluated on an outpatient basis. Causes that may need more immediate treatment or referral are listed in the section on Danger Signs below.

In general, acute cases with intolerable symptoms call for **vestibular suppression** using medications that blunt both the vestibular system and the CNS (e.g., oral meclizine 12.5–25.0 mg four times daily). Oral diazepam 2.5 mg three times daily helps vestibular suppression. Antiemetics (e.g., droperidol, odansetron [Zofran]), anticholinergics, or both assist in controlling the symptoms. Vasodilators (e.g., hydralazine, niacin, histamine, carbogen) may help relieve dizziness when a vascular disorder is suspected.

The patient should be counseled about **lifestyle changes** that include discontinuing smoking, avoiding alcohol and caffeine, restricting salt intake, and reducing life stress (12).

Vestibular exercises include maneuvers that elicit dizziness, gradually desensitizing the patient. For example, if a head turn to the right elicits dizziness, then the patient performs repeated head turns to the right until the dizziness begins, after which the patient stops and rests until the symptoms fade. The same process is repeated multiple times, and the exercises then continue with other head turns and body positions. Vestibular-suppressant medication will retard central compensation and should be used sparingly in patients undergoing vestibular exercises.

If medical management fails, **surgical treatment** can be offered. Some surgical procedures (e.g., endolymphatic sac decompression, shunting for Meniere's disease) can preserve hearing. Destructive procedures (e.g., vestibular nerve section [which can preserve hearing], labyrinthectomy [when no serviceable hearing exists]) are effective in controlling vertigo. Recently, it has been found that aminoglycoside injected experimentally into the middle ear destroys the hair cells responsible for vertigo, evidently sparing the cells responsible for hearing.

Danger Signs

Danger signs in the evaluation of patients with dizziness include the following:

- **Herpes zoster oticus (Ramsey–Hunt syndrome) with facial nerve paralysis:** requires antiviral treatment
- **Labyrinthitis (suppurative or serous):** often requires admission for control of progression and may need surgical drainage
- **Fungal infection of the labyrinth:** occurs primarily in immunocompromised individuals and requires surgical debridement and antifungal therapy
- **Temporal bone fracture with facial nerve paralysis:** may need surgical decompression of the bony canal of the facial nerve
- **Trauma accompanied by vertigo (with or without temporal bone fracture):** may need surgical exploration of the stapes
- **Trauma with unsteadiness (with or without temporal bone fracture):** may represent a subdural hematoma and may require treatment
- **Sudden vertigo and asymmetrical hearing loss:** may indicate an acoustic neuroma

- **Lightheadedness with abnormal blood glucose:** may indicate diabetes mellitus or hypoglycemia
- **Dizziness with recent onset of short-lived neurological symptoms:** may need carotid imaging and endarterectomy, especially if carotid bruits are present
- **Dizziness and palpitations:** may indicate a cardiac arrhythmia
- **Dizziness and nonspecific signs of infection and meningismus:** may indicate a CNS infection that requires treatment

Summary

Patients complaining of dizziness may have vertigo of vestibular origin, or they may be suffering from the lightheadedness or disequilibrium caused by disorders of other systems. Determining the origin of dizziness is the starting point of effective treatment.

REFERENCES

1. **Dohlman GF.** The attachment of the cupulae, otolith, and tectorial membranes to the sensory cell area. *Acta Otolaryngol.* 1971;71:89–105.
2. **McCabe BF.** The quick component of nystagmus. *Laryngoscope.* 1988;98:502–6.
3. **Fluur E.** Vestibular compensation after labyrinthine destruction. *Acta Otolaryngol.* 1960;52:367–74.
4. **Rubin W.** Nystagmography: terminology, technique, and instrumentation. *Arch Otolaryngol.* 1968;87:266–71.
5. **Stennerson RL, Van de Water SM, Systma WH, et al.** Central vestibular findings on electronystagmography. *Ear Hear.* 1986;7:176–81.
6. **Rubin W.** How do we use state-of-the-art vestibular testing to diagnose and treat the dizzy patient? An overview of vestibular testing and balance system integration. *Neurol Clin.* 1990;8:225–34.
7. **Paparella MM, Mancini F.** Vestibular Meniere's disease. *Otolaryngol Head Neck Surg.* 1985;93:148–51.
8. **Driscoll CLW, Kasperbauer JL, Facer GW, et al.** Low-dose intratympanic gentamicin and the treatment of Meniere's disease: preliminary results. *Laryngoscope.* 1997;107:83–9.
9. **Nadol JB.** Vestibular neuritis. *Otolaryngol Head Neck Surg.* 1995;112:162–72.
10. **Epley JM.** Positional vertigo related to semicircular canalithiasis. *Otolaryngol Head Neck Surg.* 1995;112:154–61.
11. **Lempert T, Tiel-Wilck K.** A positional maneuver for treatment of horizontal-canal benign positional vertigo. *Laryngoscope.* 1996;106:476–8.
12. **Cawthorne T.** The physiological basis for head exercises. *J Chart Soc Physiother.* 1944;106–7.
13. **Wall C, Rauch SD.** Perilymph fistula pathophysiology. *Otolaryngol Head Neck Surg.*

1995;112:145–53.
14. **Podoshin L, Fradis M, Ben-David J, et al.** Perilymph fistula: the value of diagnostic tests. *J Laryngol Otol.* 1994;108:560–3.
15. **Harris JP, Ryan AF.** Fundamental immune mechanisms of the brain and inner ear. *Otolaryngol Head Neck Surg.* 1995;112:639–53.
16. **Cogan DG.** Syndrome of nonsyphilitic interstitial keratitis and vestibuloauditory symptoms. *Arch Ophthalmol.* 1945;33:144.
17. **Sidorov JE, Benkovic GW, Greenfield LS, et at.** Metabolic abnormalities and vertigo. *Arch Intern Med.* 1987;147:197.
18. **Grad A, Baloh RW.** Vertigo of vascular origin. *Arch Neurol.* 1989;46:281–4.
19. **McCabe BF, Gantz BJ.** Vascular loop as a cause of incapacitating dizziness. *Am J Otol.* 1989;10:117–20.
20. **Schumacher GA.** Demyelinating diseases as a cause for vertigo. *Arch Otol.* 1967;85:93–4.
21. **Fee WEJ.** Aminoglycoside ototoxicity in the human. *Laryngoscope.* 1980;24(Suppl):1–19.
22. **Brown JJ, Baloh RW.** Persistent mal de debarquement syndrome. *Am J Otolaryngol.* 1987;8:219–22.
23. **Sloane PD, Balch RW, Honrubia V.** The vestibular system in the elderly. *Am J Otolaryngol.* 1989;10:422–9.

SUGGESTED READINGS

Drachman DA. A 69-year-old man with chronic dizziness. *JAMA.* 1998; 280:2111–8.
This article is one of the Clinical Crossroads series, detailing the evaluation and management of a man suffering from persistent dizziness.
Fitzgerald DC. Head trauma: hearing loss and dizziness. *J Trauma.* 1996; 40:488–96
This article discusses the connections between head trauma and vestibulocochlear injury, including mechanisms of injury and prognosis.
Lempert T, Tiel-Wilck K. A positional maneuver for treatment of horizontal-canal benign positional vertigo. *Laryngoscope.* 1996;106:476–8.
This article describes in detail the positional maneuvering for treating benign positional vertigo.
Ruckenstein MJ. A practical approach to dizziness: questions to bring vertigo and other causes into focus. *Postgrad Med.*1995; 97:70–81.
This article contains a broad overview of the varied causes of dizziness, with suggestions for focusing the history and physical examination on the most likely causes in each patient.
Sloane PD, Balch RW, Honrubia V. The vestibular system in the elderly. *Am J Otolaryngol.* 1989;10:422–9.
This article details some of the changes that take place in the vestibular system as the patient ages and how these affect the clinical presentation and pathophysiology.

7

Tinnitus

David A. Godin, MD
Gerard J. Gianoli, MD

Tinnitus is an auditory perception of sound that is not present in the external environment. It is common, affecting up to 7% of the U.S. population, with the incidence increasing with age. Tinnitus is usually minor and noted only in quiet environments, such as at bedtime. For some patients, however, awareness of tinnitus can result in severe dysphoria that can lead to depression and, rarely, suicide.

Most patients presenting with tinnitus describe the noise as a ringing, buzzing, or humming, whereas others report sounds such as a rhythmic ocean rumble or a chirping cricket. One half of patients with tinnitus localize sound to one ear, and the other half hear noise either from both ears or from the head in general. Twenty percent of tinnitus sufferers complain of significant effects on their quality of life, including difficulty sleeping and concentrating and problems in social interaction and daily work. Depression is often associated with tinnitus, especially in the elderly. Approximately three quarters of patients with ear disease have associated tinnitus, making common the associated otologic complaints of hearing loss, vertigo, and aural fullness.

Anatomy and Physiology

The pathophysiology of tinnitus can be divided into two main categories: para-auditory noises (arising from structures outside of the auditory system)

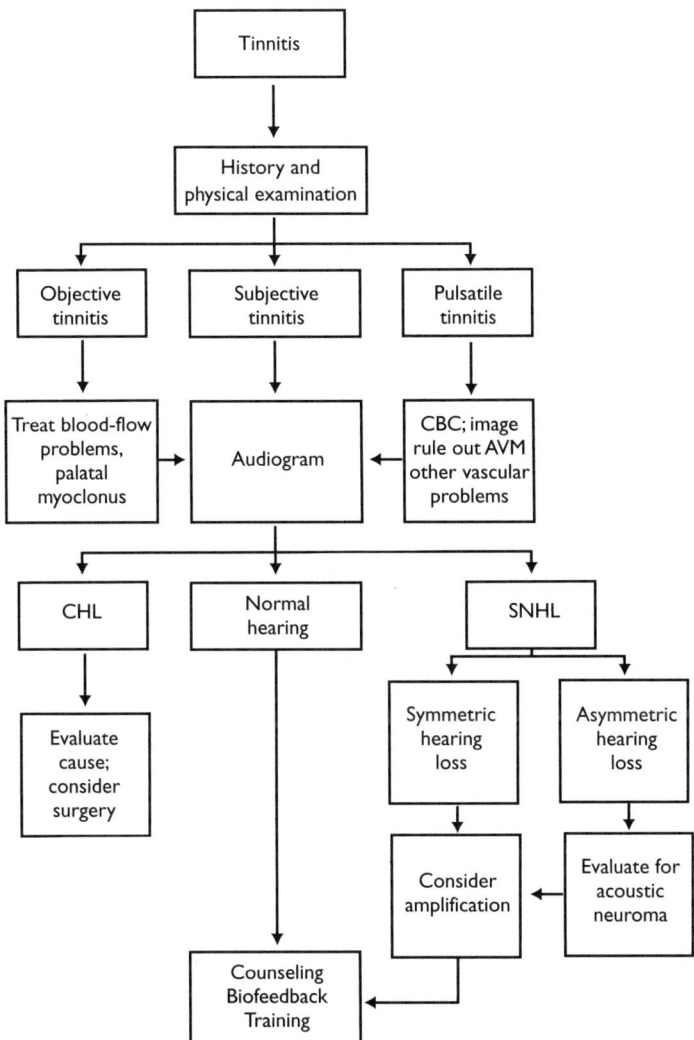

Algorithm Management of tinnitus. CHL = conductive hearing loss; SNHL = sensorineural hearing loss.

and sensorineural auditory noises (arising from structures within the auditory system [e.g., cochlea, cochlear nerve]).

Tinnitus of para-auditory origin is seen with vascular neoplasms, vascular malformations (e.g., acquired conditions such as carotid stenosis) palatal myoclonus, increased intracranial pressure (benign intracranial hypertension), and conductive hearing loss. The mechanism of tinnitus occurring with vascular disorders is thought to be mechanical energy from the increased blood flow or turbulence that is transmitted to the auditory system, which explains why this type of tinnitus is often pulsatile and changes with blood pressure. The rhythmic muscular contractions of palatal myoclonus can cause a clicking sound. Increased intracranial pressure allows transmission of pulses from Circle of Willis vessels to the cerebrospinal fluid and dural sinuses, resulting in pulsatile tinnitus. A conductive hearing loss is caused by imposing a physical change on the mechanical system of the outer or middle ear (e.g., cerumen impaction). Tinnitus results from attenuation of background sounds, making normally inaudible skull sounds audible.

Sensorineural tinnitus is associated most frequently with hearing loss, but the mechanism that causes this type of tinnitus is unknown. Theories include hyperactivity of hair cells or nerve fibers, cell injury, efferent cochlear neuron loss, or increased endolymphatic fluid pressure. Recent investigation suggests that, in some cases, the perception of sound may arise within the cochlear nucleus in the brainstem.

History

A thorough history is essential for evaluating a patient with tinnitus. Basic information includes age of onset, mode of progression, and precipitating events. The subjective history includes pitch, loudness, and location of tinnitus, although these correlate poorly with the underlying cause. Associated audiovestibular complaints (e.g., hearing loss, vertigo, aural fullness, otalgia, otorrhea) and a history of noise exposure or head trauma are also important. A dietary history can reveal heavy caffeine intake, the cessation of which may improve the tinnitus. Allergic and other forms of rhinosinusitis can contribute to eustachian tube dysfunction that worsens the patient's otologic symptoms.

The patient should be questioned about headaches, visual changes, focal neurological complaints, weight loss, possibility of pregnancy, symptoms of thyroid dysfunction, and depression (Case 7.1). Recent weight loss can be associated with a patulous eustachian tube, and the resultant transmission of pharyngeal sounds may be interpreted by the patient as a sound in the ear.

Tinnitus can interfere with sleep, work, and enjoyment of social situations. Tinnitus handicap questionnaires are available for evaluating the lifestyle effect of tinnitus. Certain medications, especially aspirin, can result in tinnitus; other drugs (e.g., aminoglycosides, antimalarials, loop diuretics) can cause hearing loss.

> **Case 7.1** **Elderly Man with Tinnitus Exacerbated by Depression**
>
> A male veteran 75 years of age complains of a constant, high-pitched "whine" that is gradually increasing in intensity. The noise increased only recently and is now keeping him awake at night. He is not aware of any hearing loss, but he does have some difficulty understanding conversational speech in noisy environments. He has hypertension, which is well controlled. He is a nonsmoker with no other known medical problems. He has had only minimal noise exposure since his combat experience in WWII. Review of systems was negative, but questioning revealed that he first began having difficulties with tinnitus keeping him awake when his wife of 52 years died 6 months previously.
>
> The physical examination is normal, with no evidence of bruits or other head and neck abnormalities. An audiogram reveals significant high-frequency hearing loss, with levels of 60 and 70 dB at 4000 Hz. Speech discrimination scores are 87% and 88%.
>
> The patient is thought to have tinnitus secondary to his hearing loss that was exacerbated by depression occurring after the loss of his wife. He is counseled about the relationship between tinnitus and hearing loss. An amplification trial is suggested, but he is not interested. However, he does agree to see a mental health professional for treatment of his suspected depression, and he responds well to counseling and a short course of mood-elevating medication.
>
> **Discussion**
>
> Sensorineural tinnitus is the most characteristic form of tinnitus encountered in the typical practice. The recent exacerbation associated with depression is common and often requires additional history to uncover. Most patients perceive that the tinnitus is the cause of sleeplessness, so the diagnosis of depression must be suspected by their physician. (Contributed by Dr. David Eibling.)

Other disease states can cause or be related to tinnitus, so past medical histories of the following may be useful: atherosclerotic carotid disease, hypertension, diabetes, thyroid dysfunction, anemia, otosclerosis, otitis media, Meniere's disease, presbycusis, multiple sclerosis, hyperlipidemia, neoplasms, and syphilis. Family history may reveal tinnitus associated with disease processes such as otosclerosis, neurofibromatosis, or familial hearing loss.

Physical Examination

The external ear and mastoid are inspected, palpated, and auscultated. Erythema, tenderness, audible sounds, and bruits are noted. The external canal is inspected with an otoscope for infection and obstruction due to cerumen, osteomas, tumors, or foreign bodies. Auscultation of the external canal may reveal objective tinnitus. This auscultation is easier to perform with a powered electronic stethoscope (Auscultear), although a regular stethoscope will suffice. Asking the patient to stop breathing during auscultation is helpful.

Pneumatic massage is used to assess tympanic membrane mobility, effusions, retractions, perforations, masses, infection, and other abnormalities. With mild eustachian tube dysfunction and minimal negative middle ear pressure, mobility of the tympanic membrane may be diminished. Asking the patient to autoinsufflate (i.e., "Hold your nose and pop your ears") often overcomes the mild eustachian tube dysfunction, returning the middle ear pressure and the tympanic membrane mobility to normal.

Tuning fork tests are performed to assess both conductive and sensorineural hearing loss. The oropharynx is evaluated, looking for palatal myoclonus or masses. The nose is inspected for masses or evidence of infection. The neck examination includes auscultation for bruits. When a bruit is found, carefully palpate for a thrill. Pulsatile tinnitus is compared with the patient's heart rate—a process that is simplified by asking the patient to mimic the sound while you palpate the pulse.

Gently applying pressure on the neck, being careful not to occlude the carotid, sometimes relieves tinnitus of venous origin. The neck is carefully palpated for any masses. Fundoscopic examination is performed to rule out evidence of increased intracranial pressure (as with benign intracranial hypertension). A complete **neurological examination** is performed with special attention to cranial nerves V, VI, VII, and VIII because they have an intimate relationship to the petrous bone within which reside the cochlea and the middle and external ear.

Differential Diagnosis

There are many classification systems for tinnitus, the most straightforward of which divides tinnitus into objective and subjective forms (Table 7.1). Objective tinnitus, which is audible to both patient and examiner, is uncommon but dramatic when encountered (Case 7.2). Sounds in this category are usually pulsating, rapid clicking, or blowing. Tinnitus noise is typically audible only to the patient, commonly occurs with intrinsic ear disease, and usually is described as ringing or buzzing. The causes of subjective tinnitus can be otologic (e.g., cerumen impaction, noise-induced hearing loss) (Case 7.3), pharmacologic (e.g., aspirin use), or metabolic (e.g., hyperlipidemia) (*see* Table 7.1).

Table 7.1 Objective and Subjective Causes of Tinnitus*

Objective Tinnitus	Subjective Tinnitus
Vascular Neoplasms	*Otologic Causes*
Glomus jugulare	Presbycusis
Glomus tympanicum	Noise-induced
Vascular Abnormalities	Cerumen impaction
Arteriovenous malformation	Middle ear effusion
Venous hums	Meniere's disease
Dehiscent jugular bulb	Otosclerosis
Hypertension	Neoplasm (e.g., acoustic neuroma)
Atherosclerotic carotid artery disease	Syphilis
Vascular loop	*Pharmacologic Causes*
High-riding carotid artery	Aspirin-containing drugs
Increased Intracranial Pressure	Aminoglycosides
Mechanical Abnormalities	Nonsteroidal anti-inflammatory drugs
Patulous eustachian tube	*Metabolic*
Palatal myoclonus	Hyper- or hypothyroid
TMJ problems	Hyperlipidemia
Multiple Sclerosis	*Depression*

TMJ = temporomandibular joint
*All forms of objective tinnitus can be included under the heading of subjective tinnitus.

Additional Diagnostic Evaluation

Investigating the causes of tinnitus using diagnostic tests can be focused by information from the history and physical examination. Audiologic evaluation is performed on all patients with tinnitus. This evaluation consists of pure-tone audiometry, speech audiometry (speech discrimination and speech-reception threshold), and impedance audiometry (tympanometry and acoustic reflex). Vestibular tests include electronystagmography, rotational studies, and posturography and are used when there is evidence of vestibular pathology in the initial work-up. With pulsatile tinnitus, a complete blood count may be warranted to rule out anemia as a contributing factor.

A variety of imaging modalities can be used to evaluate a tinnitus patient, depending on its suspected origin. Imaging is not required if the history and audiologic examination suggest uncomplicated hearing loss as the cause. High-resolution **computed tomography** of the head and temporal bone can be used to evaluate abnormal findings on physical examination. Contrast-enhanced magnetic resonance imaging of the cerebellopontile angle is helpful in excluding posterior cranial fossa tumors (e.g., acoustic neuroma). **Magnetic resonance angiography** allows visualization of vascular pathology. **Vascular studies** are indicated for the work-up of objective pulsatile tinnitus, including duplex carotid ultrasound, carotid angiography, and venography. **Electro-**

> **Case 7.2** **Woman with Objective Tinnitus Caused by an Arteriovenous Malformation**
>
> A woman 38 years of age complains of low-pitch, roaring tinnitus that is gradually increasing in intensity. The roaring fluctuates, is worse on the left side, and occasionally seems to be pulsatile. She has no history of noise exposure, familial hearing loss, associated medical problems, or dizziness. She denies otalgia, previous ear disease, and drainage. Physical examination is normal. An audiogram reveals a binaural, flat sensorineural hearing loss, with thresholds of 35 dB in her right ear and 45 dB in her left. Speech discrimination scores are 100% bilaterally.
>
> A hearing aid is fitted on her worse hearing ear. She returns 3 months later, stating that she can hear better with her aid but that the roaring has persisted. In fact, it is now so loud that her husband can hear it. Auscultation in her left ear canal and over her mastoid reveals a loud venous hum that changes in pitch with pressure of the stethoscope bell over the mastoid. Imaging shows an arteriovenous malformation (AVM) of the posterior fossa dura and temporal bone on the left, with a large draining mastoid emissary vein. She undergoes surgical excision of the dural AVM in a combined procedure with the otolaryngology and neurosurgery departments. Postoperatively, she has normal hearing and no longer requires the hearing aid.
>
> **Discussion**
>
> This case illustrates the importance of an adequate history and physical in the evaluation of tinnitus. In retrospect, this patient had been clearly describing a venous hum with a pulsatile component, yet auscultation of the skull was not performed at the initial examination. Moreover, the noise created by the venous flow resulted in "masking" of the presented sounds during the initial audiogram, leading to the false assumption that she was experiencing tinnitus due to hearing loss, when in fact she had normal hearing. (Contributed by Dr. David Eibling.)

physiologic tests, such as electromyography, are used to evaluate palatal myoclonus, and the auditory brainstem response test is used to evaluate cochlear nerve or brainstem function. Studies that are required less commonly include lumbar puncture to evaluate cerebrospinal fluid pressure (for disease processes such as benign intracranial hypertension) and allergy testing for food and environmental agents.

Management and Follow-Up

Treatment of tinnitus is difficult, and therapy is often frustrating for both patient and physician. Potentially curable causes of tinnitus are rare and include vascular anomalies, otosclerosis, otitis media, cerumen impaction, and neo-

> ### Case 7.3 Young Man with Tinnitus Caused by Noise-Induced Hearing Loss
>
> A man 22 years of age complains of high-pitched tinnitus that becomes worse at night, occasionally keeping him awake. He first noted the ringing several months ago and also has a periodic sensation of "blocked ears," worse on the left. He denies hearing loss, head trauma, or ear infection. He has no history of significant medical problems or familial hearing loss. However, he does have a history of significant noise exposure from recreational music and shooting. Furthermore, he works in a small, excessively noisy fabrication shop with stamping machines, grinders, and other equipment. He does not wear ear protection and notes occasional ear pain during shooting. He also notes that, when driving in his stereo-equipped car, he has to shout to be heard by his friends and that communication is all but impossible in the fabrication shop. In the past, he has noted tinnitus after exposure to noise, but it always ceased by the next day. Now, however, he notes that it is more or less continuously present and worse when in a quiet location. He states that his tinnitus recently became acutely louder when he was shooting his pistol next to a building that seemed to reflect the sound toward his left ear.
>
> Physical examination and an audiogram are normal, with the exception of a binaural dip in hearing thresholds at 4000 Hz to 25 dB on the right and to 40 dB on the left. Speech discrimination scores are normal. Auditory-evoked potentials are normal. He is counseled on the necessity to avoid loud noises and on the significance of hearing protection. The other three men working in the shop are contacted and advised to obtain a baseline audiogram and to use ear protection, both at work and when engaged in recreational activities. The employer was contacted and it was recommended that he enroll his employees in a hearing-conservation program.
>
> **Discussion**
>
> This young man has developed noise-induced hearing loss that is probably permanent. Although previous episodes of tinnitus most likely indicated temporary threshold shifts, the persistent nature of his tinnitus now suggests significant hair cell damage.
>
> The Occupational Health and Safety Act (OSHA) requires that all employees who work in a noise-hazardous area (defined as exposure to 85 dB averaged over 8 hours) must be enrolled in a formal hearing-conservation program. Unfortunately, not all businesses are required to comply with OSHA regulations, and it is not uncommon to find cases such as this. Education about the long-term sequelae of exposure to hazardous noise should be a part of patient wellness counseling. (Contributed by Dr. David Eibling.)

plasms. Unfortunately, most tinnitus falls into the "noncurable" category; thus, successful elimination of the symptom is elusive. Many therapies have been tried over the years, including masking, hearing aids, biofeedback, medical therapy, acupuncture, electrical stimulation, behavior modification, and surgery. None has had dramatic success.

The first and foremost treatment for tinnitus is reassurance. Once the patient has had a thorough medial evaluation that fails to reveal a specific cause for the tinnitus, the patient should be told that the tinnitus is unlikely to represent a tumor or life-endangering disease process. This is the most important aspect of managing most cases of tinnitus. Patients who are severely bothered by their tinnitus may become clinically depressed, and sleeplessness may be attributed to the tinnitus rather than to the depression. Recognizing and treating such depression is vital, but it may or may not affect the tinnitus. The management of tinnitus is outlined in the Algorithm.

Nonmedical therapy, including avoidance of loud noises, abstinence from drinking caffeinated beverages, cessation of smoking, and elimination of precipitating drugs (e.g., aspirin, nonsteroidal anti-inflammatory drugs, antimalarial agents), if possible. Other forms of therapy such as hypnotherapy, acupuncture, and yoga have shown limited success.

Masking is a technique of applying an external noise to the patient to "cover up" the tinnitus and make it inaudible. This can include simply setting the bedside clock radio between stations at night when the tinnitus is loudest (to compensate for the lack of natural masking by ambient external sounds) or using a combined hearing aid/masking unit. Masking devices provide relief for only 10% to 15% of patients. Hearing aids (with or without a masking unit) are an option for patients with associated hearing loss, because they amplify ambient noise, thereby masking the tinnitus.

Medical therapy has had limited success. The following drugs have been studied: nortriptyline, alprazolam, carbamazepine, lidocaine, procaine, tocainide, and various calcium-channel blockers. The overall evidence of tinnitus relief, however, is conflicting and limited. Lidocaine is one of the few drugs that has been proven to suppress tinnitus subjectively; however, it is limited by its short duration of action, intravenous-only route of administration (for this purpose), and potential side effects. Carbamazepine seems promising and is thought to act similarly to how it acts with trigeminal neuralgia; however, side effects and the lack of well-controlled studies have limited its use.

Biofeedback is used to approach tinnitus from a more psychological perspective. This therapy focuses on the patient's emotional reaction to tinnitus and assumes that stress plays an important role in its severity. Patients who benefit most from this type of therapy are those with the highest agitation levels due to their tinnitus. Relaxation techniques are key to this type of treatment. Self-monitoring of vital signs, body temperature, and electromyography are the most common forms of feedback. The goal in this form of therapy is not necessarily the elimination of tinnitus, but rather a better understanding and a mitigation of the factors related to the stress associated with tinnitus. Although there is no evidence from controlled studies that biofeedback works for tinnitus, some patients find it helpful. The usefulness of this modality is impaired by cost and by the fact it is not covered by medical insurance.

Habituation, one of the newest approaches to tinnitus, seems promising and involves directive counseling combined with low-level, broad-band noise produced by wearable generators. The directive counseling is designed to educate the patient about tinnitus and its possible causes. The background-noise generator facilitates habituation. According to the theory behind this therapy, masking is counterproductive because it prevents habituation. Reported results show a greater than 80% symptomatic improvement; however, habituation therapy has not been investigated under controlled experimental conditions and is not currently covered by third-party payers.

Surgery plays a role in some cases of tinnitus, such as that caused by cerebellopontile-angle lesions, neoplasms, vascular abnormalities, otosclerosis, infectious complications, and other causes of conductive hearing loss. Lumbar-peritoneal shunting can help with tinnitus that is caused by elevations in intracranial pressure resulting from benign intracranial hypertension. Tinnitus associated with Meniere's disease occasionally can be relieved by surgery. Surgery (e.g., cochlear implantation, cochlear nerve sectioning) has been studied in only a very small subset of patients.

Appropriate follow-up for patients with tinnitus depends on the underlying cause. A patient with an unremarkable examination and normal audiologic studies may be followed yearly with an annual audiogram if there are no further complaints. The patient with a defined underlying disease process, worsening symptoms, or severe lifestyle disruption should be followed more closely.

Danger Signs

Tinnitus is rarely an emergency; however, when it presents with a symptom that suggests intracranial pathology (e.g., unilateral vestibular weakness, focal neurologic deficits, severe headaches, visual changes, and profuse vomiting), emergent treatment is warranted. Tinnitus that is accompanied by uncontrolled ear infections, abnormalities on otoscopy, head and neck masses, bruits, thrills, or other suspicious lesions should prompt a thorough evaluation. Because tinnitus is relatively common, the primary danger is the temptation for the physician to skip to the work-up stage and proceed to patient reassurance. Every patient with persistent tinnitus deserves, at minimum, an accurate audiologic evaluation and, if interaural hearing asymmetry is present, an auditory brainstem response test and/or magnetic resonance imaging.

REFERENCES

1. **Jastreboff PJ, Gray WC, Gold SL.** Neurophysiologic approach to tinnitus patients. *Am J Otol.* 1996;17:236–40.
2. **Sismanis A, Starorn, MA, Sobel M.** Objective tinnitus in patients with atherosclerotic carotid artery disease. *Am J Otol.* 1994;15:404–7.
3. **Wiggs, WJ, Sismanis A, Laine FL.** Pulsatile tinnitus associated with congenital central nervous system malformations. *Am J Otol.* 1996;17:241–4.
4. **Ito J, Sakakihara J.** Tinnitus suppression by electrical stimulation of the cochlear wall and by cochlear implantation. *Laryngoscope.* 1994;104:752–4.
5. **Pulec JL.** Cochlear nerve section for intractable tinnitus. *Ear Nose Throat J.* 1995;74:468–76.
6. **Newman CW, Jacobson GP, Spitzer JB.** Development of the tinnitus handicap inventory. *Arch Otolaryngol Head Neck Surg.* 1996;122: 143–8.
7. **Jastreboff, PJ, Sasaki CT.** An animal model of tinnitus: a decade of development. *Am J Otol.* 1994;15:19–27.
8. **Sadlier M, Stephens SDG.** An approach to the audit of tinnitus management. *J Laryngol Otol.* 1995;109:826–9.
9. **Haginomori S, Makimoto K, Araki M, et al.** Effect of lidocaine injection on EOAE in patients with tinnitus. *Acta Otolaryngol.* 1995,115:488–92.
10. **Sismanis A, Smoker WRK.** Pulsatile tinnitus: recent advances in diagnosis. *Laryngoscope.* 1994;104:681–8.
11. **Mason J, Rogerson D.** Client-centered hypnotherapy for tinnitus: Who is likely to benefit? *Am J Clin Hypn.* 1995;37:294–9.
12. **Tyler RS, Babin RW.** Tinnitus. In Cummings CW, Fredrickson JM, Harker LA, et al. *Otolaryngology Head and Neck Surgery*, 2nd ed. St. Louis: CV Mosby; 1993:3031–53.
13. **Meyerhoff L, Cooper JC.** Tinnitus. In Paparella MM, Shumrick DA, Gluckman JL. *Otolaryngology.* Philadelphia: WB Saunders; 1991:1169–1179.

SUGGESTED READINGS

Jastreboff PJ, Gray WC, Gold SL. Neurophysiologic approach to tinnitus patients. *Am J Otol.* 1996;17:236–40.
This article reviews the neurophysiology of this symptom complex and discusses the physiology and mechanics of habituation treatment.

Merchant SN, Rauch SD, Nadol JB Jr. Meniere's disease. *Eur Arch Otorhinolaryngol.* 1995;52:63–75.
This article provides an up-to-date review of the vast literature about this often-puzzling disease. Details include the natural history, pathogenesis, diagnosis, and treatment.

Seidman MD, Jacobson GP. Update on tinnitus. *Otolaryngol Clin North Am.* 1996;29: 455–65.
This article gives a good basic overview of tinnitus and includes a thorough review of the varying origins of this subjective symptom, detailing approaches to treatment.

SECTION II

SINONASAL DISEASE

8

Nasal Obstruction

Eric F. Pinczower, MD

Nasal obstruction is common and often self-treated. The typical patient seeks a physician's advice only after home remedies and over-the-counter treatments have failed. Most patients have mild problems, such as upper respiratory infections, minor septal deviation, nasal valve collapse, or even an exaggerated normal nasal cycle. Some have more serious problems, such as allergic rhinitis, vasomotor rhinitis, nasal polyposis, major anatomical obstructions, benign neoplasms, or infections (e.g., sinusitis). Few patients have an aggressive neoplasm or infection. Early identification and treatment of these serious problems are essential to prevent considerable disfigurement or death.

The goal of this chapter is to present the internist with a systematic approach for diagnosing common causes of nasal obstruction and for recognizing the signs of aggressive or life-threatening infections or neoplasms.

Anatomy and Physiology

The anatomy of the nose and nasal cavities is extraordinarily complex and intimately involved with the structural anatomy of the face, skull base, cranial cavity, orbits, eyes, hard and soft palates, oral cavity, oropharynx, and nasopharynx. The nose's functions include olfaction, air filtration, and humidification, and it has an integral part in voice production as well. Normal nasal passages are narrow, with most of the space taken up by the turbinates and

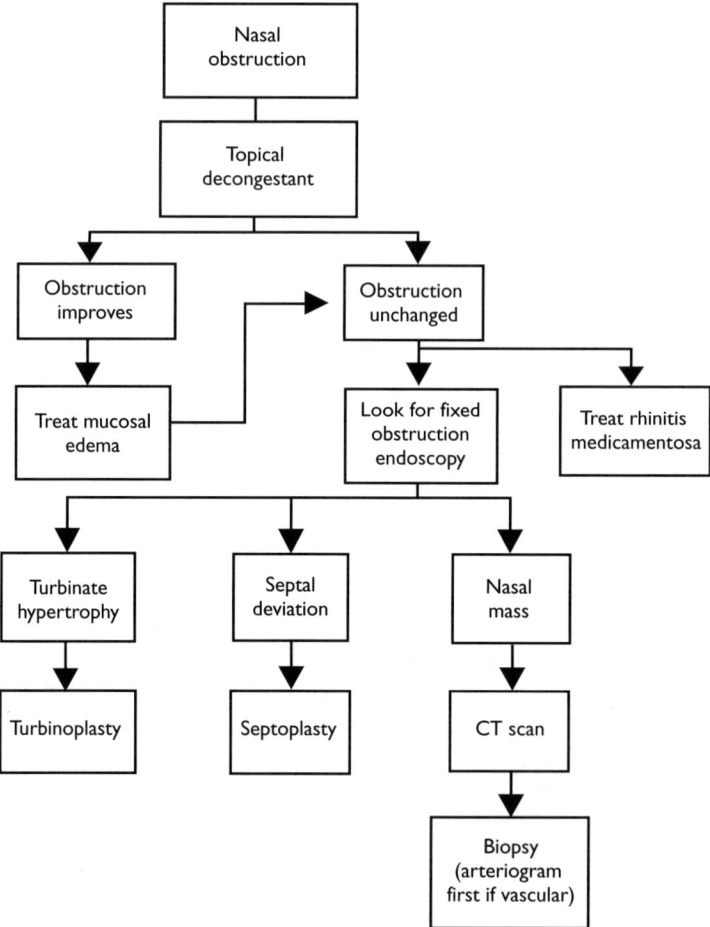

Algorithm Management of nasal obstruction. CT = computed tomography.

septum. This maximizes the filtration function and is important for the sensation of normal airflow. Abnormally patent passages give the sensation of nasal obstruction. Nasal airflow is probably not laminar in most cases, yet it is important that the nasal passage deliver enough resistance to provide a sensation of smooth airflow. In adults, the nose contributes two thirds of total airway resistance, most of which is in the anterior one third of the nose at the nasal valve.

The nasal valve is at the location of this smallest cross-sectional area in the nose, between the anterior nasal septum and the lower border of the upper lateral nasal cartilage. This is at the level of the anterior tip of the inferior turbinate. Obstruction in this area can be duplicated by gently pushing medially in the alar groove above the alar rim (Fig. 8.1). Septal deviations in this area, although subtle, may cause an obstruction that is noticeable to the patient. Similarly, a floppy or narrow valve also may be symptomatic.

Airflow through the nasal passages can be approximated by Poiseuille's law for laminar flow, which states that airflow resistance is inversely proportional to the fourth power of the radius. Thus, small changes in size can have huge differences in airflow.

The nasal airway is not static. Various physiologic and pathophysiologic events can change the cross-sectional area. The most dramatic of these events is turbinate engorgement, which occurs in most individuals on a 2- to 6-hour cycle, switching from left to right sides. The combined nasal cross-sectional area of the two sides remains essentially the same, so most people do not usually notice. This nasal cycle is thought to be important in maintaining a clean mucosal blanket. Frequently, patients can identify their own nasal cycles, but most are satisfied with reassurances that this is a normal phenomenon. Occasionally, the nasal cycle produces paradoxical nasal obstruction. For example, if a patient has a narrow left airway secondary to septal deviation, then he or she may notice obstruction only when the normal nasal cycle narrows the right side.

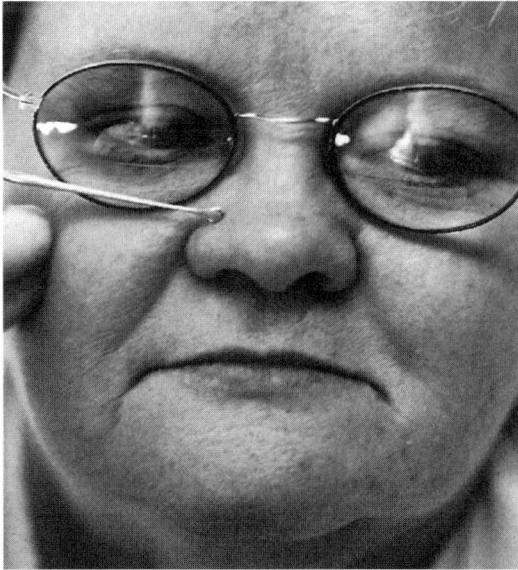

Figure 8.1 The examiner pushes inward on the alar groove. Inside this area is the nasal valve, typically the smallest cross-sectional area in the nose. (Courtesy of Dr. Karen H. Calhoun.)

Other causes of turbinate engorgement include rebound from vasoconstrictors (i.e., rhinitis medicamentosa) (Case 8.1), postural engorgement due to venous congestion while lying down, and inflammation and increased vascular permeability from irritants or an allergic response.

Nasal airflow can be measured accurately with rhinomanometry (Fig. 8.2). Patient complaints about obstruction need to be addressed regardless of the nasal airflow generated. Accurate measurement may be essential in medicolegal cases and when convincing patients with psychogenic obstruction that they do indeed have adequate airflow.

The nasal septum is usually straight with wide and narrow aspects that interdigitate with the turbinates' bulges and grooves. The airstream in a normal nose is approximately 1 to 3 mm wide, and 150 to 200 cm^2 of mucosal membrane is available to humidify and clean the airstream. The septum itself is divided into three parts: the anterior quadrilateral cartilage, the posterior bony vomer, and the superior perpendicular plate of the ethmoid (Fig. 8.3). Unless they are severe, posterior septal deviations do not cause symptomatic nasal obstruction.

The lateral nasal wall is an astonishingly complex structure that contains the openings into the paranasal sinuses, including the ethmoid and maxillary sinuses. The lateral nasal wall houses the turbinates and their mucosal coverings and even the nasolacrimal apparatus that drains tears from the eye (Fig. 8.4). The nasolacrimal duct drains out of the lateral nasal wall beneath the in-

Case 8.1 Man with Rhinitis Medicamentosa

A man 34 years of age complains of worsening nasal obstruction that is present most of the time. No medication seems to help. The rest of his history is unremarkable; specifically, there is no history of allergic-type symptoms or epistaxis.

Physical examination reveals beefy red mucosa that fails to respond to decongestant spray. Further questioning elicits a reluctant admission of the use of an over-the-counter topical vasoconstrictor, which he began using during a severe upper respiratory infection approximately 8 months ago. He has had no history of nasal obstruction before that.

The patient is educated on the process of rhinitis medicamentosa. He is assured that stopping the nasal spray use is necessary but worries about how he will be able to breathe, especially at night. He is given prescriptions for a nasal steroid spray, oral decongestant, and Medrol Dosepak.

On a return visit in 2 weeks, the patient has stopped using the topical vasoconstrictor successfully. Six weeks later, his nasal obstruction is resolved completely, even after cessation of his topical nasal steroid spray and oral decongestant.

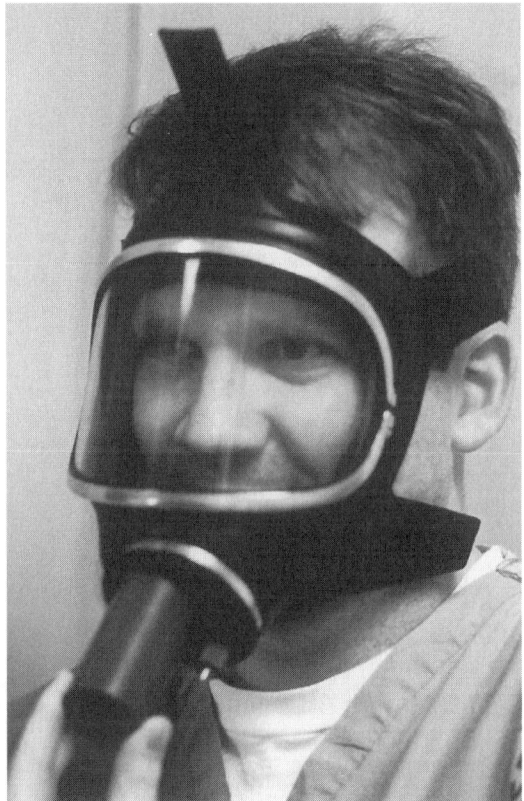

Figure 8.2 Patient with mask in place for anterior rhinomanometry. The pressure transducer is placed in one nostril, and airflow is detected from air movement through the other nostril only. (Courtesy of Dr. Karen H. Calhoun.)

ferior turbinate. Tears draining through this duct can cause irritation, contributing to mucosal edema and nasal obstruction.

As mentioned previously, turbinates and their hypertrophy are a potential source of nasal obstruction. The inferior turbinate is based solely on the lateral nasal wall, whereas the middle and superior turbinates are formed at least partially from the superior part of the nasal cavity, hanging down from the skull base. Hypertrophy or swelling of the inferior turbinate is the most likely source of inflammatory or allergic obstruction because it most directly affects the valve area.

Turbinate turgidity is guided partially by parasympathetic/sympathetic tone. The "fight or flight" response opens the nasal passages. Vasomotor rhinitis is thought to be at least partially caused by a preponderance of

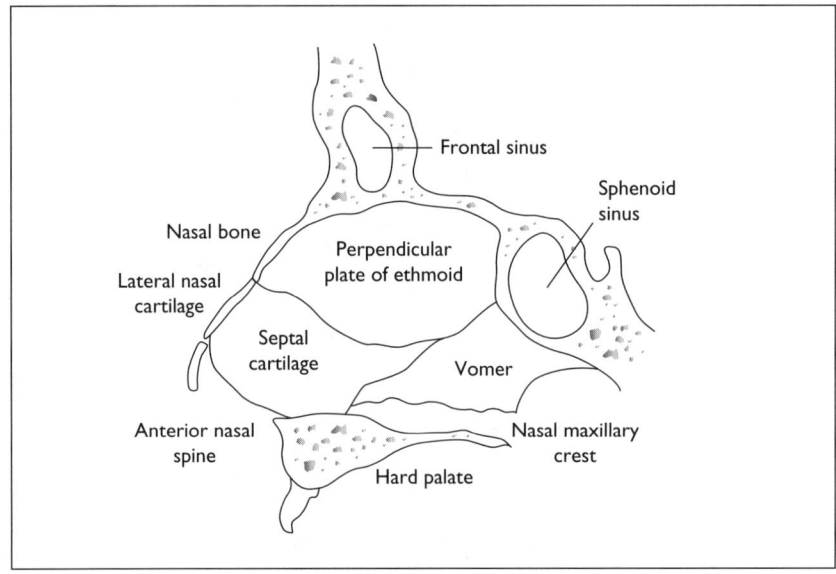

Figure 8.3 The three different parts of the septum (lateral view).

parasympathetic tone. Hypothyroidism also causes nasal congestion via a predominate effect on parasympathetic tone. Other common hormonal causes of obstruction are estrogen related; hence, premenstrual and pregnant women may complain of nasal congestion. Estrogen-containing oral contraceptives also may cause nasal obstruction.

History

From the history alone, one can gain much important diagnostic information about the cause of nasal obstruction. (Causes of nasal obstruction are listed in Table 8.1.) Age of presentation, duration of the complaint, systemic symptoms, and provoking factors are frequently enough to narrow the differential diagnosis immediately. For example, a patient who has nasal obstruction, itchy eyes, and asthma when exposed to cats is easily identified as suffering from allergic rhinitis. Similarly, it is often easy to identify patients with upper respiratory infections, vasomotor rhinitis, and rhinitis medicamentosa from history alone. Patients are questioned about allergic triggers; previous surgery; trauma; use of nasal sprays, cocaine, or other intranasal drugs; and the presence of epistaxis or drainage. Patients with nasal obstruction also may complain of snoring. The single most important historical factor that suggests

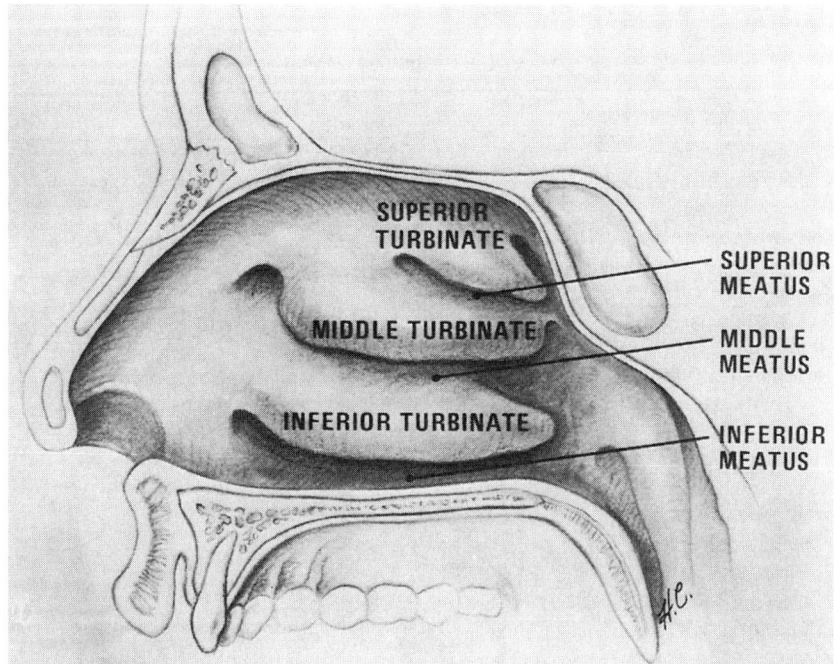

Figure 8.4 Lateral nasal wall. The major landmarks of this anatomically complex area are shown. (Republished with permission from Goode RL. *Diagnosis and Treatment of Turbinate Dysfunction SiPac.* Alexandria, VA: American Academy of Otolaryngology Head and Neck Surgery; 1996.)

a potentially dangerous nasal obstructive disorder is laterality. A patient with a nasal obstruction that changes from side to side over a 1- to 6-hour period is probably just identifying his or her own nasal cycle. Bilateral obstruction usually implies systemic or inflammatory disease, although bilateral symptoms also can occur with large nasopharyngeal or nasal cavity growths. However, unilateral obstruction (especially when progressive) should alert the physician to the possibility of neoplasm. The most common presenting sign of nasal or ethmoidal neoplasm is unilateral nasal obstruction with or without drainage. Occupational risk factors for sinonasal neoplasms include woodworking, radiation exposure, and heavy-metal exposure (especially nickel).

Symptoms and signs that indicate the process has escaped the confines of the nasal cavity are especially concerning and should alert the physician to the possibility of an aggressive disease process. These include proptosis, cheek swelling, palate distortion, dental loss, cranial neuropathies (especially fifth-nerve symptoms), and ocular motility disturbances. Anosmia is usually secondary to obstruction but may imply an intracranial or skull-base neoplasm with direct involvement of the first cranial nerve or its tract (*see* Chapter 33).

Table 8.1 Causes of Nasal Obstruction

Causes	Special Features
Traumatic	
Nasal fracture	Swelling, deviation
Nasal septal fractures	Sharp edges
Nasal septal hematoma	Massive purplish swelling; must be recognized and treated promptly
Inflammatory	
Viral upper respiratory illness	Short onset
Allergic rhinitis	Itchy eyes and nose, bluish turbinates
Vasomotor rhinitis	Cold induced
Rhinitis medicamentosa	Vasoconstrictor abuse
Rhinosinusitis (bacterial)	Pus
Wegener's granulomatosis	Associated pulmonary and otologic findings; high levels of angiotensin-converting enzyme
Neoplastic	
Benign	
Nasal polyps	Usually bilateral
Fibromas	Usually unilateral
Papilloma	Usually unilateral
Infectious papilloma	Usually unilateral
Juvenile nasopharyngeal angiofibroma	Unilateral; found in adolescent boys; epistaxis
Malignant	
Squamous cell cancer	New onset, unilateral; pain; cranial nerve palsies
Adenocarcinoma	New onset, unilateral
Melanoma	New onset, unilateral
Lymphoma	New onset, unilateral
Esthesioneuroblastoma	New onset, unilateral
Other	
Psychogenic	Diagnosis of exclusion
Foreign body	Found in pediatric or cognitively impaired patients
Crying	Unrecognized depression
Non-airflow states	Such states include long-term intubation, tracheostomy, and laryngectomy

Epistaxis and pain also are symptoms that warrant concern. In contrast to the previous example of the patient with nasal allergies, consider the possibility of juvenile nasopharyngeal angiofibroma in young men with progressive unilateral obstruction and epistaxis or with slowly progressive bilateral nasal obstruction (Case 8.2) (*see* Chapter 14).

Other important points when taking a history include facial irradiation, trauma, and dysthesias; possible foreign body; and the rate of progression of any of these complaints.

> **Case 8.2 Young Man with Juvenile Nasopharyngeal Angiofibroma**
>
> A man 19 years of age presents with left-sided nasal obstruction and epistaxis of several years' duration. He is referred to you by a colleague who noted an intranasal mass on the left. The referring physician attempted a biopsy of the mass in his office, resulting in such severe hemorrhaging that it was controlled only by placing an anterior and posterior pack, which have since been removed. The patient is otherwise healthy.
>
> Nasal endoscopy shows a posterior left-sided mass, covered in smooth reddish mucosa. Flexible endoscopy through the right nostril reveals that the mass is protruding into the nasopharynx. Because of the patient's age, gender, and previous history, you suspect a vascular lesion, probably a juvenile nasopharyngeal angiofibroma. CT and MRI scans show a small vascular tumor confined to the nose and nasopharynx. The treatment options are presented to the patient and his parents. They decide on surgery, with a preceding arteriography and embolization.
>
> On the day before the planned surgery, the neuroradiologist performs arteriography and embolization. The next day, via a combined transnasal/transoral approach, the tumor is removed completely, with a total blood loss of only 600 cm^3. The patient makes an uneventful recovery.

One also should bear in mind that nasal obstruction is a sensation that may or may not correlate with a narrowed airway or a limitation in nasal airflow. In fact, patients with overly patent airways often complain of nasal obstruction. This complaint is common in patients with atrophic rhinitis, large nasoseptal perforations, or after overzealous turbinate-reduction surgery.

Physical Examination

Simple observation of the patient can provide valuable information. Allergic shiners, bluish infraorbital swelling, mouth breathing, posttraumatic deformities, extraocular motion defects, and facial asymmetry all can provide clues. Intraoral examination may demonstrate loose teeth or deformity from tumors. Trismus (i.e., the inability to open the mouth widely) may imply tumor extension into the masticator muscles. A complete head and neck neurological examination must be performed when an invasive process is suspected, because nasal and paranasal tumors often spread to cranial nerves at the skull base. Facial swelling, proptosis, and trismus imply extension of the process into the face, orbit, and pterygoid musculature, respectively.

If the patient does not have an obvious source of nasal obstruction, (e.g., obvious nasal allergies that respond to treatment, nasal upper respiratory infection that resolves with time, elimination of symptoms after foreign-body removal) a complete head and neck examination is necessary to evaluate nasal obstruction.

Because anterior rhinoscopy is the most important and probably the most difficult element of the examination, the technique of performing it should be practiced. The patient should be positioned at the same height as the examiner. A coaxial light source (e.g., head mirror, headlight) should be focused properly in the patient's nose. If a light source is unavailable, an otologic speculum may be used to examine the nasal cavity. The speculum should be held in the examiner's nondominant hand, with the dominant hand used to control the patient's head or kept free to use other instruments as necessary. Patients need to be examined both before and after administration of a topical vasoconstrictor, such as phenylephrine or oxymetazoline. Because of the potential cardiovascular effects, these agents should be used with caution. Persistent engorgement of the inferior turbinate after application of a vasoconstrictor is often indicative of permanent turbinate hypertrophy. Accordingly, a patient with such a disorder may benefit from turbinate surgery.

With anterior rhinoscopy, one should be able to evaluate for septal deviation, turbinate hypertrophy, or obvious changes in the mucosa (Fig. 8.5). Pus or necrotic tissue may be evident, and nasal masses may be seen. The middle meatus is the most common location for both nasal polyps and neoplasms, so location alone is not diagnostic. With a unilateral mass, a firm diagnosis is needed before instituting management. With bilateral disease and an appropriate history of allergy or sinusitis, one can make the diagnosis of polyposis safely. If these polyps do not respond promptly to medical treatment (usually with nasal or oral steroids), then a biopsy may be required to rule out neoplasms (Case 8.3). Surgery may be indicated in cases in which the nasal obstruction is bothersome to the patient or causes chronic or acute sinusitis. Very pale or necrotic mucosa in immunocompromised or diabetic individuals may be secondary to invasive fungal disease from aspergillosis or mucormycosis. Immediate surgical intervention may be required to prevent significant morbidity or death. In immunocompetent hosts, allergic fungal sinusitis may be present. Surgical debridement may be required to alleviate symptoms.

Rhinomanometry is a diagnostic tool that some physicians use in their clinical practices to evaluate nasal obstruction. Rhinomanometry determines nasal passageway resistance by measuring nasopharyngeal pressure and nasal airflow rates. In adults, the nose contributes two thirds of total airway resistance. With rhinomanometry, the resistive areas are defined accurately. This resistance is then divided into three areas: 1) the vestibule,

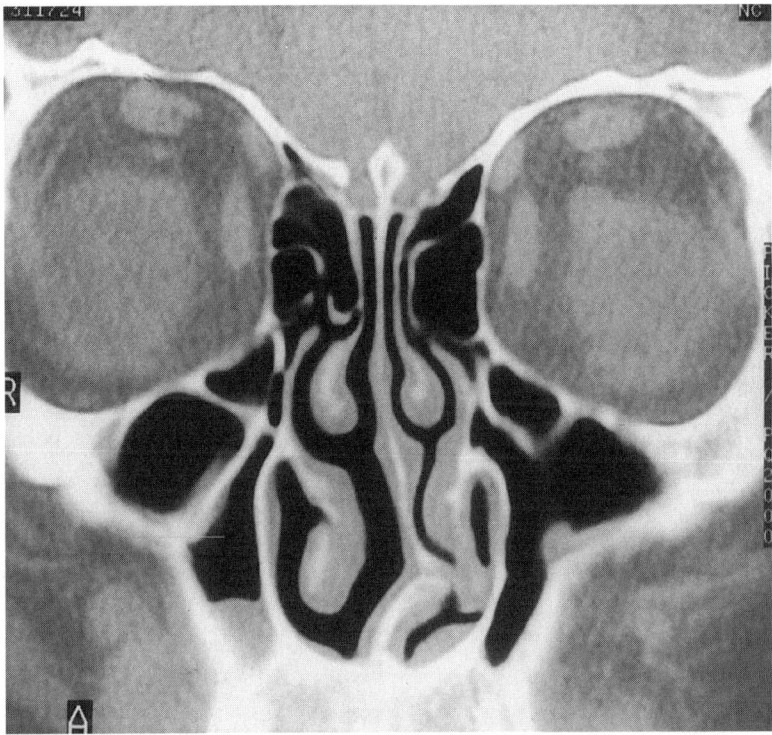

Figure 8.5 Coronal computed tomography showing a very deviated septum. The inferior turbinate on the side away from the deviation is moderately hypertrophied.

which contributes approximately one third of the resistance (primarily on inspiration); 2) the valve, which is the major resistive area; and 3) the passage itself, which has minimal effects. Most nasal resistance occurs with the valve where the anterior tip of the inferior turbinate approaches the septum. For this reason, patients with septal deviations, anterior turbinate hypertrophy, or nasal valve collapse all can have significant obstruction. The Cottle test of gently tugging on the cheek laterally next to the nasal valve frequently relives nasal obstruction and indicates the nasal valve area as the likely source of nasal obstruction.

Additional Diagnostic Evaluation

Because nasal obstruction usually is caused by the physical obstruction of the nasal airway, it is important to evaluate the entire nasal airway fully.

> **Case 8.3** **Woman with Nasal Obstruction Caused by Polyps**
>
> A woman 43 years of age presents with anosmia and nasal obstruction. The symptoms have been present for several years but seem worse recently. She has a slightly hyponasal voice. She has been tried on various allergy medications, without significant relief of symptoms. She is otherwise healthy and takes no other medications.
>
> On nasal endoscopy, both nasal cavities are found to be filled with pale gray glistening polyps, leaving only a small airway along the nasal floor. CT scan shows some mucoperiosteal thickening in her maxillary and anterior ethmoid sinuses but no opacification or other abnormalities. University of Pennsylvania Smell Identification Test (a scratch-and-sniff test with a closed-set, forced-choice format) reveals minimal ability to identify odors.
>
> A 2-month trial on topical nasal steroids yields minimal improvement. You discuss further treatment options with the patient, including oral steroids (and the usually temporary nature of the improvement with these) and surgery. The patient decides on surgery.
>
> After an uneventful nasal polypectomy, her nasal obstruction and sense of smell are much improved.

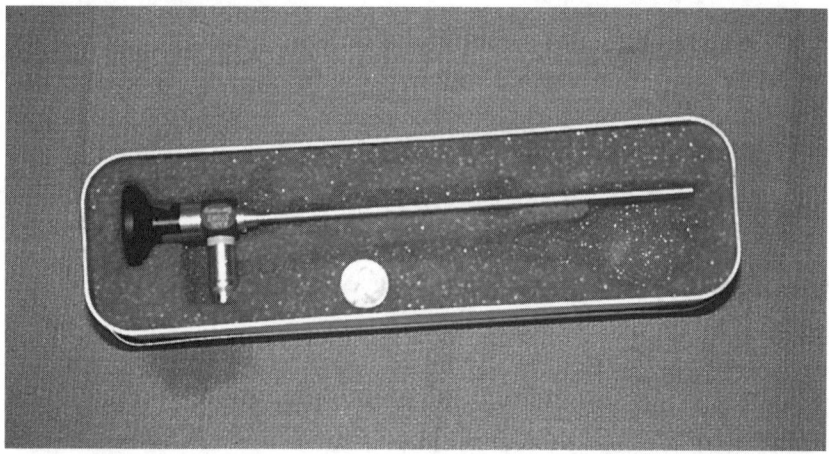

Figure 8.6 The type of nasal endoscope commonly used in office settings.

Rigid nasal endoscopy provides a clear view of the entire nasal cavity and nasopharynx (Fig. 8.6); however, it cannot reveal submucosal masses or lesions within the maxillary or ethmoid sinuses. Computed tomography (CT) is usually the radiologic study of choice. For the evaluation of sinonasal disease, coronal CT scans are most helpful because they clearly demonstrate the relationship of sinonasal pathology to the sinus base and the orbits; they also clearly demonstrate bony erosion versus remolding with erosion as the likely sign of malignant sinonasal disease (Fig. 8.7). Axial CT scanning is helpful in the evaluation of the nasopharynx. Patients with serous otitis, nasal obstruction, epistaxis, neck mass, or any combination of these may have nasopharyngeal cancer and need both a mucosal (endoscopy) and submucosal (CT scanning) evaluation (Fig. 8.8). Any patient with new onset of unilateral obstruction, epistaxis, or pain should be suspected of having a paranasal neoplasm until proven otherwise. In addition, coronal imaging should be considered before the biopsy of any lesion from the high nasal cavity or middle meatus to prevent inadvertent injury to an encephalocele.

Magnetic resonance imaging (MRI) usually is reserved for patients with known sinonasal tumors. The MRI scan is useful for treatment planning because it can accurately discriminate between a tumor and postobstructive inflammatory disease (i.e., sinusitis) secondary to a tumor.

All unilateral nasal masses require biopsy, whereas bilateral nasal polyposis—if it rapidly responds to treatment—does not. Most patients with nasal masses (other than obvious small papillomas) should undergo CT before

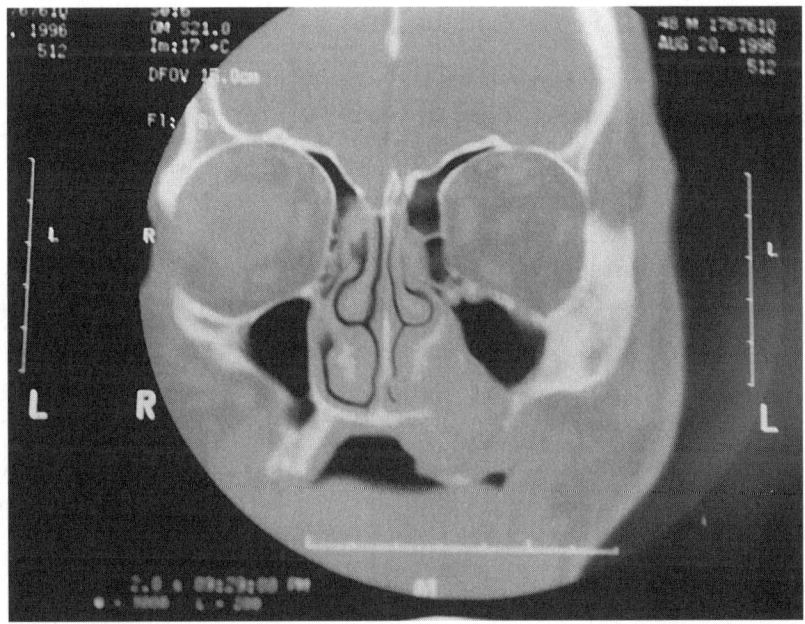

Figure 8.7 Coronal computed tomography scan showing a mass (squamous cell carcinoma) eroding the floor of the left maxillary sinus. (Courtesy of Dr. Christopher Rassekh.)

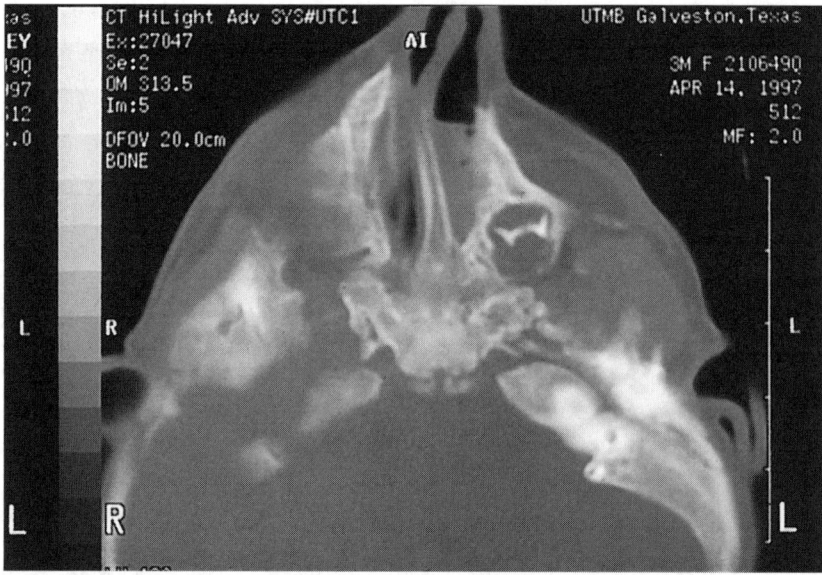

Figure 8.8 Axial computed tomography scan showing choanal atresia (i.e., failure of development of the posterior nasal aperture). This congenital condition usually is diagnosed in early childhood; however, occasionally, a unilateral case is not diagnosed until adulthood.

biopsy. Because one of the possible diagnoses is juvenile nasal angiofibroma (the biopsy of which can result in the rapid loss of a liter or more of blood), it is recommended that one determine whether the mass has characteristics that suggest intense vascularity before any biopsy is performed. A mass that appears vascular may need to undergo arteriography before biopsy. The biopsy of such masses usually is performed in the operating room.

Management and Follow-Up

The management and follow-up of nasal obstruction depends on the underlying diagnosis. The source of acute obstruction always must be identified if it does not resolve spontaneously. For example, chronic obstruction is less worrisome if it is not progressive. No patient complaint of nasal obstruction should be dismissed as being psychogenic without at least a full nasal endoscopy and CT scan, because the consequences of a missed early sinonasal neoplasm are tragic. The management of nasal obstruction is summarized in Table 8.2 and in the Algorithm.

Table 8.2 Management of Nasal Obstruction

Etiologic Disorder	Management
Traumatic disruption	
Acute	Surgical reduction
Chronic	Surgical reconstruction
Allergic rhinitis	Steroid nasal spray, sodium chromo? spray, H_1-selective blockers, systemic desensitization, turbinate surgery
Vasomotor rhinitis	Turbinate reduction, parasympathetic blockade (topically)
Rhinitis medicamentosa	Discontinuation of topical decongestant, topical steroid spray, Medrol Dosepak
Neoplasm	
Benign	Surgical resection
Malignant	Surgical resection with radiation therapy
Foreign body	Surgical removal

Danger Signs

The danger signs in patients who complain of nasal obstruction relate primarily to the signs and symptoms of neoplasms, including persistent anosmia, serous otitis, neck mass, repeated epistaxis, unilateral nasal obstruction, proptosis, cheek swelling, trismus, palate distortion, dental loss, and cranial neuropathies. The presence of any of these symptoms suggests that an imaging study (usually a CT scan) could be helpful in ruling out or detecting a sinonasal neoplasm.

Summary

Nasal obstruction is a frequent complaint among patients seen by internists. Although most of these patients have minor problems, the rare patient will have an extremely serious disease that requires prompt recognition and treatment. A high index of suspicion must be maintained, and no patient should be dismissed without a firm diagnosis or a complete work-up, including nasal endoscopy and CT scanning.

SUGGESTED READINGS

Blokmanis A. Endoscopic diagnosis, treatment, and follow-up of tumours of the nose and sinuses. *J Otolaryngol.* 1994;23:366–9.
    This article discusses the diagnosis and treatment of nasal tumors in the era of endoscopic nasal surgery. These techniques are particularly useful for benign tumors. Their use for malignant tumors is more limited, but diagnostic mapping and biopsies are possible.

Graf P, Hallen H, Juto JE. The pathophysiology and treatment of rhinitis medicamentosa. *Clin Otolaryngol.* 1995;20:224–9.

Discontinuing topical vasoconstrictors and beginning topical steroid sprays led to the resolution of the abnormal mucosal reactivity of rhinitis medicamentosa over 6 weeks.

Grymer LF, Illum P, Hilberg O. Bilateral inferior turbinoplasty in chronic nasal obstruction. *Rhinology.* 1996;34:50–3.

Patients with nasal obstruction and inferior turbinate hypertrophy were treated with surgical turbinoplasty. Over 90% of the patients experienced subjective symptom improvement. Objective measurements documented improvements in minimum cross-sectional area.

Jacobsen MH, Larsen SK, Kirkegaard J, Hansen HS. Cancer of the nasal cavity and paranasal sinuses: prognosis and outcome of treatment. *Acta Oncologica.* 1997;36:27–31.

This article details extensive experience with sinonasal cancers, including presenting symptoms, diagnosis, evaluation, treatment, and long-term follow-up. The overall 5-year local control rate was 48%.

9

Allergic Conditions of the Ear, Nose, and Throat

Richard L. Mabry, MD

Disorders of the ear, nose, and throat are commonly encountered by practitioners in virtually all fields of medicine. Allergy can contribute significantly to many of these disorders. Thus, it is wise for the non-otolaryngologist to have at least a passing knowledge of otolaryngic allergy. What follows is an overview of the subject. (For further details, readers may consult texts that deal more fully with the subject [1,2].)

Diagnosis of Allergy

History and Physical Examination

It has been said that the diagnosis of allergy is made primarily by history; this is mostly correct. The development of symptoms (detailed below in the sections on specific allergies) during specific seasons and/or circumstances suggests the presence of allergy. Physical examination findings may further support this presumptive diagnosis. The role of allergy "tests" is to determine the presence or absence of allergen-specific immunoglobulin E (IgE) for the suspected antigens. However, **to be significant, even a positive allergy test must correlate with symptom production when exposed to the antigen**. Otherwise, what the patient has is a positive test, not a clinically significant allergy.

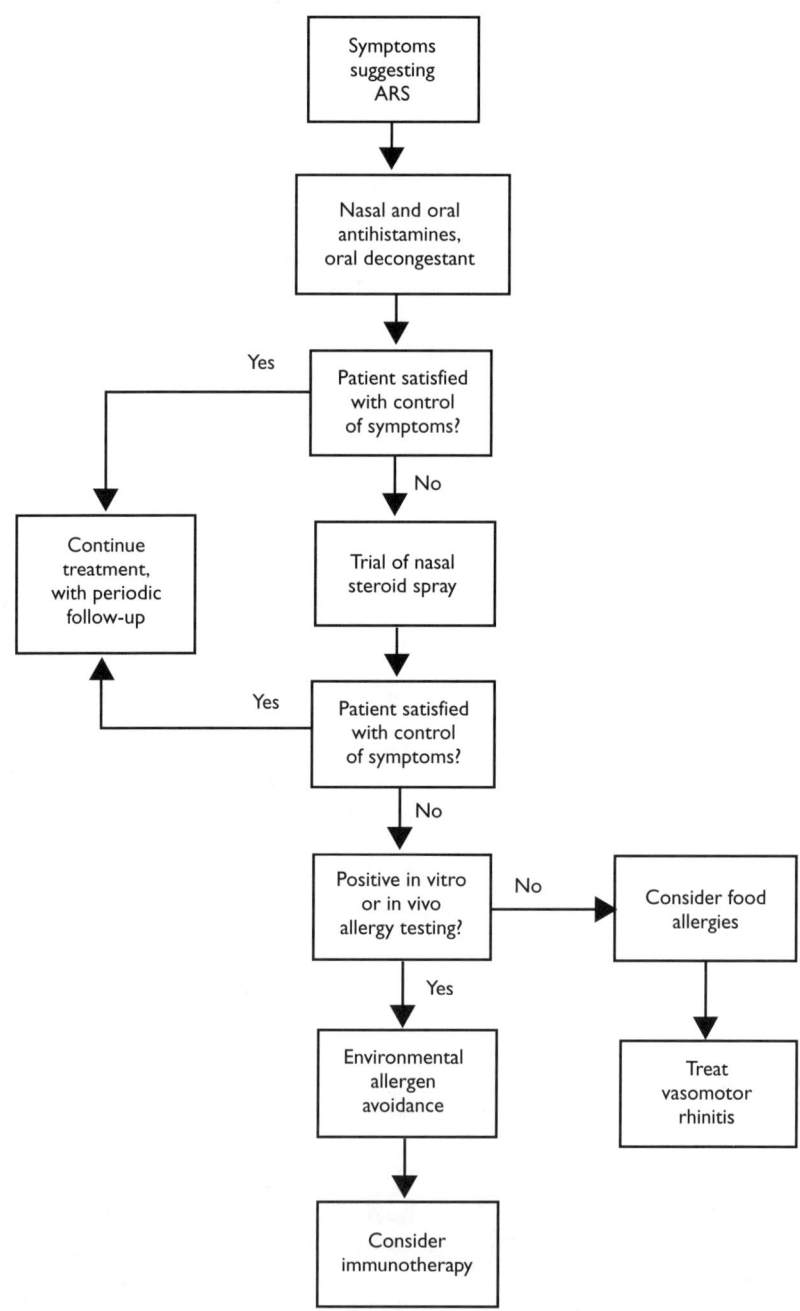

Algorithm Management of allergic rhinitis. ARS = allergic rhinosinusitis.

Determination of Specific Triggers

Allergy testing is based on the role of the IgE allergic reaction, which is specific and unique for every allergen. The presence of IgE may be demonstrated in three ways: **direct mucosal challenge**, **skin testing** (in vivo), and **direct assay from a blood sample** (in vitro).

Mucosal challenge testing is a useful research tool for studying patients with allergy, but it has no significant clinical applicability and, thus, is not discussed here.

Skin testing has been the benchmark of allergy testing for almost a century. Numerous methods of skin testing have been described over the years. These differ primarily in the technique used to deposit the antigenic material and in the depth at which it is placed.

Scratch testing, in which the skin is scarified after the application of a drop or two of antigen, has been found to be less accurate and reproducible than other methods and, hence, is no longer recommended (3).

The technique of **prick testing** was first described by Lewis and Grant (4) in 1926, and it is still in common use today. Although there are now several variations, in each one the skin is pricked superficially with a sharp instrument. Antigen may be placed on the puncture site, or the prick may be made through a drop of antigen. The test is read after 15 to 20 minutes, noting both the **wheal** (induration) and **flare** (redness) produced. These results are compared with those of positive and negative controls administered at the same time. Numerous modifications have provided different pricking instruments, including multipronged devices. The results of the prick test are reported on a scale of 0 to 4+. Unfortunately, there is as yet no uniformity in designating a single method for reading and reporting the results of this test.

In **intradermal testing**, antigen contained in a special 0.5- or 1.0-cm^3 syringe with attached bevel needle is injected into the outermost layer of the skin to produce a well-defined wheal. As with prick testing, the reaction produced is read after 15 to 20 minutes. The wheal size is noted (in some techniques, the flare also is measured) and compared with those produced by positive and negative controls.

Intradermal skin tests generally are considered to be more sensitive than skin prick tests, but they also carry a greater risk of producing a systemic reaction by introducing a greater amount of antigen (5). For this reason, single-dilution intradermal tests are not performed unless a screening prick test for that same antigen has been negative. Another approach is to perform **sequential intradermal tests** at varying antigen concentrations, beginning with an anticipated nonreacting strength and proceeding with higher strengths until reaching a concentration that produces a positive reaction (the "end point of reactivity") (Fig. 9.1). This means of titration, called **dilutional intradermal**

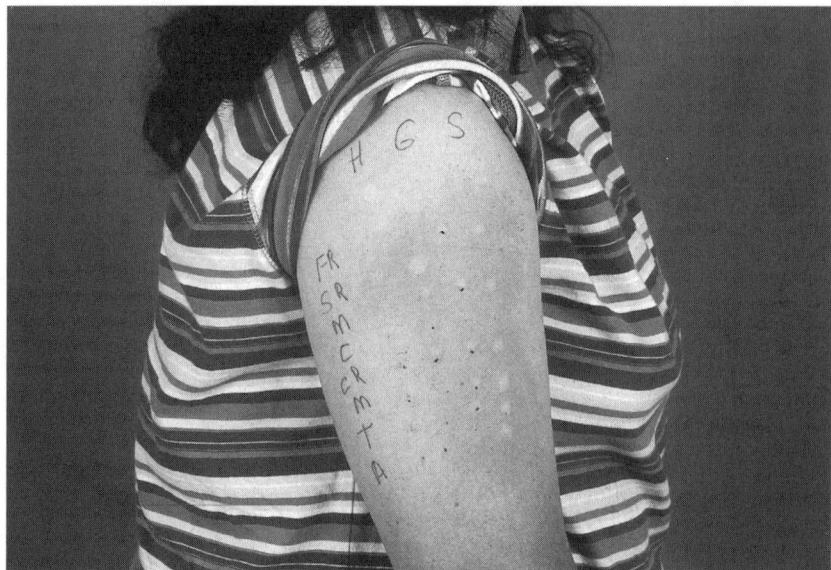

Figure 9.1 Arm showing serial end point titration testing in a very reactive patient.

testing, safely provides a determination of the exact degree of sensitivity to each antigen. It is the method of choice for most otolaryngic allergists.

Unfortunately, skin tests are affected by a number of factors, including antihistamines, tricyclic antidepressants, skin reactivity, concomitant antigen exposure, and local axonal reflexes (6). In addition, although skin testing generally is not painful, patients often are fearful of the discomfort associated with the tests. These factors have contributed to the increasing popularity of in vitro test methods.

In Vitro Testing

Although skin testing has been the benchmark for evaluating patients with inhalant allergy for almost a century, both patients and physicians have continued to seek a more accurate and comfortable method. Shortly after the characterization of IgE in 1967, Wide and coworkers (7) developed a radioimmunoassay for the detection of specific IgE antibodies in the serum. This assay was given the name **radioallergosorbent test (RAST)**. Subsequent modifications of the test, using enzymatic and other nonradioisotope markers, have been designated **enzyme-linked immunosorbent (ELISA) tests**. It was initially thought that a measurement of the total amount of IgE in the serum of a patient might provide a means of identifying allergic individuals. However, this has not been proven to be the case. Except in some rare patients, the total IgE level is rarely helpful in clinical medicine.

Assays of **allergen-specific IgE**, however, are quite specific, providing information about not only the allergens to which a patient is sensitive but also the degree of sensitivity that exists. It is possible to assess a patient's inhalant allergy status accurately by a RAST or ELISA determination of 10 to 15 significant antigens.

The **allergy dipstick test** is a simple screening test based on ELISA technology. These dipsticks, containing key inhalant allergens for the geographical area in question, are allowed to react with patient serum and various chemicals. The resulting degree of color indicates the relative amount of allergen-specific IgE in the serum. However, two caveats are necessary when using allergy dipstick tests: 1) under the terms of the Clinical Laboratory Improvement Act, they are considered "moderately complex tests," and the office using them must comply with the necessary federal requirements; and 2) although the tests are helpful for diagnosis and in planning appropriate environmental control, they may not be used as the basis for specific immunotherapy.

Other screening tests make use of several antigens bound to a common carrier (e.g., paper disc, well). This allows for a number of antigens to be assessed with a single test and, if negative, avoids the need for numerous single-antigen tests. However, if one of these screening tests is positive, specific antigens must then be assayed.

Quantitative determinations for allergen-specific IgE by either RAST or ELISA methodology now are used extensively in the diagnosis and treatment of inhalant allergy. These tests correlate well with dilutional intradermal testing and may be used as the basis for immunotherapy (9).

Ironically, the very simplicity that makes in vitro testing so popular has become a potential drawback of its use. In the past, some reference laboratories have offered the service of preparing and sending immunotherapy vials from in vitro reports to physicians for administration. This "remote practice of allergy" has been decried by all of the major organizations that represent general and otolaryngic allergy. Whether the confirmation of offending antigens is performed by either skin or blood tests, the decision as to whether it represents true allergy must be made by correlating the patient's physical findings and symptoms with the test results—a determination that requires the judgment of a physician in a face-to-face encounter with the patient.

Manifestations of Otolaryngic Allergy

External Ear

The most common allergic manifestation involving the external ear is **contact dermatitis** (Fig. 9.2). Patients who wear pierced earrings that contain nickel or chromium frequently develop weeping, red, pruritic lesions on

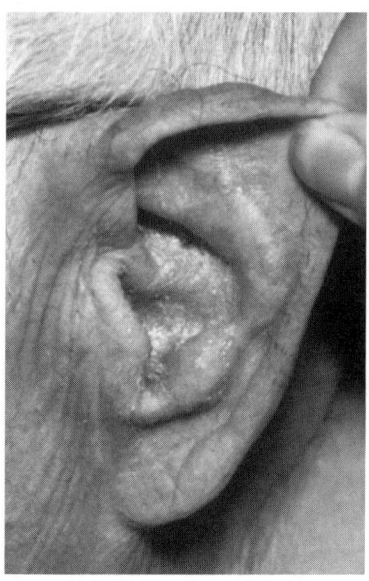

Figure 9.2 Typical contact dermatitis on the ear. (Courtesy of Dr. Berrylin Ferguson.)

the ear lobe. The diagnosis may be made by a dermatologist using patch testing, but simply having the patient switch to earrings with posts made of surgical stainless steel is often curative. A similar reaction to plastic or Silastic may occur in the ears of patients who wear hearing aids (10). Contact dermatitis may be present in other locations (Figs. 9.3 and 9.4); it has the same appearance.

Patients may develop an allergic reaction to **topically applied drugs**. The most common example is the itching, edema, and weeping of the ears that can result from the use of ear drops containing neomycin. Applying topical steroids and discontinuing the offending medication reverses these problems.

Eczema is an allergic skin disorder and may be a manifestation of an inhalant or food allergy or a contactant. Eczema generally involves multiple body areas, but the ear canal behaves like skin elsewhere, and eczematoid otitis externa is not uncommon. Topical steroid creams or drops are usually sufficient to control symptoms. Additionally, patients should avoid soaps, shampoos, hair sprays, and setting gels.

A special type of allergic external otitis is a **dermatophytid reaction** from a distant fungal infection that produces itching and desquamation of the ear canal (Case 9.1). This is a delayed hypersensitivity reaction, rather than the acute allergy seen in rhinitis. The fungi most often responsible for this are *Trichophyton*, *Oidiomycetes*, and *Epidermophyton* (a "TOE" reaction). If local measures and control of the distant fungal infection are ineffective, an otolaryngic allergist may administer specific immunotherapy (11).

Allergic Conditions of the Ear, Nose, and Throat 167

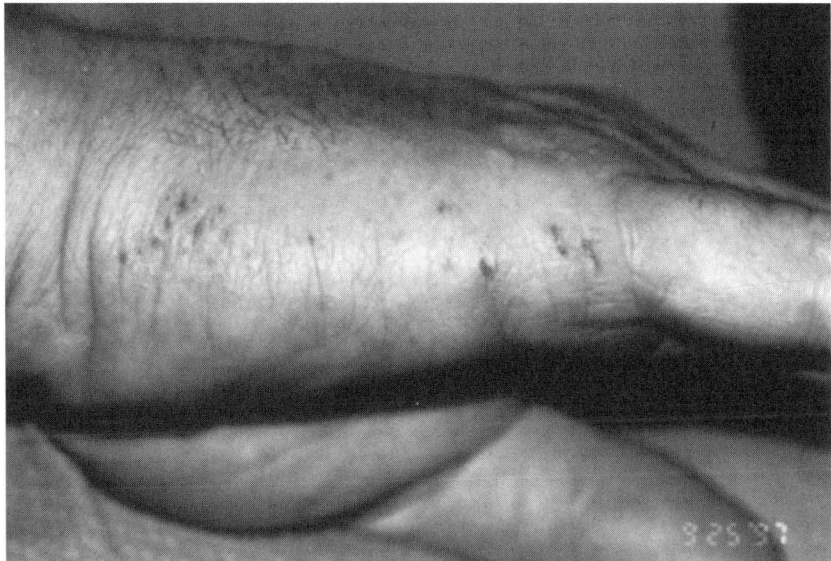

Figure 9.3 Contact dermatitis on the hand in a ragweed-allergic gardener. (Courtesy of Dr. Berrylin Ferguson.)

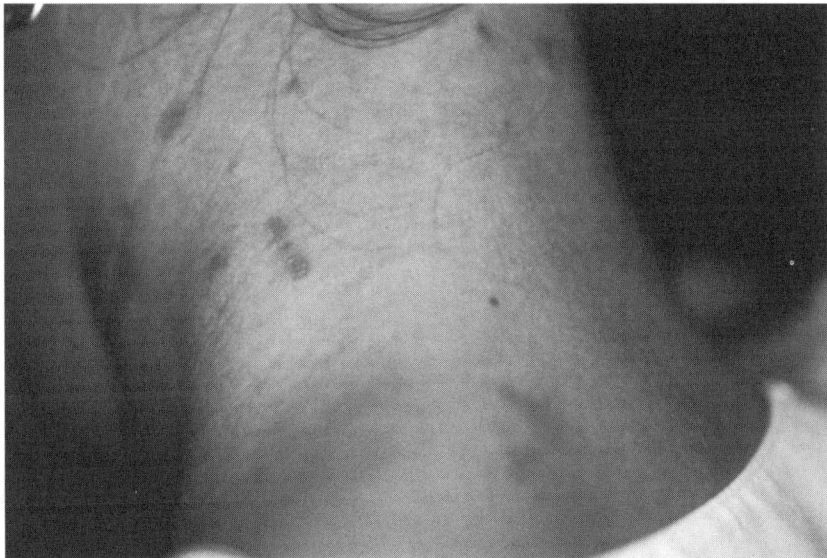

Figure 9.4 Contact dermatitis on the neck after use of a birch shampoo in a birch-allergic patient. (Courtesy of Dr. Berrylin Ferguson.)

> **Case 9.1** **Man with a Dermatophytid Reaction from a Fungal Infection at a Distant Site**
>
> A man 58 years of age presents with a 1-year history of external otitis refractory to a multiple-antibiotic preparation. Multiple cultures either show pseudomonas or are sterile. The patient has tried quinolone antibiotic ear drops and aminoglycoside ear drops with no improvement. He has had slight improvement applying cortisone creams to the ear. The patient denies any symptoms of allergic rhinitis, but you recently have heard about the id reaction in which patients have a skin eruption in the external ear canal caused by a fungal infection at a distant site. You ask the patient if he has any fungal toenail or fingernail infections. He takes off his shoes and shows you a fungal infection of the toenail (Fig. 9.5). You begin him on oral terbinafine hydrochloride (Lamisil) 250 mg/d for the next 12 weeks. He calls in 4 weeks and tells you that his ear is improving. Three months later, he reports resolution of his external ear symptoms and rash as well as his toenail infection.

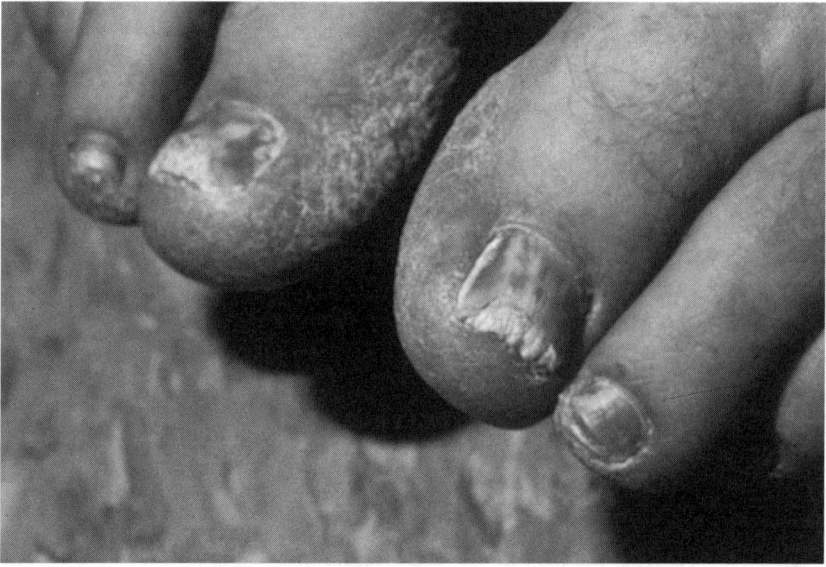

Figure 9.5 Fungal infection of the toenail. (Courtesy of Dr. Berrylin Ferguson.)

Middle Ear and Eustachian Tube

Both inhalant and food allergies have been found to correlate with eustachian tube dysfunction (12). The possible contribution of allergy to otitis media with effusion has been a source of conjecture for many years, but recent papers have supported such a connection (13–15). As a practical matter, patients with recalcitrant eustachian tube dysfunction or otitis media with effusion should be assessed for contributory abnormalities of the nasopharynx, nasal septum, turbinates, and paranasal sinuses. However, contributory allergy also should be considered.

Inner Ear

The exact cause of Meniere's disease (characterized by the triad of ear fullness and plugging, tinnitus, and vertigo) remains unclear. As early as 1923, Duke (16) suggested that allergy might play a causative role in Meniere's disease. Later work has tended to reinforce this speculation (17), although few objective studies have been carried out to support it. Howard and coworkers (18) noted a much higher incidence of inhalant allergy in patients with Meniere's disease than was found in the general population, with improvement of inner ear symptoms in a small group of patients treated with immunotherapy. Although not necessarily the first consideration, allergy evaluation should be a part of the comprehensive investigation of patients with inner ear symptoms.

Nose and Sinuses

Allergic Rhinitis

When most people speak of their "allergies," they actually mean allergic rhinitis. The symptoms of sneezing, itching, rhinorrhea, and congestion are often associated with specific seasons or circumstances, which suggests the causative allergens. For example, symptoms that begin in autumn and end with the first freeze suggest sensitivity to ragweed or other fall-related weeds. Unfortunately, most patients are allergic to multiple antigens and experience symptoms during several seasons, even throughout the year.

The patient with allergic rhinitis may present with any or all of the symptoms described above (Case 9.2). The nasal mucosa is typically boggy and more "bluish" than red or pink. Clear rhinorrhea and postnasal drainage are also prominent features of the clinical picture.

Pharmacotherapy for allergic rhinitis should proceed in a stepwise fashion, beginning with the provision of a nonsedating antihistamine (with or without a decongestant) used on an as-needed basis to control nasal allergic symptoms (*see* Algorithm). In addition, using nasal cromolyn (now available without a prescription) before an anticipated antigen exposure is helpful for many patients.

For those patients whose symptoms are not controlled by these simple measures, **topical nasal corticosteroids** are the next logical therapeutic step. However, it is important to realize that topical preparations must be used properly to be effective (19). First, because they must be able to penetrate to the nasal mucosa, these drugs may be ineffective in patients with obstructing septal deviation, turbinate hypertrophy, or large polyp masses. Second, to be effective, nasal steroids must be used regularly throughout the patient's severe allergy season. Finally, the physician must warn the patient of potential side effects (e.g., nasal crusting, dryness, or bleeding) and must watch for the development of a septal perforation. This latter complication is seen most often when patients excoriate the septal mucosa with the tip of the nasal device or direct the medication onto the nasal septum, rather than aiming it laterally (i.e., toward the corner of the eye).

Case 9.2   **Woman with Allergic Rhinitis**

A woman 29 years of age presents with complaints of nasal obstruction, sneezing, and itchy, watery eyes that are worse in the spring and autumn but are present throughout the year. Over-the-counter allergy preparations either keep her from sleeping at night or make her so sleepy during the day that she is unable to function effectively.

On physical examination, you note pale, boggy turbinates and thick, clear mucus. The remainder of her head and neck examination is normal.

Decongestant spraying and nose blowing resolves her airway obstruction, and she can breathe clearly through her nose.

Discussion

Through the history and physical examination, the most likely diagnosis is inhalant allergic rhinitis. She is most likely allergic to perennial allergens (e.g., dust mites, mold), which accounts for the presentation of symptoms throughout the year. Allergies to tree and ragweed pollen account for the spring and fall symptoms, respectively. The options for pharmacotherapy include a nonsedating antihistamine combined with a decongestant. Although the decongestant has insomnia as a side effect, the nonsedating antihistamines (e.g., fexofenadine [Allegra], loratadine [Claritin]) will not cause the daytime sleepiness seen with over-the-counter preparations (e.g., chlorpheniramine [Chlortrimeton], diphenhydramine [Benadryl]).

Because her symptoms are chronic, not sporadic, and occur with congestion and sneezing, a nasal steroid spray is the best choice. There are over a half-dozen nasal steroid sprays available, and all have similar efficacy. Because her nose is wet and runny, a nonaqueous spray would be appropriate. If the patient prefers a fragrance-free spray, then you should prescribe budesonide (Rhinocort), triamcinolone acetonide (Nasacort), or flunisolide (Aerobid). Several studies show that nasal steroid sprays actually relieve eye symptoms just as well as do the nonsedating antihistamines to which they are compared. Azelastine (Astelin) is a newly available topical antihistamine nasal spray that, unlike oral antihistamines, also relieves congestion. It has a symptom-relieving profile similar to that of nasal steroid sprays. Rather than taking 12 hours or more to be effective, azelastine can be used for sporadic symptoms because it acts quickly; however, its side effects (e.g., mild sedation, bad taste) limit its usefulness.

Case (continued)

The patient is prescribed a nasal steroid spray and is instructed in its proper application (i.e., directing the spray laterally at the turbinates avoids coating the vessels at the anterior portion of the septum). One month later, she reports complete relief of symptoms. However, over the past few days, she is noted to have epistaxis, which resolves with digital pressure to the anterior nose. She assures you that she is using the nasal spray appropriately. The patient's anterior septum shows evidence of bleeding and scabbing bilaterally. You instruct her to stop the nasal steroid spray and place her on a nonsedating antihistamine decongestant. Several days later, she calls to say that she is having difficulty with the medication because of insomnia and that she is not getting as much relief as she did with the nasal steroid spray. Her nosebleeds, however, have stopped.

At this point you recommend that the patient undergo allergy testing to pinpoint allergens and direct environmental controls. This is performed and your suspicions are confirmed: She is highly allergic to dust mite, mildly allergic to mold, and moderately allergic to ragweed and various tree and grass pollens. Environmental controls for her bedroom are discussed extensively, including mattress covers impermeable to dust mites and the washing of bedding in hot water above 130°F on a weekly basis.

She implements these environmental controls and, 6 weeks later, calls to say that she is approximately 50% better yet is still having some mild congestion and sneezing. She is concerned that in the upcoming month (March) her symptoms will be even worse.

You recommend that she start allergy shots because she is not getting effective symptomatic relief with environmental controls and medication. Allergy shots are commenced and she is able to advance without any difficulty. She requires a nonsedating antihistamine without decongestants during the spring, and by the summer she is noting quite a bit of improvement in her baseline symptoms and has no need for medication. She continues to advance her allergy shots on a weekly basis without difficulty until late August, when the allergy-injection site begins to flare, along with induration of greater than 3 cm.

You realize that the ragweed pollen counts are quite high, so you reduce the dose of the weekly shot during the ragweed season. She does fine on this regimen and, in November, begins re-escalation of her immunotherapy without difficulty. Within 1 year, she is on maintenance. Thereafter, she does well on almost no medication except for an occasional nonsedating antihistamine in the spring and fall. Over the course of 3 years, her allergy shots are decreased in frequency. After 3 years, she stops her allergy shots altogether, with no further symptoms.

Discussion (continued)

This case outlines the importance of environmental control. The role of allergy shots in patients who are receiving incomplete relief from medication is their potential, ultimately, to cure the hypersensitivity in some patients. The pros and cons of nasal steroid sprays, nasal antihistamine sprays, oral antihistamines, and decongestants are discussed elsewhere in this chapter.

Some controversy continues to exist about the possible systemic effects of topically applied nasal steroids. For example, adrenal suppression has been reported after normal doses of intranasal budesonide or fluticasone (20). Investigation continues as to the magnitude of this problem for both nasal and inhaled corticosteroids (21). Meanwhile, the clinician should be guided by a few simple rules: 1) prescribe topical steroids only after a failure of lesser measures, 2) taper to the lowest effective maintenance dose once therapeutic effect is noted, and 3) follow the patient to watch for side effects and to ensure that a continuation of the medication is necessary.

The management of allergic rhinitis may involve environmental control with specific testing to determine the incriminating antigens. This allows the physician to counsel patients accurately about avoidance measures. Such testing also can be used as the basis for definitive immunotherapy.

Rhinosinusitis

Patients with recurrent or chronic rhinosinusitis (a term that is replacing the older "sinusitis") often have contributory allergy. Before surgery is undertaken in patients with this problem, intensive medical management should be instituted, including efforts to control the contributory allergy. Management is usually begun with an orally administered, broad-spectrum antibiotic that is effective against β-lactamase–producing bacteria for 3 weeks. This regimen may allow patients to avoid surgery and may materially enhance postoperative results in those who do undergo surgery (22).

Allergic Fungal Sinusitis

This unique type of sinusitis seems to be caused by a hypersensitivity reaction to fungal organisms that come in contact with the nasal and sinus mucosa (23) (Case 9.3). Patients with allergic fungal sinusitis are immunocompetent, are most often adolescents or young adults with pansinusitis and polyposis, and have undergone previous surgery without benefit. Allergic symptoms are present in the vast majority of patients with allergic fungal sinusitis; approximately one third of these patients have asthma, and they are not aspirin-sensitive. Computed tomography scans show pansinusitis (often unilateral) and polyposis, frequently with a heterogeneity and scattered hyperdense areas.

At **surgery**, in addition to polyps and pansinusitis, one or more sinuses are generally filled with allergic mucin—a tenacious, rubbery material that is light green to black in color. Histologically, this material contains numerous eosinophils and Charcot–Leyden crystals (degenerating eosinophils). Fungal stains show the presence of noninvasive hyphae. Fungal cultures may or may not be positive.

In addition to surgery, **medical treatment** of these patients has been primarily with topical and systemic corticosteroids. However, more recently, immunotherapy (for both relevant fungal and nonfungal antigens)

> **Case 9.3** **Young Woman with Allergic Fungal Sinusitis**
>
> A woman 19 years of age with a long history of allergic rhinitis, for which she has never seen her local doctor, presents with a 4-month history of nasal airway obstruction (almost complete on the right side, partial on the left). For the past month she has noted right eye swelling and occasional double vision.
>
> Her physical examination is remarkable for right eye proptosis. She has complete occlusion of the right nose and almost complete occlusion on the left with nasal polyps. Translucent green mucin is noted. You order a computed tomography scan (Fig. 9.6), which shows remodeling of the ethmoid frontal sinuses, erosion of the lamina papyracea, and heterogeneity of the soft tissue masses within the sinus cavities. These clinical findings are characteristic of allergic fungal sinusitis.
>
> The patient is taken to the operating room within the next several weeks and undergoes endoscopic removal of nasal polyps and tenacious mucin using a microdebrider (Fig. 9.7). The pathologic specimens are sent to a laboratory with instructions to perform special fungal stains. Cultures are sent for fungus evaluation, and it grows out as *Bipolaris*. The histopathology examination reveals that the mucin contains many eosinophils with Charcot–Leyden crystals. On special fungal stains, hyphae are seen in the mucin but not in the nasal polyps or in the tissue.
>
> The patient is managed with a high-dose prednisone taper over the 10 days following surgery. She has no complications. Her vision immediately returns to normal, and she is able to breathe through her nose without difficulty immediately after surgery. She is seen on follow-up once per week, at which time her nose is debrided of crust, and she continues to improve. One month after surgery, allergy skin testing reveals that she is allergic to multiple pollen inhalants and seven of nine molds tested. You recommend that she begin allergy shots to prevent a recurrence of her allergy fungal sinusitis. She also is kept on nasal steroid sprays until her immunotherapy is advanced through maintenance. You continue to see her every 3 months, and she does well.
>
> **Discussion**
>
> Mabry and coworkers (24) recently have shown that fungal-containing immunotherapy is important in preventing recurrent allergic fungal sinusitis.

has been shown to be extremely effective in preventing a recurrence of this otherwise recalcitrant disease, making the use of systemic corticosteroids unnecessary (24).

Polyps

At one time, nasal polyps were thought to represent an allergic manifestation; however, recent writings have tended to minimize the role of allergy in polyp formation (25). Localized allergy without systemic allergic manifestations also

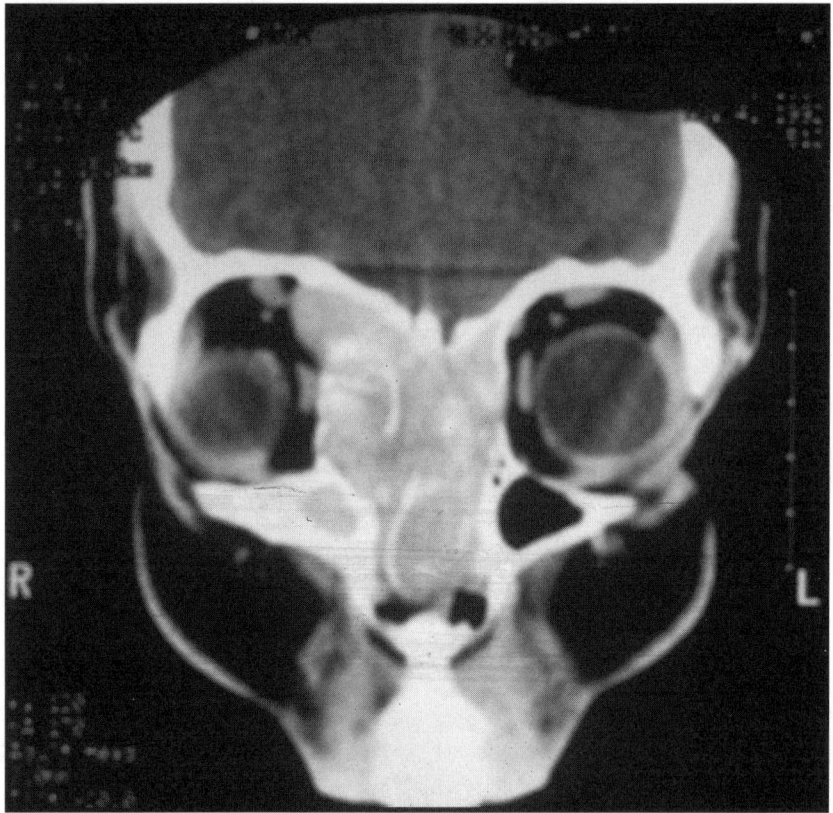

Figure 9.6 The "double density" or heterogeneity of the opaque areas on this coronal computed tomography scan is typical of allergic fungal sinusitis. (Courtesy of Dr. Berrylin Ferguson.)

has been postulated to be involved in the pathogenesis of polyps in some patients (26). Patients with nasal masses (e.g., polyps) usually require imaging studies and often need biopsies for tissue diagnosis.

Throat

The most common allergic manifestation of the throat is chronic postnasal drainage, which is generally associated with complaints of a "raw" throat. Other symptoms are habitual throat clearing (because of mucus accumulation) and "clucking" sounds (caused by the patient opposing the soft palate and posterior pharynx to relieve the chronic itching of these membranes).

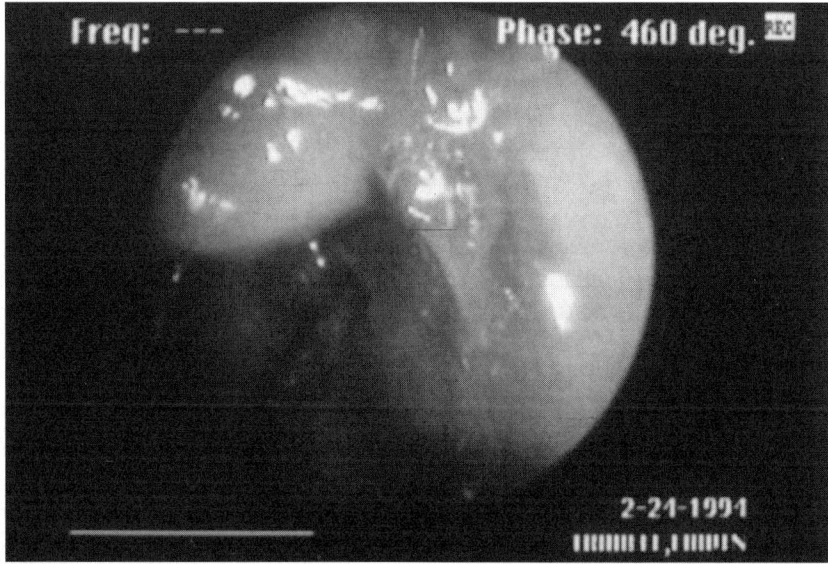

Figure 9.7 Thick inspissated pus (sometimes called "peanut butter" because of its stickiness and viscosity) is characteristic of allergic fungal sinusitis. (Courtesy of Dr. Berrylin Ferguson.)

Allergic patients may complain of hoarseness, either chronic or recurrent. Corey and coworkers (27) have described vocal nodules, subglottic edema, polypoid mucosal changes, and mucus bridging in allergic patients with laryngeal complaints.

Treatment with Immunotherapy

The best treatment of inhalant allergy is **avoidance and environmental control**, which is admirable in concept but often impractical in execution. **Pharmacotherapy** can offer symptom relief with antihistamines, decongestants, cromolyn, corticosteroids, and anticholinergic sprays. However, for patients whose symptoms are unrelieved by pharmacotherapy and for whom avoidance is not a viable option, immunotherapy should be considered.

Immunotherapy is the administration of controlled amounts of the antigens to which the patient is allergic to bring about immunomodulation. The mechanisms through which this is achieved have been postulated to lower specific IgE levels, to increase production of a "blocking" IgG antibody, or to have an effect on the T cells.

When immunotherapy is based on a prick test, single-dilution intradermal test, or both, the antigens are incorporated into the mixture at an initial arbitrary level (~1:100,000–1,000,000 weight per volume), with injections given on a weekly or twice-weekly schedule. The dose is titrated upward over a long period (sometimes months in duration) until a very high concentration (e.g., 1:50 weight per volume) is administered; however, the schedule can be modified if severe local or systemic reactions occur (28).

Immunotherapy administered after dilutional intradermal testing is characterized by incorporating the relevant antigens into the initial treatment vial at the "end point" concentration (i.e., the smallest amount of antigen required to produce a safe, positive response). Because the relationship between this type of skin test and the modified RAST test is well known, the same adjustments can be made when immunotherapy is based on most allergen-specific in vitro determinations (29). However, when immunotherapy is based on RAST, an initial skin test from the treatment vial is required as an added safety measure. When the concentration of antigens administered is adjusted individually in this fashion, a salutary effect on symptoms is often noted in 3 to 6 months. Treatment doses are advanced progressively to levels that have been shown to produce long-term immunologic and symptomatic improvement. The average duration of immunotherapy is 3 to 5 years, at which time most patients can discontinue their injections without a return of symptoms (unless an overwhelming antigen exposure occurs) (30).

It must be stressed that **immunotherapy carries a risk of anaphylaxis (31) and should be administered only under the immediate supervision of an appropriately trained specialist; dose advancement should occur only in settings in which anaphylactic reactions can be treated adequately** (32).

Summary

The internist often can make a provisional diagnosis of upper respiratory allergy based on the symptoms described by the patient and by the season or circumstances in which they appear. Pharmacotherapy with antihistamines, decongestants, cromolyn, and topical corticosteroids may offer adequate relief. However, referral to a specialist is warranted for the patient in whom avoidance is impossible or impractical and who obtains inadequate relief from conventional pharmacotherapy or requires near-constant medication to function adequately. An otolaryngologist can assess for complicating factors, such as chronic infections of the sinuses, nonallergic rhinitis, and mechanical obstruction by septal deviation or turbinate hypertrophy. Specific testing defines the triggering antigens and allows more appropriate counseling about avoidance measures. Testing also permits immunotherapy, which ultimately may allow the patient to live a more normal and productive life.

REFERENCES

1. **King HC.** *An Otolaryngologist's Guide to Allergy.* New York: Thieme; 1990.
2. **King HC, Mabry RL, Mabry CS.** *Allergy in ENT Practice: A Practical Guide.* New York: Thieme; 1998.
3. **Council on Scientific Affairs of the American Medical Association.** In vivo diagnostic testing and immunotherapy for allergy. *JAMA.* 1987;258:1363–7.
4. **Lewis T, Grant RT.** Vascular reactions of the skin to injury. *Heart.* 1926;13:219–25.
5. **Gordon BR.** Allergy skin tests and immunotherapy: comparison of methods in common use. *Ear Nose Throat J.* 1990;69:47–62.
6. **Mabry RL.** *Skin Endpoint Titration: History, Theory, and Practice.* Round Rock, TX: Meridian Biomedical; 1993:8–12.
7. **Wide L, Bennich H, Johansson SGO.** Diagnosis of allergy by an in vitro test for antigen antibodies. *Lancet.* 1967;2:1105–7.
8. **Lehr AJ, Mabry RL, Mabry CS.** The screening RAST: Is it a valid concept? *Otolaryngol Head Neck Surg.* 1997;117:54–5.
9. **Fadl R.** Experience with RAST-based immunotherapy. *Otolaryngol Clin North Am.* 1992;43–60.
10. **Derebery MJ, Berliner KL.** Allergy for the otologist. *Otolaryngol Clin North Am.* 1998;31:157–73.
11. **Ward WA Jr.** Molds: good news–bad news. In Krause HF (ed). *Otolaryngic Allergy and Immunology.* Philadelphia: WB Saunders; 1989:78–84.
12. **Derebery MJ, Berliner KL.** Allergic eustachian tube dysfunction: diagnosis and treatment. *Am J Otol.* 1997;18:160–5.
13. **Bernstein JM.** Role of allergy in eustachian tube blockage and otitis media with effusion: a review. *Otolaryngol Head Neck Surg.* 1996;114:562–8.
14. **Fireman P.** Otitis media and eustachian tube dysfunction: connection to allergic rhinitis. *J Allergy Clin Immunol.* 1997;99:S787–97.
15. **Hurst DS.** Association of otitis media with effusion and allergy as demonstrated by intradermal skin testing and eosinophil cationic protein levels in both middle ear effusions and mucosal biopsies. *Laryngoscope.* 1996;106:1128–37.
16. **Duke WW.** Meniere's syndrome caused by allergy. *JAMA.* 1923;81:2179–81.
17. **Derebery MJ.** Allergic and immunologic aspects of Meniere's disease. *Otolaryngol Head Neck Surg.* 1996;114:360–5.
18. **Howard BK, Mabry RL, Meyerhoff WL, Mabry CS.** Use of a screening RAST in a large neuro-otologic practice. *Otolaryngol Head Neck Surg.* 1997;117:653–9.
19. **Mabry RL.** Pharmacotherapy of allergic rhinitis: corticosteroids. *Otolaryngol Head Neck Surg.* 1995;113:120–5.
20. **Knutsson U, Stierna P, Marcus C, et al.** Effects of intranasal glucocorticoids on endogenous glucocorticoid peripheral and central function. *J Endocrin.* 1995;144:301–10.
21. **Lipworth BJ.** New perspectives on inhaled drug delivery and systemic bioactivity. *Thorax.* 1995;50:105–10.

22. **Davis WE, Templer JW, Lamear WR, Davis WE Jr.** Middle meatus antrostomy: patency rates and risk factors. *Otolaryngol Head Neck Surg.* 1991;104:467–72.
23. **Manning SC, Vuitch F, Weinberg AG, et al.** Allergic aspergillosis: a newly recognized form of sinusitis in the pediatric population. Laryngoscope 1989;99:681–685.
24. **Mabry RL, Marple BF, Folker RJ, Mabry CS.** Immunotherapy for allergic fungal sinusitis. *Otolaryngol Head Neck Surg.* 1998;119:648–51.
25. **Slavin RG.** Allergy is not a significant cause of nasal polyps. *Arch Otolaryngol Head Neck Surg.* 1992;118:771.
26. **Shatkin JS, Delsuphe KG, Thisted RA, Corey JP.** Mucosal allergy in the absence of systemic allergy in nasal polyposis and rhinitis: a meta-analysis. *Otolaryngol Head Neck Surg.* 1994;111:553–6.
27. **Corey JP, Gungor A, Karnell M.** Allergy for the laryngologist. *Otolaryngol Clin North Am.* 1998;31:189–205.
28. **Lawlor GL Jr, Fischer TJ, Adelman DC.** *Manual of Allergy and Immunology*, 3rd ed. Boston: Little, Brown; 1995:89–93.
29. **Tandy JR, Mabry RL, Mabry CS.** Correlation of modified radioallergosorbent test scores and skin test results. *Otolaryngol Head Neck Surg.* 1996;115:42–5.
30. **Gordon BR.** Immunotherapy basics. *Otolaryngol Head Neck Surg.* 1995;113:597–602.
31. **Tinkelman DG, Cole WQ III, Tunno J.** Immunotherapy: a one-year prospective study to evaluate risk factors of systemic reactions. *J Allergy Clin Immunol.* 1995;95:8–14.
32. **Cook PR, Farias C.** The safety of allergen immunotherapy: a literature review. *Ear Nose Throat J* 1998;77:378–88.

SUGGESTED READINGS

Derebery MJ, Berliner KL. Allergic eustachian tube dysfunction: diagnosis and treatment. *Am J Otol.* 1997;18:160–5.

This retrospective review studied 151 patients with eustachian tube dysfunction presenting to a tertiary otology practice. These patients had clinical histories that suggested allergic problems and underwent allergy testing and treatment. Over 70% had improvement in the symptoms of ear fullness, and over 80% had an improvement in allergy symptoms and general well-being.

Mabry RL. Pharmacotherapy of allergic rhinitis: corticosteroids. *Otolaryngol Head Neck Surg.* 1995;113:120–5.

This article reviews the forms of corticosteroids used in the treatment of allergic rhinitis. It presents guidelines for use, describes the differences among the different preparations currently available, and discusses the potential side effects.

Tinkelman DG, Cole WQ III, Tunno J. Immunotherapy: a one-year prospective study to evaluate risk factors of systemic reactions. *J Allergy Clin Immunol.* 1995;95:8–14.

This article followed a year-long prospective study of systemic reactions encountered in a busy allergy clinic in which one reaction occurred approximately every 1600 patient visits. Reactions were more common during dose escalation than during maintenance therapy. All severe reactions occurred within 30 minutes of injection. Asthma was not an additional risk factor for developing a systemic reaction.

10

Rhinosinusitis

D. Gregory Farwell, MD
Eric F. Pinczower, MD

Rhinosinusitis and related symptoms are among the most common presenting complaints of patients in the United States. In 1991, there were 11.6 million office visits for rhinosinusitis. The 1992 estimated direct costs from rhinosinusitis were $2.4 billion, and more than 13 million prescriptions for antibiotics were written. During the years 1990 to 1992, the number of restricted-activity days caused by rhinosinusitis were 73 million, a 50% increase from the 50 million in the period from 1986 to 1988 (1). It is clear that rhinosinusitis plays an important role in our national health and in the cost of heath care.

The vast majority of rhinosinusitis is self-limited or is easily treated by a combination of decongestants, antihistamines, and antimicrobial therapy. Occasionally, acute infections may develop into complicated infections or chronic rhinosinusitis. Our ability to diagnose and treat rhinosinusitis has improved dramatically in the past 20 years. One of the advances that have contributed to this is the use of computed tomography (CT). CT helps diagnose anatomical causes of rhinosinusitis, localizes disease, and provides a road map for surgical intervention. Another advance has been in nasal endoscopy, which has contributed to both the diagnosis and management of sinonasal disease. The combination of CT scan and nasal endoscopy has led to the understanding that the ethmoid/middle meatal complex is the key to most cases of rhinosinusitis and their management.

Facial pain, pressure, headache, nasal congestion, nasal drainage, and postnasal drip are the typical indications of acute sinusitis. Visual abnormalities, ocu-

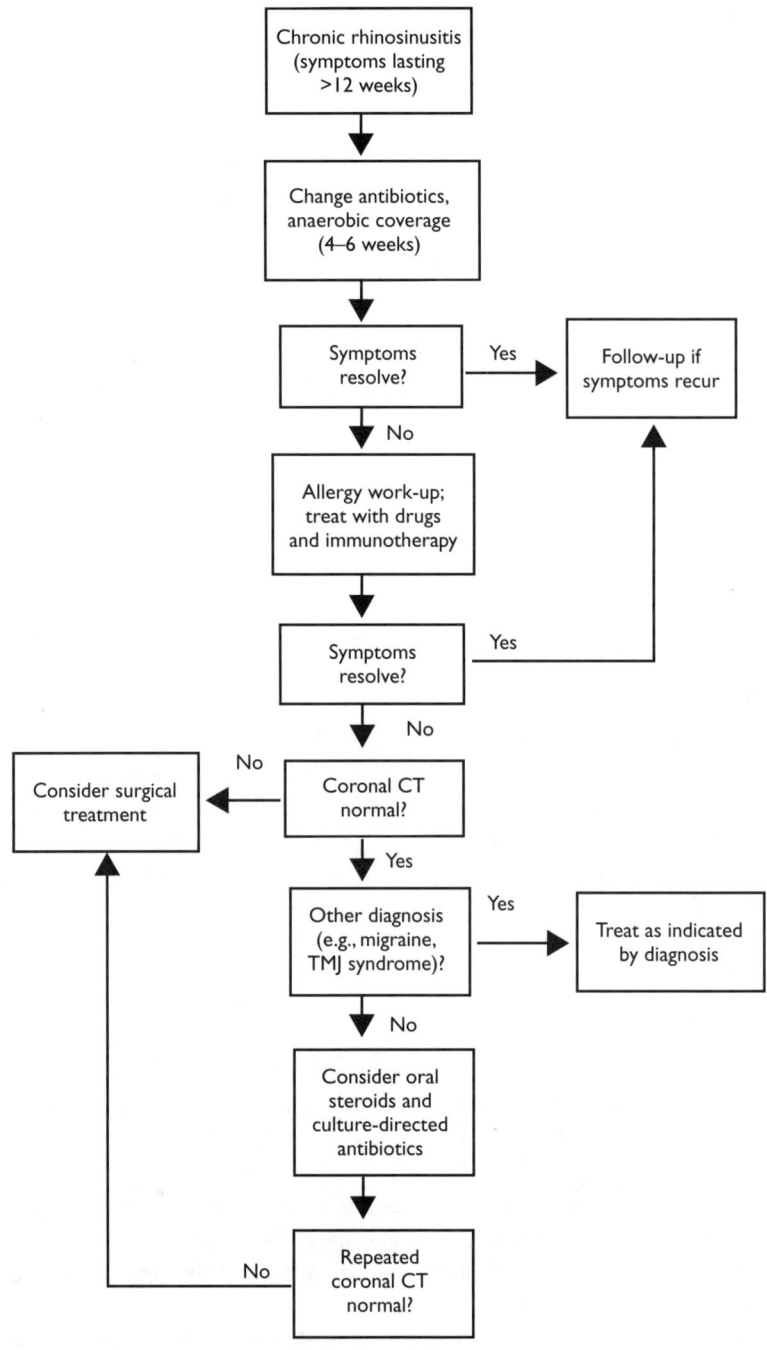

Algorithm Management of chronic rhinosinusitis. CT = computed tomography; TMJ = temporomandibular joint.

lomotor disturbances, occipital or vertex headaches, facial swelling, and altered mental state indicate advanced or complicated disease. Constitutional symptoms (e.g., fever, malaise, fatigue) are common. The inciting event in the development of rhinosinusitis is blockage of the normal sinus drainage routes, which may be caused by viral respiratory infection, allergy, or even a foreign body. When this occurs, acute rhinosinusitis may develop. *Acute rhinosinusitis* is defined as inflammation of the sinuses that lasts up to 4 weeks. The major and minor factors of sinusitis are described in Table 10.1. Patients with two major factors or one major and two minor factors are most likely to have acute rhinosinusitis (2). Acute rhinosinusitis is most frequently an acute bacterial infection that follows a viral upper respiratory tract infection. Symptoms of upper respiratory tract infections that last longer than 10 days are a strong indication that acute rhinosinusitis may be present. Case 10.1 illustrates the usual presenting symptoms and history associated with acute rhinosinusitis.

Chronic rhinosinusitis refers to disease that persists beyond 12 weeks. A history of two major or one major and two minor factors strongly supports a diagnosis of chronic rhinosinusitis (2) (*see* Table 10.1). Nasal congestion, facial pain, postnasal drip, headache, and fatigue are common symptoms. Other less-common presenting complaints are halitosis, persistent cough, and a foul-smelling nasal cavity. Patients with these symptoms often suffer from depression. The etiology of chronic rhinosinusitis is diverse; the role of bacterial infection is less universal. Differentiating true chronic sinus disease from chronic fatigue syndromes and the somatic components of depression may be challenging.

Recurrent acute rhinosinusitis is defined as symptoms and physical findings consistent with acute rhinosinusitis that either worsen after 5 days or persist beyond 10 days. Each episode lasts approximately 1 to 2 weeks, and patients have four or more episodes per year. Between episodes, patients are asymptomatic. *Subacute rhinosinusitis* refers to a condition of minimal-to-moderate symptoms of sinus inflammation that persist for more than 4 weeks but less than 12 weeks (2).

Table 10.1 Factors Associated with the Diagnosis of Rhinosinusitis

Major Factors	Minor Factors
Facial pain or pressure	Headache
Facial congestion or fullness	Fever (in all nonacute disorders)
Nasal obstruction or blockage	Halitosis
Nasal discharge or purulence or discolored postnasal drainage	Fatigue
	Dental pain
Hyposmia or anosmia	Cough
Purulence in nasal cavity on examination	Ear pain, pressure, or fullness
Fever (in acute rhinosinusitis only)	

Republished with permission from Lanza DC, Kennedy DW. Adult rhinosinusitis defined. *Otolaryngol Head Neck.* 1997:117:S1–11.

> **Case 10.1** **Woman with Acute Rhinosinusitis**
>
> A woman 36 years of age complains of severe pain in her right cheek and her right maxillary molars. Her dentist told her yesterday that she had no dental caries or abscesses that could be causing the pain, which began last week just as she was getting over an upper respiratory infection. She has not run a fever and does not have a cough, sore throat, or ear discomfort. She says she hardly blows her nose at all but feels as if something is dripping down the back of her throat that almost makes her nauseated at times. She is having problems with nasal obstruction at night.
>
> Her physical examination is normal, except for her nose in which anterior rhinoscopy reveals markedly erythematous mucosa, worse on the right than on the left. After her nose is sprayed with a decongestant anesthetic, nasal endoscopy reveals edematous erythematous mucosa on the left side. On the right, a thin trickle of pus can be seen dripping along the lateral nasal wall from under the anterior end of the middle turbinate.
>
> A diagnosis of acute sinusitis is made, and the patient is begun on amoxicillin, pseudoephedrine, and guiafenesin. She also is instructed to use oxymetazoline nasal spray twice daily for 3 days only. On her follow-up visit 2 weeks later, she reports that her symptoms began to improve in 2 days and that she is back to normal except for a continuing slight postnasal drip.

Anatomy and Physiology

The paranasal sinuses originate early in the embryologic development of the fetus. They begin as outpouchings of the nasal cavity into the facial bones. The maxillary and ethmoid sinuses begin development during the prenatal stage and are present at birth. At approximately 3 years of age, frontal and sphenoid sinuses begin to form. They are rudimentary until 5 or 6 years of age. The sinuses grow and enlarge in conjunction with the growth of the facial skeleton. The maxillary, ethmoid, and sphenoid sinuses reach full growth by puberty; the frontal sinuses continue to expand and grow into adulthood. The drainage system of the frontal, maxillary, and anterior ethmoid sinuses coalesce in the region of the middle meatus. Anatomical variations, mucosal thickening, and external compression of this "osteomeatal complex" can lead to blockage of the normal drainage pattern that results in mucosal stasis and infection (Fig. 10.1).

The mucosal drainage pattern of the maxillary sinus defies gravity. Normal mucociliary flow is in a circular direction around the sinus. Mucus exits the maxillary sinus by ascending high along the medial wall to the infundibulum and then out the middle meatus (3). For that reason, altered mucociliary clearance (secondary to genetic disease, mucosal damage, mucosal irritation, or anatomical variations) plays a lead role in the stasis of sinus

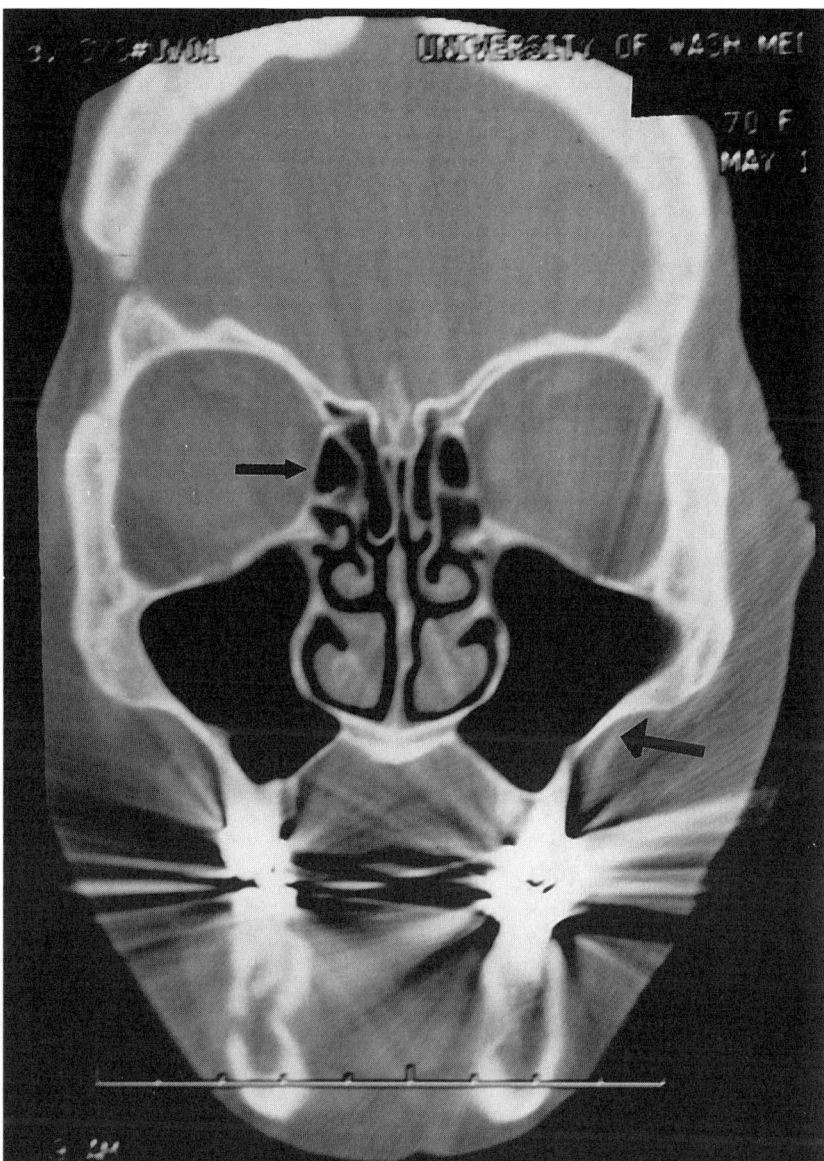

Figure 10.1 Normal sinus computed tomography scan. Note the maxillary sinus (*large arrow*), ethmoid sinuses (*small arrow*), septum, turbinates, and orbits.

contents and infection (Fig. 10.2). Allergy, with the production of histamine and other vasoactive molecules, impairs sinus drainage by producing cellular edema and an inflammatory infiltrate. Once the normal mucus of the sinuses becomes thickened or stagnant, the typical respiratory flora of the nose may proliferate in this rich culture media. This may lead to infection, with purulence that is either retained within the sinuses or discharged through the nares. Immunodeficiency states of the mucosa can lead to an overgrowth of microbial flora in the nose with secondary infection, often with atypical organisms (*see* Chapter 32).

History

The importance of a history of **facial pain** in rhinosinusitis cannot be underestimated. One must accurately determine the precise character of this presenting problem. Duration, intensity, location, and exacerbating factors provide insight into the cause of the patient's complaint.

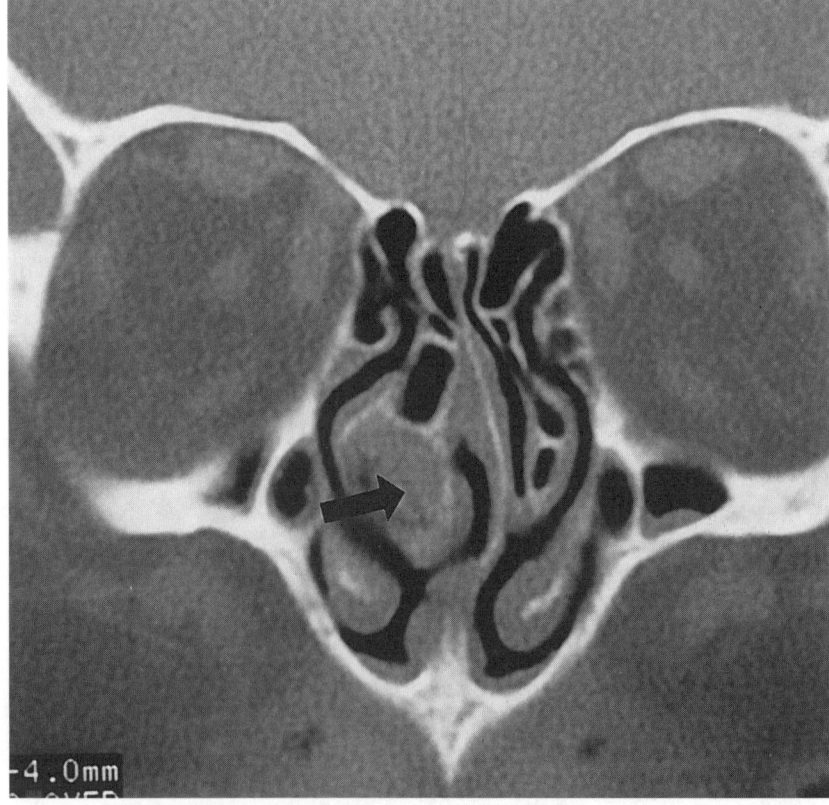

Figure 10.2 Abnormal nasal anatomy. Note that the patient's right middle turbinate has a concha bullosa (*arrow*). This patient also has a septal deviation toward the left. These anatomical abnormalities may contribute to blockage of the normal sinus drainage.

In acute rhinosinusitis, patients complain of persistent facial pain and headache. Usually, there is a preceding viral infection of the upper respiratory tract. The location of the pain—whether retro-orbital, facial, or vertex—can give some clue as to the involvement of the different paranasal sinuses. Occipital or vertex pain is associated commonly with sphenoid rhinosinusitis, whereas nasal or cheek pain with tooth tenderness is a common presentation of maxillary rhinosinusitis. Rhinosinusitis-related pain is characterized as a boring, throbbing, deep-seated pain that lasts for hours to days and is worsened by positional or barometric changes. In contrast, migraine headaches present as severe, unilateral, pulsatile, incapacitating pain that may last for hours to days. Migraines are often associated with nausea and emesis, photophobia, and a prodromal aura. All of these are uncommon with rhinosinusitis. Pain from the temporomandibular joint (TMJ) presents as an intermittent, recurrent aching in the area of the TMJ or retro-orbital regions and may extend into the temporal region.

Nasal congestion is a symptom that helps differentiate among the above entities. Rhinosinusitis is frequently associated with chronic congestion. Long-standing nasal congestion may be caused by a septal deviation or nasal polyposis. Each of these may contribute to the development of rhinosinusitis. Chronic allergic rhinitis, with swollen, edematous mucosa presents as nasal congestion. This swelling of the mucosa may predispose to obstruction of the sinus drainage patterns, which may then lead to the development of rhinosinusitis. Vascular headaches also may be associated with ipsilateral nasal congestion.

Nasal discharge is frequently associated with rhinosinusitis. The characteristics of the nasal discharge are important in determining the underlying cause. Thick, green nasal discharge is a common finding in acute rhinosinusitis. Clear nasal discharge is seen more frequently in allergic or vasomotor rhinitis. Patients with migraines also may have an associated watery discharge from vasomotor rhinitis.

Visual changes such as diplopia, altered visual acuity, and painful eye movements may be indications of complications from acute rhinosinusitis. They also may be associated with the prodrome of a migraine headache. Inflammation of tooth roots through the thin layer of maxillary bone overlying the maxillary molars may cause tooth pain. In contrast, painful trismus is associated more commonly with the inflammation of the TMJ capsule or the mastication muscles. Trismus also may be a sign of an advanced sinonasal malignancy.

Epistaxis is seen occasionally in acute rhinosinusitis. It is characterized by blood-tinged mucus. Persistent epistaxis warrants careful evaluation to rule out malignancy.

Physical Examination

The physical examination concentrates on the head and neck and cranial nerves. The external auditory canal and tympanic membrane are examined for infection or effusion, which may be an indication of eustachian tube dysfunction caused by a nasopharyngeal process. Malignancy of the external canal or middle ear, although rare, also may present as facial pain and should be looked for on routine otoscopy.

The face is inspected for swelling, asymmetry, or masses. Discoloration or breakdown of overlying skin may indicate an underlying mass. The eyes are examined for chemosis or proptosis. Extraocular muscle function is determined. Additionally, the fundus should be inspected for evidence of increased intracranial pressure or retinal abnormalities. The **cranial nerve examination** may reveal complications of rhinosinusitis, such as subperiosteal orbital abscess, mucocele, or intracranial extension (6) (Figs. 10.3 and 10.4). Ophthalmoplegia with gaze restriction, alteration in visual acuity, and diminished trigeminal sensation indicates the development of the disease outside the sinus. Diagnosis and monitoring of the progression of these findings and any cranial neuropathies is critical in the early treatment of rhinosinusitis. Early imaging with either CT or magnetic resonance imaging (MRI) is required.

The nasal cavity is inspected with **anterior rhinoscopy** to determine the condition of the mucosa. The nature of nasal discharge also is characterized. Edematous mucosa with watery nasal discharge is seen in allergic conditions.

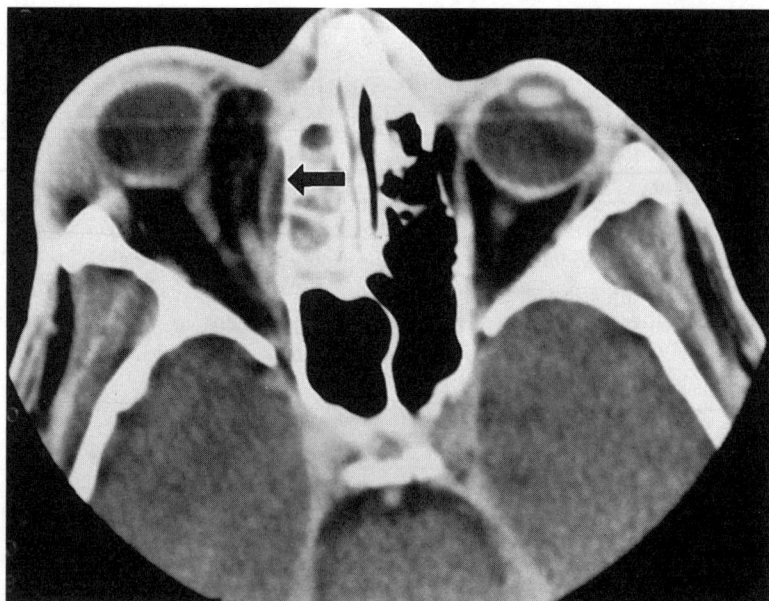

Figure 10.3 Subperiosteal abscess (arrow) in right orbit secondary to ethmoid sinusitis. Note 1) the soft tissue density along the lamina papyracea adjacent to the infected ethmoid air cells, and 2) the edema in the periorbital soft tissues.

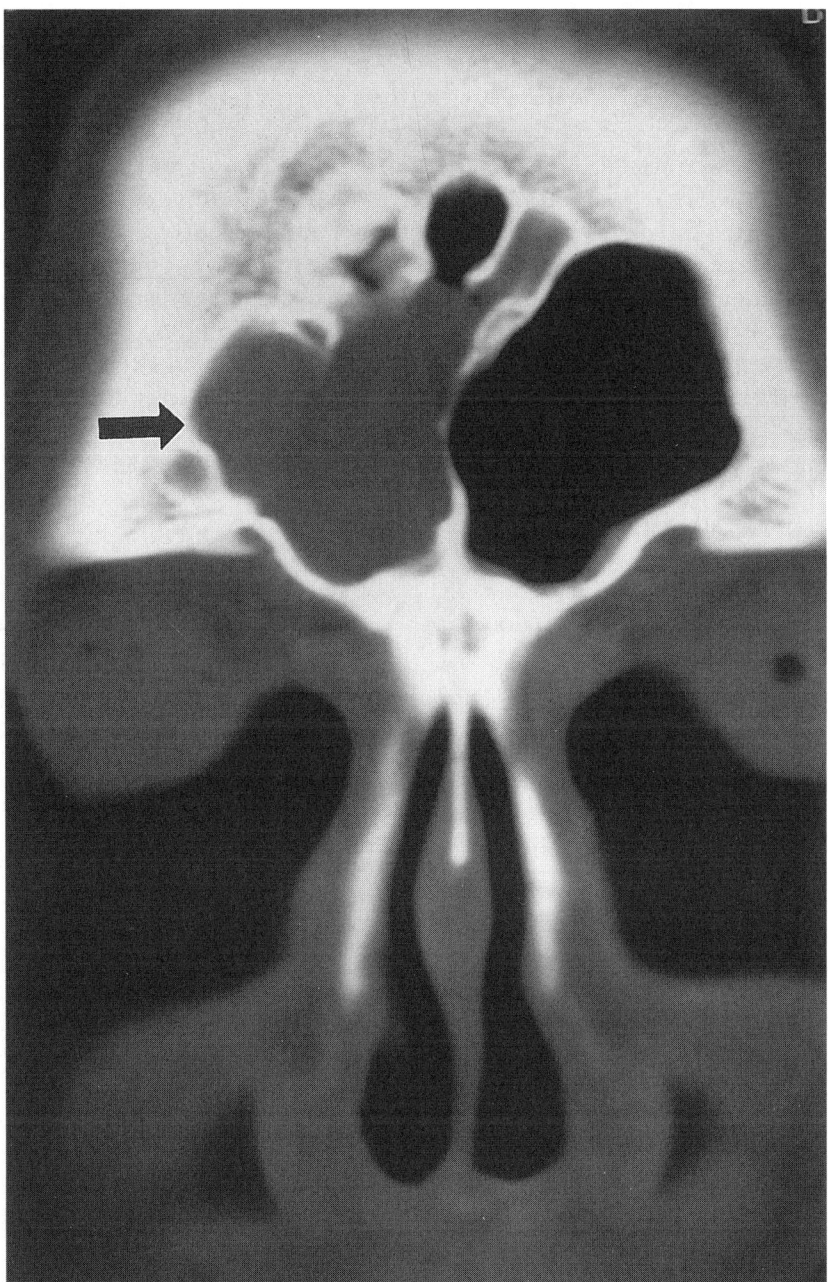

Figure 10.4 Frontal mucocele. The right frontal sinus is obliterated with a mucocele (*arrow*) that nearly fills the sinus cavity.

Erythematous, cobblestoned nasal mucosa with purulent, colored secretions is seen in infectious rhinosinusitis. Evaluating the nasal cavities of immunosuppressed patients is more difficult; patients with diabetes, lymphoproliferative disorders, or AIDS or those on chemotherapy are at greater risk for atypical or fungal infections. Nasal mucosa that appears dark or black on anterior rhinoscopy may be an indication of fungal infection, most commonly mucormycosis and aspergillosis. Very pale mucosa also may indicate fungal infection. Infection in these patients may progress rapidly. **The presence of abnormal mucosa on nasal examination in an immunocompromised patient is an emergency that requires possible surgical intervention** (7).

An **examination of the oral cavity and dentition** should be performed on every patient who complains of facial pain. The teeth and alveolar ridges are examined for signs of periodontal disease, periapical abscess or evidence of odontogenic tumors that might present with similar symptoms to rhinosinusitis. The presence of a "bite line" on the buccal mucosa, tender palpation of the pterygoids, trismus, and painful palpation of the TMJ may indicate a diagnosis of TMJ syndrome.

Differential Diagnosis

The differential diagnosis of sinonasal symptoms are listed in Table 10.2 (*see also* Chapter 23). The sinuses are innervated by the trigeminal nerve. Inflam-

Table 10.2 Differential Diagnosis of Sinus-Type Symptoms

Infectious Disorders	Neoplasms
Acute rhinosinusitis	Sinonasal
Chronic rhinosinusitis	Intracranial
Recurrent acute rhinosinusitis	
Subacute rhinosinusitis	**Neuropathic Disorders**
Fungal rhinosinusitis	Trigeminal neuralgia
Dental infection	Sphenopalatine neuralgia
Vascular Cephalgia	**Trauma**
Migraine headache	Facial trauma
Cluster headache	
Tension headache	
Other	**Psychological Disorders**
	Depression
Inflammatory Disorders	
Temporomandibular joint syndrome	
Temporal arteritis	

mation or disease of any structure innervated by the nerve or in close proximity to the nerve may result in similar sensations. When the common symptoms (e.g., nasal congestion, purulent rhinorrhea, facial pain, headache for >10 days) are present, acute rhinosinusitis is easy to diagnose. Chronic rhinosinusitis has a much more difficult cohort of ailments within the differential diagnosis. Among the more frequently related diagnoses are TMJ syndrome and migraine headaches.

Temporomandibular joint syndrome is thought to be secondary to malocclusion, tooth grinding, and/or arthritic inflammation of the TMJ capsule. The key diagnostic elements are obtained by a careful history. Trauma, tooth grinding, stress, or malocclusion all point to a possible diagnosis of TMJ syndrome. A careful examination that focuses on palpating the joint, the pterygoid musculature, and the patient's oral cavity helps eliminate or confirm the diagnosis of TMJ.

Vascular headaches (cephalgia), including migraine, are commonly misdiagnosed as rhinosinusitis. Vascular headaches are frequently associated with an **aura** and are often characterized by severe, incapacitating pain and photophobia. Other symptoms that may be associated with vascular cephalgia include dizziness, nausea, and emesis. The attacks usually last for hours and are more frequent in patients with high stress levels. Patients are typically asymptomatic between attacks and often respond to vasoactive drugs, such as sumatriptan (Imitrex) and methysergide (Sansert). Combinations of caffeine and acetaminophen also work well (4).

Sinonasal neoplasms are rare but must be considered in all new-onset facial symptoms. Unilateral obstruction, epistaxis, or pain that does not respond quickly to antibiotics or decongestants may be the presenting sign of a neoplasm. These symptoms are found more frequently in elderly patients. Squamous cell carcinoma, adenocarcinoma, juvenile nasopharyngeal angiofibroma, and primary bony tumors of the maxilla and teeth have all been misdiagnosed as rhinosinusitis. The possibility of malignancy is evaluated effectively by CT of the sinuses in patients whose symptoms persist despite adequate medical treatment. CT is preferred because it demonstrates bony architecture better than does MRI.

The patient's general health is essential when considering the differential diagnosis of predisposing and causative factors in rhinosinusitis. Coexistent illnesses such as mucosal-transport disorders (e.g., primary ciliary dyskinesia), genetic illnesses (e.g., cystic fibrosis), mucosal immunosuppression (e.g., immunoglobulin-A deficiency), and general immunosuppression (e.g., chemotherapy, lympho- and hemoproliferative disorders) are all risk factors for rhinosinusitis.

Anatomical obstructions, either congenital or posttraumatic (e.g., deviated septum, ostiomeatal polyps, bone spurs) can disturb normal sinus drainage and predispose a patient to acute and chronic rhinosinusitis (5) (Fig. 10.5).

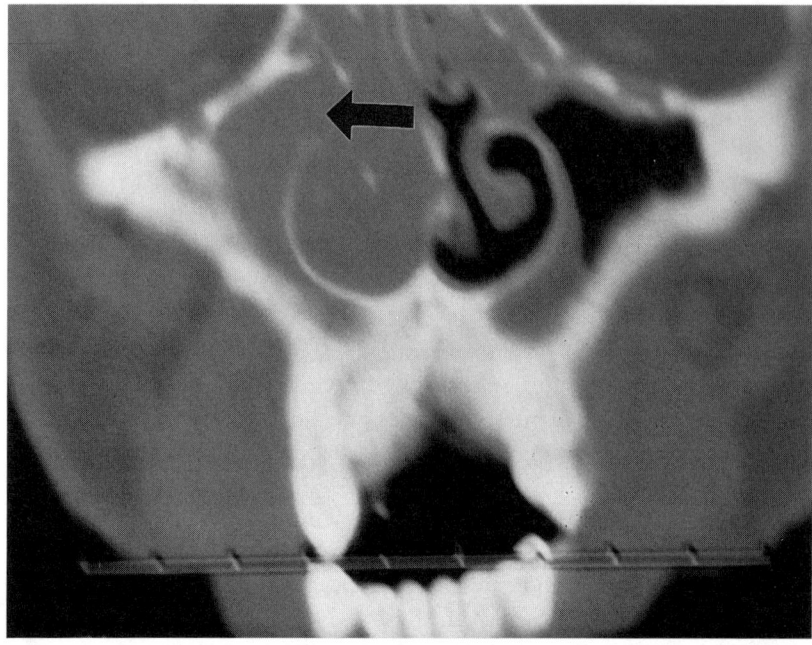

Figure 10.5 Rhinosinusitis. Note the inflammation and obstruction of the osteomeatal complex on the left (*arrow*). Additionally, the left and right ethmoid sinuses, right maxillary sinus, and nasal cavity are filled with mucosal edema and mucopurulence.

Additional Diagnostic Evaluation

Radiography

Radiographic evaluation of the paranasal sinuses and nasal endoscopy are the most important adjuvants to the history and physical in the work-up of patients with facial pain and symptoms of rhinosinusitis. Plain radiography, which has limited benefit in the diagnosis of air-fluid levels of the maxillary sinuses, has been supplanted by CT as the radiographic study of choice for the paranasal sinuses. The ethmoid sinuses are the most common site of rhinosinusitis involvement, but plain films routinely underestimate the extent of ethmoid disease and provide little of the anatomical detail needed for surgical planning (8). The Waters-view plain film of the sinuses demonstrates opacification of the maxillary sinuses and the presence of air-fluid levels.

Computed Tomography

Screening coronal CT scans provide far superior anatomical detail than do plain radiographs. In some centers, they can be completed for a price similar to that of a full plain-film series of the sinuses. A full coronal CT examination is necessary for surgical planning, especially in revision cases. Axial CT cuts are complementary and assist in the diagnosis of disease and in surgical planning.

Imaging with CT rarely is required for the diagnosis and treatment of acute rhinosinusitis. Only when impending complications are suspected, or when therapy is not adequate for patients, should CT imaging be performed. In chronic disease, aggressive medical therapy should be performed *before* obtaining CT images, allowing CT to demonstrate the irreversible component of the patient's sinus disease. Coronal scans are superior to axial scans when imaging the ostiomeatal complex and the relationship of the sinuses to the orbits and brain (9).

Magnetic Resonance Imaging

The use of MRI delineates the extent and spread of sinonasal tumors as well as the regional and intracranial complications of sinus disease. MRI also can help in the diagnosis of fungal concretions due to their low intensity or signal void on T2-weighted images (9). MRI is also useful in differentiating between tumor and retained secretions, which may determine resectability. The anatomical detail obtained with MRI is usually not necessary for the diagnosis of rhinosinusitis. Its lack of bony detail is a disadvantage when evaluating the skull base and bony borders of the paranasal sinuses. Because of the detail that MRI is able to reveal, otherwise healthy patients frequently demonstrate mucosal disease within the sinuses. **In an asymptomatic, healthy patient, mucosal inflammation seen on MRI is not significant.**

Nasal Endoscopy

Nasal endoscopy is a technique that has greatly improved our understanding of nasal physiology and our ability to diagnose and follow accurately the ailments of the nasal cavity and paranasal sinuses (Fig. 10.6). Endoscopy allows excellent visualization of the mucosa, anatomical abnormalities, and the presence and nature of secretions; it also allows direct evaluation of the ostiomeatal complex in far greater detail than the view seen on anterior rhinoscopy. The nasopharynx and the eustachian tubes can be inspected more easily and completely with endoscopy than with previous techniques, including mirror nasopharyngoscopy. The information provided by nasal endoscopy helps differentiate rhinosinusitis from other ailments associated with facial pain and nasal congestion.

Cultures

Cultures of the sinuses are difficult to obtain using blind nasal-swabbing techniques. For Food and Drug Administration drug trials, the standard is antral

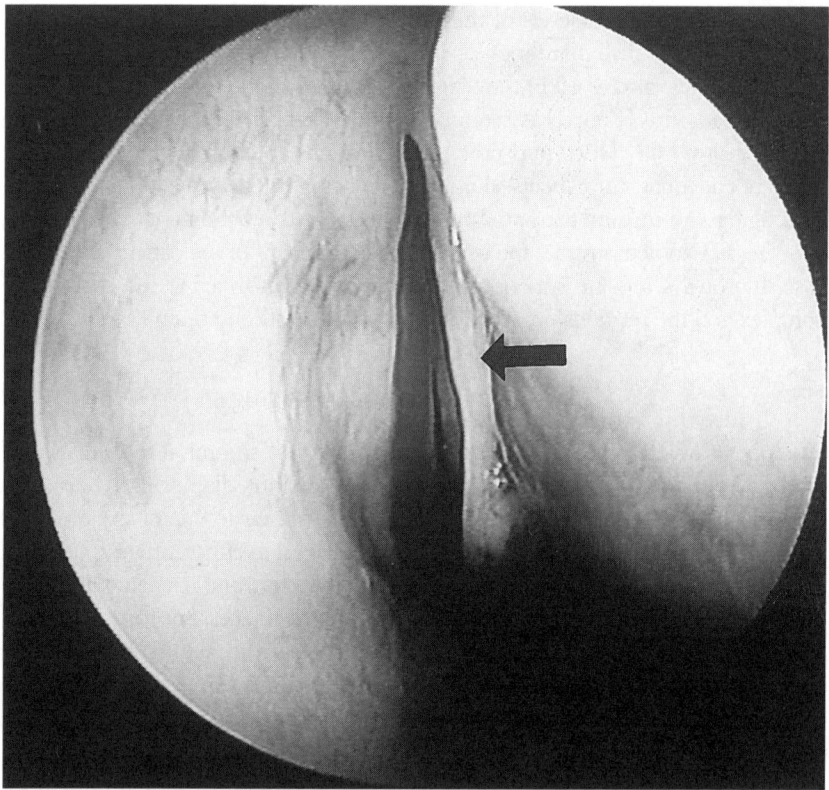

Figure 10.6 Normal middle meatus endoscopy. Note the middle turbinate (*arrow*) and the middle meatus. There is normal-appearing mucosa with no purulence.

puncture; however, this technique is generally unnecessary in the treatment of community-acquired infections. Antral aspiration is used in patients with suspected nosocomial rhinosinusitis or rhinosinusitis that has resulted in complications or in those who fail to respond to adequate therapy. Other techniques such as endoscopy-guided middle meatal cultures have been demonstrated to be reliable for obtaining more representative cultures (10). Whatever method is used to obtain it, the culture should be transported quickly to the laboratory and evaluated for aerobic and anaerobic organisms (11).

Management and Follow-Up

The microbiology of rhinosinusitis has changed little over the years; however, what *has* changed is the development of widespread resistance to commonly prescribed antimicrobials. **Acute rhinosinusitis** is caused primarily by *Streptococcus pneumoniae* and *Haemophilus influenza*. Less frequently seen are *Moraxella catarrhalis*, beta-hemolytic *Streptococcus* organisms, and *Staphylococcus aureus*. In approximately one third of acute rhinosinusitis, the microbiology reveals a mixed infection with two or more causative bacteria. Anaerobic bacteria are rarely associated with acute rhinosinusitis. The most common anaerobe involved is *Peptostreptococcus*. *Pseudomonas aeruginosa* and enteric bacteria are the usual causes of nosocomial acute rhinosinusitis.

Chronic rhinosinusitis is most frequently caused by *S. aureus*, coagulase-negative *Staphylococcus* organisms, *S. pneumoniae*, anaerobes (e.g., *Peptostreptococcus*, *Fusobacterium*, *Proteus* species), *P. aeruginosa*, and *H. influenza*. Although the bacteriology of chronic sinusitis has not been elucidated definitively, in 25% to 67% of cases the primary pathogen is an anaerobic organism. Several studies have demonstrated that there seem to be more anaerobic sources of chronic maxillary rhinosinusitis than chronic ethmoid rhinosinusitis. It is speculated that this may be due to a greater degree of occlusion of the normal drainage patterns of the maxillary sinuses, forming a relatively more anaerobic environment (12). In immunosuppressed patients, fungal sources of rhinosinusitis are recognized more frequently (12,13).

Antibiotic Therapy

The frequent use of antibiotics in the treatment of patients who present with rhinosinusitis has contributed to the emergence of resistant organisms. Once universally susceptible to penicillin, 45% to 50% of *S. pneumoniae* strains in some communities are now estimated to be resistant to the drug. *H. influenza*'s resistance to ampicillin has been reported to be as high as 30% in type-B strains and 15% in non–type-B strains. Eighty-five percent of *Moraxella* strains now produce beta-lactamase; thus, infection with this organism is unlikely to be cured by penicillin or narrower-spectrum cephalosporins. Most anaerobes are extremely resistant to many of the commonly prescribed antimicrobials (14).

Antibiotic use should be tailored with the above statistics in mind. A 10- to 14-day course is an effective duration of therapy. The current treatment guidelines recommend amoxicillin at the standard dosage (1.5–3.5 g/d) as first-line therapy for mild infections in patients who have not been treated with antibiotics within a period of 4 to 6 weeks. High-dose amoxicillin (3.0–3.5 g/d) or amoxicillin/clavulanate should be used for mild infections in patients who have been treated previously or for moderate infections in patients who have not been treated previously (15). Cefpodoxime proxetil, cefuroxime axetil, cefprozil, levofloxacin, gatifloxacin, or moxifloxacin are reasonable alternatives. Macrolides are no longer recommended as first-line therapy except as an alternative to amoxicillin alone for mild infections in previously untreated patients

(15). Because of bacterial resistance, there is an increasing likelihood of antibiotic failure. A second class of antibiotics may need to be substituted, or therapy might have to be continued for a longer duration. In complicated, immunocompromised patients, the bacterial source is often atypical and frequently resistant to commonly prescribed antibiotics. Occasionally, broader-spectrum antimicrobials (e.g., imepenam, vancomycin) and antifungals (e.g., amphotericin) are required.

In chronic rhinosinusitis, bacteria are less likely to be cultured. Polymicrobial infections with aerobes and anaerobes are common when cultured. As mentioned previously, *P. aeruginosa*, *S. aureus*, and anaerobic bacteria are isolated frequently. Treatment with antibiotics requires a broader spectrum and a longer duration for cure. For that reason, it has been suggested that antibiotic use in chronic rhinosinusitis be guided by culture results. Treatment should be directed toward coagulase-positive and coagulase-negative *Staphylococcus* and *Streptococcus* species. The current recommendation for therapy for chronic disease is 4 to 6 weeks (*see* Algorithm). Antibiotic choices similar to those used in the treatment of acute rhinosinusitis are appropriate in most cases. Clindamycin or metronidazole may be a reasonable addition to antimicrobial therapy, because a higher percentage of anaerobic bacteria causes chronic rhinosinusitis. Intravenous antibiotics with antipseudomonal therapy (e.g., ceftazidime, ciprofloxacin) also have been used in resistant or recalcitrant chronic rhinosinusitis (12).

Corticosteroid Therapy

Corticosteroid use in the treatment of rhinosinusitis has increased significantly. **Topical nasal corticosteroids** (e.g., beclomethasone, triamcinolone, fluticasone, budesonide) via nasal inhalation has been used routinely for patients with allergic rhinitis, nasal polyps, and rhinosinusitis (Case 10.2). Newer formulations have reduced the dosing of many of these medicines to daily administration. Because of the mechanism of the action of corticosteroids, their effect is gradual over a few days. With maintenance use, the effect continues in the long term. Corticosteroids decrease tissue inflammation and edema and decrease tissue eosinophilia by stabilizing vascular membranes. This reduction in interstitial edema helps to maintain open sinus ostia and decreases the postobstructive sinus infection.

Oral corticosteroids have been used successfully in the treatment of patients with chronic rhinosinusitis and nasal polyposis. They are most effective in treating patients with an allergic component to their rhinosinusitis. Oral corticosteroids must be used with care and caution because of the systemic nature of the dosing and the widespread effects that corticosteroids demonstrate in many organ systems.

> **Case 10.2 Woman with Allergic Rhinitis**
>
> A woman 45 years of age presents with a history of intermittent episodes of sinusitis, requiring treatment with antibiotics for resolution. These used to occur only in the autumn but recently have been occurring more frequently, with five infections during the past year. She is just finishing the antibiotics from her most recent infection. She also has mild asthma and notes increased wheezing whenever she has an infection. Between acute infections, she notes copious watery rhinorrhea, much sneezing, and itchy, watery eyes.
>
> She is started on a nasal steroid spray and a second-generation nonsedating antihistamine combined with an oral decongestant. Six weeks later, her symptoms have improved but are still bothersome. She undergoes testing for inhalant allergies, which shows marked sensitivity to dust mites, several molds, and ragweed.
>
> The patient makes extensive alterations in her home to decrease her environmental exposure to dust mites and molds. She continues on the above medications and is pleased when she returns 4 months later, in December, pointing out that she has gone through an entire fall season without an episode of sinusitis or any asthma flare-ups.

Decongestants

Topical decongestants (e.g., oxymetazoline) are used for the short-term treatment of acute rhinosinusitis. By shrinking the nasal mucosa, decongestants encourage drainage of the sinuses through the natural ostia, allowing purulent secretions to escape and air to enter the sinuses. Pain and pressure are relieved, speeding up symptomatic recovery. Care must be taken to minimize the use of topical decongestants to avoid the rebound phenomenon of rhinitis medicamentosa, in which the nasal mucosa becomes sensitized to the decongestant. Stopping the use of the decongestant results in a rebound phenomenon of increased swelling with increased obstruction. In general, three days of oxymetazoline per acute rhinosinusitis episode is recommended. Systemic decongestants (e.g., pseudoephedrine) also can be used to shrink nasal mucosa and to encourage sinus drainage. The use of these medications is associated infrequently with rebound nasal congestion, and they need to be used cautiously in patients with hypertension or other cardiac disorders (16).

Antihistamines

Systemic antihistamines, although often helpful in allergic rhinosinusitis, may thicken secretions and actually impair the drainage of an acutely infected sinus. Newer formulations of antihistamines (e.g., fexofenadine, loratadine, cetirizine) are less likely to thicken the secretions because of their more selective antihistamine effects. They may provide symptomatic relief in allergic rhinosinusitis. In contrast, mucolytics (e.g., guiafenesin) have been shown to increase vagal stimulation, resulting in increased mucus secretion. Thinner secretions often allow relief of nasal congestion symptoms. Physical maneuvers such as nasal saline irrigations may be helpful in the treatment of rhinosinusitis by assisting in the reduction of congestion and by flushing secretions and irritants out of the nasal cavity.

Topical Nasal Sprays, Topical Cromolyn Sodium, and Antifungal Therapy

Topical nasal sprays that contain the anticholinergic ipratropium bromide have been shown to alleviate nasal congestion by reducing glandular hypersecretion. Although no studies have been performed to evaluate their role in acute rhinosinusitis, their efficacy in reducing symptoms of the common cold suggests they may be a useful adjunctive therapy for the symptoms of rhinosinusitis (12).

Topical cromolyn sodium acts by stabilizing mast cells, reducing degranulation and the release of vasoactive and inflammatory mediators. It has minimal effects in the treatment of acute rhinosinusitis. In allergic rhinitis, it may reduce ostial occlusion and resultant rhinosinusitis by decreasing inflammation and edema of allergic rhinitis.

Antifungal therapy may be used as an adjunct to surgical treatment for fungal infections of the paranasal sinuses. As mentioned previously, acute fungal infections of the paranasal sinuses in immunocompromised patients are surgical emergencies that require prompt intervention to minimize disability and mortality (*see* Chapter 32).

Topical administration of antibiotics has been used by some physicians. Further investigations may indicate whether this form of therapy should be adapted.

Surgical Therapy

Surgical therapy is reserved for patients with recalcitrant disease or complications of acute or chronic infections. The vast majority of sinus surgery now is being performed endoscopically. The major indication is the treatment of chronic rhinosinusitis. The goal of endoscopic sinus surgery is to reverse the anatomical obstruction of the critical drainage patterns of the paranasal sinuses. Attention to the ostiomeatal unit involving the common drainage ports of the anterior ethmoid, frontal, and maxillary sinuses is the key to successful treatment. This can be performed using the surgical endoscopes with minimal risk.

There are **three general techniques** of endoscopic sinus surgery. Each one attempts to maintain the functional drainage of the sinuses; thus, the term *functional endoscopic sinus surgery*. These techniques are tailored to the individual's symptoms and anatomy and range from the most limited of procedures to more extensive resections as dictated by the patient's disease.

With the **minimally invasive approach**, the ostiomeatal complex is opened by removing a small amount of uncinate and ethmoid bulla bone to enlarge the drainage siphon of the ostiomeatal region (17). A slightly more extensive approach is the **Messerklinger approach**, which is based on the knowledge that most rhinosinusitis manifests itself in the anterior ethmoid sinuses. By opening the ostiomeatal complex and the anterior ethmoid sinuses, the vast majority of anatomical obstructions can be relieved.

The most extensive approach to ethmoid sinus surgery is the **Wigand procedure**. In this procedure, the skull base is carefully identified posteriorly in the sphenoid and posterior ethmoid sinuses. Then, using the skull base as a reference point, the ethmoid sinuses are exenterated completely, and the ostia of the maxillary sinuses and nasofrontal region are enlarged. This more extensive approach is used most commonly when the patient has failed other surgical approaches (18). In the United States, a combination of the above procedures is customized for the individual's anatomy and symptom complex.

The introduction of **microdebrider surgical instruments** has greatly aided the surgeon's ability to remove diseased tissue, obstructing bone, and inflammatory polyps with less blood loss and better visualization. Likewise, next-generation **telescopes and video monitors** have increased the resolution of the surgical field during the procedure. Newer advances in sinus surgery include the use of **intraoperative computer-aided and image-guided systems** (9). These are designed to assist in patients who have had previous surgical procedures and, thus, a lack of normal landmarks. They also help in patients with anatomical anomalies.

Septoplasty (i.e., straightening a deviated septum either by removing the deformed cartilage or weakening and resetting the cartilage) is an important adjunct to sinus surgery (Case 10.3). In patients in whom a deviated septum is impinging on the ostiomeatal unit, a septoplasty often dramatically reduces the recurrence of infection, improves the nasal airway, and reduces nasal congestion.

Polypectomy is a procedure in which inflammatory polyps are removed to open the nasal cavity and the paranasal sinuses. Typically, medical management is attempted first, including topical nasal steroids, systemic steroids, antibiotics, and avoidance of the environmental stimulants that are frequently responsible for their development. When the patient's life is affected significantly by the nasal congestion and/or recurrent rhinosinusitis associated with

> **Case 10.3** **Man with Chronic Sinusitis Caused by a Bony-Cartilaginous Spur**
>
> A man 65 years of age presents with a several-year history of facial pressure and nasal obstruction. He carries a presumed diagnosis of chronic sinusitis and currently is being treated with a nasal steroid spray and a second-generation nonsedating antihistamine. His hypertension precludes regular use of an oral decongestant. He reports that the facial pain (which is centered in his medial left cheek, around his left eye, and in the lower midsection of his forehead) is becoming worse, occurring daily, not responding to aspirin or ibuprofen, and seriously interfering with his enjoyment of life. Past allergy testing showed no major inhalant allergies. He is just finishing a course of antibiotics and feels that it has resulted in little improvement.
>
> Nasal endoscopy reveals a septum that is anteriorly straight but contains a major bony-cartilaginous spur just opposite the middle turbinate on the left, pressing the middle turbinate toward the lateral nasal wall. The mucosa on the left side of the nose is mildly inflamed, and scant clear rhinorrhea is present. There are no other abnormalities.
>
> Because the patient has had little symptom relief with aggressive medical therapy, surgical treatment is considered. A full CT scan is obtained, which shows mild mucoperiosteal thickening in the left maxillary and anterior ethmoid sinuses and blockage at the left ostiomeatal complex. The patient undergoes a septoplasty, endoscopic enlargement of the maxillary antral ostium, and opening of the anterior ethmoid cells on the left. Four weeks after surgery, the patient notes that his daily headaches are gone.

polyposis, and the polyps are not responsive to medical management, surgery is frequently indicated. Polypectomy has been made faster and safer by the introduction of the microdebrider. Vigorous postoperative care and monitoring is essential because polyps are prone to recur; postoperative topical steroid use has been helpful in reducing this recurrence. Polyps associated with cystic fibrosis and Sampter's triad (aspirin sensitivity, nasal polyposis, and asthma) are associated with higher recurrence rates (20).

Although usually avoided in the treatment of acute rhinosinusitis, surgical therapy is required occasionally. Acute infection that does not respond to antibiotic therapy may benefit from **maxillary sinus tap and lavage**, which can be performed in the office or at the bedside; however, it often causes significant discomfort. Subperiosteal abscesses or more extensive involvement of the orbits may require surgical drainage either through an endoscopic approach or a more traditional external ethmoidectomy approach. The external ethmoidectomy approach is through a small incision between the medial canthus and the bridge of the nose. Isolated sphenoid rhinosinusitis may present with cranial neuropathies, especially ophthalmoplegia, severe headache, and visual complaints. It requires urgent drainage, which usually can be performed endoscopically. Intracranial extension of rhinosinusitis, whether subdural, epidural, or intraparenchymal, is an indication for urgent evaluation, neurosurgical consultation, and possible surgical intervention.

Chronic infection may result in the development of mucoceles or infected mucoceles (mucopyocele). These, in turn, may result in clinical symptoms due to mass effect or local inflammatory effects. They require drainage, which may be performed through an endoscopic or open approach. Chronic infection that does not respond to appropriate medical therapy may be amenable to endoscopic sinus surgery. Persistent ethmoid disease may require revision surgery through an open approach as previously mentioned.

Chronic frontal sinus disease may require obliteration of the sinus for permanent treatment. Frontal sinus **obliteration** is an operation in which the anterior table of the frontal sinus is removed. The mucosa is stripped and drilled away, and then the sinus is filled with fat to "obliterate" the sinus, rendering it nonfunctional and preventing the recurrence of frontal sinus infection. Although patients may be hesitant to undergo this procedure because of the large scalp incision, it is extremely well tolerated. Another option for frontal sinus disease is the **Lothrop procedure**, in which the anterosuperior septum is resected (either endoscopically or through an external approach) and the frontal ostia are expanded into a single large opening to improve drainage from the frontal sinus.

Maxillary sinus disease that does not respond to endoscopic surgery may require an open approach through a **Caldwell–Luc procedure**, which is an opening in the canine fossa of the anterior maxillary sinus well above the upper tooth roots. Through this approach, diseased mucosa, polyps, or tumors can be biopsied or removed.

All sinus surgery involves risk. The greatest risk is to surrounding structures, including the eye (blindness, diplopia), dura (cerebrospinal fluid leak), brain (encephalopathy), and intracranial vessels (stroke). Anatomical knowledge, preoperative imaging, and direct visualization of the operative field are all essential for safe and effective sinus surgery. Even in the best hands, up to 20% of patients who require sinus surgery may ultimately require reoperation.

Danger Signs

The most frequently encountered problem in the management of rhinosinusitis and facial pain is failure of the patient to improve. In the acute episode, failure to improve may indicate resistant bacteria, fungal disease, extension of the infection, or misdiagnosis. When this occurs, a change of antibiotics, CT imaging of the sinus or head, and nasal endoscopy should be considered. Proptosis may indicate a subperiosteal or orbital abscess that requires intravenous antibiotics and possible surgical drainage. Any change in cranial nerve status (e.g., ophthalmoplegia, anesthesia of the trigeminal nerve, alteration in visual acuity, dysphagia) suggests extension of the infection and mandates urgent imaging and referral. Likewise, change in mental status may indicate intracranial involvement and mandates urgent evaluation and treatment.

Patients with immunosuppression or other medical problems (especially diabetes mellitus) who present with facial pain should be examined carefully for signs of dusky nasal mucosa and fungal rhinosinusitis. Mucosa that is anesthetic on examination may indicate fungal infection. In these patients, acute sinusitis should be treated aggressively because it could progress rapidly through a complicated course. Management of the patient's blood sugar level and immune status is important in controlling the disease. Facial pain that is atypical in presentation should be evaluated for neoplastic involvement of the foramen rotundum and ovale. Additionally, patients with persistent pain and epistaxis should be evaluated carefully for signs of neoplasm within the nasal cavity.

REFERENCES

1. **National Center for Health Statistics.** Data from the National Health Survey, No. 184, Series 10. Vital health statistics. In *Current Estimates from the National Health Interview Survey* Hyattsville, MD: USDHHS, PHS, CDC, and NCHS; 1992. (DHHS publication [PHS] 93-1512.)
2. **Lanza DC, Kennedy DW.** Adult rhinosinusitis defined. *Otolaryngol Head Neck.* 1997:117:S1–11.
3. **Lanza DC, Kennedy DW.** Current concepts in the surgical management of chronic and recurrent acute sinusitis. *J Allergy Clin Immunol.* 1992;90:505–10.
4. **Skaer TL.** Clinical presentation and treatment of migraine. *Clin Ther.* 1996; 18:229–45.
5. **Lund VJ.** Bacterial sinusitis: etiology and surgical management. *Pediatr Infect Dis J.* 1994;:S58–62.
6. **Wagenmann M, Naclerio RM.** Complications of sinusitis. *J Allergy Clin Immunol.* 1992;3:552–4.
7. **Morrison VA, Pomeroy C.** Upper respiratory tract infections in the immunocompromised host. *Semin Respir Infect.* 1995;10:37–50.
8. **Kennedy DW.** Overview. *Otolaryngol Head Neck Surg.* 1990;5:847–54.
9. **Zinreich SJ.** Rhinosinusitis: radiologic diagnosis. *Otolaryngol Head Neck.* 1997;117: S27–34.
10. **Klossek JM, Dubreuil L, Richet H, et al.** Bacteriology of the adult middle meatus. *J Laryngol Otol.* 1996:110:847–9.
11. **Ferguson BJ, Mabry RL.** Laboratory diagnosis. *Otolaryngol Head Neck.* 1997;117: S12–26.

12. **Benninger MS, Anon J, Mabry RL.** The medical management of rhinosinusitis. *Otolaryngol Head Neck.* 1997;117:S41-9.
13. **Brook I.** Microbiology and management of sinusitis. *J Otolaryngol.* 1996;25:249-56.
14. **Baquero F, Loza E.** Antibiotic resistance of microorganisms involved in ear, nose, and throat infections. *Pediatr Infect Dis J.* 1994;1(Suppl 1):S9-14.
15. **Sinus and Allergy Health Partnership.** Antimicrobial treatment guidelines for acute bacterial rhinosinusitis (ABRS). *Otolaryngol Head Neck.* 2000;5(Suppl):S32.
16. **Mabry RL.** Therapeutic agents in the medical management of sinusitis. *Otolaryngol Clin North Am.* 1993;26:561-70.
17. **Setcliff RC.** Minimally invasive sinus surgery: the rationale and the technique. *Otolaryngol Clin North Am.* 1996;1:115-24.
18. **Lusk RP.** Endoscopic approach to sinus disease. *J Allergy Clin Immunol.* 1992;90:496-504.
19. **Metson R, Gliklich RE, Cosenza M.** A comparison of image guidance systems for sinus surgery. *Laryngoscope.* 1998;108:1164-70.
20. **Lanza DC, Kennedy DW.** Current concepts in the surgical management of nasal polyposis. *J Allergy Clin Immunol.* 1992;90:543-5.

SUGGESTED READINGS

Anon J, Mabry RL. The medical management of rhinosinusitis. *Otolaryngol Head Neck.* 1997;117:S41-9.

This article reviews the pathophysiology, microbiology, and natural history of sinusitis. It suggests development of individualized treatment plans based on the variables of symptom duration and severity.

Mabry RL. Therapeutic agents in the medical management of sinusitis. *Otolaryngol Clin North Am.* 1993;26:561-70.

This article reviews the recent developments in pharmacotherapy for treatment of sinusitis. There is an emphasis on the risk-benefit ratio of each medication.

Wagenmann M, Naclerio RM. Complications of sinusitis. *J Allergy Clin Immunol.* 1992;3:552-4.

This review presents the complications of sinusitis. The orbital complications occur primarily in children, can result in permanent visual loss, and require immediate aggressive therapy for satisfactory resolution. Intracranial complications unfortunately often cause few early symptoms. As with orbital infections, early recognition and usually surgical treatment are essential components of successful treatment.

11

Epistaxis

Darryk W. Barlow, MD

Epistaxis is a common and often self-limiting disease that affects men and women equally. Anterior bleeding is most common in young adults. Posterior bleeding (i.e., bleeding that originates in the posterior part of the nasal cavity) is more common in older adults who have associated vascular disease and hypertension. Epistaxis is more common during the winter; it is aggravated by low humidity, upper respiratory infection, and allergy.

Anatomy and Physiology

The nasal cavity is lined with pseudostratified, ciliated, columnar epithelium that is attached firmly to the underlying basement membrane. Specialized olfactory epithelium is found on the superior turbinate, the superior septum, and the cribriform plate. The nasal mucosa is thin, richly vascularized, and well innervated. Mucosal glands provide a protective layer of mucus. Nasal dryness from low humidity or infection causes desiccation, cilia loss, and mucosal injury, with subsequent inflammation, crusting, and bleeding.

The nasal cavity receives its blood supply from branches of the external and internal carotid arteries (Fig. 11.1). The facial and internal maxillary arteries provide the most nasal blood supply. The superior labial artery (a

Epistaxis 203

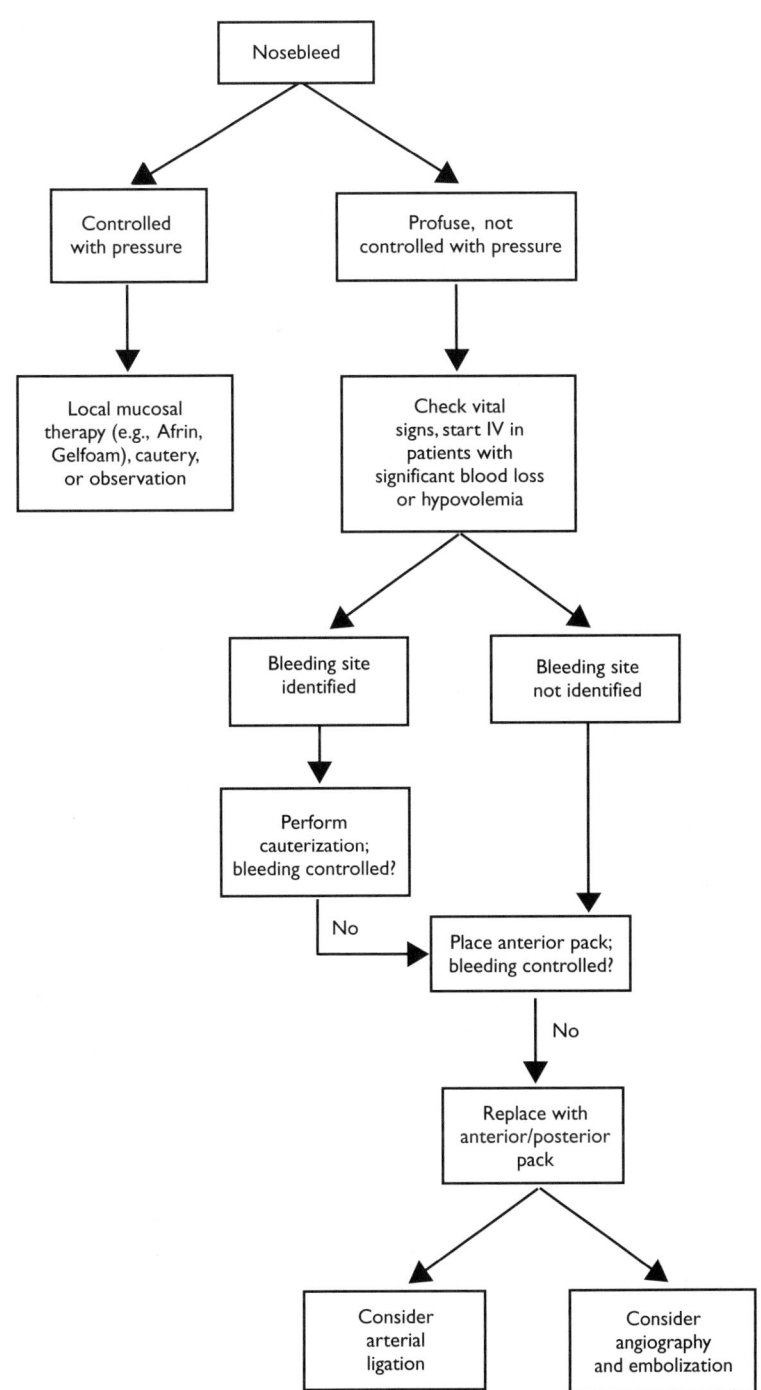

Algorithm Management of epistaxis.

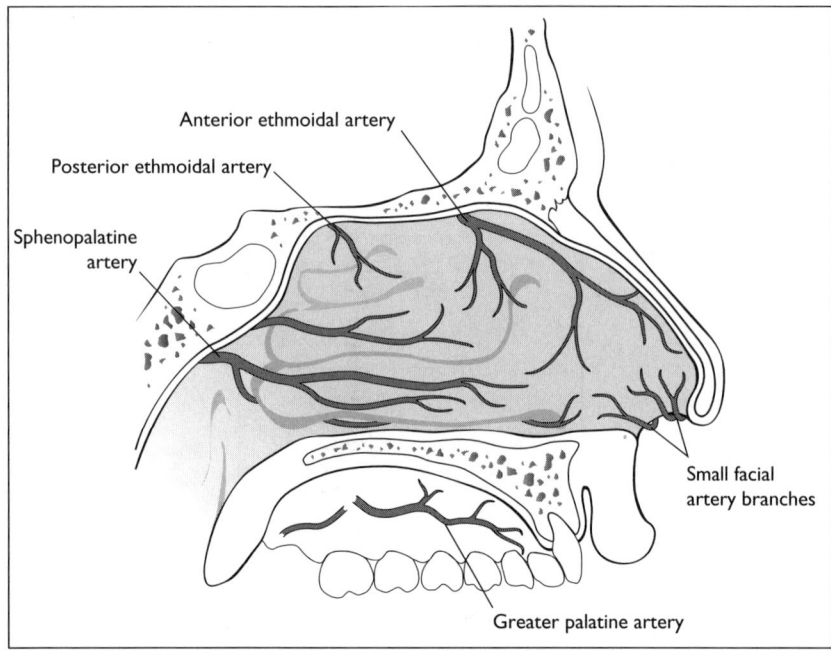

Figure 11.1 Blood supply of the nasal cavity. Both the internal and external carotid systems supply the nasal mucosa.

branch of the facial artery) has a septal branch that supplies the anterior nasal septum and vestibule. An alar branch supplies the nasal ala (Fig. 11.2). The internal maxillary artery supplies the posterior superior alveolar artery, the infraorbital pterygoid canal, and the pharyngeal and descending pharyngeal arteries within the pterygopalatine fossa. It then terminates in the sphenopalatine artery, which enters the posterior nose and divides into septal branches. These arteries are all important sources of epistaxis.

The ophthalmic artery is the first major intracranial branch of the internal carotid artery. It arises at the level of the anterior clinoid process and cavernous sinus. Within the orbit, the ophthalmic artery branches to form the anterior and posterior ethmoid arteries, which course medially and exit the orbit through separate foramina in the lamina papyracea. The larger anterior ethmoid artery supplies the anterior ethmoid air cells, the anterior third of the lateral nasal wall, and the septum. The posterior ethmoid artery supplies the posterior ethmoid cells, superior turbinate, adjacent septum, and anastomoses with sphenopalatine artery branches (Fig. 11.3).

Two areas of the nose are frequently associated with epistaxis. Most anterior epistaxis originates at Kiesselbach's plexus (or Little's area; on the anterior septum at which the branches of the sphenopalatine, anterior ethmoid, and superior labial

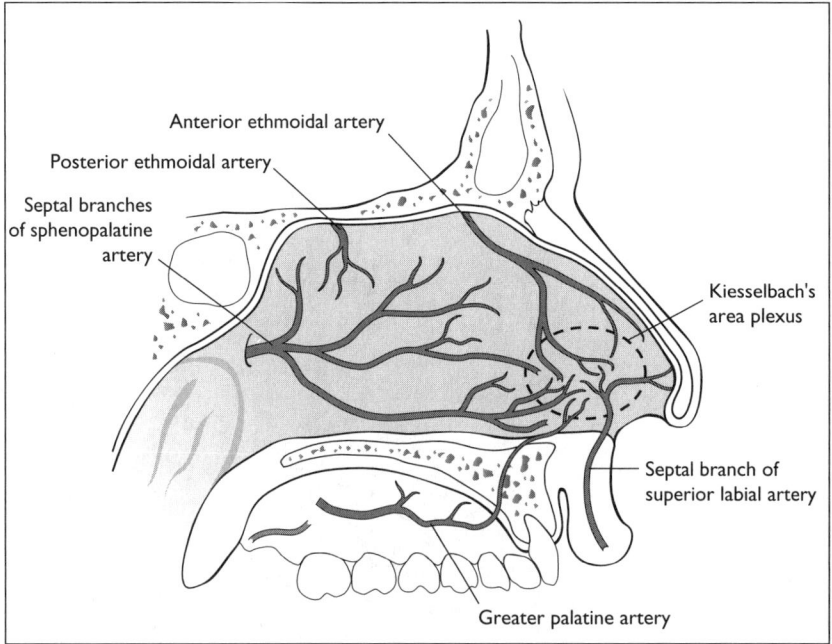

Figure 11.2 Blood supply of the nasal septum.

arteries anastomose). Most posterior bleeding originates at Woodruff's plexus (behind the middle turbinate at which the sphenopalatine artery enters the nose).

History

Severe, active epistaxis requires prompt control of the hemorrhage before thorough questioning. Once the patient is stable, a directed history is obtained. Age, onset of bleeding, amount of blood loss, site (e.g., anterior or posterior; right, left, or bilateral), precipitating factors (e.g., trauma, infection, surgery), previous history of bleeding, other medical problems (e.g., cardiovascular, pulmonary, liver, hematologic), medications (e.g., nonsteroidal anti-inflammatory drugs [NSAIDs], Coumadin), family history of bleeding disorders, and overall general health are all important in determining the cause.

Physical Examination

As with an acute hemorrhagic event, the patient's vital signs and stability should be determined. (*See* the section on Management and Follow-Up for

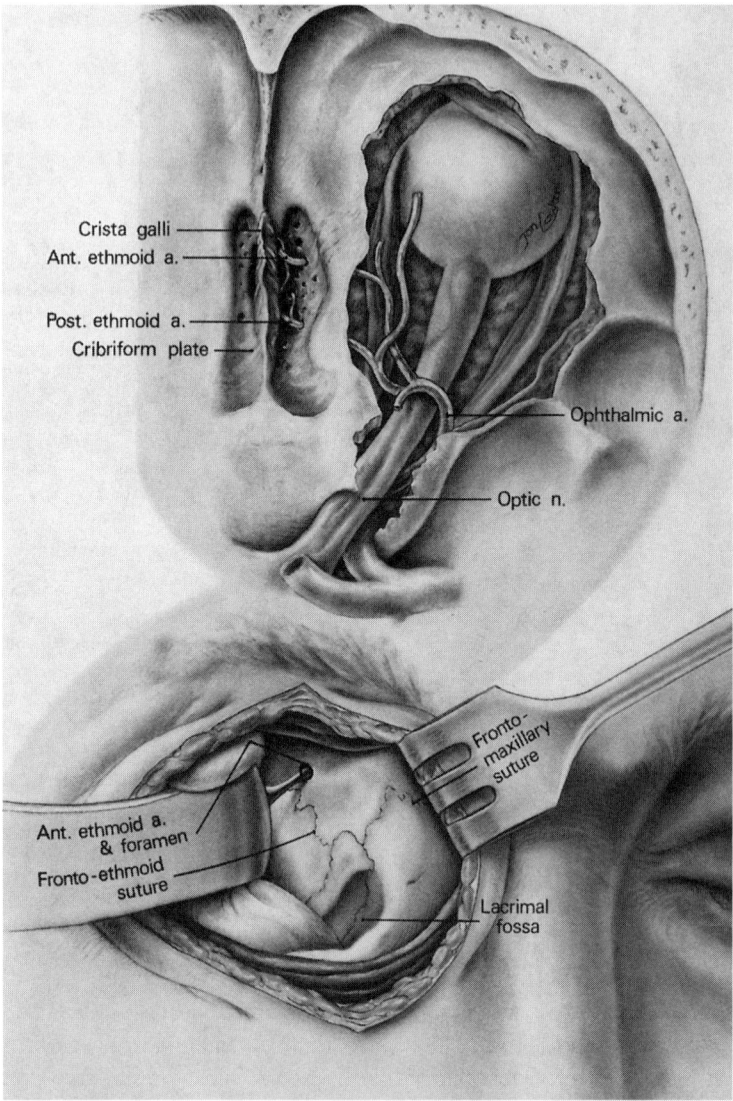

Figure 11.3 Top, View of the orbit from above after removal of the bony roof. **Bottom,** The approach for ligation of the ethmoid arteries. (Republished with permission from American Academy of Otolaryngology–Head and Neck Surgery.)

how to proceed if the patient is hemodynamically unstable.) To determine the site of the bleeding, proper preparation is important. The patient should be gowned and made comfortable. The physician and assistant must follow universal body-fluid precautions, including wearing gloves, gowns, masks, caps, and eye protection. Necessary ancillary equipment includes adequate lighting (a quality headlight frees up both hands), nasal speculum, Yankauer suction, Frazer-tip suction (#10-12), tongue depressors, bayonet forceps, local anesthetic (e.g., 1% lidocaine with 1:100,000 epinephrine) and a topical vasoconstrictor and anesthetic (e.g., oxymetazoline plus lidocaine, tetracaine, or cocaine). Anesthetic and vasoconstrictive agents are soaked on cotton pledgets (1 cm x 3 cm) (Fig. 11.4).

A complete head and neck examination is performed; then the nose is examined. Inform the patient that your examination may cause the bleeding to begin again due to the removal of the blood clot or mucus crust. If the nasal cavity is occluded with blood clot, have the patient forcefully blow his or her nose into a handful of tissue. Carefully evaluate the nasal cavity for the site of bleeding, infection, trauma, septal deviation, perforation, tumor, or other abnormality. Active bleeding and mucosal edema can obstruct visualization. Topical vasoconstriction and anesthesia can be obtained with pledgets soaked in oxymetazoline plus 4% lidocaine or 4% cocaine. Vital signs should be monitored carefully. The pledgets are placed along the nasal floor, septum, and superior nasal vault bilaterally. After 5 to 7 minutes, remove the pledgets and reevaluate. Successful management depends on identifying the bleeding site.

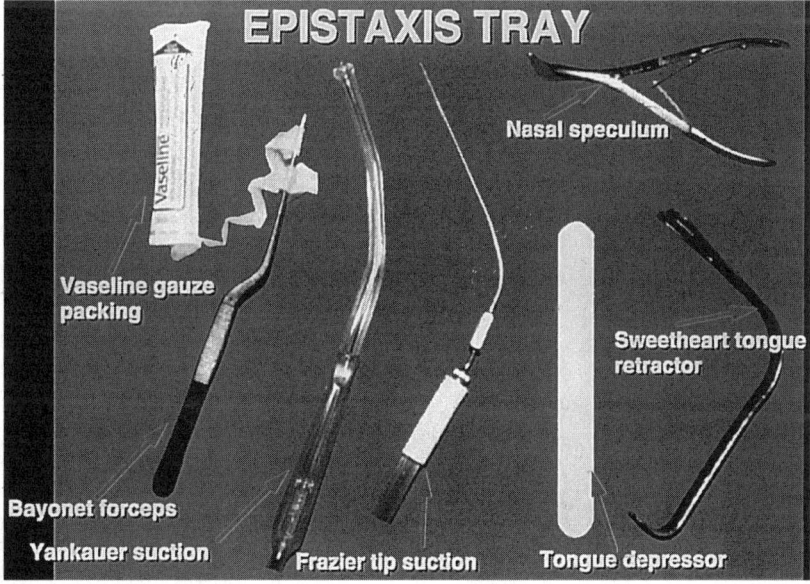

Figure 11.4 Some of the basic instruments required for treating epistaxis. (Republished with permission from Chin KN, Kennedy DW. *Epistaxis*. Alexandria, VA: American Academy of Otolaryngology–Head and Neck Surgery; 1998.)

Additional Diagnostic Evaluation

A self-limited, isolated episode of bleeding is usually just that, and an extensive work-up to determine the exact cause is not indicated. Severe or recurrent epistaxis warrants a systematic search for the cause (Case 11.1). A complete blood count is obtained in patients with severe or recurrent bleeding to assess anemia, platelet count, or other abnormalities. Depending on the degree of hemorrhage, serial hematocrit determinations are indicated. If there is evidence of a coagulopathy, a coagulation profile (i.e., prothrombin time, partial thromboplastin time, and fibrinogen level) is indicated. The usefulness of a bleeding time is controversial. Facial or sinus radiographic studies are helpful in selected cases of facial trauma, infection, or suspected neoplasm. Paranasal sinus computed tomography or magnetic resonance imaging is indicated if a tumor is identified or suspected (Fig. 11.5).

Case 11.1 Man with Long-Standing Hypertension Who Has Recurrent Epistaxis

A man 63 years of age has a 3-week history of intermittent epistaxis occurring from both nostrils, and it seems to him to be getting worse. He had an episode the previous night that he describes as having "blood all over the place." It took approximately 20 minutes for the bleeding to stop. You discuss the weather with him, noting that it is colder earlier than usual this year and that most people had to start using their furnaces about a month ago. The remainder of his history is normal, except for long-standing, well-controlled hypertension.

Anterior speculum examination reveals prominent small vessels on the anterior septum bilaterally. To minimize the chance of developing a septal perforation, you cauterize only the right side (last night's bleeding came from this side; also, the vessels look bigger). After additional topical anesthesia, you use a silver-nitrate stick to cauterize the area. You instruct the patient to use a topical antibiotic ointment at the entry of his nostril twice per day.

You explain to the patient that the forced dry air in his house's heating system is probably responsible for the drying in his nasal mucosa. You recommend the use of a bedside vaporizer during the night, if not a humidifier for the whole house.

He returns for follow-up 2 weeks later. He has had just one or two short episodes of epistaxis, both on the right side. Your examination reveals well-healed mucosa on the right and unchanged prominent vessels on the left anterior septum. You anesthetize and cauterize these without difficulty.

Phone follow-up a month later reveals that his new humidifier is working well and that he has had no further problems with epistaxis.

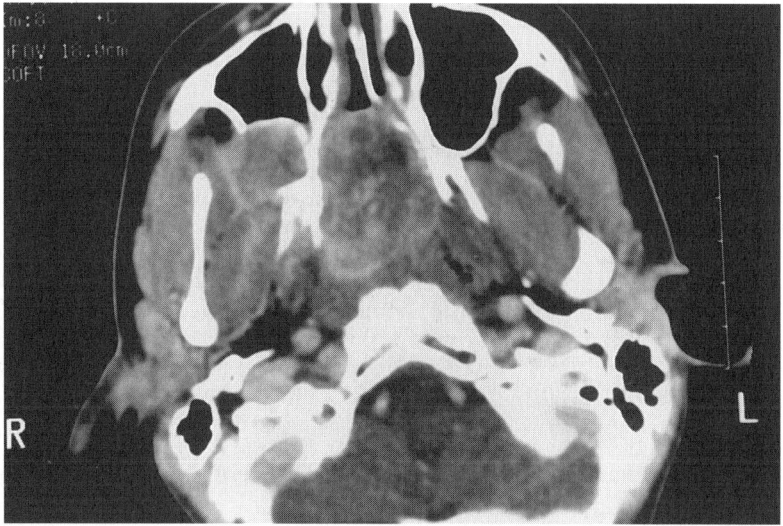

Figure 11.5 Computed tomography scan showing an angiofibroma that occupies part of the nasal vault. These tumors occur in adolescent males and present with unilateral nasal obstruction and epistaxis. (Courtesy of Dr. Christopher Rassekh.)

Differential Diagnosis

The local and systemic causes of epistaxis (Table 11.1) are discussed below.

Local Causes

Direct trauma to the nose, with or without nasal bone or septal fracture, can lacerate the mucosa. The resulting bleeding is usually anterior and self-limiting. Extensive facial and skull-base fractures can be accompanied by severe epistaxis, which can be difficult to control. Digital trauma, or "picking" the nose, is also a frequent cause, even in adults. Other traumatic local causes of epistaxis are frequent sneezing or hard nose-blowing.

Upper respiratory infections, sinusitis, and allergy can cause mucosal inflammation, dryness, crusting, and bleeding. Environmental irritants, volatile chemicals, cocaine, and topical vasoconstrictors can cause epistaxis. Anatomic defects (acquired or congenital) can cause turbulent airflow and subsequent mucosal irritation and hemorrhage. Septal perforations are frequently accompanied by inflammation, crusting, and bleeding. Postoperative epistaxis is a complication of septoplasty, rhinoplasty, repair of nasal or facial fractures, and sinus surgery.

Unilateral obstruction, odoriferous purulent rhinorrhea, and epistaxis often are due to a nasal foreign body. This is most common in adult mentally

Table 11.1 Causes of Epistaxis

Local	Systemic
Trauma (e.g, fracture, digital [nose-picking], nose plugs)	Arteriosclerosis
	Hypertension
Infection or inflammation	Drugs (NSAIDs, anticoagulants)
Surgery	Blood dyscrasias
Septal deformity	Systemic toxic (heavy metals)
Foreign body	Hereditary hemorrhagic telangiectasia (Osler–Weber–Rendu disease)
Toxic chemical	
Neoplasm	Alcohol and tobacco use
Granulomatous disease	Idiopathy

NSAIDs = nonsteroidal anti-inflammatory drugs.

handicapped patients and in young children (2–5 years of age). Batteries and organic material should be removed promptly.

Nasal cavity tumors can present with unilateral symptoms of obstruction and with purulent or bloody drainage (Case 11.2). Common sinonasal tumors include inverted papilloma, hemangioma, adenoid cystic carcinoma, squamous cell carcinoma, melanoma, and nasopharyngeal carcinoma. Severe or posterior bleeding in adolescent boys can result from juvenile nasopharyngeal angiofibroma. Diffuse crusting, friable granulation tissue, and septal perforation are clinical signs of granulomatous disorders. Wegener's granulomatosis, sarcoidosis, tuberculosis, and syphilis can present with epistaxis. Diagnosis requires a high index of suspicion.

Systemic Causes

Atherosclerotic changes and hypertension are frequently associated with epistaxis in the elderly (Case 11.3). With aging, vessel walls become less elastic, resulting in poor vasoconstriction and, thus, bleeding that can be severe and persistent. Coagulopathies are another cause of epistaxis. A history of easy bruising, severe bleeding from minor trauma, or a family history of a bleeding disorder warrants further investigation. Hereditary diseases include several forms of hemophilia and von Willebrand's disease. Epistaxis also can occur with alcoholism, chronic liver disease, immunodeficiency, thrombocytopenia, and other lymphoproliferative disorders.

Blood-clotting abnormalities are major side effects of medications such as NSAIDs, Coumadin, heparin, chloramphenicol, carbenicillin, and dipyridamole. Hereditary hemorrhagic telangiectasia (Osler–Weber–Rendu disease) is an autosomal-dominant disorder with characteristic cherry-red telangiectasias throughout the mucosal and cutaneous surfaces of the body. In

Case 11.2 — Teenage Boy with Juvenile Nasal Angiofibroma Manifested as Epistaxis

A boy 13 years of age is brought to you by his parents. They are very concerned about the two bad nosebleeds he has had over the past several weeks. Each episode took them several hours to control, and they almost made a trip to the emergency room with the last one (2 days ago). Both nosebleeds were primarily from the left nostril, although some blood seemed to come from the right nostril, too, during the last episode. The rest of the boy's history is unremarkable.

After a basic head and neck examination, you anesthetize the boy's nose and examine his nasal cavities with a rigid endoscope. You find a large reddish-brown mass filling the posterior nasal cavity on the left. You ask him how he could possibly breathe on that side, and he says, "Doc, I haven't gotten a good breath of air through that side of my nose in more than a year." On the right side, you think there is a similar mass at the posterior edge of the septum.

Computed tomography shows a highly vascular mass filling the left nasal vault and approximately one third of the nasopharynx. Arteriography is consistent with a juvenile nasal angiofibroma and shows no intracranial extension. The interventional radiologist successfully carries out embolization of the feeding vessels. The next day, the patient is taken to the operating room, where a transpalatal approach to the tumor is undertaken. The tumor is resected with a total blood loss for the entire procedure of less than 600 cm^3. The patient's postoperative recovery is uneventful.

Case 11.3 — Elderly Woman with Hypertension with Profuse Active Epistaxis

You are called by the local emergency department physician about a woman 76 years of age whose epistaxis he cannot control. He has intravenous fluid in place, is running lactated Ringers' solution, and is waiting for the hematocrit results. He also has requested typing and screening for two units of packed red blood cells.

When you get to the emergency department, you discover a frail, frightened patient, actively bleeding from both nostrils. She has a long history of hypertension that has been well controlled but has had gastroenteritis for the past week or so and thinks she vomited up most of the pills as soon as she took them. Her blood pressure is now 220/130, and her internist is also in the emergency department working on controlling her blood pressure.

After placing an anterior and posterior pack, you admit the patient to the hospital, assigning her supplemental oxygen, hydration, antibiotics, mild sedation, and bed rest. Two days later, she has had no further bleeding. In the treatment room, you slowly remove the packing. Endoscopic examination of her nose shows only mild mucosal irritation. After a half-day of observation, she is discharged. Follow-up in your office a week later shows well-controlled blood pressure and no further bleeding.

this disease, the vessel walls lack muscular contractile elements, resulting in structural weakness and the development of arteriovenous fistulae. Patients typically present after puberty with recurrent spontaneous epistaxis. The severity is due to lack of muscular elements that promote vasoconstriction in the vessel wall (4).

Ten percent of epistaxis is idiopathic, with no specific cause ever having been determined despite extensive evaluation.

Management and Follow-Up

Successful management of epistaxis requires an organized approach. Epistaxis can be frightening; the stress response often results in elevated blood pressure and increased bleeding. Be calm and reassure the patient.

Vital signs should be monitored closely. Patients with significant blood loss, active bleeding, or signs of hypovolemia require intravenous-fluid resuscitation with lactated Ringer's solution. The hematocrit should be checked. Blood that is typed and screened or cross-matched early in the course of epistaxis ensures readiness of suitable blood if transfusion is required. Supplemental oxygen and electrocardiography monitoring are indicated in patients with signs or symptoms of hypoxia or a history of coronary artery disease.

Nasal bleeding can be classified by the bleeding site. Fortunately, in most cases, the bleeding site is anterior and responds to conservative treatment. Severe epistaxis, usually posterior in origin, is potentially life threatening.

Treatment of anterior epistaxis is begun with topical vasoconstriction. Topical medication (e.g., Afrin) can stop many mild nosebleeds. It can be sprayed either directly into the nose or onto a cotton ball (until saturation) that is then placed in the nostril. In either case, the nostril is pinched shut firmly and held for 5 to 10 minutes.

Identifying and treating an underlying cause of epistaxis can prevent bleeding or make it easier to control. Treatment of uncontrolled hypertension diminishes the chances of troublesome epistaxis. Epistaxis can be anticipated in patients on Coumadin, heparin, or other blood thinners. Epistaxis is more prevalent in the winter months when dry, heated, indoor air can desiccate the nasal mucosa. Prophylactic use of nasal saline spray or gel and indoor humidification can prevent nosebleeds.

Isolated, minor bleeding (most commonly from Kiesselbach's plexus on the anterior septum) can be controlled with silver-nitrate–stick chemical cautery. Alternately, a hand-made cotton applicator (i.e., a small amount of cotton wrapped around a small metal probe) can be used to apply phenol (88%–100%). Chemical cautery requires a dry field and does not work on an actively bleeding vessel (5). Application of cautery to similar places on both sides of the septum can compromise the blood supply to the cartilage in between, possibly resulting in a septal perforation.

If the bleeding continues, endoscopy may identify a specific source located more posteriorly in the nose that can be cauterized.

Follow-up includes antibiotic ointment (e.g., Bactroban, Bacitracin) that is applied liberally in the nostrils at least three times per day. Frequent use of saline nasal spray and home humidification is helpful for dry, irritated mucosa. The patient is instructed to avoid hard nose-blowing and to sneeze with the mouth open to prevent dislodging a healing crust.

Electrocautery is helpful with a larger bleeding vessel seen most commonly with **posterior epistaxis**. This requires specialized equipment and deep local or general anesthesia (6) (Fig. 11.6).

If the bleeding cannot be controlled with cautery or if the site cannot be identified, then an anterior nasal pack may be required (Fig. 11.7). Various packing materials are available. Dissolvable packing such as oxidized cellulose (e.g., Surgicel, Oxycel), microfibrillar collagen (e.g., Avatene), or absorbable gelatin sponge (e.g., Gelfoam) does not require removal. This is especially useful in anxious patients or in those with coagulopathy in which packing removal can cause mucosal injury and restart the bleeding. Treatment should be individualized to the patient.

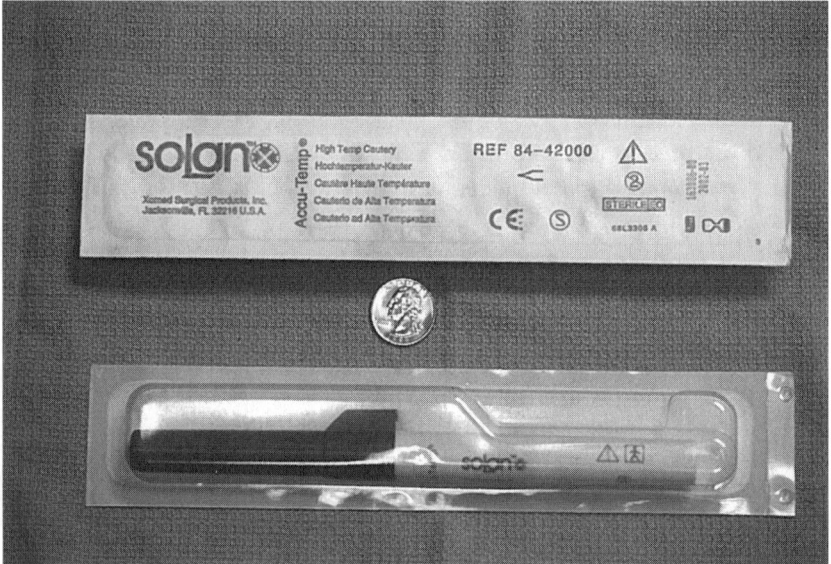

Figure 11.6 A disposable electrocautery unit can be very helpful in treating epistaxis. The nasal mucosa must be anesthetized before use.

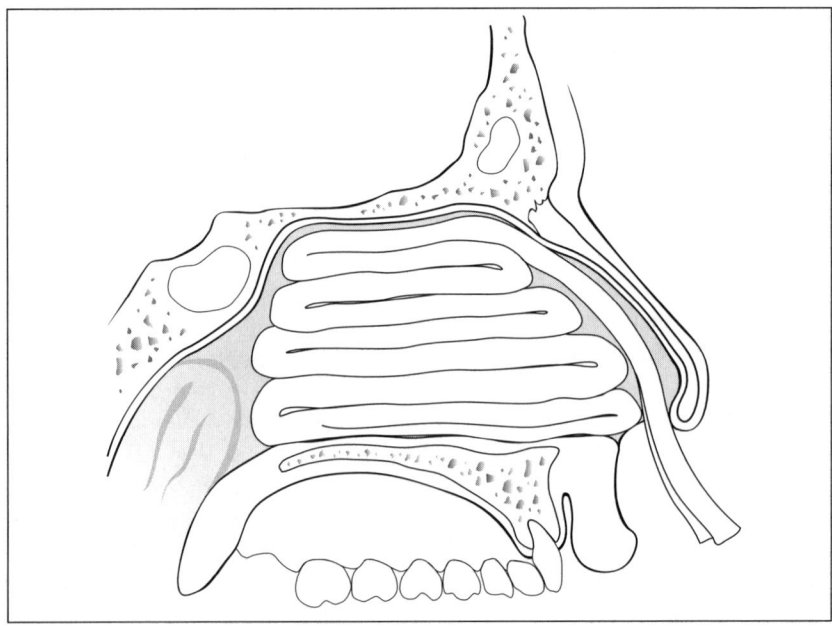

Figure 11.7 Traditional anterior pack, with layer upon layer of Vaseline-impregnated gauze, filling the anterior nasal vault.

Expanded methylcellulose nasal tampons come in various sizes and shapes and are useful if the pack can be placed directly against the bleeding site. After placement in the nose, the rigid pack is expanded with saline, 1% lidocaine with 1:100,000 epinephrine, or oxymetazoline (e.g., Afrin) that has been dripped onto the sponge to provide additional vasoconstriction and anesthesia. In patients with a septal spur, it may be less traumatic to insert the pack after expansion (7).

Petroleum-jelly strip gauze (1.5 in x 72 in) is effective if placed properly. Coated with antibiotic ointment (e.g., Bactroban, Bacitracin) before insertion, the gauze is placed with direct vision and is layered from the nasal floor to the superior nasal vault. Care should be taken not to injure the septal or turbinate mucosa. The quality of placement is more important than the quantity of packing used—regardless of the material, a poorly placed pack does not stop bleeding. Patients with packing usually receive broad-spectrum oral antibiotics to prevent sinusitis and potentially reduce the chance of toxic shock syndrome, which can result from toxin-producing *Staphylococcus aureus* (8). Nasal packing is painful, and analgesic medication is often required.

Stable patients can be discharged. Patients with significant anemia, poor control of other medical conditions (e.g., hypertension, cardiovascular disease), or no assistance at home (especially frail, elderly patients) should be admitted for observation. Limited physical activity and stress avoidance are important in preventing recurrent bleeding. Aspirin or NSAID use should be discontinued until the site of bleeding has healed completely.

The nasal packing should be removed in 3 to 7 days, depending on the patient, and the nasal cavity should be reexamined.

Posterior epistaxis is often severe and usually cannot be controlled with anterior nasal packing. Treatment options include the following (Figs. 11.8 and 11.9; *see also* Fig. 11.3):

1. Traditional anterior/posterior nasal pack (tonsil pack placed in the nasopharynx in combination with an anterior strip-gauze pack)
2. Inflatable balloon pack (#12-16 French Foley catheter with 30-cm^3 balloon, a double-balloon device, or expanded methylcellulose anterior/posterior pack)
3. Endoscopic cautery
4. Surgical ligation of the internal maxillary, anterior ethmoid, and/or posterior ethmoid arteries
5. Angiographic embolization

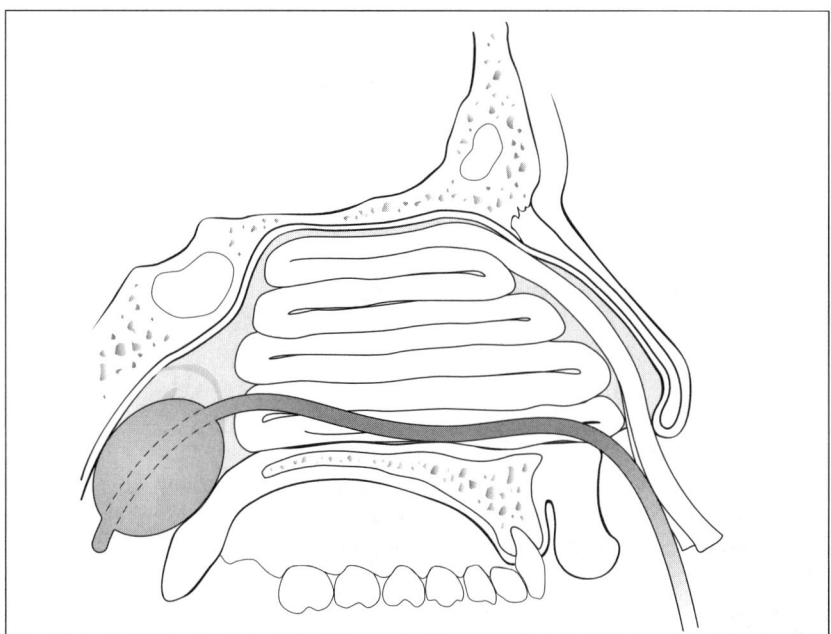

Figure 11.8 The traditional posterior pack is placed in the nasopharynx, providing a firm structure against which gauze packing in the posterior nasal vault can be applied.

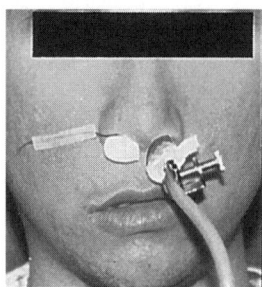

Figure 11.9 Patient with a posterior pack in place. (Republished with permission from Chin KN, Kennedy DW. *Epistaxis*. Alexandria, VA: American Academy of Otolaryngology Head and Neck Surgery.)

Controversy exists over which treatment is more effective and in what order they should be performed. Each technique has potentially serious complications. Please refer to the referenced articles for descriptions of each technique (6,9–17).

The Algorithm outlines the management of epistaxis.

Danger Signs

Epistaxis is potentially life threatening. Patients with a history of a large amount of blood loss, profuse active bleeding, or both need immediate intervention (*see* Case 11.3). Vital signs should be monitored closely. Signs of hypovolemia include tachycardia, hypotension, tachypnea, and agitation. Patients with these signs require prompt intravenous-fluid resuscitation with lactated Ringer's solution. Blood should be typed and cross-matched because a transfusion may be required if hemorrhaging becomes severe. Hypoxia is treated with supplemental oxygen, and electrocardiograph monitoring is used in patients with coronary artery disease.

Patients who present with anemia (i.e., hematocrit < 38%) or a posterior bleeding site or who require a blood transfusion are more likely to need **surgical intervention** for management (9).

REFERENCES

1. **Montgomery W.** Surgery of the nose. In Montgomery W (ed). *Surgery of the Upper Respiratory System*, vol. 1, 2nd ed. Philadelphia: Lea & Febiger; 1989:321.
2. **Lepore M.** Epistaxis. In Bailey BJ (ed). *Head and Neck Surgery–Otolaryngology*, vol. 1, 1st ed. Philadelphia: JB Lippincott; 1993:428–45.
3. **Abelson T.** Epistaxis. In Paparella MM, Shumrick DA, Gluckman JL, Meyerhoff WL (eds). *Otolaryngology*, vol. 3, 3rd ed. Philadelphia: WB Saunders; 1991:1831–40.
4. **Haye R, Austad J.** Hereditary hemorrhagic teleangiectasia–argon laser. *Rhinology*. 1991;29:5–9.
5. **Toner JG, Walby AP.** Comparison of electro- and chemical cautery in the treatment of anterior epistaxis. *J Laryngol Otol.* 1990;104:617–8.

6. **O'Leary-Stickney K, Makielski K, Weymuller EA Jr.** Rigid endoscopy for the control of epistaxis. *Arch Otolaryngol Head Neck Surg.* 1992;118:966–7.
7. **Pringle MB, Beasley P, Brightwell AP.** The use of Merocel nasal packs in the treatment of epistaxis. *J Laryngol Otol.* 1996;110:543–6.
8. **Jones J, MacRae DL.** Toxic shock syndrome. *J Otolaryngol.* 1990;19:211–3.
9. **Barlow DW, Deleyiannis WB, Pinczower EF.** Effectiveness of surgical management of epistaxis at a tertiary care center. *Laryngoscope.* 1997;107:21–4.
10. **Spafford P, Durham JS.** Epistaxis: efficacy of arterial ligation and long-term outcome. *J Otolaryngol.* 1992;21:252–6.
11. **Singh B.** Combined internal maxillary and anterior ethmoidal arterial occlusion: the treatment of choice in intractable epistaxis. *J Laryngol Otol.* 1992;106:507–10.
12. **Elden L, Montanera W, Terbrugge K, et al.** Angiographic embolization for the treatment of epistaxis: a review of 108 cases. *Otolaryngol Head Neck Surg.* 1994;111:44–50.
13. **McFerran DJ, Edmonds SE.** The use of balloon catheters in the treatment of epistaxis. *J Laryngol Otol.* 1993;107:197–200.
14. **Montgomery W, Reardon E.** Early vessel ligation for control of severe epistaxis. In Snow J (ed). *Controversies in Otolaryngology.* Philadelphia, PA: WB Saunders; 1980:315–9.
15. **Ward P.** Routine ligation of the internal maxillary artery is unwarranted. In Snow J (ed). *Controversies in Otolaryngology.* Philadelphia, PA: WB Saunders; 1980:320–6.
16. **Wang L, Vogel D.** Posterior epistaxis: comparison of treatment. *Otolaryngol Head Neck Surg.* 1981;89:1001–6.
17. **Cannon CR.** Effective treatment protocol for posterior epistaxis: a 10-year experience. *Otolaryngol Head Neck Surg.* 1993;109:722–5.

SUGGESTED READINGS

O'Reilley BJ, Simpson DC, Dharmeratnam R. Recurrent epistaxis and nasal septal deviation in young adults. *Clin Otolaryngol.* 1997;21:12–4.

This article determines that epistaxis often occurs on the side toward which a septum is deviated, possibly due to turbulent airflow patterns and mucosal drying.

Srinivases V, Patel H, John DG, Worsley A. Warfarin and epistaxis: Should warfarin always be discontinued? *Clin Otolaryngol.* 1997;22:542–5.

This article concludes that, with appropriate treatment of epistaxis and maintenance of the INR within the therapeutic range, discontinuation of anticoagulants because of epistaxis is rarely needed.

Viducich RA, Blanda MP, Gerson LW. Posterior epistaxis: clinical features and acute complications. *Ann Emerg Med.* 1995;25:592–6.

This article provides an excellent summary of the complications that occur with posterior epistaxis and its treatment.

12

Nasal Fractures

J. David Kriet, MD
Craig S. Murakami, MD

The prominent position of the nose as the most anterior structure of the mid-face makes it one of the most commonly injured facial structures. Fractures of the nasal skeleton typically result from altercations, sporting injuries, and motor vehicle accidents. Because associated injuries may be present, a thorough evaluation of the patient with nasal injuries is necessary. Additionally, because some of these patients become involved in lawsuits, accurate, detailed documentation is important.

Anatomy and Physiology

The superior one third of the nose is composed of paired nasal bones superiorly. The lower two thirds of the nasal skeleton is formed by the paired upper lateral and lower lateral (or alar) cartilages. The lateral nasal wall includes the ascending or nasal process of the maxilla. Additional internal support is provided by the nasal septum, which is formed anteriorly by the quadrangular cartilage, posterosuperiorly by the perpendicular plate of the ethmoid, posteroinferiorly by the vomer, and inferiorly by the maxillary crest. Nasal fractures may involve either the bony or cartilage structure of the nasal framework and are classified as either displaced or nondisplaced based on the degree of movement at the fracture site (Fig. 12.1). The degree of displacement correlates with the amount of force sustained at the time of the injury.

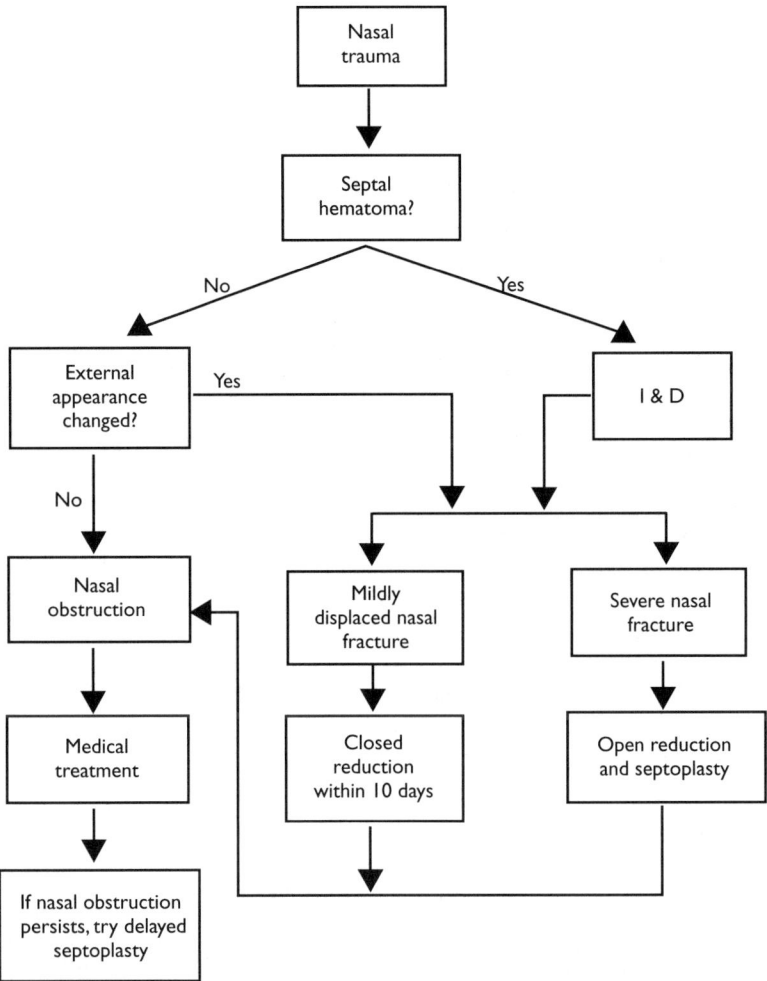

Algorithm Management of nasal trauma. I&D = inclusion and drainage.

History

The patient usually presents with pain and swelling after a blow to the nose or face. The swelling continues to evolve and increases over the next 24 to 48 hours. Epistaxis usually occurs at the time of injury, resolving spontaneously or with direct pressure. **Epistaxis can be life threatening**, however, and may require nasal packing or surgery to control the hemorrhage (*see* Chapter 11).

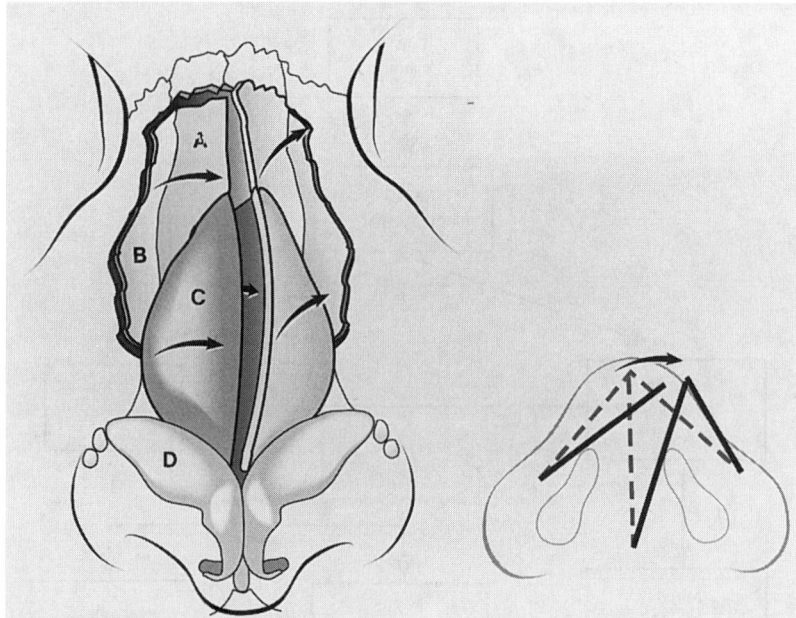

Figure 12.1 Frontal and base views of nasal fracture that is displacing bony and cartilaginous framework to the left. Arrows indicate direction of force. A = nasal bone; B = ascending process of maxilla; C = upper lateral cartilage; D = lower lateral cartilage.

The patient should be questioned about the mechanism of injury, loss of consciousness, change in visual acuity, and diplopia. Watery rhinorrhea could signal a leak of cerebrospinal fluid (CSF). Mild nasal congestion is common after a nasal fracture. Total nasal obstruction, however, is unusual and may indicate an associated severe fracture of the septum or a septal hematoma. If the patient presents days or weeks after an injury with fever, chills, and increasing nasal pain or swelling, be suspicious of a septal abscess, which ultimately causes permanent destruction of the nasal cartilaginous support (saddle-nose deformity). Rarely, a septal abscess can lead to life-threatening complications, including meningitis, cerebral abscess, subarachnoid empyema, and cavernous sinus thrombosis. Always inquire about tetanus immunization status.

Inquire also about subjective malocclusion or numbness of the face or teeth; if present, this suggests maxillary fractures. Finally, ask the patient whether the appearance of his or her nose has been altered by the trauma. A comparison with a preinjury photograph or driver's license picture is often helpful.

Physical Examination

Examination begins with a general head and neck examination to detect associated or more serious injuries (*see also* Chapter 26). Inspect and palpate the facial skeleton, noting any bony step-off, ecchymoses, or lacerations (Fig. 12.2). Because of the close proximity of the nose to the eyes, a basic **eye examination** should be performed. Visual acuity is assessed using a finger count as a minimum and, if any abnormal visual findings are present, a near card or Snellen chart. A **hyphema** or **corneal injury** can be recognized while assessing pupillary size, shape, and response. Management by referral to an ophthalmologist of these ocular emergencies takes precedence over treating the nasal fracture. **Extraocular motility** may be restricted with an associated orbital fracture. Similarly, traumatic **telecanthus** can be seen with a naso-orbitoethmoid fracture (Fig. 12.3). Palpate the upper dental, mid-face, and malar regions and inspect the patient's occlusion to avoid missing a mid-face fracture.

A focused **nasal examination** should be performed. Inspection of the external nose reveals any swelling, lacerations, ecchymoses, depression, deviation, or instability. Palpation of the nasal skeleton may reveal point tenderness or bony crepitus at the fracture site. Any laceration should be inspected for exposed cartilage or bone (Fig. 12.4). Viewing the nose from below and looking up into the nostrils may reveal a displacement or distortion of the nasal tip.

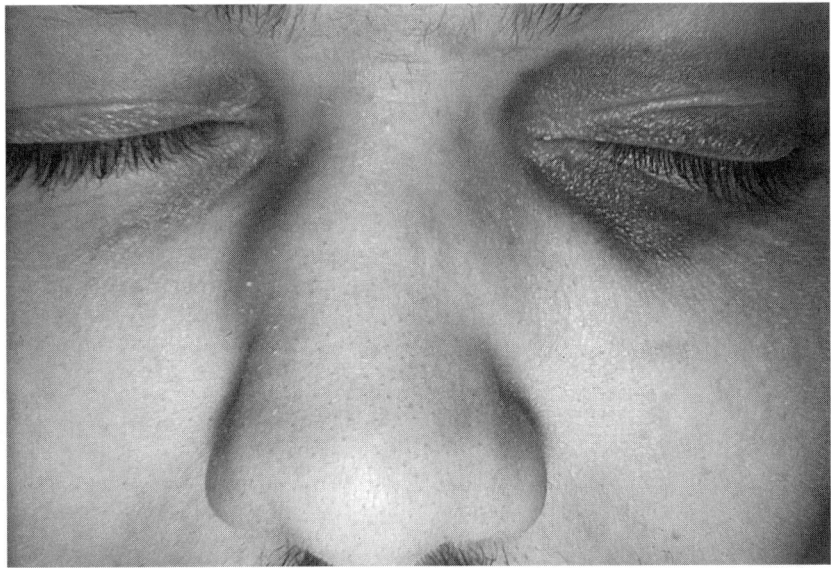

Figure 12.2 A patient with an acute nasal fracture, showing swelling and ecchymosis. (Courtesy of Dr. David E. Eibling.)

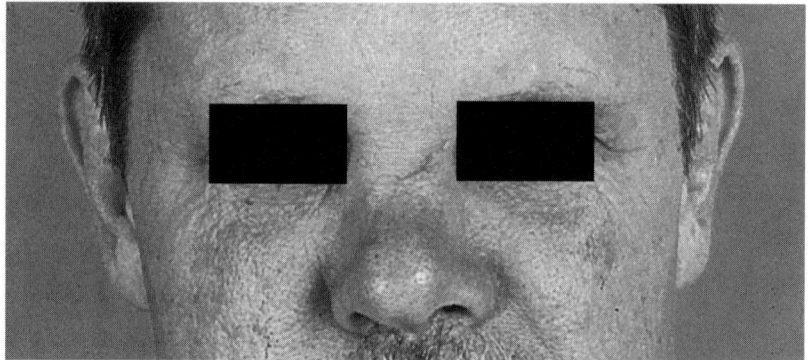

Figure 12.3 Increased intercanthal distance typical of traumatic telecanthus. (Courtesy of Dr. Karen H. Calhoun.)

Visualize the nasal cavity with a nasal speculum and head mirror (or headlight). Note any nostril asymmetry, displacement of the caudal septum, or obvious obstruction or septal deviation. Decongest the nostrils with oxymetazoline or phenylephrine (Neo-Synephrine) and repeat the examination after waiting an adequate time for the medication to take effect (usually 5 minutes is sufficient). In addition to providing increased visualization of the intranasal structures, the decongestant helps decrease any minor epistaxis present. Of utmost importance is the inspection of the nasal septum. The shearing forces associated with the nasal injury may be sufficient to strip the mucoperichondrial attachments from the underlying septum. This can result in a submucoperichondrial septal hematoma. Septal hematomas are most common in children and may occur in the absence of a bony nasal fracture (Fig. 12.5). A septal hematoma is manifested by a swollen or thickened nasal septum that feels boggy when palpated with a cotton-tip applicator. The hematoma devascularizes the cartilaginous septum, eventually resulting in resorption of cartilage. This loss of septal support leads to a saddle-nose deformity (Fig. 12.6). The differential diagnosis of nasal fractures is shown in Table 12.1.

Additional Diagnostic Evaluation

Nasal radiographs are often obtained in the emergency department setting. Although they may demonstrate a fracture, nasal radiographs provide little additional information over that which can be obtained through careful history and physical examination. The radiographs certainly do not assist in treatment planning. Conventional radiographs have been advocated for medicolegal docu-

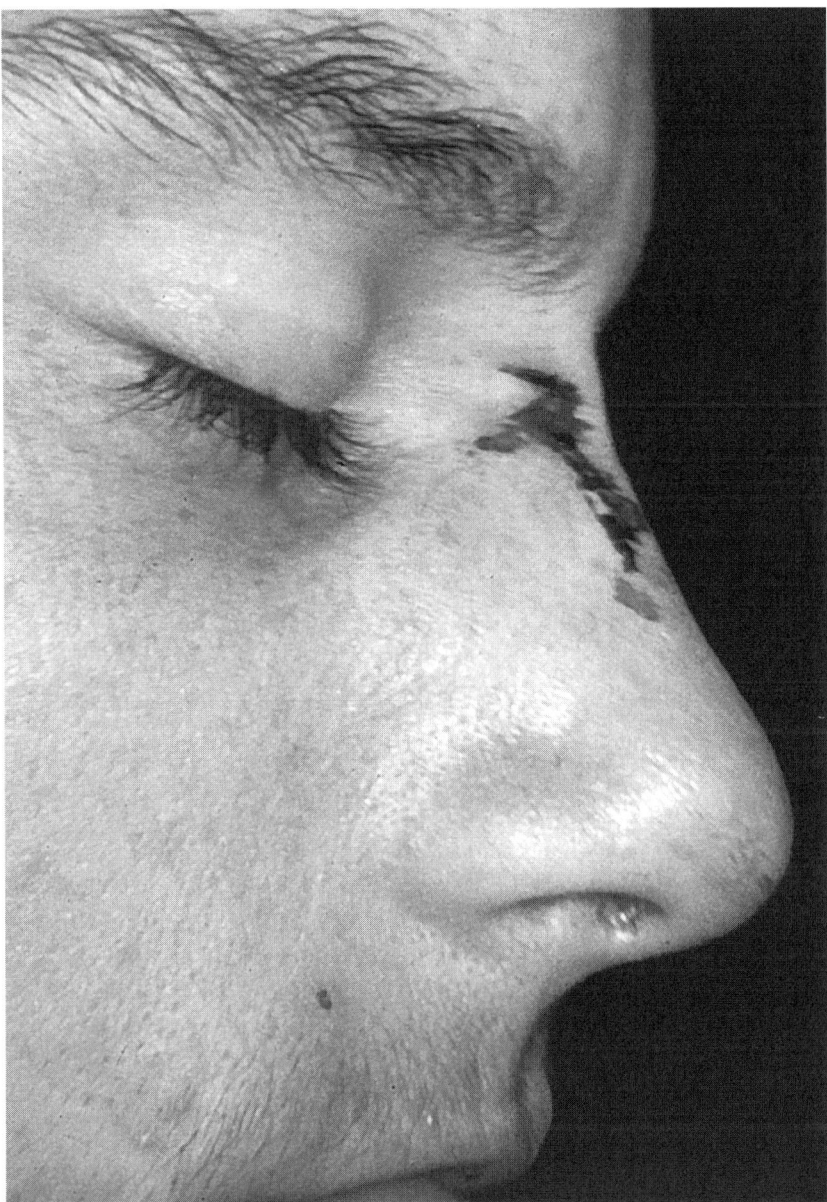

Figure 12.4 Complex nasal fracture, with lacerations exposing nasal cartilage and bone. (Courtesy of Dr. David E. Eibling.)

mentation purposes; however, because up to 50% of nasal fractures heal with a fibrous union, **a plain radiograph cannot reliably differentiate between an**

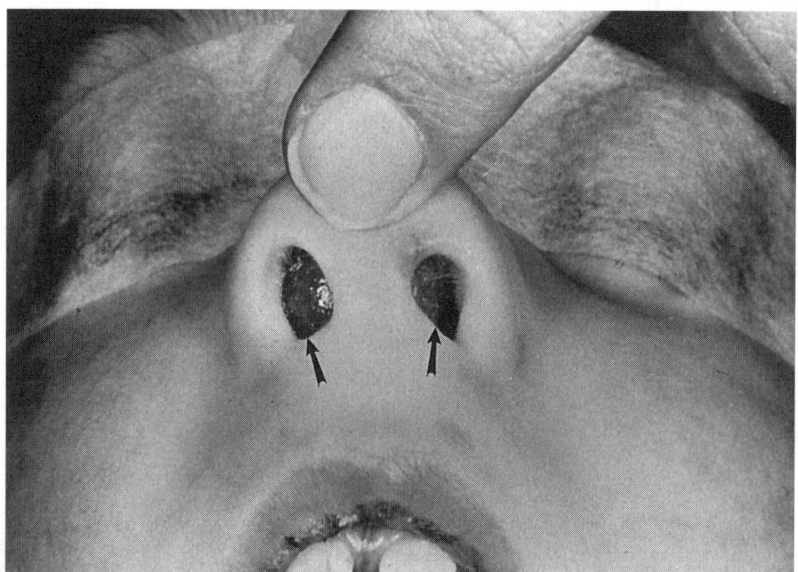

Figure 12.5 Minor nasal trauma with nasal obstruction. Arrows indicate an untreated septal hematoma.

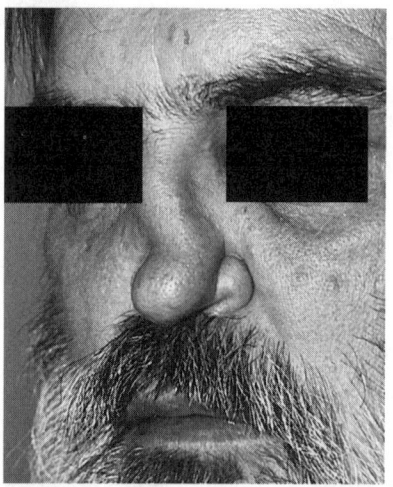

Figure 12.6 Saddle-nose deformity after untreated septal trauma.

old and a new fracture. This limits its usefulness, even for medicolegal purposes. If the history and examination raise concerns for associated facial or orbital fractures, then axial and coronal computed tomography of the facial skeleton should be performed to provide information about the integrity of the facial skeletal framework.

Table 12.1 Differential Diagnosis of Nasal Fractures

Isolated soft tissue injury	Septal hematoma or abscess
Nasal fracture	Acute sinusitis
Mid-face fracture	Nasal polyps
Naso-orbitoethmoid fracture	Neoplasm

Management and Follow-Up

Initial management is supportive once septal hematoma or other more serious injuries are ruled out. **Gauze pads (4 in x 4 in) soaked in ice water** should be applied to the periorbital region during the first 24 hours after injury, providing symptomatic relief of discomfort and helping to **minimize subsequent swelling**. Ice-cold gauze pads are preferred over an ice pack because applying the latter might cause additional displacement of the nasal fracture. **Topical decongestants** can help reduce nasal congestion due to inflamed nasal mucosa; however, their use should be limited to 3-days' duration to avoid rebound nasal congestion. The use of decongestants should not replace direct visualization of the septum to rule out a septal injury.

If the patient has a mildly displaced nasal fracture and presents before developing significant edema, he or she may be a candidate for immediate closed reduction (Case 12.1). Closed reduction involves intranasal and external manipulation of the nasal bones, which is performed using topical and local anesthesia. Severe nasal fractures, however, usually involve the septum and require open reduction and septoplasty. Open reduction involves direct

---

Case 12.1 **Man with a Displaced Nasal Fracture Requiring Immediate Closed Reduction**

A man 45 years of age runs into your office, clutching a bloody towel to his nose. He explains that he fell, hitting his nose on a street curb, and thinks he may have broken his nose. Once he is settled in an examination room, you note that the bleeding has stopped. Because this injury took place less than an hour ago, there is still minimal swelling, and you can see a marked crookedness to his nasal dorsum that is quite different from his usual appearance. You happen to catch your surgical colleague just as he is leaving for lunch; he examines the patient, concurs with your diagnosis of nasal fracture, and suggests immediate closed reduction of the fracture. In the treatment room, he anesthetizes the nose and is able to manipulate the displaced nasal bone into a more normal position. He puts a splint on the patient's nose and asks him to return in several days for follow-up. One week later, the splint is removed, and the patient is satisfied with the functional and cosmetic results.

> **Case 12.2** **Man with a Suspected Hematoma or Abscess After Nose Injury**
>
> A man 24 years of age was playing in a softball tournament two days ago and was hit in the nose with a bat. He was not too concerned because he says that he had broken his nose before. He comes to you today, however, because he is unable to breathe through his nose. On physical examination, you note ecchymosis in both inferior orbital areas and tenderness to palpation on the nasal bone. When you look in the nose, there seems to be a mass near the front of the nose on both sides. Suspecting a septal hematoma or abscess, you start the patient on broad-spectrum antibiotics and ask a specialist colleague to see the patient. She concurs with your diagnosis and drains the hematoma, leaving the nose with loose packing. One week later, the splint is removed, and the patient is happy with functional and cosmetic result. On 10-year follow-up, there is no evidence of dorsal saddling.

exposure of the nasal bones. **Nasal fractures should be reduced within 7 to 10 days after the edema has partially subsided. Bony reduction after this time is often not possible because the facial bones heal quickly.** Open reduction with osteotomies is then required for nasal bone repositioning. CSF rhinorrhea is indicative of a more severe facial skeletal injury (*see* Chapter 26).

Danger Signs

Fever, chills, increasing nasal pain, and surrounding nasal erythema may indicate the beginning of an infection that can lead to intracranial complications. A thickened or boggy nasal septum may indicate a septal hematoma or abscess (Case 12.2). Visual changes or a widened intercanthal distance can occur with naso-orbitoethmoid or other complex facial fractures. Watery rhinorrhea may indicate a CSF leak. Untreated CSF leaks may lead to meningitis. Persistent epistaxis (especially brisk, bright-red, brief bleeding) can occur with posttraumatic aneurysms or fistulas and should be investigated with arteriography.

SUGGESTED READINGS

Canty PA, Berkowitz RG. Hematoma and abscess of the nasal septum in children. *Arch Otolaryngol Head Neck Surg.* 1996;122:1373–6.
  This article details the occurrence of septal injuries and describes evaluation and management.

Daw JL, Lewis VL. Lateral force compared with frontal impact nasal fractures: need for reoperation. *J Craniomaxillofacial Trauma.* 1995;1:50–5.
  This article discusses the biomechanical forces operant in nasal fractures and the differential injuries resulting from different vectors of force.

Illum P. Legal aspects in nasal fractures. *Rhinology.* 1991;29:263–6.

This article contains a good discussion of the medicolegal dilemmas and pitfalls in treatment of nasal fractures.

Pollock RA. Nasal trauma: pathomechanics and surgical management of acute injuries. *Clin Plast Surg.* 1992;19:133–47.

This article is a concise review of mechanisms of injury and the surgical treatment of these injuries.

Stranc MF, Robertson GA. A classification of injuries of the nasal skeleton. *Ann Plast Surg.* 1979;2:468-474.

This article details a useful classification system for describing nasal injuries.

SECTION III

Upper Aerodigestive Tract

13

Mucosal Lesions of the Oral Cavity, Tongue, and Oropharynx

Elizabeth A. Blair, MD
David E. Eibling, MD

The oral cavity, tongue, and oropharynx have multiple functions, including taste, speech, mastication, and deglutition. Disorders in this region can range from inconvenient to life threatening. In addition to primary mucosal disorders such as tumor or infection, over 70% of systemic disorders can present with or develop manifestations on the mucosal surfaces of the head and neck.

Anatomy and Physiology

Forming the opening to the oral cavity, the lips are muscular folds covered with skin externally, labial mucosa internally, and vermilion at the transition zone. Richly endowed with both sensory and motor nerves (cranial nerves V and VII), the lips have a tremendous effect on speech, swallowing, communication, and facial expression. The mucosa of the lips extends laterally to form the buccal mucosa and line the inside of the cheeks. The buccal and labial mucosa should be smooth and pink. The opening of the parotid duct (Stensen's duct) pierces the buccal mucosa adjacent to the upper second molars. The mucosa extends superiorly and inferiorly to cover the maxilla and mandible, forming the gingiva. The sulcus between the lips or the cheek and the alveolus is termed the *labiogingival* or *buccogingival sulcus*. In some races, the gingiva may exhibit physiologic hyperpigmentation.

The roof of the oral cavity is formed by the hard and soft palate. The hard palate constitutes the anterior two thirds of the palate and is formed by one anteromedial (premaxillary) and two lateral palatine processes that fuse early in development. It is covered with a densely adherent mucosa that has a rough appearance (rugae). Minor salivary glands are located on the palate near the posterior margin and produce mucin. Failure of the lateral processes to fuse results in a cleft palate and in persistent communication between the nasal and oral cavities. Failure of the premaxilla to fuse is associated with a cleft lip and palate.

The soft palate separates the posterior nasal airway or nasopharynx from the oropharynx. Its lateral attachments merge with the tonsillar pillars, and its central raphe ends in the uvula. The soft palate is a dynamic muscular structure with a complex role in speech and swallowing, controlling the flow of air, liquids, and food. Defects in soft palate function (e.g., due to congenital clefts, surgical excision, and neurological diseases) are manifested clinically by hypernasal speech and regurgitation of liquids into the nose while drinking (rhinolalia).

The tongue is a mass of interdigitating muscles (the genioglossus, hyoglossus, and styloglossus) covered with a thin mucosa ventrally and with a thicker epithelium dorsally that is richly endowed with touch and taste receptors. The anterior two thirds of the tongue, derived from ectoderm, extends from the tip to the V-shaped groove known as the terminal sulcus. The posterior end of the "V" marks the foramen cecum (i.e., the origin of the thyroid gland). The posterior one third of the tongue, derived from endoderm, is the base of tongue and extends inferiorly into the vallecula, just anterior to the epiglottis. A variable amount of lymphoid tissue (the lingual tonsil) is located on the tongue base. The tongue base is not visible on routine oral examination without the use of specialized instrumentation but is easily palpable in a cooperative patient.

Filiform papillae (the most common variety of papillae) are distributed uniformly over the tongue, giving it a rough or raspy feel. Their function is primarily mechanical (e.g., for licking ice cream cones). The fungiform papillae (mushroom-like red structures dispersed through the filiform papillae) are more common on the anterior tongue and function as special sensory epithelium. The anterior fungiform papillae detect "sweet," and the lateral ones detect "salt." The circumvallate papillae (the largest of the "taste buds") are located posteriorly behind the terminal sulcus.

The floor of the mouth is bounded posteriorly by the tongue, laterally and anteriorly by the lingual surface of the mandible, and inferiorly by the mylohyoid and geniohyoid muscle sling. The floor of the mouth is covered with a thin, loose mucosa that extends from the ventral tongue to join the adherent gingiva on the lingual surface of the mandible, and it is divided by the lingual frenulum in the midline. The submandibular glands are situated below the posterior floor of the mouth, and the main excretory ducts (Wharton's ducts) transverse anteriorly under the mucosa and exit at the sublingual caruncula adjacent to each side of the lingual frenulum. The sublingual glands are posterior and lateral to the frenulum and are superior to the submandibular glands in the loose areolar submucosa of the floor of the mouth. These glands may drain through several small accessory ducts that are in close proximity to the submandibular duct. Occasionally, they drain into the submandibular duct itself.

History

The details of the duration, character, and location of the specific oral cavity symptoms are often key to arriving promptly at the correct diagnosis. History of risk exposure (e.g., smoking, snuff dipping, tobacco chewing [Fig. 13.1], or alcohol use), previous similar episodes, occupational hazards, and predisposition to infection should be noted. Patients should be asked about bleeding, changes in sensation (dental and mucosal), pain, alterations in speech or swallowing functions, and changes in taste. The patient's past medical and surgical histories are important, including trauma, previous procedures, and current and recent medications. Symptoms that may suggest malignancy are listed in Table 13.1.

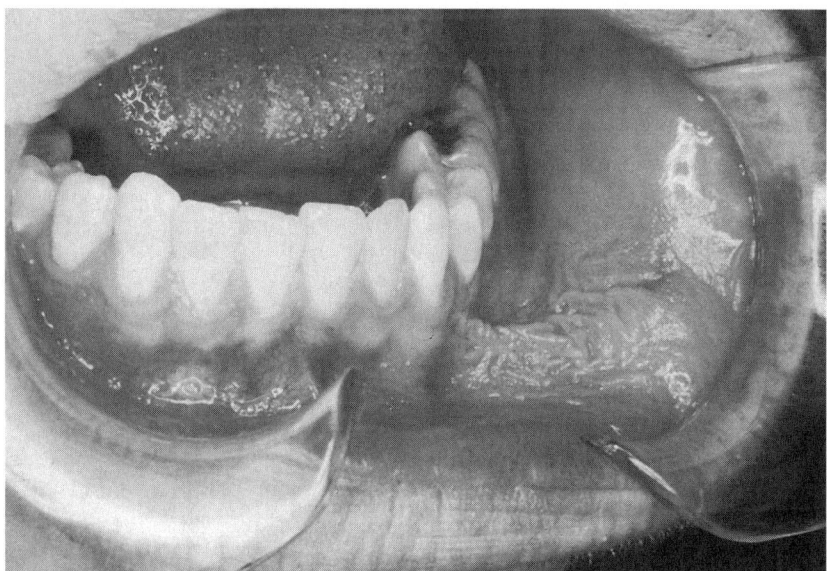

Figure 13.1 Snuff-dipper's leukoplakia. This mucosal change is due to the constant irritation of "quid" being held in the buccogingival or buccolabial sulcus. The epithelial changes usually return to normal if use of the irritating substance is discontinued.

Table 13.1 Danger Signs Suggestive of Oral Cavity Cancer

Pain	Halitosis
Nonhealing sore	Changes in the ability to chew, swallow, or breathe
New localized or generalized swelling	Bleeding
Changes in the gross appearance of mucosal surfaces	Weight loss

Oral lesions seldom present with bleeding, which is most commonly seen with gingivitis, severe tonsillitis, malignancy, hemangioma, and clotting disorders. Common causes of oral pain are aphthous and traumatic ulcers. Malignant tumors of the tongue base or tonsil often present with referred pain to the ipsilateral ear (often with minimal local complaints). **A patient over 40 years of age who has persistent unilateral throat pain with ipsilateral ear pain is presumed to have pharyngeal cancer until proven otherwise.**

The alteration of normal oral bacteria resulting from antibiotic or steroid use may lead to stomatitis, glossitis, gingivitis, or pharyngitis caused by yeast, fungal, or antibiotic-resistant bacterial infections. A particularly severe form of autoimmune stomatitis is associated with Stevens–Johnson syndrome, which is often caused by drugs such as sulfonamides. Chemotherapy drugs and radiation therapy both can cause a severe stomatitis or mucositis. Vitamin deficiencies, such as a lack of B_{12} or folic acid, also can present as stomatitis or with a burning tongue. Patients with stomatitis should be questioned about their diet, use of dental pastes and mouth washes, industrial exposures, and exposure to communicable diseases.

Many systemic infectious processes can be associated with oral signs. Syphilis may appear in the oral cavity as a chancre or mucous patch, gonorrhea as acute pharyngitis, and venereal warts as oral and pharyngeal papillomas. Infectious mononucleosis often presents as severe membranous tonsillitis. Patients with AIDS can have aphthous ulcers, histoplasmosis, or Kaposi's sarcoma of the oral cavity.

Physical Examination

Personal protective gear should be used when performing an oral cavity examination. Modified eyeglass lenses may be necessary for the presbyopic examiner to permit close inspection without abandoning eye protection. With a bright overhead (e.g., dental) light or headlight for illumination, the examiner should use two tongue blades to inspect the gums, buccal mucosa, mouth floor, tongue sides and underside, pharynx, palate, tonsils, and major salivary duct orifices. A hand-held illumination device (e.g., otoscope, flashlight) makes the detection of subtle abnormalities and small lesions nearly impossible. In a very sensitive patient, topical anesthetic may be required to suppress the gag reflex and permit a good oral examination. A laryngeal mirror is useful when examining the roof of the mouth and the lingual surfaces of the gingiva and teeth.

Palpation is necessary for a complete examination. One gloved hand is used to hold the tongue forward with a gauze square while the other hand palpates the tongue, assisting in the detection of invisible submucosal malignant lesions (especially those of the tongue base). Bimanual examination of the cheeks and floor of mouth aids in the diagnosis of salivary gland disease, salivary duct stones, and disorders of the submental and submandibular lymph nodes. When masses or lesions are identified, they must be palpated and the relationship to surrounding structures noted. Palpation assists in determining the extent of the lesion and often whether it is localized or infiltrating.

The openings of the parotid glands (Stensen's ducts) are on the buccal mucosa opposite the second maxillary molar; the openings of the submandibular ducts (Wharton's ducts) are on the anterior floor of the mouth adjacent to the frenulum. When the patient has symptoms of sialadenitis, it is helpful to dry these openings with gauze and then to massage the affected gland to see if clear saliva, pus, or nothing emerges from the opening. Impacted stones may be visible or palpable at the duct orifices (Fig. 13.2).

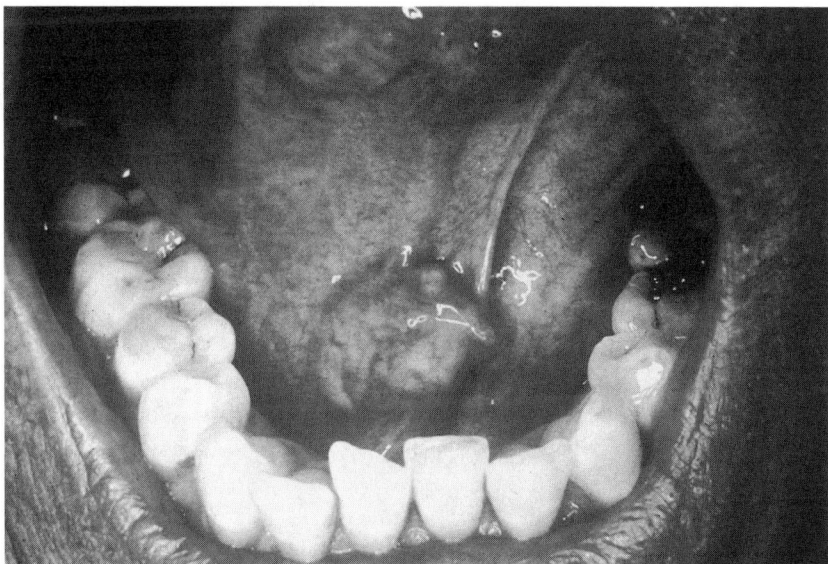

Figure 13.2 Salivary stone impacted at the orifice of Wharton's duct in a patient with swelling of the ipsilateral submandibular gland. These stones can be removed easily by incising the duct over the stone.

The submandibular glands usually are just under the anterior body of the mandible, wrapping around the posterior border of the mylohyoid muscle. With aging and loss of mandibular bulk, these may become ptotic or they may sag, descending farther into the neck. The patient may suddenly notice the swelling and seek evaluation, thinking that the gland is a tumor. However, ptotic submandibular glands are usually in similar positions on both sides of the neck, and bimanual palpation will confirm the diagnosis. Examination of the oral cavity also should include bilateral palpation of the neck and adjacent structures as addressed in Chapter 20.

Additional Diagnostic Evaluation

With a few exceptions, radiologic studies are not used in the diagnosis of oral cavity lesions. Plain radiographs may be helpful in confirming the diagnosis and location of a sialolith (salivary gland stone) that is causing recurrent obstruction with pain or infection. **Dental radiographs**, especially panoramic views (e.g., Panorex studies) may be helpful in diagnosing expansive or destructive lesions that originate in the mandible. These radiographs also may help in delineating the extent of periodontal and periapical decay. **Computed tomography (CT)** is most useful in evaluating larger or infiltrating masses and is best at evaluating bone involvement. CT is also helpful in identifying obstructing stones. **Magnetic resonance imaging (MRI)** is most useful in estimating the extent of soft tissue disease in lesions of the tongue base and for defining vascular lesions. Unfortunately, metal in the mouth (e.g., fillings, implants, braces) creates a scatter effect on CT scans and an image void on MRI scans, which can limit their usefulness. **Ultrasound** is occasionally useful in cystic disorders of the neck, mouth floor, and tongue, especially as an adjunct to **fine-needle–aspiration biopsy (FNAB)**, which is helpful in the diagnosis of submucosal oral and oropharyngeal lesions.

In FNAB, the needle is passed into the lesion many times while applying gentle negative pressure on a syringe that is relaxed while the needle is withdrawn. The material in the needle is immediately placed on a slide and air dried or treated with a cytologic preservative. Some physicians perform FNAB in their own clinics, whereas others require a cytopathologist to perform the aspiration biopsy. Aspiration by a cytopathologist allows for an immediate preliminary diagnosis.

Differential Diagnosis

The differential diagnosis of oral cavity lesions is extensive. Table 13.2, although lengthy, is incomplete but forms the basis of the following discussion.

Table 13.2 Differential Diagnosis of Oral Cavity Lesions

Anatomic Aberrations and Inherited Conditions

Cleft uvula, soft palate, hard palate, and upper lip
Lip pits
Median rhomboid glossitis
Geographic tongue
Fissured tongue
Lingual thyroid
Lateral pharyngeal bands
Fordyce spots
Palatal torus
Mandibular torus
Migratory glossitis
Black hairy tongue
Elongated styloid process
Exostoses

Systemic, Allergic, and Autoimmune Disorders

Aphthous ulcers
Behçet's syndrome
Sjögren's syndrome
Pemphigoid
Melkersson–Rosenthal syndrome
Gingival hypertrophy, gingivitis, epulis associated with hormonal changes (e.g., pregnancy, puberty, effects of birth-control medication)
Giant cell epulis associated with hyperparathyroidism
Oral candidiasis associated with diabetes
Pernicious anemia
Mucosal ulcerations associated with Crohn's disease and ulcerative colitis
Necrotizing sialometaplasia
Lichen planus

Medication-Induced Conditions

Chemotherapy mucositis
Radiation mucositis
Stevens–Johnson syndrome
Gingival hyperplasia
Xerostomia
Angioneurotic edema

Infectious Lesions

Herpes zoster and simplex
Mononucleosis
Kawasaki disease
Streptococcal tonsillitis
Vincent's angina
Oral syphilis
Conditions of immune suppression (suppression)
Candidiasis (thrush)
Actinomycosis
Tuberculosis
Histoplasmosis

Trauma and Acquired Conditions

Leukoplakia
Erythroplakia
Buccal linea alba
Oral burns caused by caustic ingestions
Ulcers
Mucocele
Ranula
Lacerations

Benign Neoplasms

Pyogenic granuloma
Epulis
Granular cell myoblastoma and fibroma
Parapharyngeal space mass
Dental tumor—odontogenic (from tooth structures)
Hemangiomas
Lymphangiomas
Cystic hygromas
Weber–Rendu–Osler syndrome

Local Conditions—Malignancies

Squamous cell carcinoma
Salivary gland carcinoma
Lymphoma
Plasmacytoma
Mucosal melanoma
Kaposi's sarcoma

It is important to note that, for many of these conditions, there are also systemic manifestations and that oral cavity lesions must be evaluated in the context of associated signs and symptoms.

Diagnosis and Management of Specific Oral Lesions

Anatomic Aberrations and Inherited Conditions

Lip pits are squamous epithelium–lined tracts arising near the midline of the lower lip at the junction of mucosa and skin (some extend more than 1 cm into the lip) that are found exclusively in patients with cleft deformities. These pits tend to become infected and may require excision.

A short lingual frenulum (**ankyloglossia**, or "tongue tie") can interfere with the mobility of the tongue's tip. In most cases, this is managed in infancy and is encountered rarely in adults.

Unusual configurations of the uvula are not uncommon. A cleft uvula requires no treatment; however, an elongated uvula occasionally requires excision due to precipitation of pharyngeal symptoms. An enlarged uvula may be caused by chronic irritation from heroic snoring, infection (Quincke's disease), or angioneurotic edema.

Median rhomboid glossitis (Fig. 13.3) is an oval area in the midline of the tongue that is devoid of papillae; it is associated with candidiasis. **Migratory glossitis** ("geographic tongue" or "wandering rash of the tongue") appears in young and middle-aged adults (Fig. 13.4); occasionally, there is a mild burning sensation. Treatment is symptomatic, including topical anesthetics and oral hygiene. **Black hairy tongue** is caused by elongated papillae on the dorsum of the tongue that become stained (often with the smoke of tobacco products) (Fig. 13.5). Some of the above lesions may be associated with oral candidiasis and may respond to antifungal treatments.

A deeply **fissured tongue** ("scrotal tongue") occasionally is encountered, often in members of a family (Fig. 13.6). It is more common in patients with Down's syndrome, and forms part of Melkersson's syndrome (i.e., recurring angioneurotic edema, Bell's palsy, and fissured tongue). Treatment is directed toward removal of trapped debris within the fissures to prevent associated inflammation. The tongue may be brushed or otherwise mechanically cleaned periodically.

A maroon-colored, smooth, rounded mass on the dorsum of the tongue posterior to the circumvallate papillae may represent **lingual thyroid**; a *thyroid scan is diagnostic*. This may simply be thyroid tissue and should not be removed until a functioning thyroid gland is found in the neck. These masses may cause dysphagia and, occasionally, respiratory obstruction.

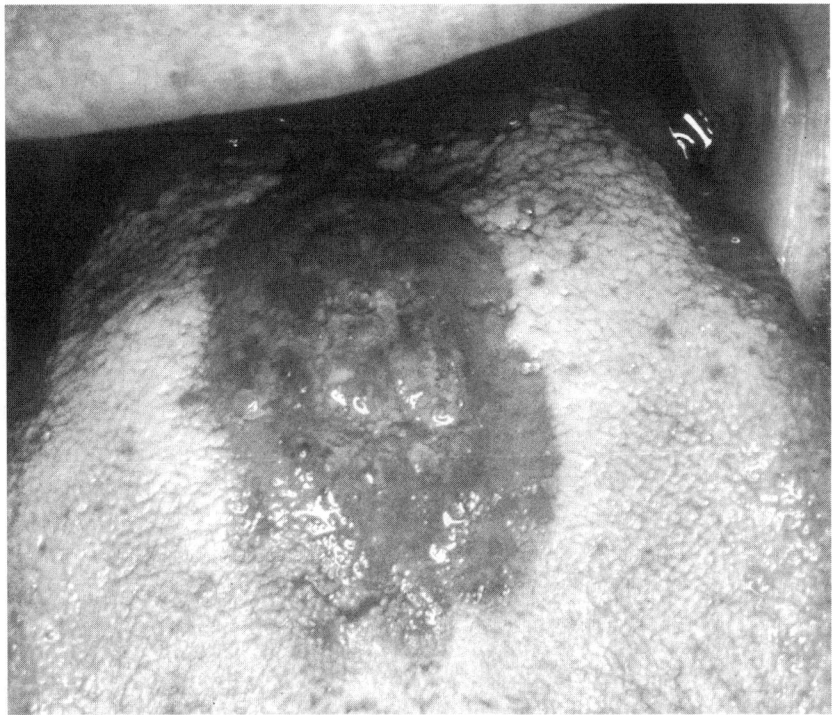

Figure 13.3 Median rhomboid glossitis. A benign lesion in the midline of the tongue that is devoid of papillae. The lesion usually harbors an overgrowth of candidiasis.

Fordyce spots are ectopic sebaceous glands that appear as yellow granulations on the buccal mucosa near the molar teeth (Fig. 13.7). The condition is benign and requires no treatment.

An **elongated styloid process** (defined as a process exceeding 2 cm in length) occasionally can result in symptoms (usually sore throat with referred otalgia [Eagle's syndrome]). Diagnosis is made by reproducing the pain on palpation of the tonsil fossa and is confirmed with radiographs that demonstrate an elongated styloid process. *Care must be taken not to miss a carcinoma that might be causing the symptoms.* Treatment is resection of the styloid process.

Lateral pharyngeal bands are lymphoid aggregates within the sides of the oropharynx posterior to the tonsillar fossae. They can become inflamed and appear as mildly red, papular lesions on the pharyngeal mucosa, a condition sometimes referred to as *granular pharyngitis*. If they are responsible for chronic symptoms, the lesions can be removed by laser vaporization or surgical excision.

Benign **exostoses** occur on the mandible and hard palate, can attain significant size, and are of no clinical significance. Occasionally, a **torus mandibu-**

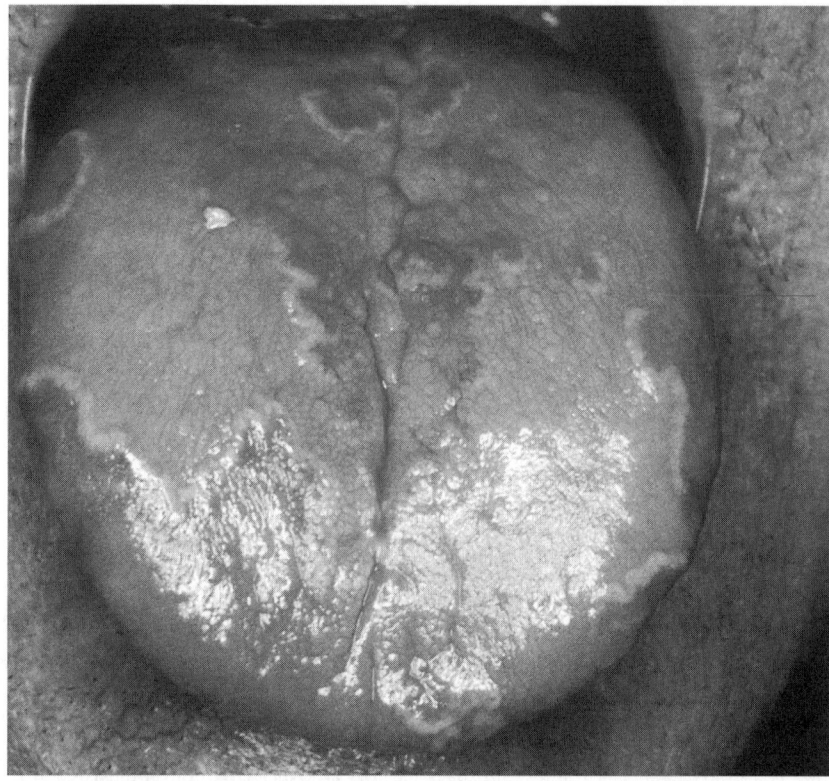

Figure 13.4 Geographic tongue or migratory glossitis consists of migrating areas of epithelium that are denuded of papillae. The cause is unknown and no treatment is necessary.

laris (Fig. 13.8) or **torus palatinus** (Fig. 13.9) can interfere with dentures. Treatment is surgical removal.

Systemic, Autoimmune, and Allergic Conditions

Canker sores, or **recurrent aphthous ulcers**, are common; nearly everyone has had them (Fig. 13.10). The ulcers present as small rounded patches of red-bordered yellowish exudate less than 1 cm in diameter and are painful. They often seem to be associated with stress, occur either singularly or in "crops," and usually last for approximately 1 to 2 weeks (Case 13.1). In women, their presence may correlate with the menstrual cycle. Oral aphthous ulcers may occur with **pernicious anemia, folic acid or B_{12} deficiency, malabsorption syndromes**, and **inflammatory bowel disease**. Treatment is problematic and aimed at reducing symptoms. Local therapy usually is not effective in the

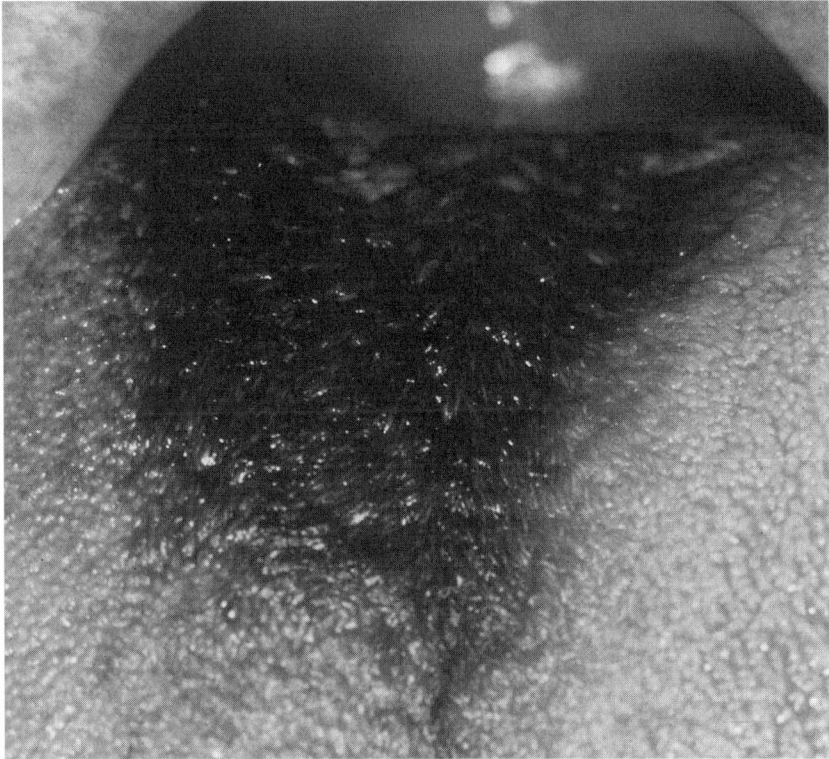

Figure 13.5 Black hairy tongue. Hyperkeratotic papillae become elongated and are stained with food and tobacco, resulting in an appearance of hair growing on the dorsum of the tongue. No treatment is necessary.

treatment of these ulcers, but symptomatic relief may be afforded by applying topical steroids in Orabase, topical analgesics, or oral Benadryl. Antimetabolite agents are temporarily effective in severe cases. Immunologic stimulation using a series of bacterial vaccines has received some recognition. Thalidomide has been reported to be effective in treating severe recurrent aphthous stomatitis; however, its teratogenic record mitigates its use.

Behçet's syndrome consists of recurring aphthous stomatitis, urogenital ulceration, and inflammation of the eye (iridocyclitis [e.g., uveitis, retinal vasculitis, optic nerve atrophy]) that affects middle-aged men of Mediterranean descent. Patients are at risk for joint arthritis, acneiform skin lesions, gastrointestinal perforations, and meningomyelitis. Diagnosis is difficult to make. Effective treatment remains elusive, but success has been reported with thalidomide, colchicine, cyclophosphamide, cyclosporine, acyclovir, chlorambucil, and steroids.

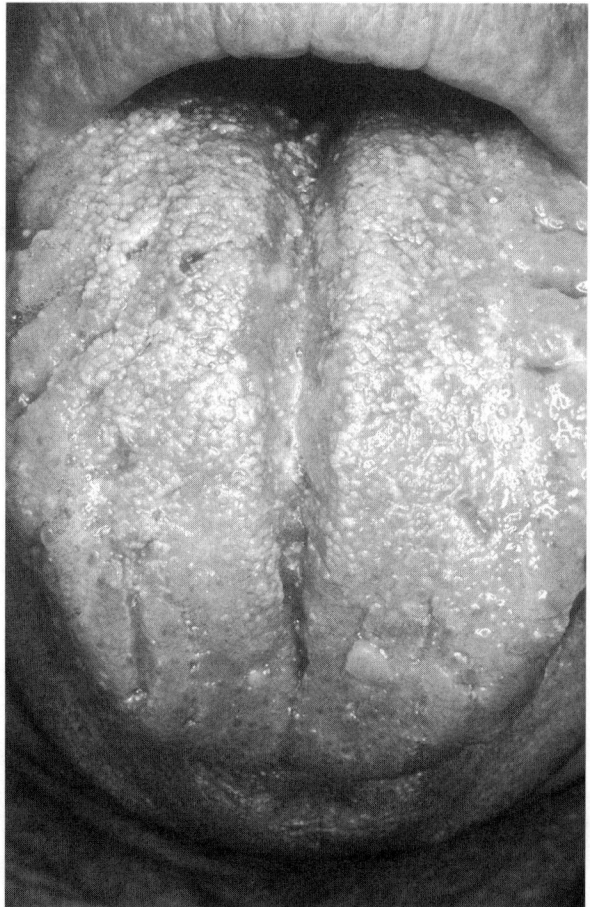

Figure 13.6 Fissured tongue or scrotal tongue is encountered in less than 10% of the normal population. It seems to be genetic and is found most commonly in elderly patients. It also may be associated with geographic tongue (see Fig. 13.4).

Patients afflicted with **Sjögren's syndrome** have generalized salivary and lacrimal gland dysfunction and present with xerostomia and dry eyes. The xerostomia may be associated with dental disease, atrophic glossitis, black hairy tongue, or candidiasis. Thick saliva also can block the major salivary ducts, causing recurrent submandibular or parotid gland sialadenitis. Salivary gland enlargement, especially parotid swelling, may become marked. Diagnosis is via serologic tests (SS-A and SS-B); if the diagnosis is uncertain, biopsy of a minor salivary gland may be necessary. Xerostomia can be treated with saliva substitutes; the treatment of thrush and black hairy tongue is with

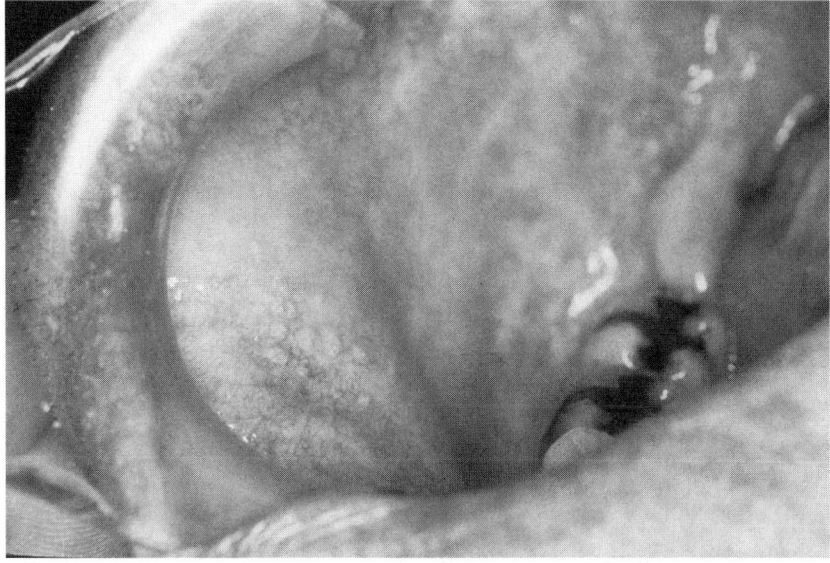

Figure 13.7 Fordyce's spots are benign ectopic sebaceous glands that appear most commonly on the buccal mucosa.

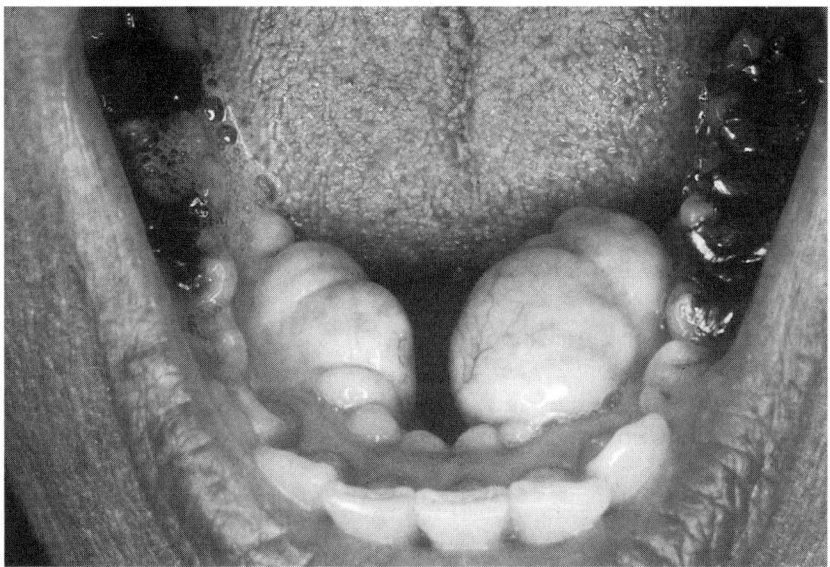

Figure 13.8 Torus mandibulari are benign bony projections that occur on the lingual (medial) aspect of the mandible. No treatment is necessary.

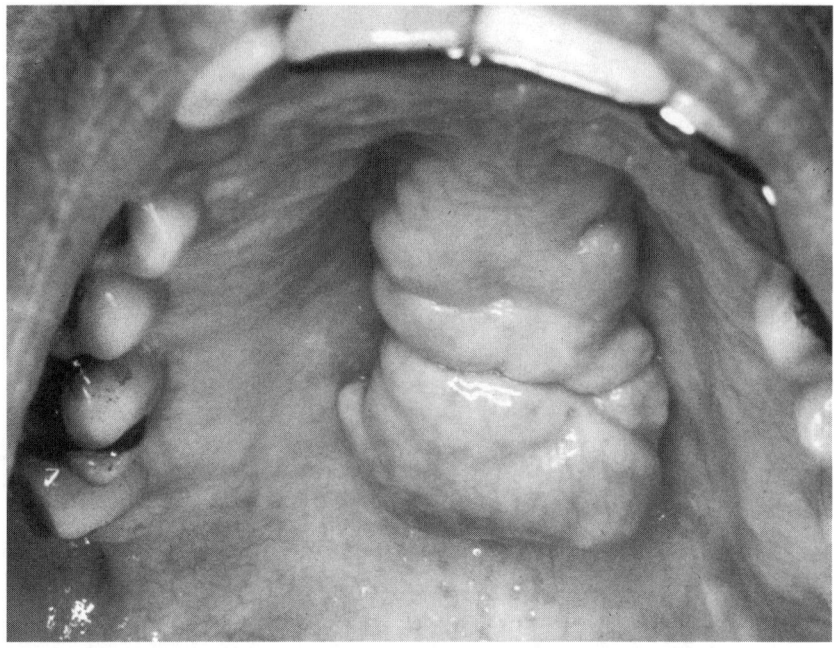

Figure 13.9 Torus palatinus is a hard bony protuberance in the midline of the palate. It is of no consequence but may require removal to facilitate fitting of dentures.

cleansing and antifungal preparations. Major, recurring salivary gland infections occasionally require surgical resection.

The combination of a deeply furrowed tongue, recurrent facial angioneurotic edema, and recurrent facial paralysis constitutes **Melkersson–Rosenthal syndrome**. It is more common in women, and histology demonstrates granulomas that are suggestive of tuberculosis or sarcoidosis.

Pemphigus and **bullous pemphigoid** can occur in the oral mucosa and present with bloody or serous bullae of the mucous membranes of the mouth, tongue, and oropharynx. Diagnosis is by biopsy with immunofluorescent staining of basement membrane.

Pregnancy, puberty, and birth-control medication may be associated with **gingival hypertrophy** and **gingivitis**. An epulis can occur in association with pregnancy and commonly occurs on the gingiva. A **giant cell epulis** is a maroon-colored, sessile lesion ("brown tumor") associated with **hyperparathyroidism**. This lesion resolves after control of the hyperparathyroidism.

Oral candidiasis may be associated with **diabetes mellitus**.

Patients with **Crohn's disease** often have oral manifestations that include mucosal ulcerations similar to aphthous ulcers (Fig. 13.11). Differentiating these ulcers from the more common aphthous ulcers may be difficult.

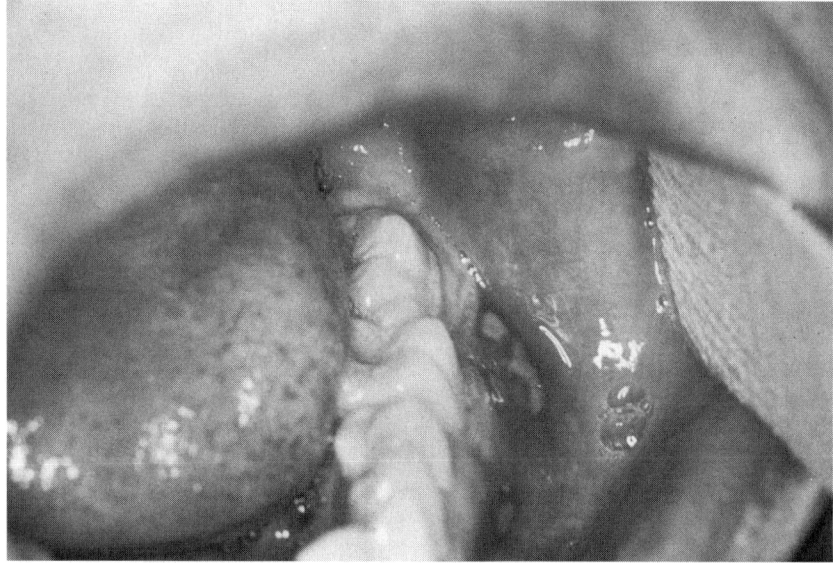

Figure 13.10 Multiple aphthous ulcers (canker sores) are common and quite tender. Symptomatic treatment can be offered; however, no treatment is known to hasten healing or prevent recurrences.

Case 13.1 Young Woman with Recurrent Aphthous Ulcers Associated with Stress

A female college student 19 years of age comes to the student health center complaining of mouth ulcers. She has no history of significant medical illnesses but is currently preparing for final exams and is having "boy trouble."

Physical examination reveals five ulcers involving the gingiva, labial mucosa, and underside of her tongue. The largest is 0.5 cm in diameter; all are white with a surrounding halo of erythema and swelling. They are exquisitely tender. There is minimal nontender adenopathy with several 1-cm nodes palpated in the anterior jugular chain.

She is given a bottle of 2% lidocaine viscous and topical triamcinolone in Orabase and is reassured. She improves after final exams and vacations with her family. However, she returns several months later with an exacerbation.

Discussion

This is a common presentation for recurrent aphthous ulcers. In nearly every case, the ulcers occur in "crops" and result from some form of stress. Biopsy is not required, and treatment is supportive. Patients must understand that treatment is for comfort only and not likely to result in cure.

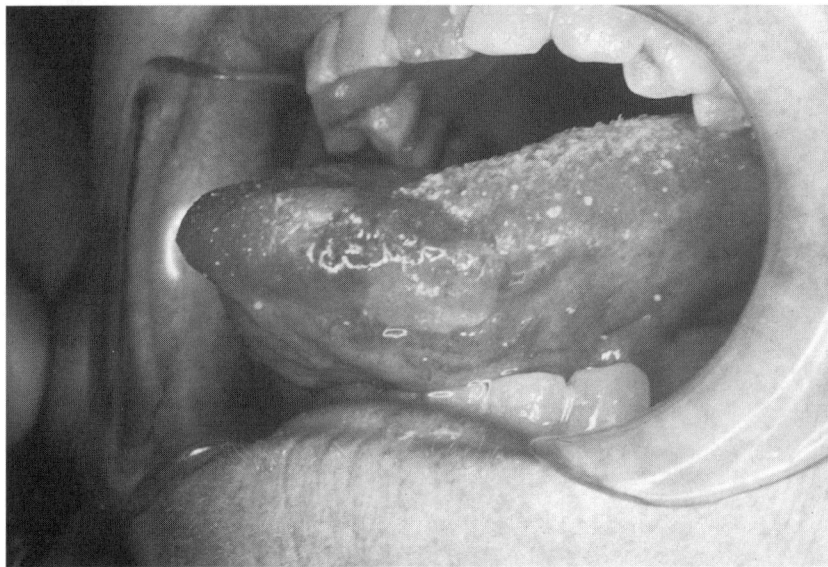

Figure 13.11 Crohn's disease can present as oral ulcers.

Necrotizing sialometaplasia occurs on the palate in adults and presents as ulcerated, irregular lesions with surrounding inflammation that are believed to result from prolonged exposure to tobacco and alcohol. They resemble carcinoma. Biopsy demonstrates metaplasia of minor salivary glands surrounded by inflammation. This disease is self-limiting and resolves without treatment.

Lichen planus can occur on the tongue or buccal mucosa. The lesions consist of smooth areas of mucosa separated by lacy threads of hypertrophic mucosa (Fig. 13.12) and may ulcerate, mimicking discoid lupus erythematosus. Persistent, ulcerated, mucosal lichen planus is termed *erosive lichen planus* and can progress to squamous cell carcinoma in some cases. There is convincing evidence that the disorder responds to systemic and topical steroids.

Infectious Processes

Viral Conditions

The initial **herpes simplex** infection occurs with varying degrees of severity in infancy and childhood, remaining dormant in mucosal cells thereafter. Recurrences manifest as a vesicular skin rash ("cold sore") or as mucosal ulcerations (Fig. 13.13) when host resistance diminishes (e.g., with emotional stress, menstrual cycle, febrile episodes, severe fatigue, underlying immunosuppres-

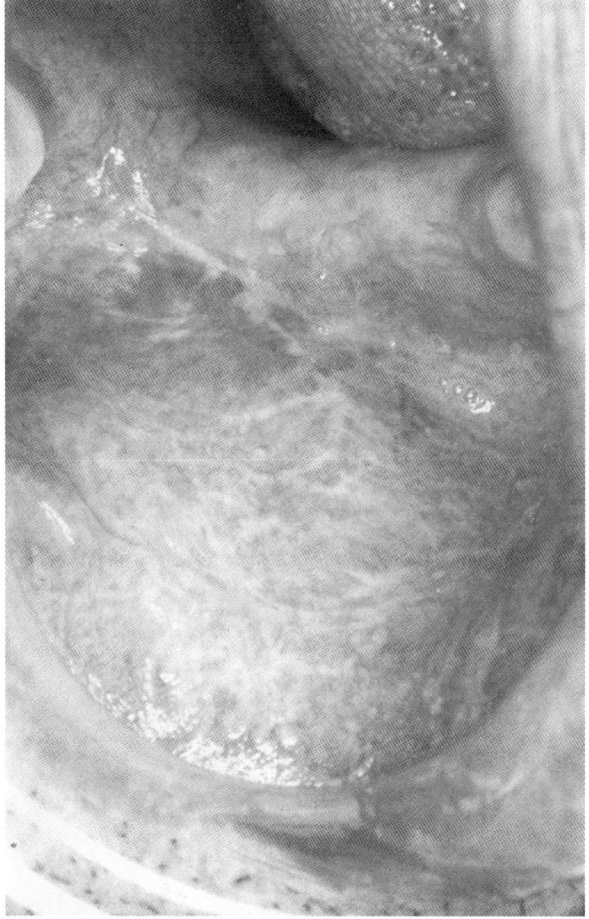

Figure 13.12 Lichen planus is commonly encountered on the buccal mucosa and characteristically presents as a reticulated pattern of white lines. Inflammation is usually minimal at this stage.

sion). Successful treatment with acyclovir is possible if administered early in the course. Topical steroids also may provide some symptomatic relief by reducing inflammation.

Oral **herpes zoster**, encountered less commonly than herpes simplex, represents mucosal or dermal manifestations of the varicella (chicken pox) virus lying dormant in the cells of the somatic nervous system and emerging during periods of impaired host resistance. Grossly similar to aphthous stomatitis and herpes simplex, the eruptions are unilateral and correspond with specific sensory nerve distribution (Fig. 13.14).

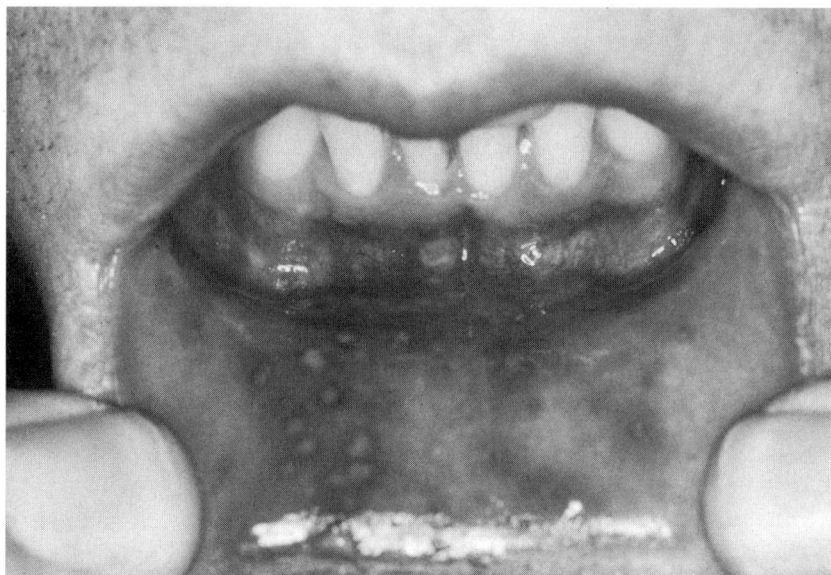

Figure 13.13 Herpes simplex begins as a vesicular eruption that ulcerates, resembling multiple aphthous ulcers.

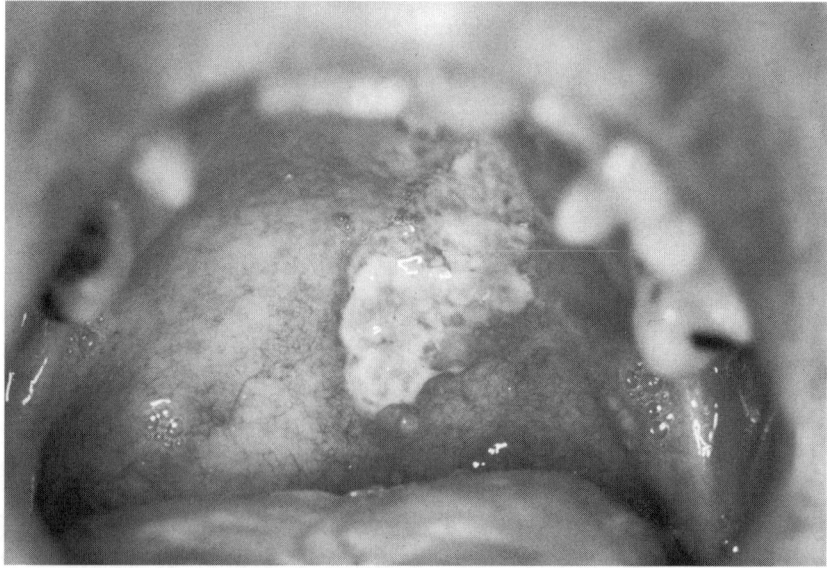

Figure 13.14 Herpes zoster is indistinguishable from herpes simplex except that the eruption lies within the distribution of a single sensory nerve.

Infectious mononucleosis can range from mild coryza to prolonged systemic disease and is commonly encountered in teenagers and young adults; however, it may occur in the very young and elderly. Exudative tonsillitis with associated adenopathy is its most prevalent feature. A positive culture for group A beta-hemolytic streptococci is not uncommon and can confuse the diagnosis. Mononucleosis tonsillitis does not respond to antimicrobial agents, and this response failure is an indication to rule out the disease using laboratory studies. The monospot may be negative initially, and bacterial superinfection can result in a leukocytosis. If the clinical picture suggests mononucleosis in the absence of corroborative laboratory determinations, the tests should be repeated in 3 to 5 days. A morbilliform rash develops in 20% of patients treated with ampicillin or its congeners, confirming the diagnosis. Patients with severe symptoms usually respond rapidly to steroids. If tonsillar swelling threatens the airway and does not respond to medical management, emergency tonsillectomy may be required.

Kawasaki disease, caused by the coxsackie virus, produces a mouth and tongue that are sore and dry, cervical adenopathy, desquamated volar skin surfaces, conjunctivitis, and malaise. More common in adolescents and in young adult men, Kawasaki disease is self-limiting (running its course in 2 weeks) and is treated symptomatically. Because there is a threat of coronary artery aneurysm with this disease, treatment with salicylates is required and should be begun within 4 days of onset to prevent cardiac complications.

Acute bacterial tonsillitis usually is caused by group A beta-hemolytic streptococci (Fig. 13.15). Debris in tonsillar crypts become colonized, resulting in local tissue sepsis with systemic symptoms of fever, chills, malaise, severe pharyngeal discomfort, and referred otalgia. The tonsils are swollen, red, and partially covered by a yellowish exudate, and the breath is fetid. Cervical (jugulodigastric) lymph nodes are often enlarged and tender. Penicillin is the drug of choice, with a macrolide substituted in patients allergic to penicillin.

Resistant organisms such as *Haemophilus influenzae* or *Branhamella catarrhalis* (and now even some group A streptococci species) have been reported in acute tonsillitis and require appropriate antibiotics. Superinfection with resistant anaerobic bacteria can also follow prolonged antibiotic exposure and may warrant a trial of a specific antibiotic. Frequent infections suggest the need for tonsillectomy, which is also indicated for recurrent peritonsillar abscess, unilateral tonsillar enlargement that suggests a lymphoma or other malignancy, and tonsil hypertrophy that results in sleep apnea.

Vincent's angina, or "trench mouth," initially begins as an inflammation of the gums that can spread to the oral and pharyngeal mucosa. It is caused by a symbiotic infection of a spirochete and a bacterium, usually encountered in patients who are smokers or may be immunosuppressed and who have

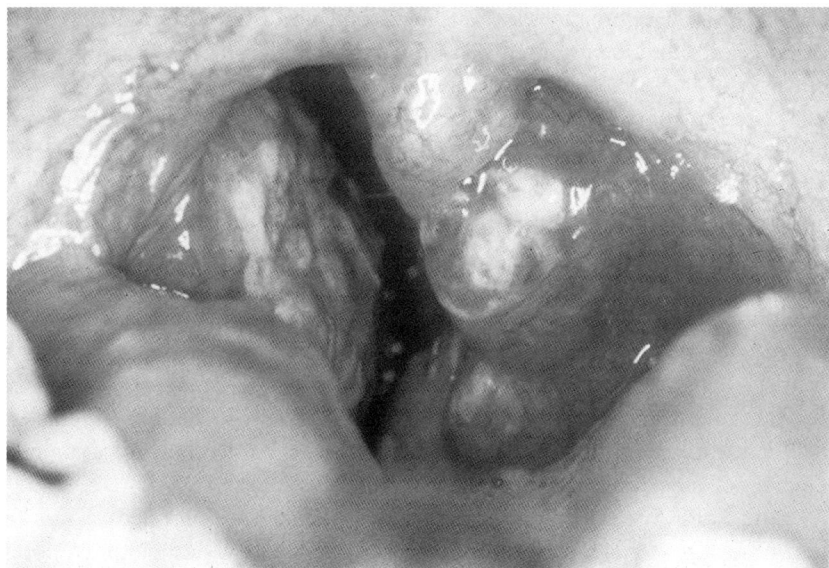

Figure 13.15 Acute follicular tonsillitis develops due to microabscesses in the tonsillar crypts.

poor oral hygiene. Treatment is with a program of vigorous oral care, antibiotics, and lifestyle changes.

Primary syphilis can present as an oral lesion (Fig. 13.16), although it is rarely encountered (or recognized). The lesion, sometimes called a "mucous patch," heals spontaneously, often delaying treatment of the systemic infection. A darkfield examination can suggest the diagnosis. Treatment is with high doses of penicillin or erythromycin as appropriate for the genital form.

Aphthous stomatitis, oral lichen planus, oral lymphomas, leukemia, and candidiasis frequently occur in patients with **AIDS**. Oropharyngeal and esophageal **candidiasis** usually respond to fluconazole (Diflucan), and refractory cases can be treated with an oral suspension of amphotericin B. Nausea, vomiting, and abdominal pain are reported side effects, and oral ulceration can occur from herpetic or cytomegalovirus infection. Also common in patients with AIDS is **hairy leukoplakia**, an unusually vigorous form of leukoplakia, and **Kaposi's sarcoma** (*see* section on Malignant Tumors below).

Squamous papillomas of the oropharynx are very common and usually appear on the free edge of the soft palate or uvula as soft, nontender, fleshy masses. These masses represent infection with the human papilloma virus. Although not considered premalignant, they should be removed to rule out the possibility that they represent early malignancy.

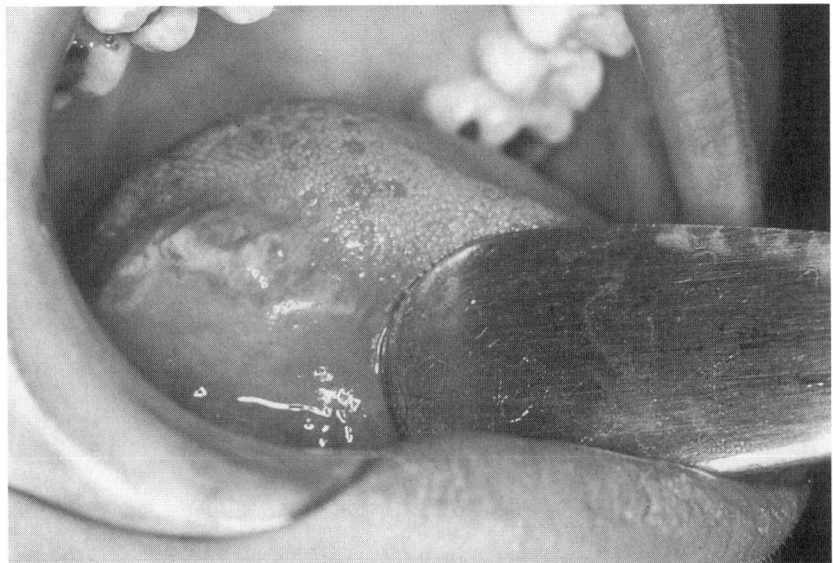

Figure 13.16 Syphilitic chancre can present in the oral cavity and can be confused with malignancy.

Fungal and Mycotic Infections

Pathologic overgrowth of *Candida albicans* (oral **thrush** [Fig. 13.17]) is commonly encountered in patients who use inhaled or intranasal steroids. The practice of routinely rinsing the mouth after inhaled steroid use will reduce the incidence of these conditions. Candidiasis also may be associated with prolonged antibiotic therapy or with immunosuppression. "Swish and swallow" antifungal agents or oral troches are usually effective. The effectiveness is maximized by prolonging the contact of the topical agent in the oral cavity. Systemic therapy includes imidazole compounds for severe cases.

Dental prophylaxis, gingival surgery, root canal, or dental extractions sometimes precede **cervicofacial actinomycosis**. This disease presents with a nearly painless, enlarged swelling of the perimandibular lymph nodes that eventually become cystic. Systemic symptoms are rare, and the diagnosis is established when surgical drainage yields yellow aggregates of fungal debris (sulfur granules). Treatment is with incision and drainage, dental hygiene, and prolonged (several months) therapy with high-dose antibiotics.

Oropharyngeal **tuberculosis** is unusual and is seen only in the elderly or immunocompromised patients. Lesions are single or multiple irregular, circumscribed, highly contagious ulcers that may be either painful or painless.

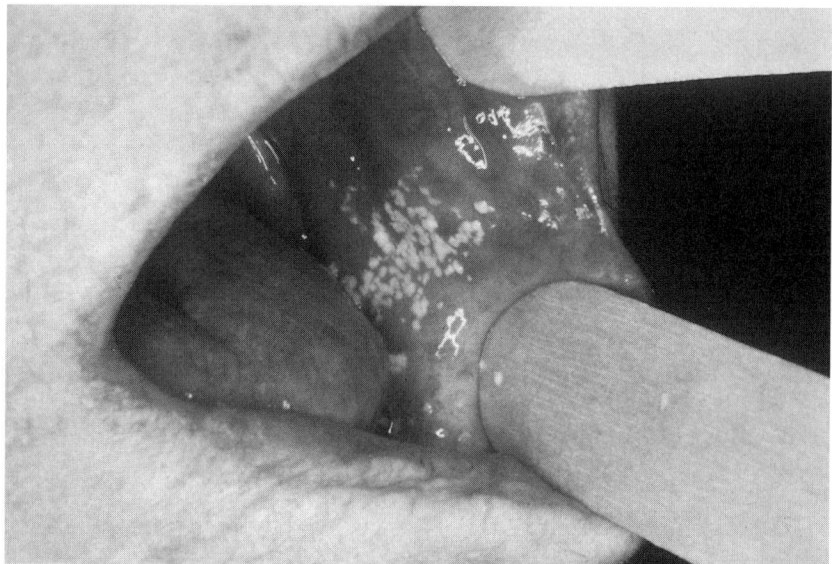

Figure 13.17 Candidiasis, or thrush, is commonly encountered in immunocompromised patients or those using inhaled or intranasal steroids. Topical therapy usually will suffice, although systemic therapy occasionally will be required.

Cervical lymphadenopathy is common. Diagnosis requires a high level of suspicion and is often delayed, resulting in inadvertent infection of health care personnel. Treatment is culture directed with appropriate antituberculosis drugs.

Histoplasma capsulatum often infects the immunocompromised and can present with oral ulcerations. Treatment is with amphotericin B or ketoconazole.

Medication-Induced Conditions

Chemotherapy-induced mucositis commonly accompanies the treatment of various malignancies (Fig. 13.18). Radiation of the oral cavity also produces **radiation mucositis** (Fig. 13.19). When both chemotherapy and radiation are used concomitantly, the condition is even more severe. Mucositis, which may be a dose-limiting side effect of these therapies, is manifested by widespread ulcerations that may involve every mucosal surface of the oral cavity (Case 13.2). Management is difficult, dental care is essentially impossible, and narcotics are often required for pain. Local treatment with various recipes is possible, but pain will persist until the ulcers heal.

Stevens–Johnson syndrome is a painful autoimmune inflammation of the oral and circumoral tissues that occurs after treatment with specific drugs

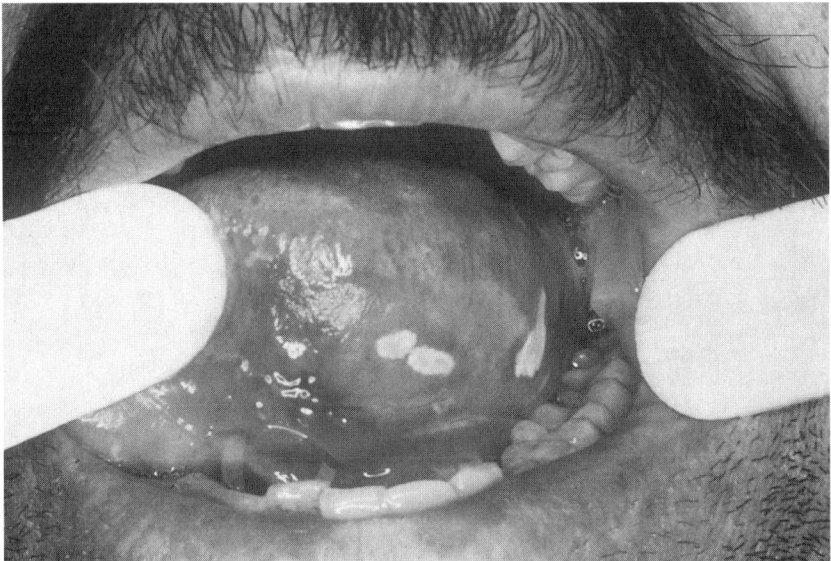

Figure 13.18 Stomatitis due to chemotherapy is common and may be a major component of chemotherapeutic toxicity for some patients.

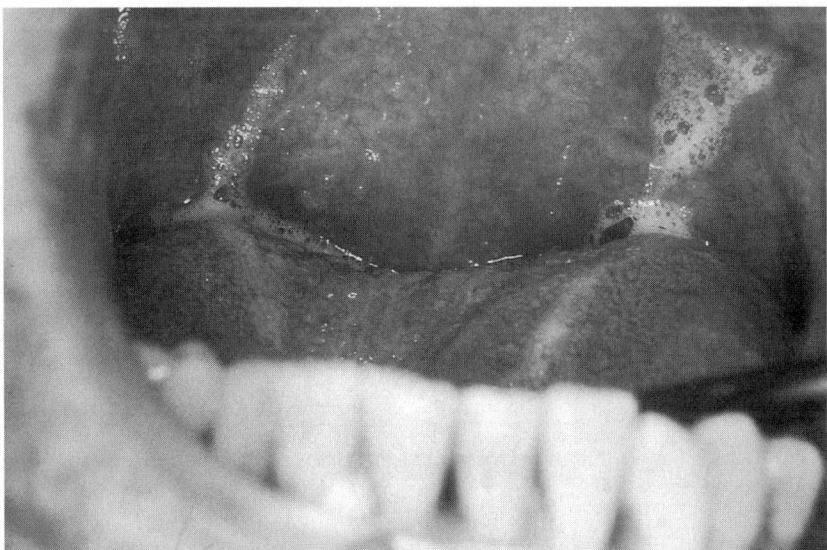

Figure 13.19 Mucositis following radiation treatment is due to the effect of radiation on both the mucosa and the reduced salivary flow. Topical anesthetics and moisturizing agents are helpful, but the condition may be so severe that supplemental enteral feedings are required.

> **Case 13.2 Man with Chemotherapy Mucositis**
>
> A man 56 years of age develops acute myelocytic leukemia and you treat him with CHOP (cyclophosphamide, hydroxydaunomycin, Oncovin, and prednisone). Five days after the first course of treatment, the patient calls the office to report that he cannot eat because of mouth ulcers. He has tried over-the-counter preparations but still is unable to eat. You call in prescriptions for "magic swizzle" and codeine elixir to his pharmacy. When he returns for his routine blood tests, his pain has largely improved, with obviously healing ulcers.
>
> **Discussion**
>
> Mucositis is commonly encountered in patients receiving chemotherapy. The extent of the ulcerations correlates with the neutrophil nadir. At times, the pain is so severe that oral intake is impossible, and alternative means of feeding and hydration may become necessary. Symptomatic therapy should be offered; various topical "recipes" are available. One favorite recipe (often called "magic swizzle") consists of Benadryl, liquid antacid, and lidocaine viscous.

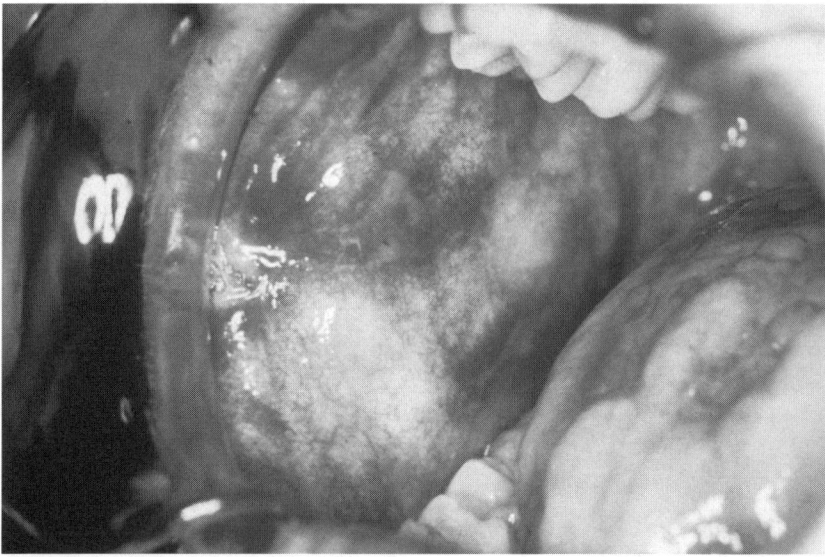

Figure 13.20 Steven–Johnson's syndrome is part of a generalized reaction and is often due to administered drugs.

(e.g., sulfonamides, phenytoin) (Fig. 13.20). The oral manifestations occur in association with the cutaneous process. This is a potentially serious condition and is treated by discontinuing the offending agent and administering topical and systemic steroids. Intravenous hydration also may be necessary.

Various psychoactive medications (e.g., tricyclic antidepressants, phenothiazines, lithium, antimetabolite agents [fluorouracil, adriamycin, and methotrexate]) result in reductions in salivary flow that lead to **xerostomia** with stomatitis and oropharyngitis. Dry nasal mucosa and xerostomia also accompany treatment with isotretinoin (Accutane). Phenytoin, calcium-channel blockers, and cyclosporin can cause gingival hyperplasia.

Angioneurotic edema is submucosal edema of the mouth, lips (Fig. 13.21), tongue, palate, or pharynx. It may be due to an allergic response, a familial error of metabolism, or an idiosyncratic response to therapy with an angiotensin-converting–enzyme (ACE) inhibitor. It is critical to note that this condition can occur rapidly and can progress, causing airway obstruction. Black patients are more likely to be affected than are white patients. Treatment is with Benadryl, epinephrine, and steroids. Tracheotomy may be necessary because intubation may not be possible. Cases have been reported to occur after prolonged use of ACE inhibitors; hence, a history of long-term administration does not rule out angioneurotic edema due to ACE inhibitors. Interestingly, some patients initially present with a "sentinel event" of minimal swelling and localized pain before the development of dramatic life-threatening swelling. These patients should be switched to an alternative antihypertensive. (*See* Chapter 18 for more information on this topic.)

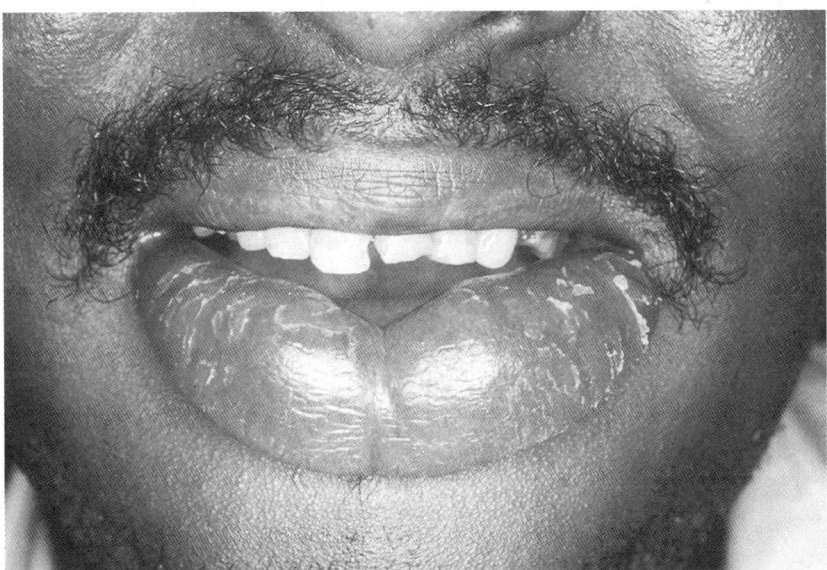

Figure 13.21 Angioneurotic edema of the lip due to the use of angiotensin-converting–enzyme inhibitors. If the tongue or pharynx is involved, tracheotomy may be necessary.

Traumatic and Acquired Disorders

Leukoplakia and Erythroplakia

Epithelial changes due to chronic irritation (usually from tobacco products) are acquired mucosal lesions of the oral cavity and oropharynx that are common in adults. These changes are considered premalignant, and early identification can facilitate the early detection of malignancy or perhaps warrant lifestyle intervention to reduce the probability of progression to malignancy (Case 13.3). *Leukoplakia* refers to the gross appearance of a "white patch" (Fig. 13.22), whereas the term *erythroplakia* refers to a "red patch." Normal mucosa is pink and smooth, and both leukoplakia and erythroplakia are associated with changes not only in color but also in surface texture. These disorders often coexist in the same region, a condition often referred to as *nodular leukoplakia*. The degree of mucosal atypia, ranging from hyperkeratosis without dysplasia through the range of mild, moderate, or severe dysplasia to in situ carcinoma and frank invasive carcinoma cannot be determined by inspection; biopsy is required. Leukoplakia is more apparent on inspection but has a relatively low probability of representing malignancy or severe dysplasia on biopsy. However, biopsy of erythroplakia will demonstrate severe dysplasia or malignancy approximately 50% of the time. Hence, although it may be appropriate to follow leukoplakia if the suspicion for

---

Case 13.3   Young Man with Leukoplakia Associated with Tobacco Use

An auto repairman 24 years of age comes in for routine health maintenance. He is essentially healthy but has been using smokeless tobacco daily since age 10. Oral cavity examination reveals a rough, white area of mucosa in his anterior labiogingival sulcus. On questioning, he admits that the location is the same one that he uses for his "quid." The leukoplakia is wrinkled but is not associated with any areas of erythroplakia. No other oral cavity abnormalities were noted and there were no palpable neck nodes.

You discuss the abnormality in detail with the patient, as well as the need for tobacco cessation. He is lost to follow-up but returns 5 years later with his new wife and young child. He is no longer using smokeless tobacco but is now smoking two packs per day. His oral cavity mucosa has returned to normal, but there is generalized mild erythema. He is not interested in discussing tobacco cessation.

Discussion

Leukoplakia due to smokeless tobacco is reversible if the patient discontinues the irritant. Unfortunately, this young man, like many others, did not abandon tobacco. He merely switched the delivery device when his wife objected to its use. He remains at risk for the development of tobacco-related disease and should be followed for life.

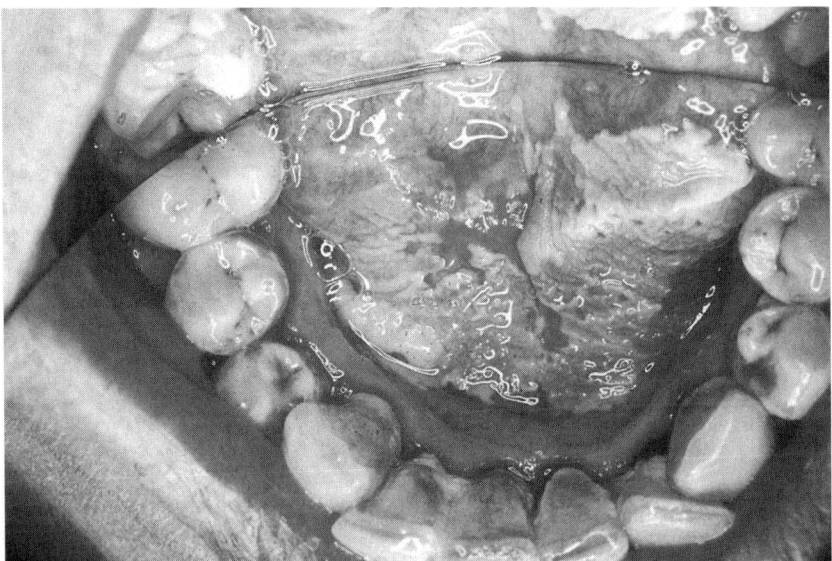

Figure 13.22 Leukoplakia denotes a "white patch" that is generally accepted to be a premalignant lesion. Biopsy is indicated to rule out dysplasia.

malignancy is low, areas of erythroplakia (or nodular leukoplakia) must be biopsied. Because identification of erythroplakia is difficult (particularly in the patient with extensive mucosal changes due to tobacco and alcohol use), staining with toluidine blue may enhance visualization of involved areas.

A line of hyperkeratosis called **buccal linea alba** is often noted on the buccal mucosa along the bite line. Wide variability between individuals is probably related to variations in individual oral habits, such as sucking on cheek tissues during periods of stress. This condition is benign and requires no treatment.

Caustic ingestions characteristically result in oral burns (Fig. 13.23). Often, these are the only injury because the patient rapidly expectorates the material before swallowing. Unfortunately, because the risk of serious injury (or death) due to burns of the esophagus and stomach is much greater, esophagoscopy is mandatory. (*See* Chapter 30 for further details on this subject.)

Oral Cavity Trauma

Trauma to the oral cavity is common and may be associated with facial injuries. As with all trauma of the head and neck, careful attention to the cervical spine is mandatory. Accurate alignment of the vermilion border is the key to repairing lip lacerations successfully. Adequate debridement and removal of dead tissue and foreign material are critical. The orbicularis oris muscle must be approximated, as well as the skin and mucosa.

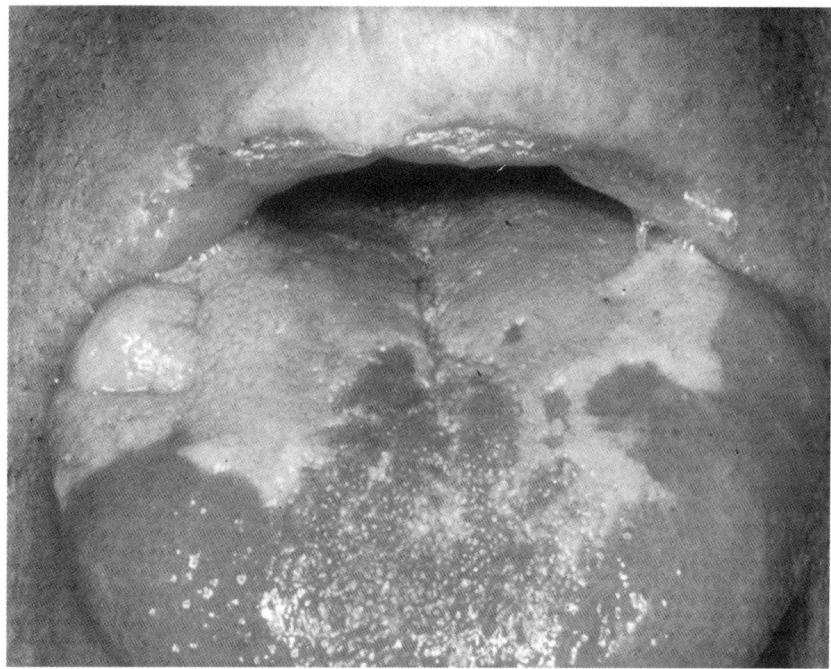

Figure 13.23 Caustic ingestions can result in oral cavity burns. Esophageal or gastric injury is much more likely to be significant; hence, esophagoscopy is warranted.

The tongue is difficult to suture effectively because of the thin, friable mucosa that is stretched over mobile striated muscle that has poor suture-holding characteristics. Most small lacerations of the tongue are best allowed to heal without sutures; however, massive lacerations require suturing to prevent permanent deformity. An injured tongue can become edematous, threatening the airway. Major contusions require airway monitoring for up to 48 hours.

Patients with diabetes and hemophilia and those who are immunocompromised require careful monitoring for signs of airway insufficiency and sepsis after oral trauma. Bacteremia is assumed in oral or lingual lacerations; hence, **patients with known heart-valve disease or joint prostheses may require antibiotic prophylaxis.**

Benign and Malignant Neoplasms

Benign Tumors

Tumors of the oral cavity are not uncommon and can represent either benign or malignant growths. A good rule of thumb is to consider biopsy for all unrecognized lumps encountered during the examination. However, many of

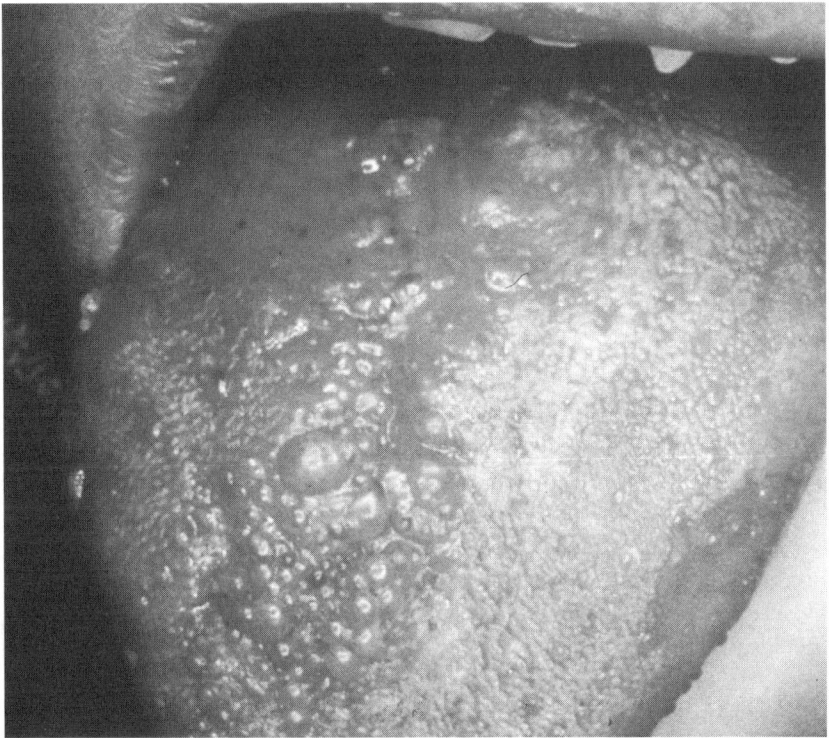

Figure 13.24 Lymphangioma of the tongue in this patient has resulted in macroglossia.

these masses represent common benign conditions; if recognized as such, biopsy is not necessary.

Soft cystic **mucoceles**, which often occur on the lips and may be traumatized, are the result of a blocked minor salivary gland duct. Treatment is excision or marsupialization, typically under local anesthesia.

Hemangiomas can occur in the oral cavity or pharynx. They are unusual and occasionally require excision. Large, dilated lymphatic channels can appear as **lymphangiomas** or **cystic hygromas** (Fig 13.24). Although more common in children, these benign tumors can occur in adults. Because they tend to enlarge, they are best excised.

Patients with **Weber–Rendu–Osler syndrome** (hereditary hemorrhagic telangiectasias) have friable mucosal and cutaneous telangiectases that can bleed with minimal or no trauma, resulting in chronic blood loss and iron deficiency anemia. These lesions may appear on the lips, mouth, nose, and entire gastrointestinal tract. Lesions that cause recurrent bleeding may be ablated with lasers or cautery or, if they involve thin mucosa, replaced with skin grafts. (*See* Chapter 11 for a more detailed description of this syndrome.)

Pyogenic granulomas can arise on the skin or mucosal surface. The lesions consist of exuberant inflammatory tissue and are related to chronic trauma. Biopsy is necessary for removal and to rule out malignancy. Laser vaporization, electrodesiccation, and surgical excision are effective for removal.

Obstruction of a minor salivary duct in the floor of the mouth can lead to the formation of a **ranula**, a thin-walled cyst with an appearance resembling the "belly" of a frog (*Ranus catesbeiana*). These cysts can form on the undersurface of the tongue and in close proximity to Wharton's duct, causing problems with chewing and speaking. A plunging ranula extends through the mylohyoid muscle and presents as an ill-defined submental mass. Treatment of either variety is by surgical excision.

Granular cell myoblastomas and fibromas are benign submucosal tumors that are most often found in the anterior two thirds of the tongue. Surgical excision is the treatment of choice.

Parapharyngeal masses present as asymptomatic, painless masses in the lateral wall of the oropharynx that result in deviation of the tonsil and anterior pillar toward the midline. These masses may achieve considerable size, becoming large enough to cause symptoms of fullness in the throat and dysphagia, and are usually either salivary gland tumors (often extending from the deep lobe of the parotid) or nerve tumors (arising from nerves in the region). (*See* Chapter 21 for further discussion of benign salivary neoplasms.)

Cervical osteophytes can present as obvious masses on the posterior pharyngeal wall. Finger palpation is diagnostic; if necessary, the diagnosis can be confirmed with CT or MRI.

Malignant Tumors

Oral cavity cancer is the most common form of head and neck cancer, most of which begin on the side of the tongue and the floor of the mouth. The vast majority of malignant tumors arising on the mucosal surfaces of the upper aerodigestive tract are **squamous cell carcinomas** (Fig. 13.25), whose incidence strongly correlates with **tobacco and alcohol abuse**. Other factors implicated in the development of mucosal squamous cell carcinomas are Epstein–Barr virus, human papilloma virus, Plummer–Vinson syndrome, erosive lichen planus, and leukoplakia. Symptoms may be nonexistent or listed among those in Table 13.1. Premalignant lesions, such as leukoplakia and erythroplakia, are discussed above. Squamous cell carcinoma is **locally invasive** and metastasizes early via **lymphatic spread**. The incidence of metastatic disease is greater as the primary tumor size increases. (*See* Chapter 31 for extensive discussion and representative illustrations of this disease).

More than half of all of these tumors are not detected until they are of considerable size and have metastasized to the regional lymph nodes in the neck, emphasizing the value of early detection and diagnosis. Cancer of this type

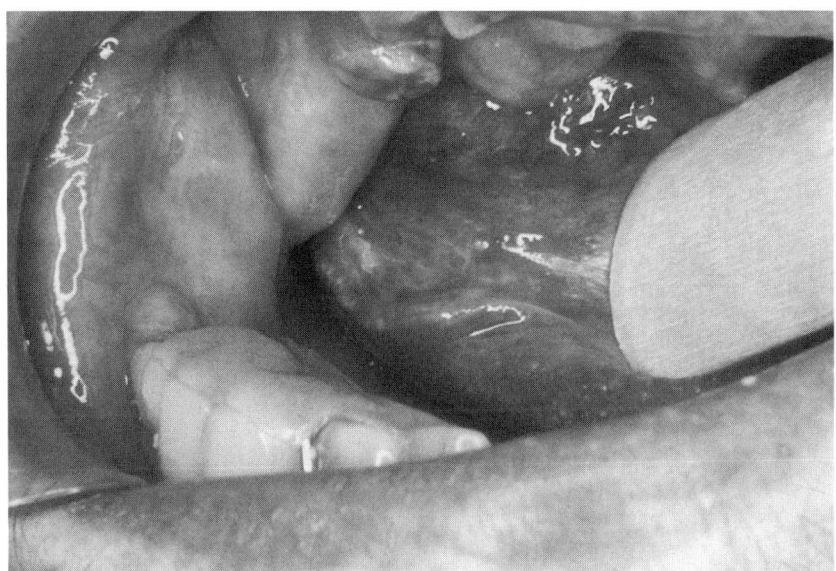

Figure 13.25 Squamous cell carcinoma of the tongue, with ulceration and induration.

that arises in the oral cavity or oropharynx is readily detectable by inspection, and **all at-risk patients should undergo an oral cavity examination as part of their routine medical care**. Examination of the nasopharynx and hypopharynx requires specialized instrumentation and expertise; however, the oral cavity is readily accessible for visual examination.

Any lesion of the mucosal surface that cannot be identified readily should be biopsied. The biopsy specimen should be obtained at the margin of the lesion to include a portion of normal mucosa. Biopsy can be performed easily with punch forceps, a skin punch, or a small scalpel. Injecting a local anesthetic that contains epinephrine not only reduces discomfort but also minimizes bleeding. Bleeding usually can be controlled easily with pressure or cauterized with a silver nitrate stick or disposable battery-powered cautery device. As in all biopsies, the site should be labeled and arrangements made to follow up on the outcome. If a biopsy specimen is returned as necrotic tissue, a new specimen must be obtained, with care taken to ensure that some normal tissue is included.

Other malignancies that occur in the oral cavity and oropharynx are cancers of the minor salivary glands, lymphomas, and a wide variety of unusual malignancies that occur infrequently. **Minor salivary gland malignancies** arise submucosally and are most likely malignant (Fig. 13.26). (*See* Chapters 20 and 21 for a more detailed discussion these neoplasms.) The submucosal

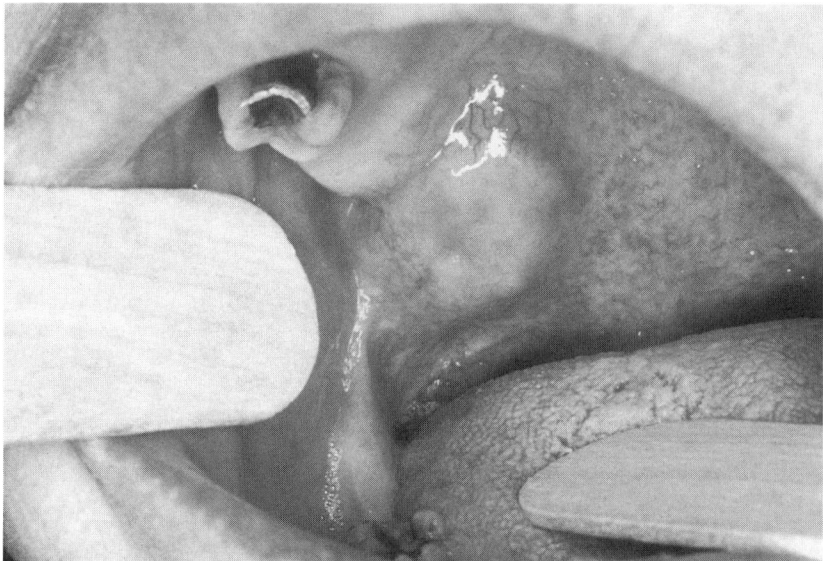

Figure 13.26 Adenocystic carcinoma of a minor salivary gland of the palate. Tumors of the minor salivary glands are usually malignant.

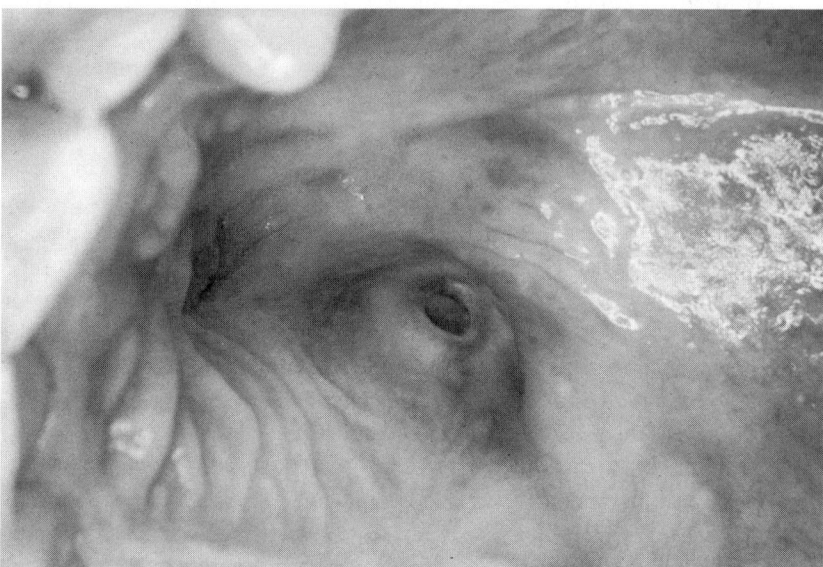

Figure 13.27 Kaposi's sarcoma in a patient with AIDS. This tumor has ulcerated, resulting in pain and bleeding; therapy should be offered.

occurrence makes biopsy more difficult than with primary mucosal cancer. **Lymphomas** usually occur in preexisting lymphoid tissue of Waldeyer's ring and may present as enlargement of the palatine or lingual tonsils. Tonsillectomy is indicated for biopsy if unilateral tonsillar enlargement is noted on routine physical examination.

Kaposi's sarcoma is an AIDS-defining tumor that frequently presents in the oral cavity. At onset, it resembles a submucosal hematoma with dark violaceous hue (Fig. 13.27). Later, it develops into a friable, fungating mass that bleeds easily. Treatment is problematic, and local care is difficult because of its friable nature.

Mucosal melanoma is rare. Treatment requires wide excision with consideration for local lymph node dissection. Unfortunately, most tumors have metastasized at the time of presentation, making the prognosis grave. However, most pigmented lesions of the oral cavity represent either amalgam tattoos (caused by inadvertent introduction of dental filling material into the submucosa during dental treatment [Fig. 13.28]) or natural mucosal pigmentation in black-skinned individuals.

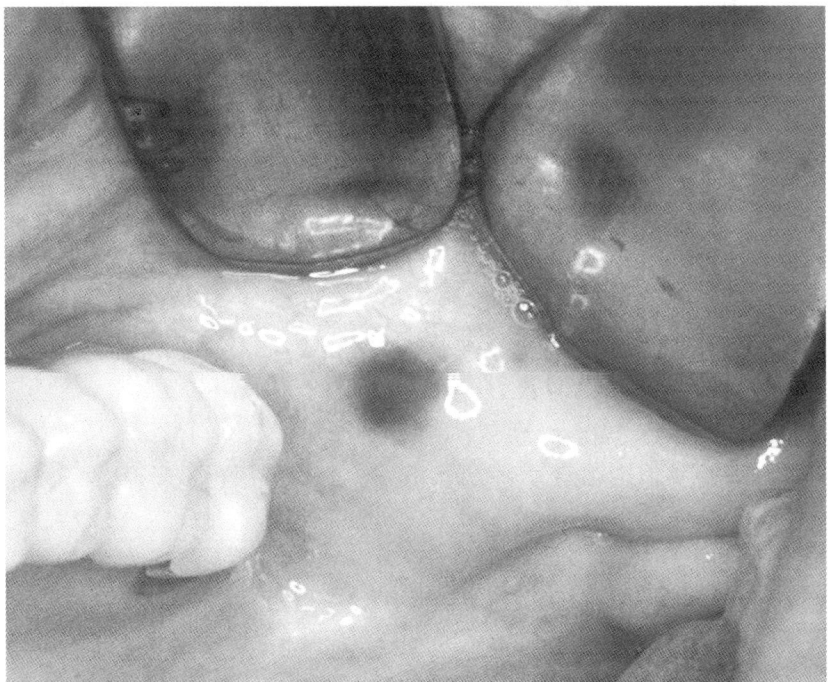

Figure 13.28 Amalgam tattoo due to implantation of dental amalgam in the submucosa is the most common cause of oral pigmented lesions. No treatment is necessary.

Summary

Mucosal and submucosal abnormalities of the oral cavity and oropharynx are common. Many of these are associated with systemic disease processes, whereas some are normal variants. Others, however, represent malignancies and must be identified early if the patient is to be cured with minimal morbidity. Patients who abuse tobacco and alcohol are at high risk for malignancy and should undergo oral cavity screening at the time of their routine medical care. Most viral infective processes are self-limiting, and symptomatic treatment is indicated. Oral lesions that accompany systemic diseases tend to parallel the systemic processes in severity and clinical course.

SUGGESTED READINGS

Bull TR. *Atlas of ENT Diagnosis*, 3rd ed. St. Louis: Mosby–Yearbook; 1995.

Colby, Kerr, Robinson. *Color Atlas of Oral Pathology*, 5th ed. Philadelphia: JB Lippincott; 1980.

Langlais RP, Miller C. *Color Atlas of Common Oral Diseases*, 2nd ed. Philadelphia: Lippincott–Williams & Wilkins; 1998.

All of these colorful books contain good photographs of a wide variety of oral lesions. Each provides a handy reference of oropharyngeal abnormalities encountered in clinical practice.

14

Disorders of the Nasopharynx

John W. Cavo Jr., MD
Eric F. Pinczower, MD

Many symptoms can be caused or worsened by nasopharyngeal disorders. These symptoms include nasal obstruction, ear discomfort, hearing changes, vocal changes (e.g., hypernasality, hyponasality, different voice resonances), bleeding (nasal or oral), and facial pain. This chapter details the anatomy of the nasopharynx and the diagnosis and treatment of nasopharyngeal disorders.

Anatomy and Physiology

The nasopharynx is a cuboidal space bounded laterally by the eustachian tube orifices. Each eustachian tube ends in the posterolateral nasopharyngeal wall surrounded by the torus tubarius and a small recess (Rosenmüller's fossa) (Fig. 14.1). Horseshoe-shaped bits of fibrocartilage (torus tubarii) lie at the medial ends of the eustachian tubes, holding the tubes closed except during swallowing and yawning. When air pressure in the middle ear exceeds atmospheric pressure (e.g., as during ascent in an airplane), the healthy eustachian tube orifice permits passive air to exit into the nasopharynx. When middle ear pressure is lower than atmospheric pressure, active opening of the eustachian tube orifice is required to equalize pressure. Swallowing or yawning (i.e., using the medial and lateral pterygopharyngeus and pharyngopalatine muscles) actively opens the orifices. The anterior boundary is the

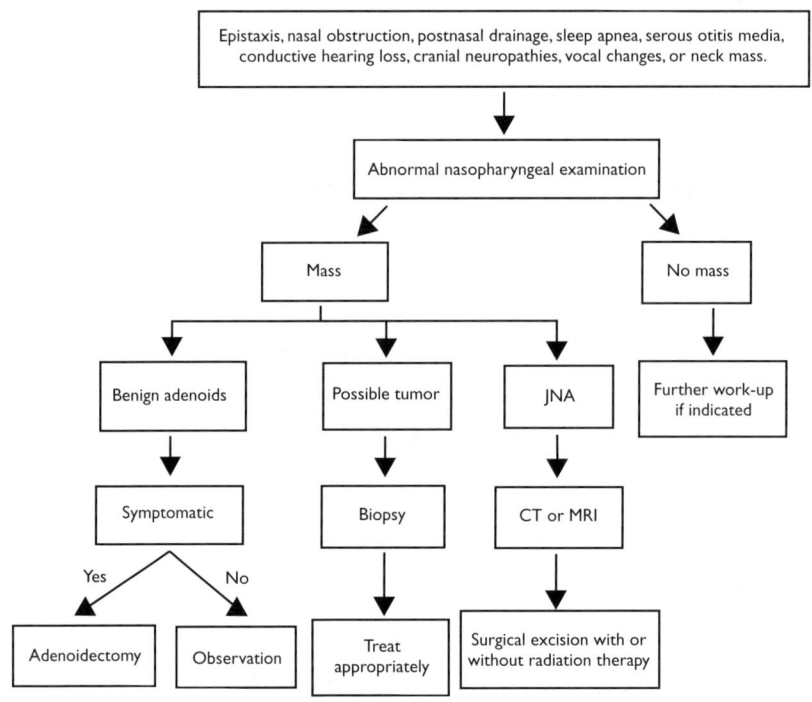

Algorithm Management of nasopharyngeal disorders. CT = computed tomography; JNA = juvenile nasopharyngeal angiofibroma; MRI = magnetic resonance imaging.

posterior choanae of the nose (Fig. 14.2), which is also the posterior end of the nasal airway. The paired choanae (one for each nasal cavity) are divided by the rigid bony posterior portion of the septum (the vomer). The posterior boundary consists of the superior pharyngeal constrictor muscles and the cervical spine (Fig. 14.3). The adenoid pad is on the posterior wall of the nasopharynx. A high midline "dimple" is the remnant of Rathke's pouch, an embryologic predecessor to the pituitary gland, at which craniopharyngiomas arise. Lower on the posterior wall, Tornwaldt's bursa—an embryologic notochord remnant—is sometimes found. The superior boundary is the clivus, which is the nasopharyngeal roof. The soft palate forms the anteroinferior nasopharyngeal wall.

History

Nasal airway obstruction is common in nasopharyngeal disorders. Patients may note a change in the voice quality when the normal resonance of the na-

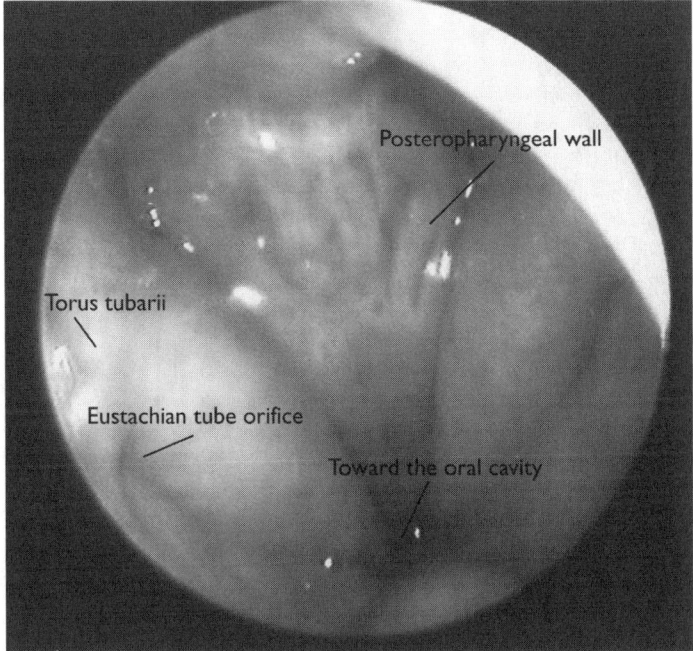

Figure 14.1 Endoscopic photograph depicting the view from the posterior nasal cavity, looking backward into the nasopharynx. The lateral bulges are the lateral pharyngeal walls; the posterior pharyngeal wall is directly ahead. The indentations at either side at the top are the Rosenmüller's fossae; the eustachian tube orifices are within them. The dark area at the bottom is the opening to the oral cavity. (Courtesy of Dr. Stephanie Cordes.)

sopharynx is lost. New-onset snoring is common with nasopharyngeal disorders. Anosmia (loss of the sense of smell) occurs when airflow is obstructed, which can cause partial loss of the sense of taste. Pain and bleeding may signal malignancy. Nasopharyngeal masses can obstruct the eustachian tube, causing middle ear serous effusion (serous otitis media) and conductive hearing loss. Epistaxis or hemoptysis can signal nasopharyngeal malignancy.

Rapid weight loss can result in patulous (overly patent) eustachian tubes, causing patients to complain of fullness in the ear that varies with respiration. These patients can obtain relief by putting their heads in a dependent position. When sitting down, they are more comfortable resting their heads on a desk or table.

Physical Examination

The traditional nasopharyngeal examination involves a head mirror or headlight. The patient's tongue is depressed, and the nasopharynx is examined

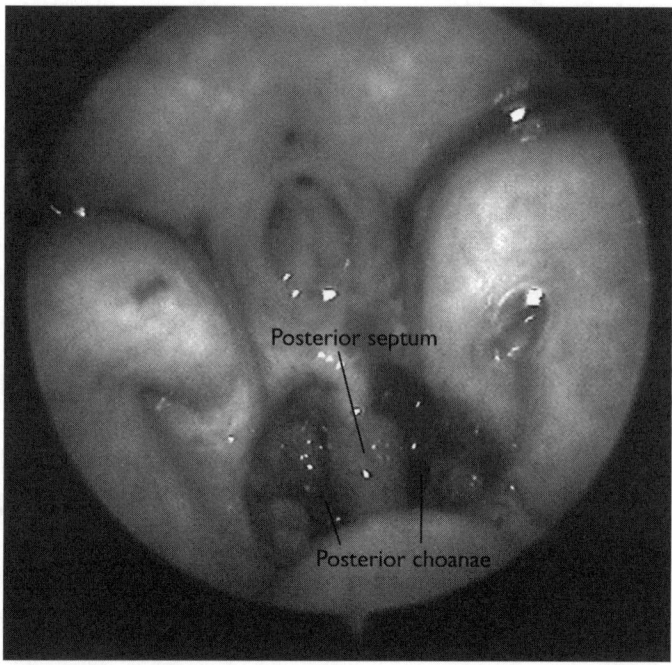

Figure 14.2 Endoscopic photograph of the nasopharynx, looking anteriorly and upward from within the nasopharynx. The central, lighter-colored, columnar structure is the posterior end of the septum. The two darker openings on either side of this structure are the posterior ends of the nasal cavities that comprise the posterior choanae. The tissue within these cavities is the posterior end of the turbinates. (Courtesy of Dr. Stephanie Cordes.)

with a small, warmed mirror (Fig. 14.4). A good view usually can be obtained by having the patient breathe simultaneously through the nose and mouth while a warmed mirror is carefully advanced beyond the palate. Having the patient say "uh *huh!*" while breathing through the nose and mouth relaxes the soft palate, permitting the best view of the nasopharynx (Fig. 14.5).

Important structures to visualize are the midline posterior end of the septum (the vomer), the torus tubarii, Rosenmüller's fossae (at which the eustachian tubes begin), the posterior wall of the nasopharynx, and the posterior ends of the inferior turbinates. The examination also may be performed using topical anesthesia and a fiberoptic or rigid nasopharyngoscope that is introduced though the nose (Fig. 14.6). It is possible to see the nasopharynx in nearly all patients unless he or she has a severely deviated nasal septum. Because the nasopharynx has a variable amount of adenoid tissue, and because many nasopharyngeal tumors are submucosal, even the most experienced examiner may find it difficult to detect some masses. If there is uncertainty after physical

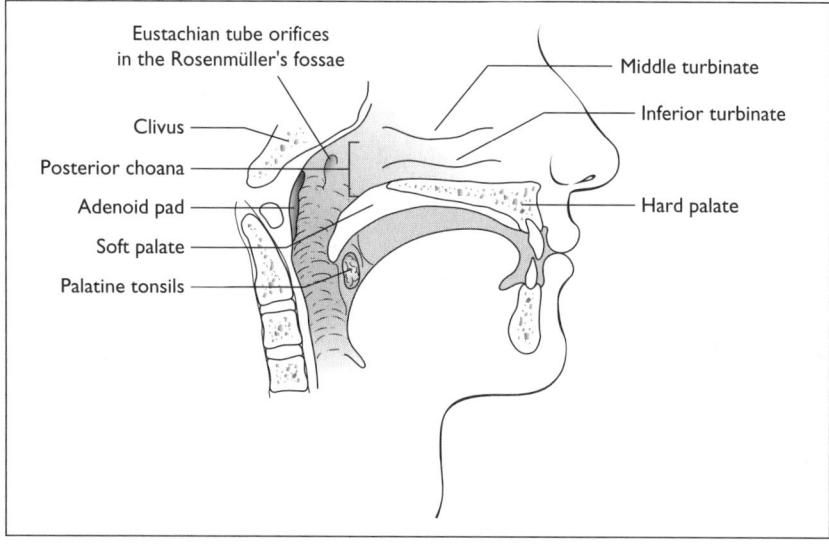

Figure 14.3 Anatomic structures surrounding the nasopharynx.

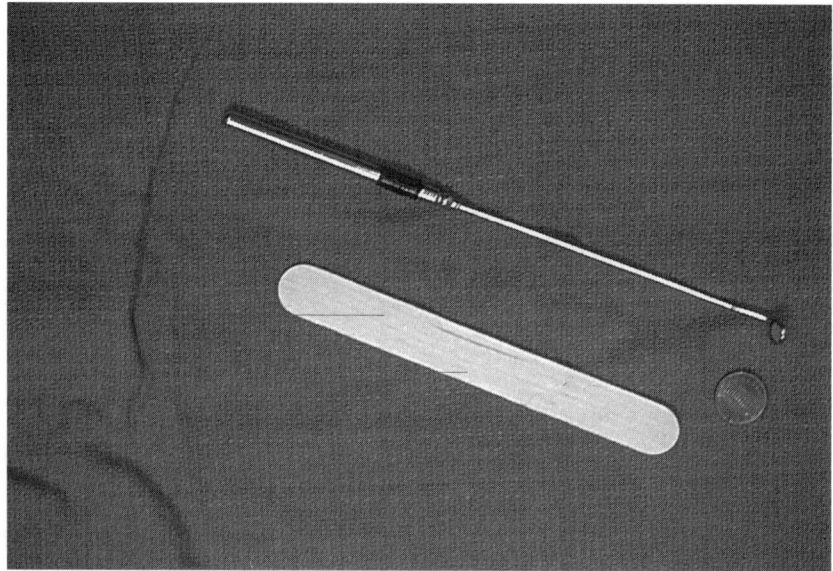

Figure 14.4 The mirror used to examine the nasopharynx is very small compared with an average-sized laryngeal mirror and a penny.

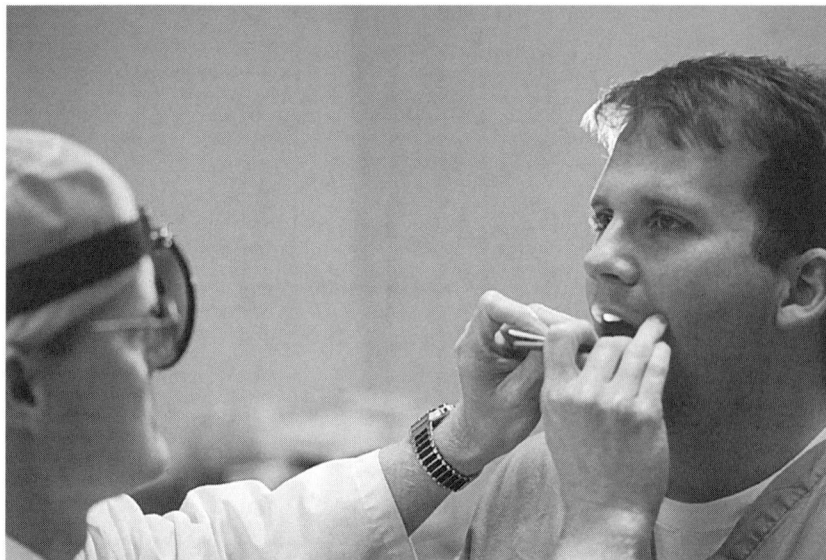

Figure 14.5 Optimal positioning for examining the nasopharynx with a head mirror and small mirror.

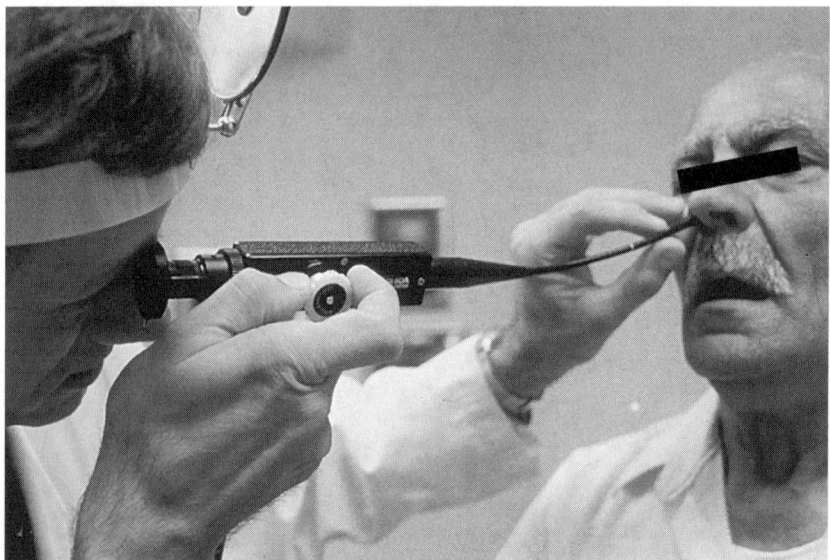

Figure 14.6 A fiberoptic endoscope being passed through the nose to examine the nasopharynx. (Courtesy of Dr. Jonas T. Johnson.)

examination, computed tomography (CT) is indicated. Digital examination of the nasopharynx is uncomfortable and is best done with the patient sedated or under general anesthesia.

Diagnosis and Management

The simplest diagnostic imaging study of the nasopharynx is the lateral soft tissue radiograph, which is used most often to define adenoid size (Fig. 14.7). CT or magnetic resonance imaging (MRI) can provide accurate images when a submucosal, sinus, orbit, or skull-base extension of a nasopharyngeal process is suspected. Scanning is mandatory when evaluating suspected malignant lesions of the nasopharynx and benign aggressive tumors (e.g., juvenile nasopharyngeal angiofibroma, tuberculosis, fungal disorders, high anterior cervical spine disorders). The differential diagnosis is shown in Table 14.1. The management of nasopharyngeal disorders is outlined in the Algorithm.

Inflammatory Conditions

Infectious mononucleosis, myxoviruses, enteroviruses, adenoviruses, respiratory syncytial viruses, rheoviruses, and coxsackieviruses frequently involve the nasopharynx. Viral infections cause myalgias, sore throats, mild fever, and malaise that typically last up to 14 days (Case 14.1). Nasopharyngeal inflammation and edema may cause eustachian tube dysfunction with subsequent serous or acute otitis media. Treatment of the viral disorders is symptomatic, using antipyretics, analgesics, topical anesthetics, mucolytics, decongestants, and hydration. Prompt treatment of bacterial infections of the nasopharynx may prevent spread to the middle ear via the eustachian tubes.

Nasopharyngeal Effects of Systemic Medical Conditions

Any disease process that causes lymphoid hypertrophy can present with nasopharyngeal symptoms secondary to adenoid hypertrophy, including a full spectrum of diseases from simple benign adenoid hypertrophy to lymphoid proliferation associated with AIDS, lymphoma, or sarcoidosis.

Sjögren's syndrome can cause a thickening of mucosal secretions and blockage in mucosa-lined ductal systems (e.g., eustachian tube), which in turn cause secondary serous otitis media and recurring otitis media. The problem is solved by inserting pressure-equalizing tubes through the tympanic membranes.

Inhalant allergies can cause mucosal edema in the nasopharynx that contributes to nasal obstruction and eustachian tube dysfunction, leading to serous otitis media. Medical management of the allergy often leads to resolu-

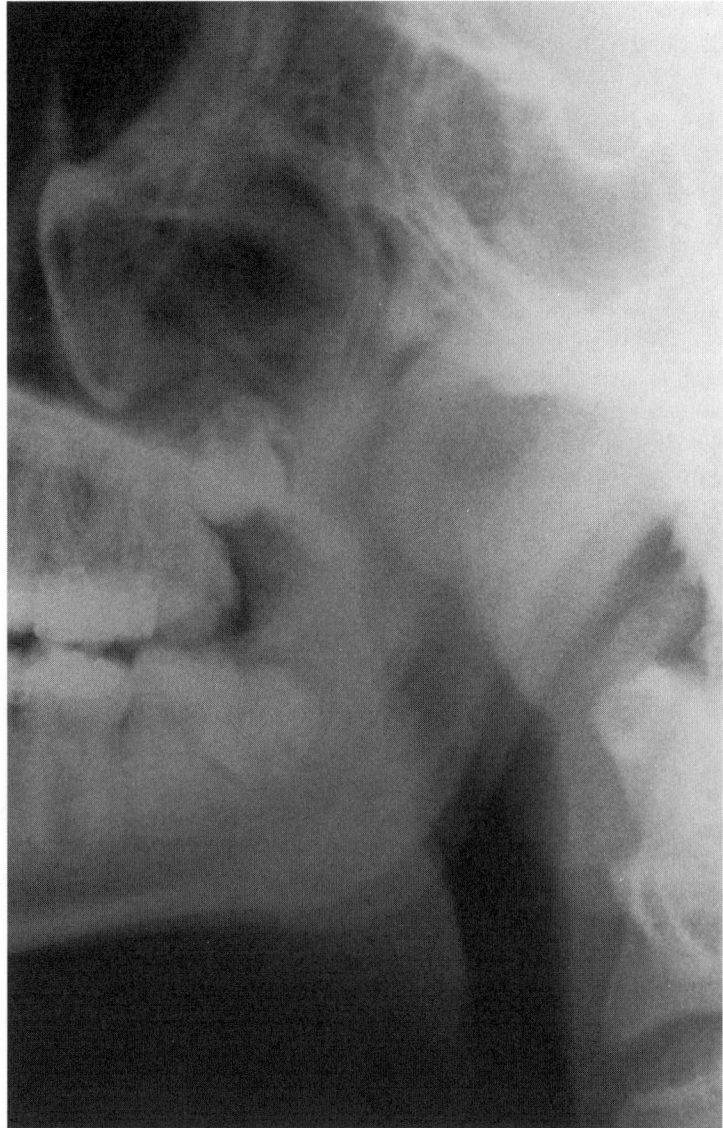

Figure 14.7 Lateral radiograph of the nasopharynx, showing the shadow of adenoid tissue.

tion of the serous otitis media; if it does not resolve, pressure-equalizing tubes can be inserted.

Fungal infections of the nasopharynx are rare, usually occurring with sinonasal fungal infection. Infection with *Mycobacterium*, *Rhinosporidium*, or *Pneu*-

Table 14.1 Differential Diagnosis of Nasopharyngeal Disorders

Inflammatory Conditions

Viral infections
Bacterial infections
Fungal infections
Tuberculosis

Systemic Medical Conditions

Inherited conditions and congenital syndromes
Choanal atresia
Tornwaldt's cyst
Rathke's pouch
Autoimmune disorders
Allergic conditions

Benign Tumors

Pleomorphic adenoma
Amyloidoma

Malignant Tumors

Squamous cell carcinoma (e.g., lymphoepithelioma, anaplastic carcinoma)
Lymphoma
Adenoid cystic carcinoma
Rhabdomyosarcoma
Metastatic disease

Local Disorders

Adenoidal hypertrophy
Patulous eustachian tube
Polyps arising from nasopharyngeal tissue
Juvenile angiofibroma

Case 14.1 Woman with Acute Nasopharyngitis

A woman 45 years of age presents with a 1-week history of upper throat pain. On additional questioning, she relates that she has had some pain associated with nasal breathing, especially when outdoors in the cold weather. She had a cold approximately 2 weeks ago; however, most of those symptoms have resolved. She is afebrile and otherwise healthy.

Nasal endoscopy reveals a beefy, red nasopharyngeal mucosa with small specks of pus. A diagnosis of acute nasopharyngitis is made.

She is treated for 10 days with a broad-spectrum antibiotic. On return visit 2 weeks later, her symptoms have resolved. Repeat endoscopy shows resolution of the mucosal erythema, with the nasopharyngeal mucosa now normal in color.

---

mocystis alerts the physician to the likelihood of acute AIDS. *Mucor* infection in a diabetes or other immunocompromised patient is a surgical emergency, because early, complete debridement dramatically improves survival. Treatment of other fungal rhinosinusitis may involve systemic antifungal medication, surgical excision of diseased tissue, and adequate drainage.

Tuberculosis can cause ulcerative lesions in the nasopharynx and may be associated with cervical adenopathy. The inflamed nodes are usually in the posterior triangle of the neck, whereas nasopharyngeal carcinoma typically is found in the apex of the posterior triangle. Nasopharyngeal tuberculosis can be seen alone and does not imply tuberculous infection elsewhere in the body.

Local Disorders

The most common benign mass in the nasopharynx is enlarged **adenoids**, which are present in almost all children. Enlarged adenoids can cause mouth breathing and hyponasal speech. With severe adenoidal hypertrophy, there may be recurring otitis media and sinusitis, chronic mouth breathing, snoring, swallowing disorders, and a general failure to thrive. The chronic mouth-breather develops a typical facial appearance—an elongated mid-face, sometimes known as adenoid facies. Adenoidal enlargement also may cause chronic epistaxis, disturbed dental development, and carrier states (e.g., *Haemophilus influenzae*, beta-hemolytic *Streptococcus*). Adenoidectomy is curative. The adenoids usually involute during late childhood; thus, symptomatic adenoid enlargement in the adult is unusual. If an adult seems to have enlarged adenoids, be suspicious of AIDS, lymphoma, or nasopharyngeal cancer. An adenoidectomy biopsy is indicated and curative.

Atrophy of the soft tissues around the eustachian tube (caused by chronic disease states, rapid weight loss, or bulimia) may result in a **patulous (overly patent) eustachian tube**. Symptoms include a feeling of pressure in the ear that varies with breathing and an annoying tendency for the patient's voice to reverberate in his or her affected ear. Sometimes relief can be obtained by regaining lost body weight or by placing pressure-equalizing tubes in the tympanic membranes; oral guiafenesin may alleviate the symptoms. In the occasional patient whose symptoms remain bothersome, consider 1) building up the tissues of the eustachian orifice with injections of emulsified Gel-foam (temporary) or Teflon paste (permanent), or 2) performing a levator tendon transfer or section.

Most **nasopharyngeal polyps** arise within the nose or sinuses, but some originate in the nasopharyngeal mucosa. **Antrochoanal polyps** extend from the maxillary sinus and can achieve a prodigious size, causing severe nasal airway obstruction. Some can be seen through the mouth, hanging down beyond the edge of the soft palate into the oropharynx. Surgical removal is curative.

Nasopharyngeal or nasal obstruction or epistaxis in the male adolescent indicates **juvenile nasopharyngeal angiofibroma (JNA)** until proved otherwise; diagnosis is confirmed by CT or MRI (Fig. 14.8). JNA originates in the pterygopalatine fissure behind the maxilla, pushing the bony septa ahead as it grows into the nasopharynx, orbit, sinuses, skull base, cavernous sinus, or

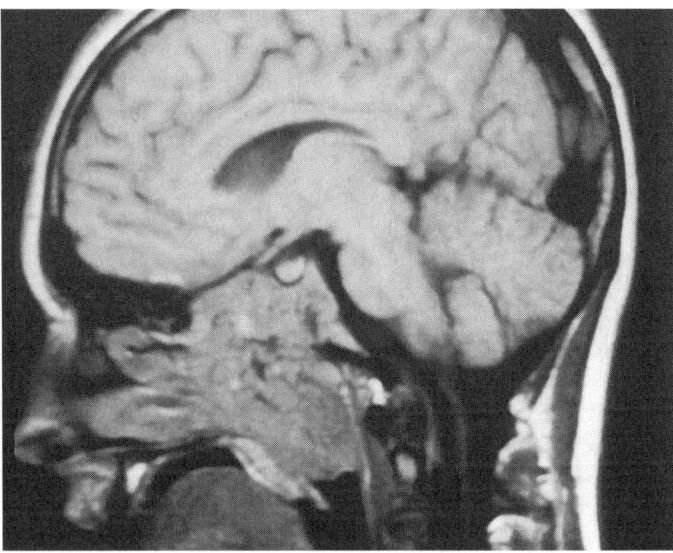

Figure 14.8 Large juvenile angiofibroma is seen in this computed tomography scan. (Courtesy of Dr. David Eibling.)

brain. Surgical excision of these highly vascular tumors is preceded by embolization of the contributing vessels. Although JNA tumors are not highly radiosensitive, radiotherapy can be useful in arresting their growth and may be the only reasonable treatment option for massive tumors.

Congenital Conditions

Choanal atresia results from failure of the buccopharyngeal membrane to cleave during embryologic development. The obstruction is bony in 90% of individuals, bilateral in 60%, more common in women, and often associated with cardiac and other deformities. Bilateral choanal atresia is life threatening in newborns (all of whom are obligate nose-breathers) and is usually diagnosed and treated in infancy. Unilateral choanal atresia may be relatively asymptomatic, causing nasal obstruction with upper respiratory infections and mild chronic unilateral rhinorrhea. Such cases may not be diagnosed until adulthood. Diagnosis is by fiberoptic examination, followed by CT for surgical planning. Treatment involves removing the bony obstruction and forming an epithelial-lined nasal passage, which may be accomplished by either transnasal or transpalatal approaches. Tornwaldt's cysts and Rathke's pouches are embryologic remnants; although rarely symptomatic, surgical excision is necessary when these are symptomatic (e.g., nasal obstruction).

Benign Nasopharyngeal Tumors

Benign lesions of the nasopharynx are rare (except for polyps, JNAs, and Tornwaldt's cysts). **Pleomorphic adenomas** arise from minor salivary glands and usually can be "shelled out" surgically. **Amyloidomas** are rare benign tumors of the nasopharyngeal soft tissue whose irregular margins may lead to confusion with a malignancy.

Malignant Tumors

The most common nasopharyngeal malignancy is **squamous cell carcinoma**. This disease is more common in men and in people from southeastern China (Fig. 14.9) (Case 14.2). The lesions typically originate in Rosenmüller's fossa in young to middle-aged adults, metastasizing to the neck when the primary tumor is still quite small. Common presenting complaints are neck mass or unilateral

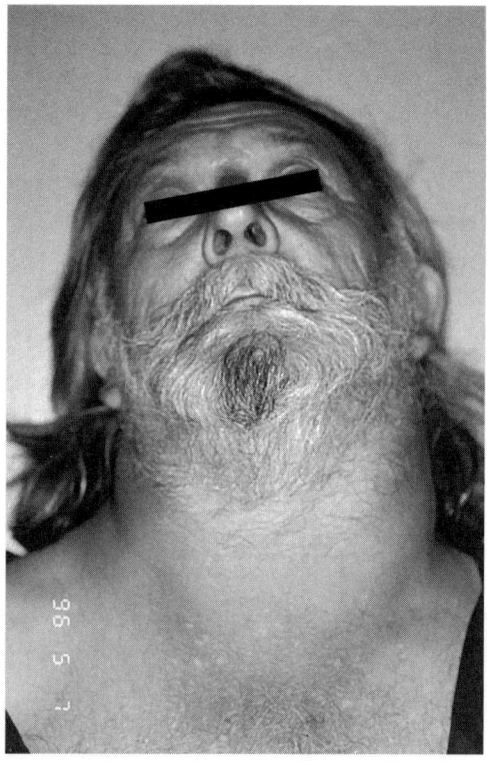

Figure 14.9 This patient developed large neck metastases from a nasopharyngeal carcinoma. (Courtesy of Dr. David Eibling.)

> **Case 14.2 Man with Squamous Cell Carcinoma That Is Manifested by a Neck Mass**
>
> A man 62 years of age presents with a 3-month history of a hard mass 4 cm in diameter approximately halfway down the posterior border of the right sternocleidomastoid muscle. It has been growing slowly and is not painful or tender. There are no other neck masses. He also relates that his hearing is "off a little" in his right ear, and he now uses his left ear when on the phone.
>
> Physical examination, including flexible fiberoptic nasopharyngoscopy, reveals no abnormalities except a serous effusion behind the right tympanic membrane.
>
> Fine-needle aspiration of the mass shows moderately differentiated squamous cell carcinoma. In the operating room, panendoscopy reveals a normal nasopharyngeal mucosa without erythema, edema, masses, ulcerations, or other lesions. Selected biopsies are taken from both of Rosenmüller's fossae and several other sites in the nasopharynx. The biopsy from the right fossa shows squamous cell carcinoma. Metastatic work-up does not reveal any further spread of tumor. The patient's diagnosis is T1N2M0 nasopharyngeal squamous cell carcinoma.
>
> He is treated with primary radiation therapy to the primary (nasopharynx) and both necks.

serous otitis media with a conductive hearing loss (due to eustachian tube blockage by the tumor); epistaxis also can be a presenting symptom. Squamous cell tumors that have a high lymphoid content are called *nasopharyngeal lymphoepitheliomas*.

The primary lesions are often painless but may cause bloody postnasal discharge. The disease spreads first to the upper retropharyngeal nodes, which are often clinically silent, and then to the ipsilateral high cervical nodes. As the disease progresses locally, cranial nerves become involved. The fifth nerve is usually the first of the cranial nerves to be affected, resulting in headaches or facial pain and decreased corneal reflexes. The glossopharyngeal, vagal, spinal accessory, hypoglossal, and abducens nerves also can be involved. Differential diagnosis includes necrotizing sialometaplasia and tuberculosis. Radiotherapy, with or without chemotherapy, is the main treatment for nasopharyngeal carcinoma. Hodgkin's disease and non-Hodgkin's lymphoma have been described as occurring primarily and secondarily in the nasopharynx.

Rare tumors of the nasopharynx include adenoid cystic carcinomas and rhabdomyosarcomas. **Adenoid cystic carcinomas (cylindromas)** extend via a perineural tissue invasion, with metastatic spread to pulmonary tissue in the form of asymptomatic large "snowball" metastatic foci. Rhabdomyosarcomas occur primarily in the nasopharynx and are aggressive malignancies seen more commonly in boys, but rarely beyond 6 years of age. **Metastasis** to the nasopharynx is rare; however, the rich lymphatic network in the nasopharynx places it at risk for metastatic disease from any distant primary tumor.

Danger Signs

The primary danger in treating nasopharyngeal disorders is missing or delaying the diagnosis of a malignancy. Signs that suggest malignancy include a hard, fixed neck mass; severe pain; epistaxis; unilateral serous effusion in the middle ear; and conductive hearing loss. Fiberoptic examination in the office often reveals a suspicious lesion in patients with these symptoms. CT usually is obtained to delineate the extent of the lesion, followed by examination under general anesthesia to biopsy and map the lesion.

Summary

The nasopharynx is a relatively clinically silent area of the head and neck. A high index of suspicion is required to avoid missing serious nasopharyngeal problems. Any patient with serous otitis media, epistaxis, nasal obstruction, or an undiagnosed neck mass needs to be evaluated carefully for possible nasopharyngeal pathology.

SUGGESTED READINGS

Derebery MJ, Berliner KI. Allergic eustachian tube dysfunction: diagnosis and treatment. *Am J Otol.* 1997;18:160–5.
  Describes how inhalant and food allergies can affect the function of the eustachian tube and how different allergy treatments can improve the patient's symptoms.

Fagan JJ, Snyderman CH, Carrau FL, Janecka IP. Nasopharyngeal angiofibromas: selecting a surgical approach. *Head Neck.* 1997;19:391–9.
  Details the considerations in surgical approaches for this disease and investigates factors that affect recurrence.

Indudharan R, Valuyeetham KA, Kannan T, Sidek DS. Nasopharyngeal carcinoma: clinical trends. *J Laryngol Otol.* 1997;111:724–9.
  Reviews the clinical presentations and initial diagnostic work-up of nasopharyngeal carcinoma.

Mukherji SK, Castillo M. Normal cross-sectional anatomy of the nasopharynx, oropharynx, and oral cavity. *Neuroimag Clin North Am.* 1998;8:211–8.
  Reviews the normal cross-sectional anatomy of these areas on CT and MRI.

Vasef MA, Ferlito A, Weiss LM. Nasopharyngeal carcinoma with emphasis on its relationship to Epstein–Barr virus. *Ann Otol Rhinol Laryngol.* 1997;106:348–56.
  Describes the geographic distribution, pathogenesis, and predisposing genetic and environmental factors of this disease.

15

Dysphagia

John W. Cavo Jr., MD
David E. Eibling, MD

Dysphagia is a common complaint and is often a significant problem for the elderly patient. The sequelae of dysphagia are weight loss, aspiration, and a reduction (or elimination) in the pleasure of eating and in the social interaction associated with meals. Dysphagia affects not only the elderly but also many other patients with a number of chronic illnesses; it may be an important early symptom in a variety of disease processes (Tables 15.1 and 15.2). Vague dysphagia also may be a complaint in some poorly defined clinical entities, such as globus hystericus. It is important to distinguish between dysphagia (difficulty swallowing) and odynophagia (painful swallowing). It is perhaps enlightening to note that, although it is technically only a symptom, dysphagia has been assigned its own ICD-9 diagnosis code. This assignation is fortunate considering that the efforts directed toward symptom management are often considerably more intensive than those directed toward the underlying disease process. At the top of the differential diagnosis list for odynophagia is tumor, and the first step in the work-up is to rule out the presence of an upper aerodigestive tumor. This chapter deals with dysphagia and its pathophysiology, evaluation, and therapeutic strategies.

Relevant Anatomy and Physiology

Dividing the swallowing function into four phases (the oral preparation, oral, pharyngeal, and esophageal phases) facilitates the discussion of normal and

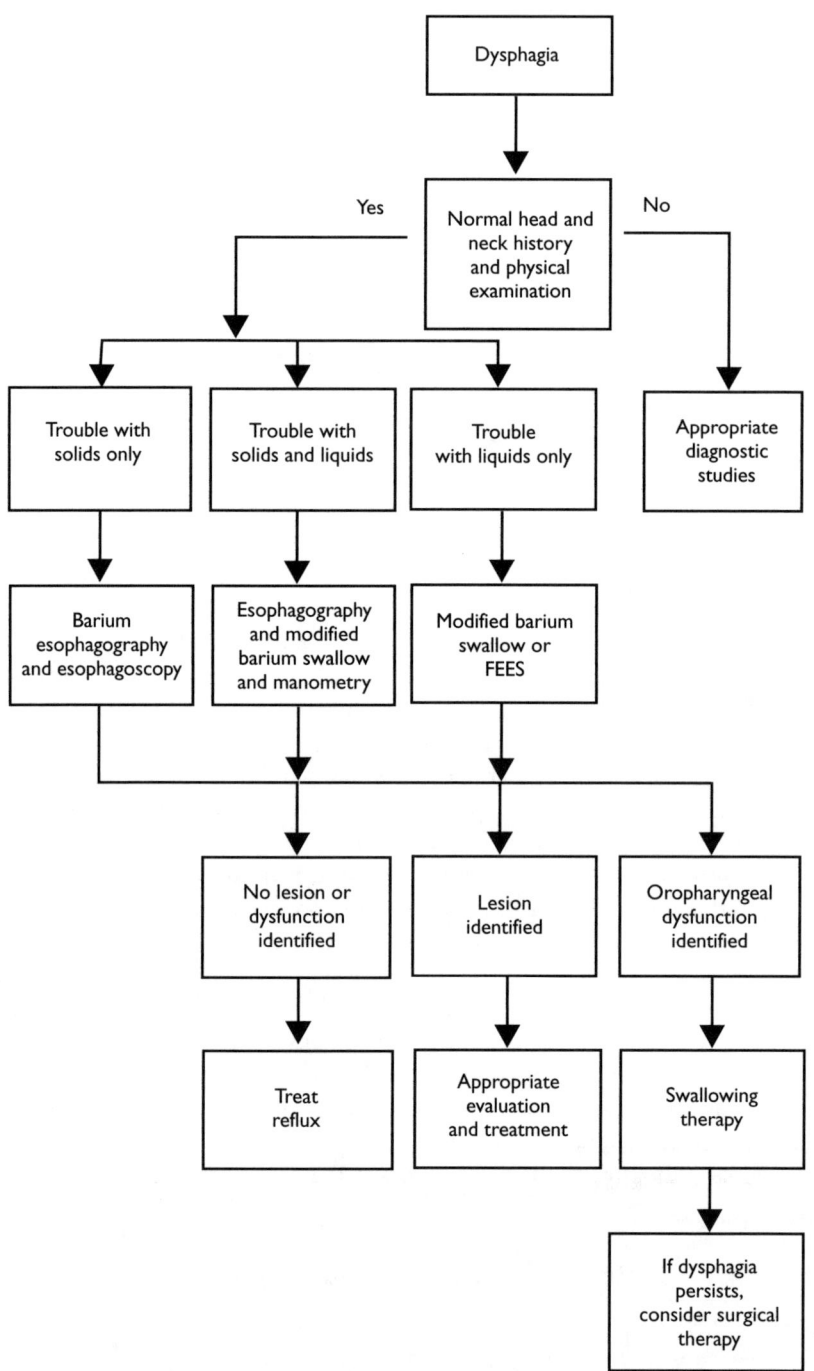

Algorithm Management of dysphagia. FEES = flexible (fiberoptic) endoscopic examination of swallowing.

Table 15.1 Systemic Causes of Dysphagia

Musculoskeletal Disorders
Osteoarthritis (especially involving the cervical spine)
Kyphoscoliosis
DISH
Ankylosing spondylitis
Pectus excavatum

Cardiovascular Disorders
Left atrial enlargement
Thoracic aneurysms
Vascular rings

Neurological Disorders
Parkinson's disease
Stroke
Myasthenia gravis
Presbyesophagus
Progressive demyelinating disorders
Oculopharyngeal syndrome

Connective Tissue and Autoimmune Disorders
Sjögren's syndrome
Scleroderma
Polymyositis rheumatica
Rheumatoid arthritis
Lupus erythematosis

General Disorders
Diabetes
Alcoholism
Pernicious anemia
Hypothyroidism

Medications
Anticholinergics
Antidepressants
Antihypertensives
Diuretics
Phenothiazines

DISH = diffuse idiopathic skeletal hyperostosis

Table 15.2 Local Problems That Cause Dysphagia

Oropharyngeal Disorders
Tongue base, palatal, and tonsillar disorders
Neoplasms
Foreign bodies
Tumor resection (e.g., palate, tongue, floor of mouth)
Cranial neuropathies

Hypopharyngeal and Cervical Esophageal Disorders
Cricopharyngeal achalasia
Zenker's diverticulum
Thyroid enlargement
Strictures
Neoplasms
Foreign bodies
Cervical spine surgery

Thoracic Esophageal Disorders
Motility disorders
Presbyesophagus
Achalasia
Intrinsic esophageal obstruction (e.g., scarring, neoplasms, foreign bodies)
Extrinsic esophageal obstruction (e.g., cardiovascular, neoplasms, musculoskeletal, mediastinal masses)

abnormal function. The mouth-to-stomach transit time, which varies with the size and texture of the food bolus, ranges from 8 to 11 seconds (most of which is required for passing through the esophagus). In a normal, young individual, the oral and pharyngeal phases each take less than 1 second.

Although the oral preparation phase is technically not part of the swallow, it is important for effective deglutition. Moreover, defects in this phase are common and may dramatically interfere with swallowing function.

Oral Preparation Phase

Food cannot be ingested by a human (compared with, say, a snake) without it first being converted from a solid to a liquid or semisolid state. Tearing and grinding solid food requires intact dentition, either natural or prosthetic. Dentition defects are common and may result in clinical sequelae that mimic dysphagia, often causing misdirected (and costly) evaluation and therapy. Intact salivary function is required for liquefying the food bolus and for lubricating and moisturizing the mucosal surfaces. Various local and metabolic factors can result in an insufficient amount of saliva, which also mimics dysphagia. Finally, mastication requires an intact structural and functional oral cavity. Surgical defects, neurological disability, and a variety of other conditions can result in defective oral cavity food preparation and subsequent dysfunctional deglutition.

Oral Phase

After it is masticated and mixed with saliva (oral preparation phase), the food bolus is formed and positioned in the middle of the tongue. The oral phase occurs when the bolus is pressed firmly against the tonsillar pillars (Fig. 15.1). This voluntary motion triggers the involuntary pharyngeal phase of swallowing. The oral phase often is disrupted significantly (a failure of swallow initiation) in patients with neurological disorders or in those who have undergone surgery for oral cavity cancer. The inability of the oral cavity to position or hold the bolus also can result in defective swallowing function by permitting oral contents to escape into the pharynx either before or after a swallow, causing leakage into the airway (aspiration).

Pharyngeal Phase

The pharynx of all mammals plays an integral part in both deglutition and respiration. In adult humans, these two functions do not normally occur simultaneously; rather, these functions use the common cavity at different times. The phase begins when the tongue pushes the bolus posteriorly into the oropharynx. The soft palate elevates, closing off the nasopharynx and preventing na-

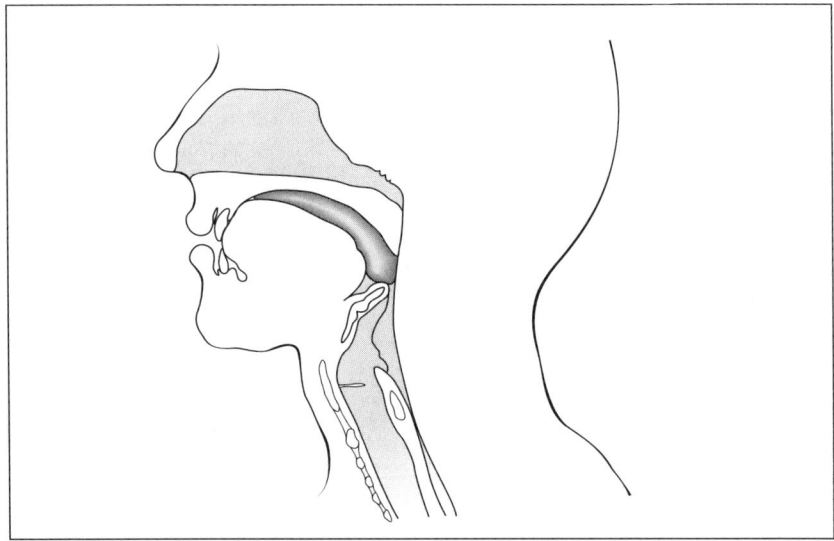

Figure 15.1 Oral phase of swallowing. The food bolus is positioned in the middle of the tongue, which then presses the bolus against the palatine arches, triggering the pharyngeal swallow. Weakness or malignancies of the tongue can affect this portion of swallowing function dramatically. (Republished with permission from Eibling DE, Johnson JT, Bacon GE. *Understanding and Treating Aspiration SiPac*. Alexandria, VA: American Academy of Otolaryngology–Head and Neck Surgery; 1993.)

sopharyngeal regurgitation. The superior constrictor muscle (an envelope of striated muscle originating at the skull base) contracts, beginning pharyngeal peristalsis. However, the primary propulsive force in this phase is the "tongue-driving force." Respiration ceases (usually during expiration), the larynx closes and elevates, and the epiglottis retroflexes, diverting the bolus around the opening of the larynx (Fig. 15.2). The larynx closes via adduction of the arytenoids as well as by their approximation to the base of the epiglottis. Vocal cord paralysis reduces the efficacy of vocal cord closure and can result in dysphagia. Bolus propulsion is enhanced by a shortening of the pharynx and by both a passive and active dilatation of the upper esophageal sphincter (cricopharyngeal muscle) caused by laryngeal elevation. The cricopharyngeal and inferior constrictor muscles then relax, permitting the food to pass into the upper esophagus. This phase lasts approximately three quarters of a second.

Esophageal Phase

The esophageal phase of swallowing begins as the cricopharyngeus muscle relaxes and as the hypopharyngeal contents pass into the thoracic esopha-

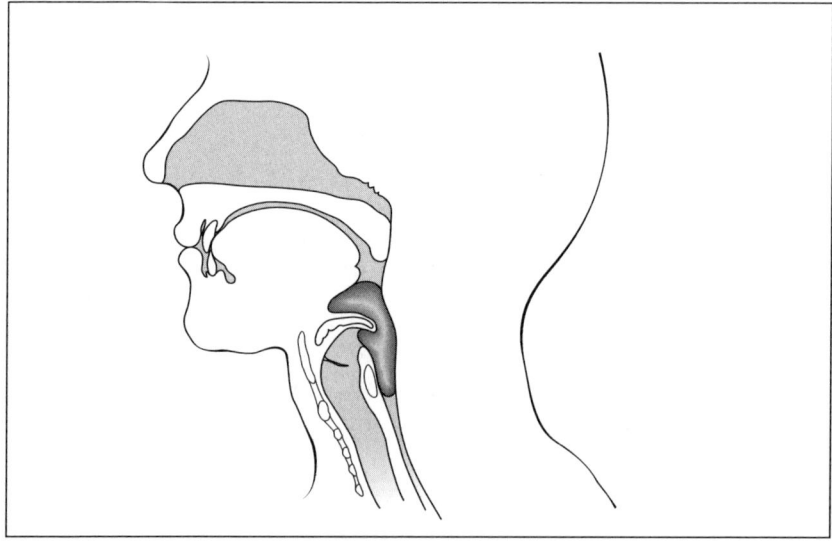

Figure 15.2 Pharyngeal phase of swallowing. The bolus is propelled inferiorly past the glottis by a combination of tongue pressure and pharyngeal muscle peristalsis. The larynx closes reflexively, and the epiglottis diverts the bolus around the glottic inlet. The larynx rises, shortening the pharynx and actively opening the cricopharyngeal muscular sphincter. (Republished with permission from Eibling DE, Johnson JT, Bacon GE. *Understanding and Treating Aspiration SiPac.* American Academy of Otolaryngology–Head and Neck Surgery; 1993.)

gus (Fig. 15.3). The food bolus is propelled 20 to 25 cm through the thoracic esophagus by a series of peristaltic contractions. As the inferior esophageal sphincter relaxes, the bolus moves into the gastric cardia. Transit through the thoracic esophagus requires approximately 6 to 9 seconds.

Differential Diagnosis

Because symptoms of dysphagia are usually nonlocalized, the differential diagnoses are typically numerous. Tables 15.1 and 15.2 list some of the more common causes of dysphagia, separating them into **local** and **systemic** disease processes. As a rule, **esophageal disorders** present with **obstructive-type symptoms**; therefore, solid foods tend to be more problematic. A barium swallow is most helpful in these cases. **Pharyngeal and oral disorders** often present with **aspiration** as manifested by coughing with liquids or aspiration pneumonitis. Modified barium swallow or functional endoscopic evaluation of swallowing under direct visualization is the best

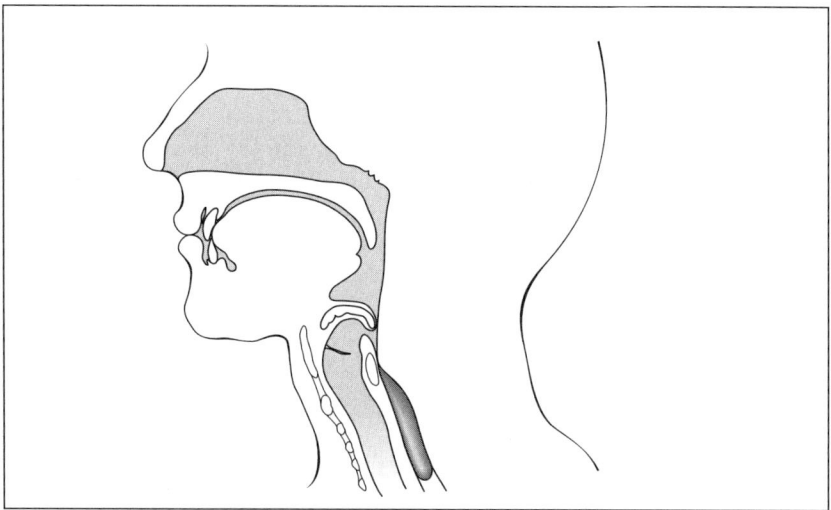

Figure 15.3 Esophageal phase of swallowing. The longest of the swallowing phases, the esophageal phase requires 6 to 9 seconds to move the bolus of food from the pharynx to the stomach. (Republished with permission from Eibling DE, Johnson JT, Bacon GE. *Understanding and Treating Aspiration SiPac.* Alexandria, VA: American Academy of Otolaryngology–Head and Neck Surgery; 1993.)

method of diagnosing the cause. However, affected sites usually are not mutually exclusive, and many patients suffer from dysphagia that involve many organ systems. Prudent physicians recognize that dysphagia may be a component of many illnesses and subsequently are aware of the potential for significant morbidity.

Systemic Conditions That Cause Dysphagia

Stroke

The most common cause of dysphagia in the general population is stroke, which affects approximately 750,000 individuals per year, with as many as 50% of these patients having some dysphagia. In most patients, however, the dysphagia resolves rapidly. The prevalence of stroke ensures that the disease (and its accompanying dysphagia) is encountered by nearly every physician who treats adults. The significance of dysphagia in the stroke patient is well known, accounting for much of the acute and chronic morbidity associated with stroke. Many patients have minimal or no symptoms and are at risk for aspiration; hence, most institutions have developed multidisciplinary dysphagia teams to evaluate and treat afflicted individuals.

Parkinson's Disease

James Parkinson himself described dysphagia as a key component of the disease that was named after him. Prospective evaluation of swallowing function demonstrates dysphagia in a high percentage of patients with early Parkinson's disease, often in the absence of any clinical complaints. Clinical progression leads to obvious dysphagia and to worsening problems with aspiration. Weakness and dyscoordination are seen on contrast, endoscopic, and manometric swallowing studies (Case 15.1). Patients begin to swallow smaller boluses and may aspirate liquids– a condition that gradually worsens with disease progression. Most patients eventually develop pneumonia, sometimes as the terminal event in the disease.

Lower Motor Neuron Disorders

Weakness, wasting, and fasciculations characterize lower motor neuron disorders such as amyotrophic lateral sclerosis and various bulbar palsies. Multiple sclerosis patients also may develop intermittent bulbar weaknesses. Postpolio syndrome is commonly associated with dysphagia. All of these disorders can result in dysphagia by affecting any of the critical muscular actions required for swallowing, including motion of the tongue and palate, laryngeal closure or elevation, and peristalsis. In most instances of lower motor neuron dysfunction, multiple swallowing actions are affected; hence, procedures that correct one specific function (e.g., vocal cord augmentation, cricopharyngeal myotomy) typically provide only limited benefit.

An unusual but occasionally encountered cause of dysphagia is Arnold–Chiari malformation with resultant vagus nerve dysfunction. Although rarely seen in adults, dysphagia may be the presenting symptom. Surgical decompression can result in significant improvement.

Muscular Diseases

Striated muscle weakness occurring with diabetes, demyelinating neuropathies, alcoholism, and polymyositis rheumatica often causes dysphagia.

Muscular dystrophies are characterized by progressive skeletal muscle weakness. The involvement of deglutition muscles causes dysphagia that sometimes worsens to aspiration. Oculopharyngeal syndrome is a type of familial muscular dystrophy that occurs primarily in French-Canadian patients in whom dysphagia is accompanied by diplopia. Hypothyroidism can cause dysphagia by either muscular weakness or thyroid enlargement with subsequent extrinsic esophageal compression.

Myasthenia Gravis

Severe weakness of the deglutition muscles is seen commonly with myasthenia gravis. Dysphagia may be the presenting symptom in myasthenia gravis; aspiration pneumonia may be the terminal event. Typically, dysphagia in

> **Case 15.1** **Elderly Man with Dysphagia Caused by Parkinson's Disease**
>
> A man 78 years of age with Parkinson's disease is spending an inordinate amount of time eating (averaging 45 minutes to 1 hour per meal) and has a "wet"-sounding voice for several minutes after meals. His disease has been slowly progressive, and he has required occasional dose adjustments of his medication (Sinemet). He is able to ambulate (shuffle) without assistance, but he has a significant resting tremor and an obviously weak voice. He has not had any episodes of pneumonia, and he denies difficulty swallowing. His family suspects that he has lost weight, but they have not been able to persuade him to get weighed.
>
> His physical examination is unremarkable, with the exception of the characteristics of Parkinson's disease. Fiberoptic laryngoscopy is normal for his age, with normal vocal cord motion but with some bowing during phonation. A flexible (fiberoptic) endoscopic examination of swallowing (FEES) demonstrates significant delay in swallowing all food consistencies, with marked residue in his pharynx following swallowing.
>
> Alternating food consistency is recommended, with emphasis on soft and semisoft foods and thickened liquids (and only minimal sips of thin liquids to clear any residue). The patient begins to work regularly with a speech pathologist at a local rehabilitation hospital as an outpatient to strengthen vocal cord and pharyngeal muscles using standard techniques. This therapy is not covered by insurance, but his family agrees to pay the $200-per-week fee. He agrees to be weighed on a periodic basis, and he is advised that if he is unable to maintain his weight he needs to make a decision about alternative feeding methods. Finally, you adjust his Sinemet dose again in an attempt to optimize therapy.
>
> **Discussion**
>
> Parkinson's disease is well recognized as a major cause of morbid dysphagia with weight loss and aspiration due to slowing and weakness of pharyngeal transit. Investigators have pointed out that swallowing function often is affected much more severely than is recognized by the Parkinson's disease patient (compared with patients with a globus) and may be the eventual cause of his or her demise. Swallowing function may vary dramatically with medication dose and timing and is often responsive to speech therapy directed at laryngeal and pharyngeal strengthening. Finally, many patients with Parkinson's disease eventually have to make a decision about whether to accept alternative feeding methods or to assume the inevitable risk of aspiration pneumonia. A few patients may elect to undergo laryngotracheal separation to continue on an oral diet, even though this procedure results in permanent tracheostomy and loss of voice.

these patients is worse later in the day and is accompanied by ill-defined fatigue. Ptosis may be present and, in combination with dysphagia, should be an indication for further investigation.

Alcoholism

An esophageal motility disorder that develops in some alcoholics is characterized by tertiary waves on manometry and on contrast studies. One must remember that alcoholics are also at increased risk for developing malignancies of the pharynx and esophagus, which may present with dysphagia (Case 15.2). Esophageal reflux and varices also can play a role in dysphagia in alcoholics.

Diabetes

Esophageal motility disorders are encountered commonly in diabetes patients, who due to their immunocompromised state are also vulnerable to esophageal candidiasis, which can cause severe odynophagia.

Sjögren's Disease and Other Autoimmune Diseases

Sjögren's disease results in secondary dysphagia due to reduced salivary flow and resultant inadequate lubrication of the food bolus. Sclerotic changes in

---

Case 15.2 Alcoholic Man with Squamous Cell Carcinoma That Presents as Dysphagia

An unemployed man 57 years of age presents with a difficulty in swallowing. He is a heavy user of alcohol and tobacco and has had a previous episode of hemoptysis for which chest radiography and bronchoscopy were negative. He admits to some weight loss as evidenced by him having moved his belt buckle two holes, but he is not sure of the exact amount of weight he had lost. He also notes some ear pain but denies having a sore throat.

Physical examination reveals normal ears and oral cavity. Indirect laryngoscopy is normal, but finger palpation of his oropharynx reveals a massive submucosal tumor that involves most of his tongue base. Computed tomography confirms the physical findings and does not reveal any adenopathy. Barium esophagography was normal. The tumor is biopsied and found to be squamous cell carcinoma.

The patient enrolls in an experimental protocol of concurrent radiotherapy and chemotherapy.

Discussion

This case illustrates that patients often confuse pain on swallowing with difficulty swallowing. Moreover, although this patient previously had undergone bronchoscopy, the tumor was submucosal and was not visualized. Adding to the difficulty in diagnosis, barium esophagography was normal because of the submucosal nature of the tumor and the emphasis on detecting esophageal pathology with this study. In the end, the physical examination, which included oropharyngeal palpation, led to the diagnosis.

the soft tissues of the upper thoracic esophagus cause dysphagia in scleroderma. Lupus erythematosus and other autoimmune diseases also can present with dysphagia.

Other Systemic Causes of Dysphagia
Pernicious anemia causes a ridge of hypertrophied soft tissue (web) on the posterior hypopharyngeal wall that can cause dysphagia (Plummer–Vinson syndrome). Patients who are immunocompromised due to a variety of causes are at risk for oral, pharyngeal, or esophageal ulcerations or infections (especially candidiasis).

Local Problems That Cause Dysphagia

Foreign Bodies
Two kinds of foreign bodies can present with dysphagia: 1) sharp foreign bodies that lodge in the upper aerodigestive tract and result in pain, and 2) blunt objects (e.g., poorly masticated meat) that become impacted in the esophagus and result in obstruction. In both instances, the history usually provides valuable information to direct the evaluation. (*See* Chapter 29 for a complete discussion of foreign body evaluation and management.)

Cricopharyngeal Achalasia
The cricopharyngeus muscle originates on the posterior cricoid cartilage and surrounds the upper esophagus, comprising most of the upper esophageal sphincter. This sphincter is opened by laryngeal elevation as the muscle relaxes, allowing the food bolus to pass into the thoracic esophagus. When the cricopharyngeus fails to relax or when laryngeal elevation is weak, the cricopharyngeus muscle acts as an obstruction. Barium studies in the lateral projection may show a bar of soft tissue indenting the posterior wall of the cervical esophagus. Mirror or fiberoptic examination may reveal pooling of saliva and/or mucus in the pyriform sinuses. Surgical division of this muscle (cricopharyngeal myotomy) often improves symptomatology and is occasionally curative. Patient selection is difficult, and the role of this procedure remains controversial, especially in neurologically impaired patients.

Zenker's Diverticulum
Long-standing cricopharyngeal dysfunction can lead to the development of a pulsion diverticulum through a congenital weakened area of the pharyngeal constrictor musculature that lies just cephalad to the cricopharyngeal muscle. Known as Zenker's diverticulum, it can become quite large and is associated with significant dysphagia for the patient. Patients often have symptoms of as-

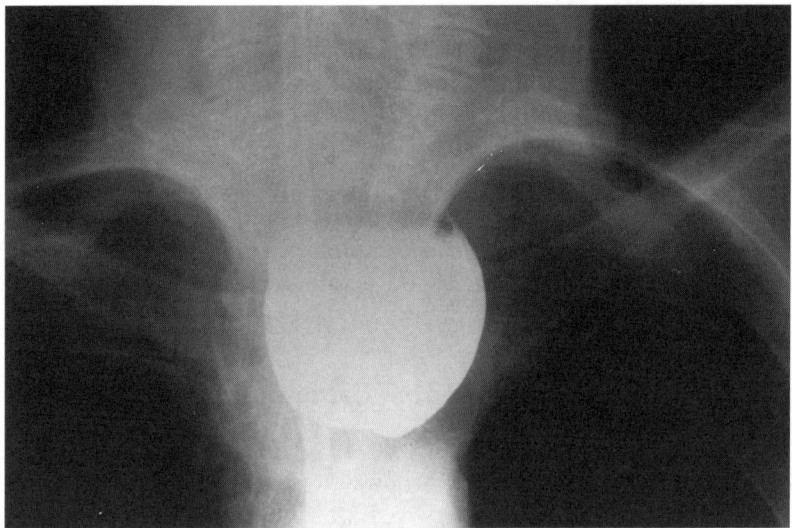

Figure 15.4 Zenker's diverticulum seen in the anteroposterior projection after barium esophagraphy has been performed. These pulsion diverticuli occur just above the cricopharyngeus muscle sphincter and respond well to surgical division of the cricopharyngeus (either endoscopic or open), with appropriate management of the diverticulum.

piration or chronic mucus production and complain classically of coughing up undigested food. Diagnosis is via radiography (Fig. 15.4), which usually demonstrates a prominent cricopharyngeal sphincter and the pouch. Flexible endoscopy is often thwarted by the endoscope's tendency to pass into the diverticulum instead of into the esophagus. Zenker's diverticulum can cause potentially life-threatening dysphagia in elderly patients and may be mistaken for cancer (Case 15.3).

Diffuse Esophageal Spasm

Patients with diffuse esophageal spasm suffer substernal, cramp-like pain. Because it may be difficult to distinguish between angina and diffuse esophageal spasm, patients who acutely present with substernal pain are evaluated routinely for both. Contrast and manometric studies demonstrate diffuse spastic activity.

Gastroesophageal Reflux Disease

Pathologic gastroesophageal reflux (GERD) has been recognized in 10% to 15% of the population. Uncomplicated GERD typically is not associated with dysphagia; therefore, dysphagia that occurs in a patient with known or suspected GERD should precipitate an investigation to discover another cause.

> **Case 15.3   Elderly Man with Zenker's Diverticulum**
>
> A man 85 years of age who resides in an assisted-living home has lost 25 lb in the past 6 months and has a "wet" vocal quality. He is a nonsmoker and only recently has been a poor eater. His past medical history is unremarkable, and it does not appear that he has suffered a stroke.
>
> Physical examination reveals significant pooling of secretions in his hypopharynx but no anatomic or neurologic abnormalities. Barium esophagography reveals a large Zenker's diverticulum.
>
> Endoscopic stapler–assisted diverticulotomy with division of the cricopharyngeus muscle is performed uneventfully. Within 1 week, the patient is eating "several times" what he did before the procedure.
>
> **Discussion**
>
> Zenker's diverticulum can result in potentially life-threatening dysphagia for the elderly (especially those in chronic-care facilities) and can mimic cancer. In most instances, barium esophagography is diagnostic. Treatment by either open or endoscopic cricopharyngeal myotomy is curative and should be offered even to frail, elderly individuals, such as the man in this case study.

GERD is caused by incompetence of the distal esophageal sphincter, which may occur in both obese and normal-weight individuals. Regurgitation of stomach contents into the distal esophagus, typically after a large meal when the patient is reclining, can cause subxiphoid pressure and discomfort. Radiographic evidence of an incompetent distal esophageal sphincter or a sliding hiatal hernia may suggest GERD but is present in only approximately one third of patients with documented reflux. Manometric studies reveal decreased distal esophageal sphincter tone. A Bernstein test helps differentiate between substernal pain caused by reflux and angina. The "gold standard" for the diagnosis of reflux is 24-hour Ph-metry. In this test, a catheter is placed in the esophagus to sample its contents continuously. A small incidence of reflux is considered normal, and the criteria for abnormal esophageal reflux are well established. It must be noted that patients with pharyngeal reflux may not have the classic symptoms of GERD. This lack of reliability has led many centers to use dual-probe Ph-metry, in which an upper probe is positioned at the level of the laryngeal inlet. However, upper-probe criteria have yet to be established.

Globus Hystericus

The sensation of a "lump" in the throat is called *globus* and is a common complaint encountered by physicians. Over half of affected patients can be demon-

> **Case 15.4** **Woman with Dysphagia That Represents Gastroesophageal Reflux Disease**
>
> A woman 45 years of age with a body mass index in the top 10% complains of a 3-year history of a "lump" in her throat. This symptom is nearly always present and occasionally awakens her from sleep. She has not had any difficulty swallowing either solids or liquids and has not had to alter her diet. She is a nonsmoker, does not drink alcohol, and denies having sore throat and otalgia.
>
> Physical examination is unremarkable, and a barium swallow reveals a hiatal hernia. A presumptive diagnosis of GERD is made.
>
> The patient is treated with phase I antireflux measures with a proton-pump inhibitor for 30 days. She returns later, stating that her globus sensation has improved significantly, and she is switched to a chronic H_2 blocker.
>
> **Discussion**
>
> This patient presented with a complaint of globus but, on further questioning, did not actually have dysphagia, nor did she have any danger signs to suggest that a serious disease was accounting for her complaint. Her physician elected to treat her empirically without confirmatory 24-hour Ph-metry, although some physicians might have elected to do so. Others might have recommended a formal esophagogastroduodenoscopy to rule out Barrett's esophagus.

strated to suffer from GERD, but a significant number do not respond to antireflux therapy (Case 15.4). One must recognize that globus is exceptionally nonspecific and occasionally may be an indication of a serious disease process. Hence, symptoms of globus without an obvious cause necessitate evaluation, with persistent symptoms requiring a repeated evaluation.

Achalasia

Achalasia is defined as distal esophageal flaccidity and a failure of the distal esophageal sphincter to relax normally to permit food to enter the stomach. Patients with this disorder present with dysphagia (often with more trouble swallowing solids than liquids) and have normal physical findings on flexible pharyngoscopy. Contrast studies demonstrate a dilated distal esophagus whose stretched length gives it a sigmoid shape. Manometric studies identify the hypotonic esophageal segment and the abnormal behavior of the lower esophageal sphincter that are characteristic of this disorder.

Cervical Spine Disease

Anterior surgical approaches to the cervical spine that require dissection and retraction of the pharynx and larynx often lead to dysphagia, probably through an interruption of the motor and sensory innervation. This dysphagia may be of short duration or may be prolonged. Avoiding excessive retraction or injury to the pharynx reduces but does not eliminate the risk of postoperative dysphagia. Injury to the recurrent laryngeal nerve during surgery also can contribute to this dysphagia. The surgical approach is from the patient's left side.

Large osteoarthritic spurs may develop on the cervical spine in patients with long-standing osteoarthritis of the spine and may impinge on the pharynx. This condition is most common in patients with diffuse idiopathic spinal hyperostosis. Although usually asymptomatic, these bony growths occasionally may become large enough to affect swallowing, usually by impairing laryngeal motion or by deflecting bolus material. Surgical resection may provide benefit for some patients; however, selecting which ones benefit is not a straightforward process, and some may become worse after surgery.

Cancer of the Larynx and Pharynx

Cancer that occurs in the upper aerodigestive tract can present with dysphagia, and it is important to recognize that these patients often complain of difficulty swallowing due to pain. The most common cancers to present with dysphagia are those of the pyriform sinus, supraglottis, tonsils, and tongue base. A typical patient with carcinoma of the upper aerodigestive tract is a middle-aged smoker and heavy drinker who is experiencing unilateral throat pain when swallowing. The pain is often constant and may radiate to the ipsilateral ear or to the mandibular angle. The physical examination is straightforward because most of these tumors can be visualized on indirect or fiberoptic examination or can be palpated with a gloved finger. Early diagnosis is the key to cure and successful rehabilitation of patients with these and other head and neck cancers. (*See* Chapter 31 for further discussion of cancer of the head and neck.)

Cancer of the Esophagus

The incidence of esophageal cancer has been rising steadily and is thought to be associated with Barrett's esophagus. Because of the insensibility and distensibility of the esophagus, identifying early cancer is problematic. Symptoms are usually vague, so an early diagnosis is unlikely. Classically, patients complain of dysphagia to solids, and the diagnosis is made by barium studies and/or esophagoscopy (Case 15.5). Because most of these tumors are at an advanced stage when they are discovered, survival is poor. It seems likely that further advances in the management of esophageal cancer will occur only when there is a better understanding of the significance of premalignant esophagitis.

> **Case 15.5** **Elderly Man with a History of Cancer Who Presents with Dysphagia to Solids**
>
> A man 65 years of age—a heavy tobacco user who underwent irradiation for early vocal cord carcinoma 6 years ago (with apparent cure)—presents with a 3-month history of increasing dysphagia to solids. After the diagnosis of his tumor, he had stopped smoking. Since then, he has been otherwise healthy, with the exception of some mild heartburn. His dysphagia initially manifested itself after he ate meat that lodged itself in his esophagus for nearly a minute before passing. After that incident, the patient has felt food "hold up" in a similar fashion several times. Consequently, he has modified his diet, is careful to chew his food completely, and tends to avoid large bites of beef and other meats. He has not experienced any weight loss, has had no voice change, and has no discomfort (except for the two or three times that food had been stuck).
>
> Physical examination was normal, with the exception of previous irradiation changes to his larynx and anterior neck skin. Barium esophagography reveals an irregularity of the esophageal mucosa just above the gastroesophageal junction. Esophagogastroduodenoscopy (EGD) reveals Barrett's esophagus involving 60% of the esophagus and a 2-cm ulcerated lesion on the anterior wall of the esophagus 3 cm above the gastroesophageal junction. Biopsy of the lesion reveals adenocarcinoma, and computed tomography staging demonstrates no evidence of transmural invasion or mediastinal or peri-aortic adenopathy. Further examination of the stomach and duodenum is normal.
>
> A trans-hiatal esophagectomy is performed, which removes not only the tumor but also the entire thoracic esophagus involved with Barrett's. The patient's esophagus is reconstructed with a gastric "pull-up," which was well tolerated. Adjunctive therapy with an investigative protocol is recommended, but the patient refuses.
>
> **Discussion**
>
> A high index of suspicion for a second cancer of the upper aerodigestive tract is required in any patient who has been treated previously for a malignancy in the region. This patient's symptoms were worrisome because his symptoms were increasing and seemed clearly to be of an obstructive nature. Even if his barium esophagogram had been interpreted as normal, the patient should be referred for an EGD. The role of routine EGD in the detection of patients with Barrett's esophagus is not well defined. Perhaps, in retrospect, this patient had a long history of symptomatic GERD that should have prompted earlier referral—there is some evidence that GERD may play a role in vocal cord cancer. Further longitudinal studies are needed.

History

The duration of the swallowing disorder, its characterization as pain or obstruction, and the sensation of its location are important for the diagnosis.

Symptoms can suggest the anatomic level of the problem. Dysphagia to solids suggests esophageal obstruction, whereas dysphagia to liquids suggests a pharyngeal disorder (usually due to a neuromuscular disease). Hypopharyngeal dysfunction causes suprasternal discomfort; esophageal dysphagia is often associated with substernal or subxiphoid pain. Distal esophageal obstructions sometimes cause pressure referred to the suprasternal area.

A history of weight loss aids in determining the significance and duration of dysphagia. Asking the patient about self-imposed dietary changes or the duration of an average meal (i.e., "How long does it take to you to eat?") often provides valuable clues to dysphagia's effects. The patient also should be asked about voice change, hemoptysis, substernal discomfort, regurgitation of food, nasal leakage of liquids, and otalgia. A history of previous surgery or trauma of the pharynx, chest, or abdomen should be sought. A history of caustic ingestion suggests esophageal stricture or a malignancy in the esophageal scar tissue. (*See* Chapter 30 for further discussion of caustic ingestion.)

The patient may have a history of a disease process that suggests the cause of the dysphagia. Spinal osteoarthritis, tuberculosis, and conditions that produce mediastinal scarring, congenital cardiovascular anomalies, and thyroid enlargement are possible causes of extrinsic esophageal obstruction. Systemic neuromuscular disorders may indicate problems with esophageal motility (e.g., ptosis of the upper eyelids due to myasthenia gravis may suggest the cause of dysphagia). Stroke patients or those suffering from progressive neurological disorders often develop dysphagia. Family history is important in Plummer–Vinson syndrome, oculopharyngeal dysphagia, and forms of muscular dystrophy. A social history of tobacco and/or alcohol use raises the suspicion for malignancy.

Some medications can be etiologic (*see* Table 15.1). Antihistamines, anticholinergics, antidepressants, and antihypertensives suppress salivary gland function, which can cause dysphagia. Phenothiazines and the anticholinergics administered with them may cause significant dysphagia (Case 15.6). The orofacial and pharyngeal dyskinesias may be so severe as to result in dysphagia; however, the accumulation of thick mucus in the hypopharynx due to reduced salivary flow is even more significant.

Physical Examination

There are often few significant physical findings in dysphagia patients, but recognizing the degree of nutrition may be helpful. A complaint of dysphagia in a patient with obvious weight loss may require a different approach than

> **Case 15.6** **Woman with Dysphagia Caused by Use of Phenothiazines**
>
> A woman 52 years of age presents with a 3-year history of chronic dysphagia. She has not had any weight loss, and she seems to have more difficulty with solids than with liquids. Her past medical history is significant for schizophrenia that has been pharmacologically well controlled for many years with thioridazine (Mellaril, a phenothiazine drug) and benztropine (Cogentin). She is a nonsmoker and does not drink alcohol.
>
> Physical examination is nearly normal, with only minimal evidence of extrapyramidal effects of the phenothiazine medication. However, all of the mucosal membranes of her oral cavity and pharynx are dry, and thick adherent mucus is visualized on her supraglottic mucosa.
>
> The patient is reassured that her symptoms and the findings are a normal response to her medications. She is advised to increase her water intake, especially between meals.
>
> **Discussion**
>
> This case illustrates one cause of swallowing dysfunction that can accompany medication, even if administered in therapeutic doses. Many medications (usually diuretics) cause changes in salivary viscosity, which is the most common dramatic effect. Major tranquilizers also can affect swallowing by inducing an extrapyramidal movement disorder of the oral cavity. She had an obvious cause for her dysphagia and had no symptoms or history to suggest other serious disease; hence, her physician elected not to proceed with further investigation (e.g., barium esophagography). This decision could be questioned by others, because it is possible that the patient could have developed another disease entity (e.g., peptic stricture).

the same complaint in an individual who is obviously well nourished. A symptomatic thyroid or other neck mass may be visible or palpable. Complete examination of the oral cavity and hypopharynx is mandatory. The presence or absence of the gag reflex is not a reliable indicator of swallowing function. Dental disease or dry mucous membranes may provide a clue to the underlying pathology. Mirror, telescopic, or fiberoptic examination is standard. Finger palpation of the tongue, pharynx, and palate may be helpful. Pyriform sinus tumors may be seen on indirect mirror examinations or on fiberoptic pharyngolaryngoscopy. Hypopharyngeal pooling of secretions is noted in patients with dysphagia due to a number of processes (either neurological or esophageally obstructive) and is not diagnostic on its own.

Systemic findings may suggest a central nervous system or neuromuscular cause of dysphagia. Occasionally, a palpable cervical node may be the site of metastatic spread of esophageal or hypopharyngeal malignancy.

Additional Diagnostic Evaluation

Contrast Studies and Radiology

Plain radiography of the soft tissues of the neck are unlikely to be beneficial in the evaluation of dysphagia, except possibly to detect foreign bodies. Unfortunately, calcifications in the larynx may be confused easily with small bony foreign bodies, limiting the usefulness of this modality. Chest radiographs should be obtained when indicated, especially if esophageal obstruction or aspiration is suspected.

Contrast studies of the pharynx and the upper esophagus are critical in the diagnosis of disorders that cause dysphagia. A barium swallow discloses the amount of time taken to complete the process, muscular coordination during swallowing, completeness of the pharyngeal clearing of contrast, and evidence of aspiration. The standard examination technique is **barium esophagography**, in which a cup of barium liquid with the consistency of a milkshake is administered during fluoroscopy. The patient ingests a volume sufficient to distend the pharynx and esophagus. Spot films are obtained at various times during the examination, and the examination usually is videotaped for subsequent study. Unfortunately, timing the spot films is difficult, and the quality of the study is highly variable. Pharyngeal abnormalities may be missed due to the rapid motion of the bolus through the pharynx. Moreover, the study usually is aborted if aspiration is encountered, and retrieving videotaped studies may be difficult in many centers. Therefore, although this examination is an excellent means for evaluating the esophagus, it is not satisfactory for identifying lesions or dysfunction of the pharynx.

Esophageal studies allow the analysis of peristaltic waves, transit times, and infringements on the esophagus by neighboring structures. One should pay particular attention to the lower esophageal sphincter. A normal lower esophageal sphincter relaxes as swallowed material approaches. Failure of the lower esophageal sphincter to open suggests achalasia, often accompanied by a dilated, sigmoid-shaped distal esophagus or a diffuse esophageal spasm. Uncoordinated tertiary esophageal contractions are often present. Barium is the best contrast medium for performing esophageal studies unless esophageal perforation or aspiration is suspected. In these cases, a water-soluble contrast medium (e.g., Gastrograffin) is preferable. However, if aspiration is likely, these substances should be avoided because they are toxic to lung tissue.

A modification of the standard barium study is now used routinely for examining patients with known or suspected pharyngeal dysfunction. This **modified barium swallow** (or "cookie swallow") tests the patient's swallowing ability, using foods and liquids of varying consistencies and volumes. The examination is videotaped (with videofluoroscopic imaging)

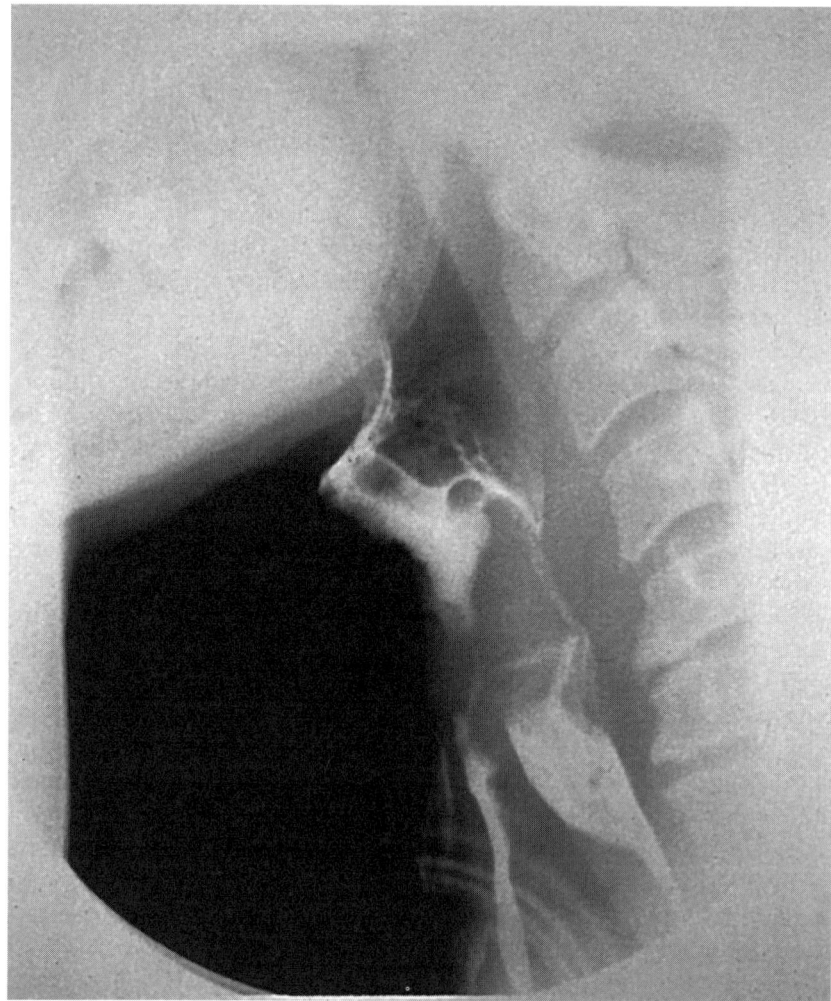

Figure 15.5 Modified barium swallow demonstrating aspiration. Optimum radiographic evaluation of pharyngeal function can be achieved with the modified barium swallow, during which small quantities of food with contrast are administered in a study performed jointly by a radiologist and a speech pathologist. Slow-motion replay can demonstrate specific abnormalities and specify maneuvers that may help alleviate some of the dysfunction. (Republished with permission from Eibling DE, Johnson JT, Bacon GE. *Understanding and Treating Aspiration SiPac*. Alexandria, VA: American Academy of Otolaryngology–Head and Neck Surgery; 1993.)

and reviewed in slow (usually frame-by-frame) motion to permit an examination of the individual components of the complex pharyngeal swallowing process. If aspiration occurs, it is of a small volume, and the examination usually can be continued to define the precise defect (Fig. 15.5). This study, performed jointly by a radiologist and a specially trained speech and language pathologist, has become the standard technique for evaluating patients with oropharyngeal dysphagia. A review of the tape by the referring physician is often useful in understanding the significance of the specific defect in swallowing function. It must be noted that both barium esophagography and the modified barium swallow have specific indications and both should be requested, because it may be necessary to examine pharyngeal *and* esophageal function. Pharyngeal abnormalities can be missed on barium esophagography, and esophageal lesions can be missed on modified barium swallow.

Endoscopic Examination of the Pharynx and Larynx

The widespread practical use of endoscopic examination of the pharynx, esophagus, and trachea has had to wait for the development of optical systems and reliable illumination. The early history of these examinations is fascinating and is best documented in the writings of Chevalier Jackson, the father of endoscopy. Over the past two decades, improved optical systems (particularly flexible fiberoptic imaging technology) have revolutionized the evaluation of the pharynx and esophagus (as well as many other lumina) and are now standard in all health care facilities (Fig. 15.6).

Flexible fiberoptic transnasal examination of the larynx and pharynx is performed easily in the office setting, requiring minimal topical anesthesia. This examination is well tolerated and should be standard in all patients with pharyngeal complaints. A modification of the examination using the test administration of food substances, called **flexible (fiberoptic) endoscopic examination of swallowing (FEES)**, is now becoming a standard means of evaluating pharyngeal function. In some instances, this latest examination technique replaces the need to perform a modified barium swallow to evaluate pharyngeal dysfunction. It is being used in an ever-increasing number of both acute and chronic care facilities. Fiberoptic examination with these smaller endoscopes is not adequate for examining the cervical or thoracic esophagus, and the pyriform sinuses often cannot be well visualized because of the instrument's inability to distend the normally collapsed lumina.

Esophagoscopy

Esophagoscopy can be performed with either rigid or flexible instrumentation. Rigid instrumentation usually requires general anesthesia and typically is reserved for procedures such as the removal of foreign bodies. Flexible fiberoptic esophagoscopy usually is performed in conjunction with an exami-

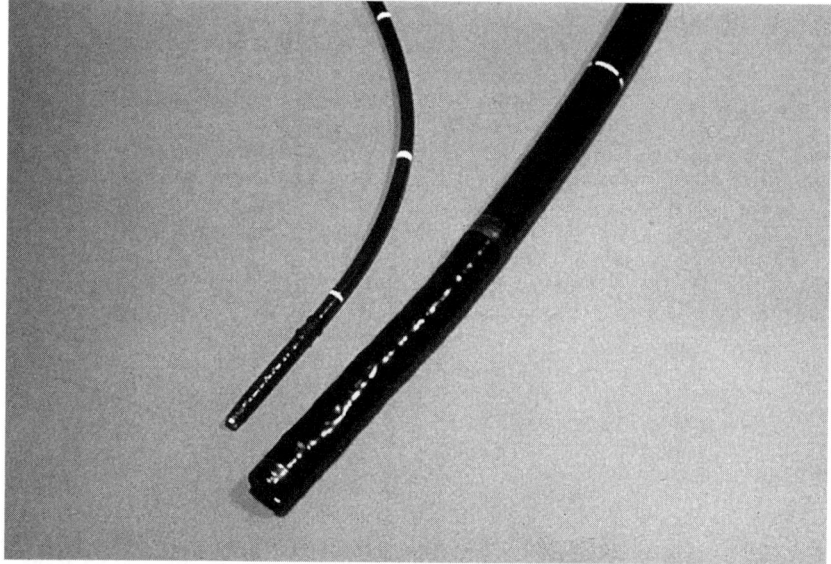

Figure 15.6 Flexible fiberoptic nasal pharyngoscope and gastroscope. Note the dramatic differences in size between the two instruments; the nasal pharyngoscope can be passed easily through the nose into the pharynx with minimal topical anesthesia, whereas the gastroscope must be passed through the mouth, requiring sedation.

nation of the stomach and duodenum and requires sedation (but not general anesthesia). Newer instrumentation permits the endoscopic removal of some foreign bodies and fiberoptic laser treatment of lesions of the thoracic esophagus. It must be noted that, because the flexible gastroscope is passed blindly through the level of the cricopharyngeal muscle, one can easily miss lesions of the tongue base, larynx, and pharynx (e.g., pyriform sinus cancer). Nevertheless, flexible fiberoptic esophagoscopy is required in patients with dysphagia. Esophagoscopy may be the only means of identifying early esophageal cancers or the presence of Barrett's esophagus, which is believed to represent a premalignant lesion. The indications for esophagoscopy vary with each institution, but there is a consensus that persistent esophageal dysphagia without a recognizable cause deserves endoscopic examination.

Manometry

Esophageal manometry is performed by placing pressure transducers in the esophagus and then monitoring pressure changes at various locations during the swallow. Its primary value is in the evaluation of disorders of the thoracic esophagus, but it also can help diagnose cricopharyngeal achalasia. Manometry can be performed simultaneously with fluoroscopy, increasing the precision of identifying the anatomic location of the manometric sensors as pressure readings are taken. Manometry should be reserved for evaluating complaints of dysphagia in patients whose radiographic and endoscopic examinations have been inconclusive. Manometric studies that detect unusual flaccidity of the thoracic esophagus with failure of the esophagogastric sphincter to relax strongly suggest achalasia. Contrast findings together with the typical manometric findings confirm achalasia. Patients with diffuse esophageal spasm usually have high intraluminal pressures during esophageal swallowing, and peristaltic waves are poorly orchestrated. Lupus erythematosus, rheumatoid arthritis, and chronic alcoholism often cause a loss of tone in the distal thoracic esophagus and diminished intraluminal pressures.

Management

Because dysphagia therapy is directed at managing the disease responsible for the dysphagia, management requires that the cause first be identified (*see* Algorithm). In most instances, therapy is intuitive. For example, foreign bodies should be removed, often emergently, to prevent the complications of perforation or aspiration of saliva. Malignancies of the oral cavity, pharynx, and esophagus require therapy (even if only palliative) to ensure adequate nutrition and management of oral secretions. Newer techniques using laser vaporization or an injected photosensitizer (photodynamic therapy) may provide significant palliation to patients with obstructing esophageal cancer. Dysphagia following therapy for head and neck or esophageal cancer is often problematic, and long-term enteral feedings with a gastrostomy may be required.

Motility disorders may respond to prokinetic agents, and dysphagia associated with GERD should be treated with antireflux medications (e.g., H_2 blockers, proton-pump inhibitors) and lifestyle alterations. These medications should be used for at least 4 weeks. Altering the pharmacologic therapy of other disorders may help in the management of drug-induced dysphagia. Frequent sips of water or agents to enhance salivation (e.g., pilocarpine) may help with dysphagia associated with reduced salivation, such as that caused by certain medications. Management of Zenker's diverticulum is via division of the cricopharyngeal muscle (with or without resection of the diverticulum) and is usually curative. Endoscopic myotomy with division of the party wall between the diverticulum and the esophagus (wherein lies the cricopharyngeus muscle) has become standard in many institutions and provides significant improvement in swallowing function without the morbidity of an open surgical procedure. Balloon dilitation of achalasia may relieve the dysphagia associated with this entity. In addition, as mentioned earlier, cricopharyngeal myotomy is occasionally curative in cricopharyngeal achalasia; however, patient selection is difficult, and the role of this procedure remains controversial.

Relief of dysphagia after administrating a cholinergic drug (e.g., edrophonium) is strong diagnostic evidence of myasthenia gravis. Dysphagia associated with Parkinson's disease may respond dramatically to alterations in anti-Parkinson's therapy. Abstinence from alcohol may be effective in correcting the symptoms and objective signs of dysphagia caused by alcoholism. Esophageal candidiasis (often found in diabetics and in those with other immunodeficiencies) is treated pharmacologically with topical (e.g., Nystatin 100,000 U per 1 cm^3 "swish and spit") and systemic (e.g., Diflucan 100 mg/d) antimycotic drugs.

Oropharyngeal dysphagia secondary to stroke, lower motor neuron disease, muscular disease, esophageal spasm, and globus may respond to alterations in dietary consistency and eating techniques. These strategies are best determined by a speech therapist who is trained in the evaluation and management of swallowing disorders. Speech therapists use a broad range of diagnostic techniques (e.g., modified barium swallow, functional endoscopic evaluation of swallowing) to ascertain the level and mechanism of the swallowing disorder. A modified barium swallow is performed under fluoroscopy, and it evaluates the swallow from the lips to the upper esophagus. By visualizing the swallow with foods of different consistency, the therapist can direct treatment toward specific sites or problems. The functional endoscopic evaluation of swallowing is a direct examination of the oral cavity, oropharynx, and hypopharynx that has been shown to be as effective as the barium swallow in diagnosing the area of concern and in directing therapy. Dysphagia that accompanies tracheostomy often is managed optimally by decannulation or valving of the tracheostomy tube. As mentioned previously, patients with dysphagia due to cervical spine disease may benefit from surgical resection; however, patient selection is problematic, with some patients' symptoms worsening after the procedure.

Dysphagia that accompanies Parkinson's disease and other neurological disorders is often associated with morbid aspiration and weight loss. Swallow function may be responsive to swallowing therapy directed at laryngeal and pharyngeal strengthening. With increased disease progression, a feeding tube or gastrostomy may be required to maintain adequate caloric intake. If aspiration becomes life threatening, laryngotracheal separation (i.e., surgical separation of the airway and digestive tract) may be necessary. (*See* Chapter 18 for more details on the management of aspiration.)

Danger Signs

Danger signs include dysphagia associated with the following:
- Weight loss
- Pain or sore throat

- History of substance abuse
- Previous esophageal or pharyngeal surgery
- Voice changes
- Otalgia
- Signs of neurological disease
- Aspiration
- Recurrent pneumonia
- Coughing with liquids
- Substernal pain
- Respiratory symptoms

Summary

Dysphagia is a common complaint that accompanies a wide variety of disease processes. It may be the only, or initial, symptom of a serious or even life-threatening disease. A history and physical examination, including endoscopic examination of the upper aerodigestive tract and contrast studies of swallowing structures and their function, reveals the cause of the dysphagia in most cases. Fiberoptic esophagoscopy often is required, and manometry and 24-hour Ph-metry may be helpful in some instances. Therapy should be directed at the cause of the problem. If required, caloric supplementation should be provided to prevent further weight loss.

SUGGESTED READINGS

Carrau RL, Murry T. *Dysphagia.* San Diego, CA: Singular Press; 1998.
> *This comprehensive text covers the full range of clinical dysphagia. It is divided into pathophysiology, evaluation, and treatment sections. Written by a multidisciplinary panel of experts, it is currently the most complete and up-to-date text that addresses dysphagia.*

Langmore SE, Schatz K, Olson N. Endoscopic and videofluoroscopic evaluations of swallowing and aspiration. *Ann Otol Rhinol Laryngol.* 1991;100:678–81.
> *This paper outlines the use of the endoscopic evaluation of swallowing in patients with dysphagia.*

Logemann J. *Evaluation and Treatment of Swallowing Disorders.* San Diego: College-Hill Press; 1983.
> *This textbook addresses the evaluation and management of oropharyngeal dysphagia in detail. Written by speech therapists, it is a particularly valuable reference for those who manage patients with dysphagia associated with neurological disease.*

Richter JE. Long-term management of gastroesophageal reflux disease and its complications. *Am J Gastroenterol.* 1997;92(4 Suppl):30–4S.
> *This recent review by a known authority addresses the problem of GERD that presents with pharyngeal and laryngeal complaints. Although dysphagia is an unusual component of GERD, this article is likely to be valuable to the practicing physician who frequently encounters patients with pharyngeal complaints.*

16

Obstructive Sleep Apnea

Kenneth B. Briskin, MD

Obstructive sleep apnea syndrome (OSAS) is a disorder characterized by excessive snoring and periodic breathing with repetitive apneas, hypopneas, and arousals that leads to fragmented sleep. OSAS has been identified as a distinct entity for the past 25 to 30 years. The prevalence seems to be greater than 1% for young men, rising to over 10% for elderly men. The specific health consequences are still being studied; however, there seems to be significant morbidity associated with OSAS. Additionally, there is evidence that OSAS patients have an increased susceptibility to cardiovascular complications (e.g., stroke, hypertension, cardiac arrhythmias, myocardial infarction), which is probably related to the hypoxemia that occurs during apneic episodes (1–3) (*see* Algorithm A). Another complication of OSAS is excessive daytime somnolence with poor work and social functioning. Impairment of alertness makes the patient susceptible to work or automobile accidents. In children, OSAS has been implicated as a cause of poor school performance, failure to thrive, and cor pulmonale.

Therapy for OSAS, which is directed at avoiding cardiovascular complications and excessive daytime sleepiness, can be divided into surgical and nonsurgical categories. These treatments, depending on the individual case and history, must be considered carefully.

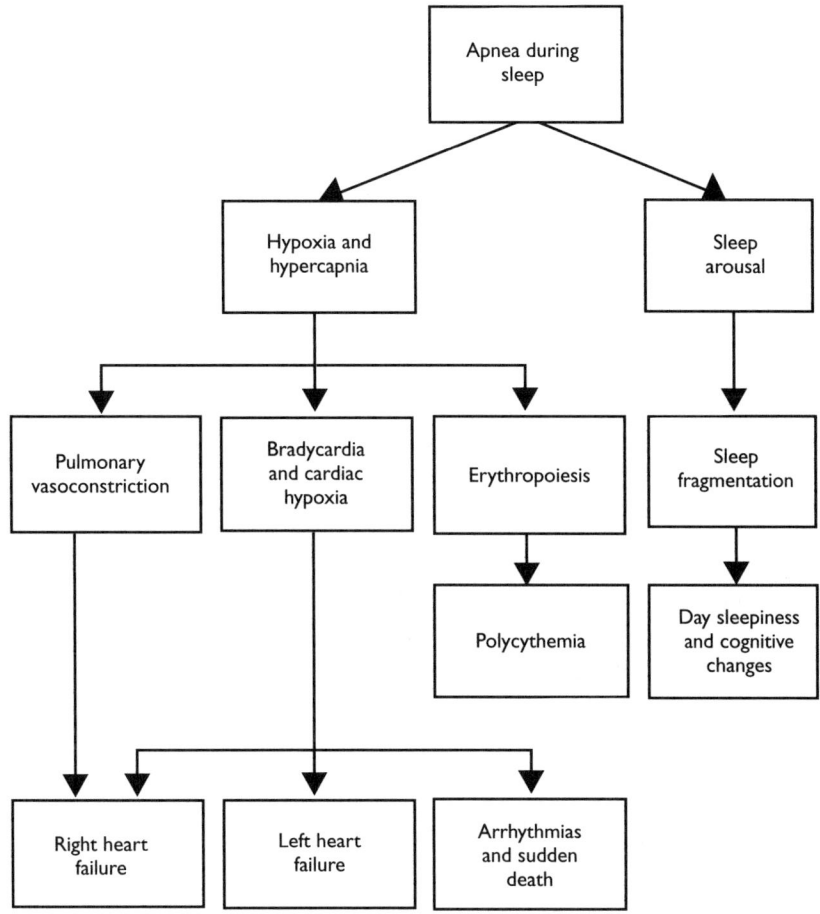

Algorithm A Medical consequences of obstructive sleep apnea.

Typical Presenting Symptoms

Patients presenting with OSAS are commonly obese, and almost one third of morbidly obese patients demonstrate significant symptoms (4). Men are affected more commonly than are women, but this may be due to a higher prevalence of obesity among men. The prototype OSAS patient is "Joe the Fat Boy" (from Charles Dickens' *Pickwick Papers*) who fell asleep whenever he sat still. This type of sleep apnea is sometimes called "Pickwickian."

Certain groups of patients, conditions, and physical abnormalities are associated with a high incidence of OSAS, including adenotonsillar hyperplasia,

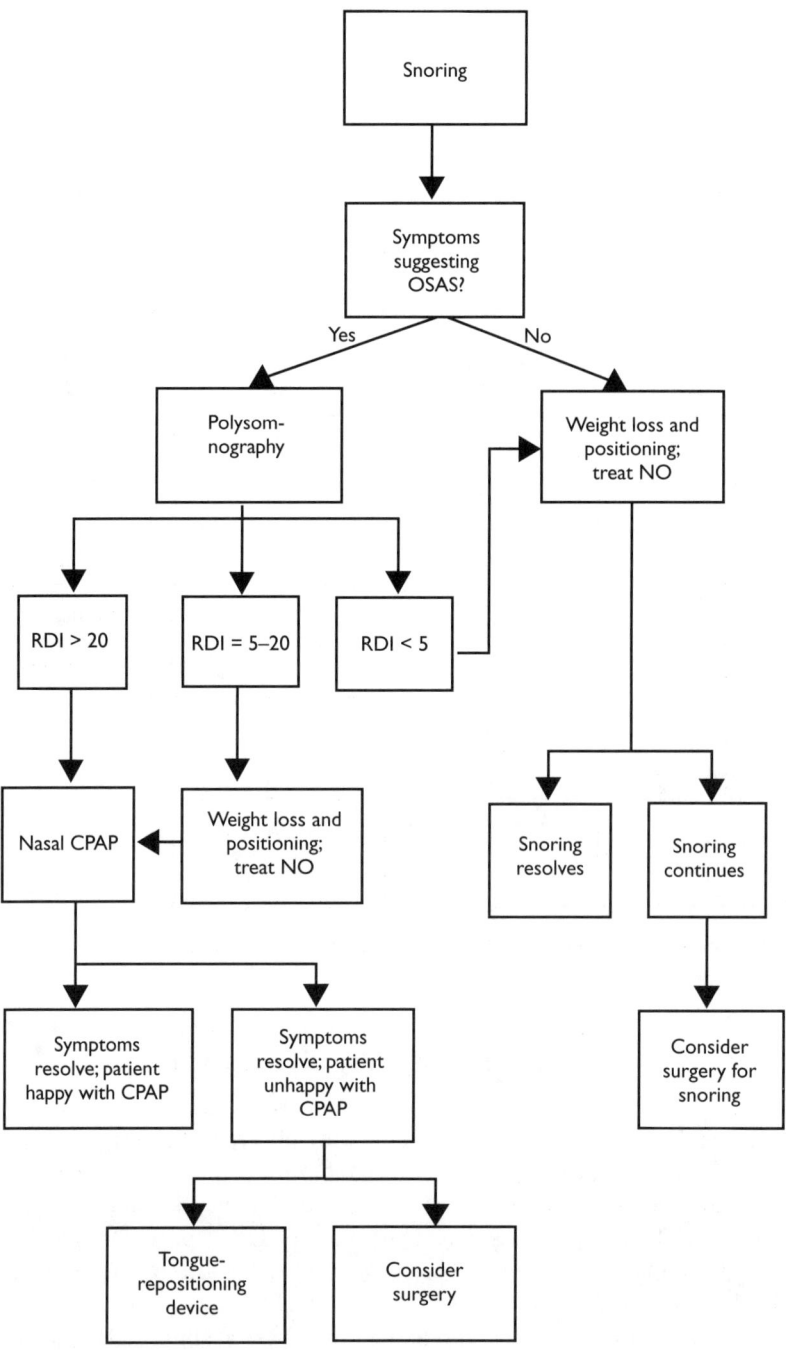

Algorithm B Management of sleep apnea. CPAP = continuous positive airway pressure; NO = nasal obstruction; OSAS = obstructive sleep apnea syndrome; RDI = respiratory disturbance index.

hypothyroidism, acromegaly, Down's syndrome, micrognathia, retrognathia, or macroglossia. Extreme hypothyroidism and marked uvular edema are rare causes. Common causes of acquired OSAS include neoplasm, oncologic resection, and radiation-induced edema or fibrosis of the upper aerodigestive tract.

Typically, patients present with a partner who complains of loud, insidious snoring (Case 16.1). Partners also may note episodes of apnea during sleep, and the patient may complain of daytime somnolence with associated sleeping while driving or working. Many patients also complain of impaired mental function and reduced libido. In children, partial airway obstruction may be identified by chronic snoring, continuous movement, and a very disorganized sleep architecture.

Other causes of daytime somnolence include insomnia related to depression, narcolepsy, restless leg syndrome, and other factors (e.g., stress, heavy meals or alcohol near bedtime, job or child care requirements).

Relevant Anatomy and Physiology

Obstructive sleep apnea syndrome has been associated most commonly with the obese Pickwickian patient. Although obese patients comprise a substantial portion of the OSAS population, the problem can affect those without the typical body morphology. True Pickwickian syndrome patients (those with hypercapnia and right-sided congestive heart failure) make up only approximately 10% of OSAS patients.

Patients with OSAS typically have airways that collapse more easily than do normal patients, leading to a partial or complete obstruction (Fig. 16.1),

Case 16.1 Weight Loss as a Treatment for Primary Snoring

A man 38 years of age presents with a 2-year history of snoring that has worsened to the point that his wife must sleep in a separate room. The patient denies daytime somnolence, and his wife has not noted any episodes in which her husband has appeared to struggle for breath while sleeping. Past medical history is significant for a recent 30-lb weight gain and tonsillectomy as a child.

Physical examination shows a moderately enlarged soft palate. The patient is diagnosed with primary snoring. Based on the history, he is not felt to have evidence of obstructive sleep apnea, so a sleep study is not obtained.

A weight loss program is recommended, which the patient successfully completes. On return 6 months later, his snoring has been substantially reduced.

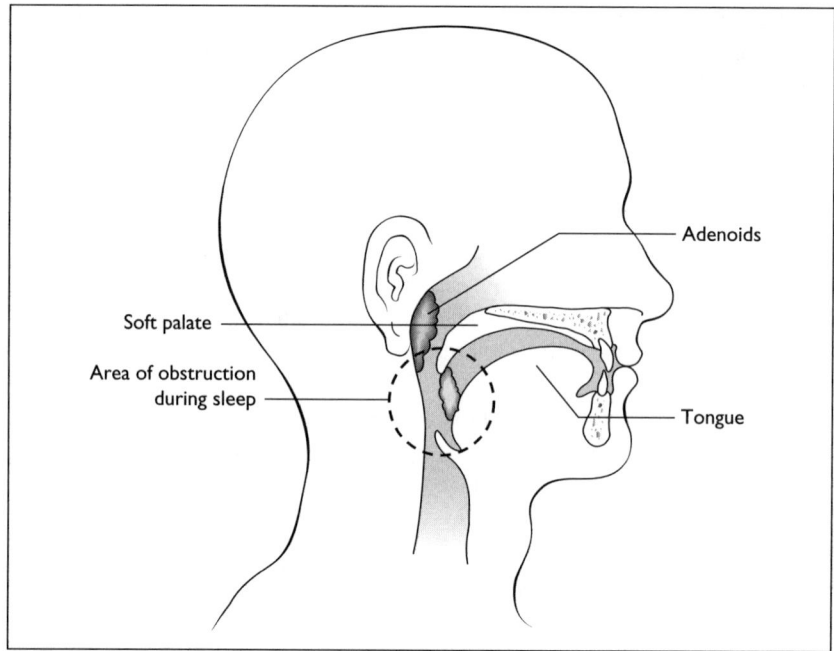

Figure 16.1 Common locations of upper airway obstruction. The posterior soft palate and uvula contribute to retropalatal obstruction, and tissue at the base of tongue contributes to retroglossal obstruction.

particularly in the absence of upper airway muscle activity (e.g., during sleep). Typically, there is less posterior airway space at the base of the tongue. The cervicofacial anomalies that cause this include a lower than normal hyoid bone; a relatively posterior or small mandible; relative macroglossia; and thickened, redundant mucosa and submucosal tissues in the oropharynx and hypopharynx.

A number of physiologic consequences are associated with the apneas. These include cessation of airflow, hypoxia, and hypercarbia. In addition to episodes of oxygen desaturation, other cardiovascular effects are common. Nocturnal cardiac arrhythmias secondary to oxygen desaturation can occur. Bradycardia is the most common arrhythmia during the apneic phase.

By monitoring the electroencephalogram and electro-oculogram, normal sleep can be divided into four stages. Stages I and II are the lighter levels of sleep, whereas stages III and IV non-REM are the deeper levels of sleep (slow-wave sleep). REM (rapid eye movement) sleep is the time of greatest airway vulnerability to collapse. Although the arousal threshold is decreased (compared with deep sleep), there is a loss of skeletal muscle tone. Some patients with mild or moderate OSAS may demonstrate significant airway obstruction only during REM or slow-wave sleep.

Many patients have marked reduction in the amount of their REM sleep. The REM periods are punctuated by severe obstructive episodes that lead to oxyhemoglobin desaturation and arousals into lighter sleep. Even if the patient has complete arousal from sleep, he or she usually resubmerges rapidly into deep sleep only to be awakened again. The patient has no recollection of these events because less than 2 minutes of wakefulness does not result in a remembered event. Successful OSAS treatment is associated with spending more time in REM sleep than is normal because of previous sleep deprivation (REM rebound).

History

Obtaining a sleep history for patients who present with sleep-related complaints is critical and often involves questioning not only the patient but also his or her bed partner. The initial interview should determine the patient's sleep habits, including appropriate length and quality, and focus on the degree of sleep deprivation and any subsequent disability.

The main complaints are snoring, gasping, and snorting. Although snoring is common in the general population, only a small percentage of patients with snoring have sleep apnea. Conversely, all patients with sleep apnea snore. This snoring can be characterized as continuous, intermittent, or positional. Milder cases of OSAS may have symptoms only while in the supine position. A history of daytime sleepiness (e.g., napping, impaired mental functioning, sleeping while driving or working) should be taken. Recent weight gain and the use of alcohol, sedatives, and medications must be explored. Other medical conditions to be reviewed include neurological disease, renal dysfunction, hypertension, cardiovascular disease, asthma, endocrine dysfunction, and gastroesophageal reflux disease. The physician should question the patient about signs of anxiety or depression. It is important to determine whether the sleep difficulty occurs all the time or only under certain conditions (e.g., while sleeping on vacation). A family history of sleep problems also should be explored. The Epworth Sleepiness Scale is a useful tool for assessing daytime sleepiness (Table 16.1).

Physical Examination

The primary goals of the physical examination are to define the overall **anatomical predisposition** for airway obstruction and to recognize focal lesions that may be corrected. The craniofacial structure of the patient should

Table 16.1 Epworth Sleepiness Scale*

Situation	Score
Sitting and reading	
Watching TV	
Sitting inactive in a public place (e.g., theatre, in a meeting)	
Being a passenger in a car for 1 hour without break	
Lying down to rest in the afternoon when circumstances permit	
Sitting and talking to someone	
Sitting quietly after a lunch without alcohol	
Sitting in a car while stopped in traffic for a few minutes	
Total	

*The patient is instructed to rate his or her chance of dozing off in each of these situations, choosing the most appropriate ranking for each of these situations (if the patient has been in a particular situation recently, he or she should make an educated guess) on the following scale: 0 = would never doze off, 1 = slight chance of dozing off, 2 = moderate chance of dozing, 3 = high chance of dozing.

be noted. Significant abnormalities that contribute to upper airway resistance may be seen in both adults and children. Any **craniofacial abnormality** that produces an underdeveloped maxilla or mandible can lead to significant obstruction. This can include patients with Treacher Collins syndrome, Pierre Robin syndrome, or Down's syndrome. Many patients are mouth-breathers, a condition attributable to nasal airway obstruction caused by turbinate hypertrophy, septal deviation, or adenoid hypertrophy.

Examining the oral cavity and oropharynx can provide excellent clues as to the cause of the patient's condition. There may be an elongated soft palate and uvula with surrounding folds of redundant mucosa. Retrognathia, micrognathia, or macroglossia can contribute to all of the patient's symptoms. Upper airway obstruction from hypertrophy of the tonsils and adenoids must be assessed, especially in the pediatric patient.

To evaluate the upper airway fully, a **fiberoptic laryngoscopy** should be performed. This examination should focus on the degree of obstruction at different levels (including the nasopharynx and oropharynx), observing the movement of the pharyngeal walls, palate, and base of tongue. These observations help determine whether surgical intervention can alleviate the obstructive symptoms.

Differential Diagnosis

The differential diagnosis of obstructive sleep apnea includes any other disorder that causes excessive daytime sleepiness. The two most common are **sleep de-**

privation and **periodic movement syndromes**. Periodic leg-movement disorder, often accompanied by restless leg syndrome, is often recognized by the patient's sleeping partner. The cause of sleep disorders may be differentiated by polysomnography (*see* section on Additional Diagnostic Evaluation below).

Additional Diagnostic Evaluation (Laboratory Tests)

Polysomnography can confirm patient complaints of poor sleep and can provide the most objective, reproducible means of determining whether sleep-related abnormalities are contributing to the cause of the patient's symptoms (Fig. 16.2). This test characterizes sleep stages and records respiratory events, cardiac arrhythmias, oxyhemoglobin desaturations, and muscular abnormalities.

Apnea is defined as a cessation of respiration for longer than 10 seconds. Hypopnea is a respiratory event characterized by the reduction of air flow by 50%. The **respiratory disturbance index (RDI)** reflects the total number of apneas and hypopneas per hour of sleep and is used to report the results of polysomnography. An RDI of greater than 5 is abnormal. Severe cases of OSAS usually have an RDI greater than 40. Oxyhemoglobin is another critical measurement of the sleep study. Desaturations of less than 85% are highly significant, and any desaturations of less than 60% represent severe obstructive apnea.

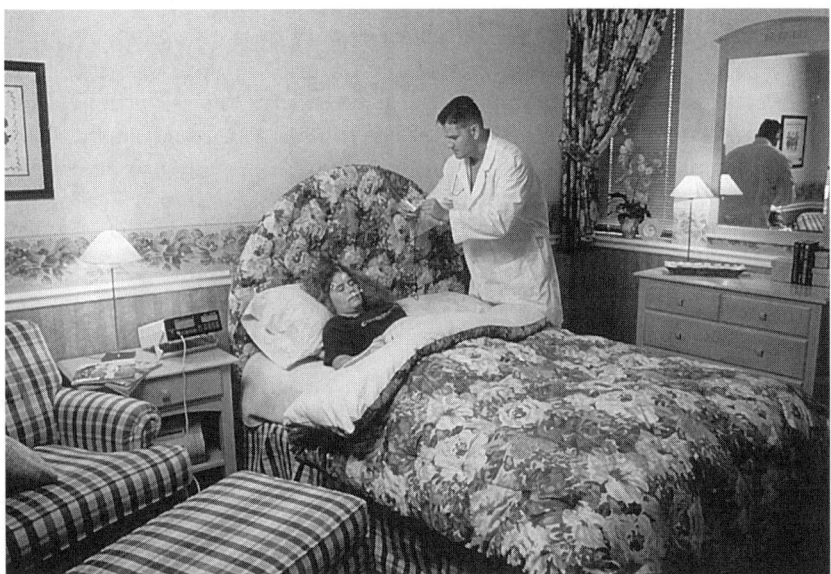

Figure 16.2 Patient undergoing polysomnograhy in a sleep laboratory. (Courtesy of Dr. Samuel Kuna.)

Some laboratories use the **multiple sleep latency test** to differentiate OSAS daytime tiredness from narcolepsy. Typically, this test is performed during the day and consists of a series of four to five naps, 2 hours apart. Narcolepsy is accompanied by short-onset sleep (an onset of less than 5 minutes is considered pathologic).

Other tests are less useful but may provide insight into secondary abnormalities. An electrocardiogram and chest radiograph may reveal cor pulmonale if the OSAS is long-standing. Thyroid function tests may reveal underlying hypothyroidism that requires hormone replacement. Soft-tissue films of the neck are useful in obtaining cephalometric data for planning surgical intervention.

Management

Treatment options may be divided into surgical and nonsurgical methods (Table 16.2) (*see* Algorithm B). Treatment is often dependent on the patient's history.

Nonsurgical Management

Patients with OSAS should **avoid sedating substances at night**, including sleeping pills, alcohol, and sedating antihistamines.

Weight loss is effective in decreasing the number of apneic events, the extent of arterial oxygen desaturation, and the amount of sleep disruption in patients with OSAS. The relationship between weight loss and improvement in the number of apneas and hypopneas is not linear; a large improvement in OSAS can occur with rather minimal weight loss in some patients. The number of ap-

Table 16.2 Management of Obstructive Sleep Apnea

Nonsurgical Treatment	Surgical Treatment
Weight loss	Uvulopalatopharyngoplasty
Continuous positive airway pressure	Laser-assisted uvulopalatoplasty
Topical or systemic medication for nasal obstruction	Radiofrequency fibrosis
	Palatal advancement
External nasal dilator adhesive strips	Palatal flap
Internal nasal dilator devices	Genioglossal advancement
Mechanical devices	Hyoid advancement
Tongue-retaining devices	Midline glossectomy
	Bimaxillary advancement
	Inferior sagittal mandibular osteotomy
	Hyoid suspension
	Tonsillectomy
	Adenoidectomy

neas decreases by approximately 50% with a 10% weight loss. Unfortunately, voluntary loss of weight is difficult for many patients, and maintaining such a weight loss is a significant problem. Patients seem to be most successful with weight loss when they are supervised carefully in structured programs. Weight loss is used generally as an adjunct to other methods of treatment.

The most common nonsurgical treatment is nasal **continuous positive airway pressure** (CPAP) (Fig. 16.3). CPAP produces positive pressure within the upper airway to counteract the subatmospheric collapsing pharyngeal pressure. This procedure prevents collapse of the airway that would otherwise occur with inspiration. CPAP is effective when used correctly (Case 16.2); however, its success is hampered by poor compliance in many OSAS patients. Generally, objective compliance is reported at 50% or less in patients who undergo CPAP. Discomfort of the device, nasal dryness or bleeding, and traveling with the device are cited as reasons for noncompliance (Case 16.3). Newer machines are easier to use and are less obtrusive (Fig. 16.4). Improvements in compliance are associated with smaller, more comfortable masks; in-line hu-

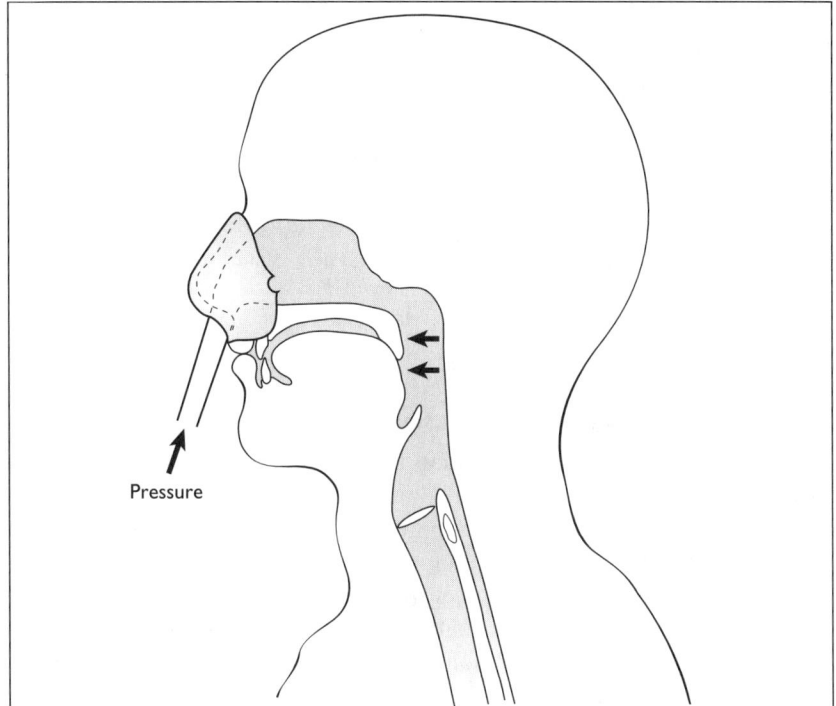

Figure 16.3 Nasal continuous positive airway pressure. This diagram shows how the pneumatic splinting of the retroglossal and retropalatal areas diminishes upper airway collapse.

> **Case 16.2** **Use of Continuous Positive Airway Pressure in the Treatment of Sleep Apnea**
>
> A woman 26 years of age complains of a choking sensation and frequent awakening at night and sleepiness while driving. On entering the examination room, you note that she is dozing in her chair. She is 5'4" and 195 lb and has attempted to lose weight for the past 4 years.
>
> Physical examination shows a large soft palate and minimal tonsillar tissue. Fiberoptic examination shows redundant mucosa in the hypopharynx. A sleep study shows desaturations to 72% and an RDI of 35.
>
> A CPAP trial during the sleep study reduces the RDI to 8 and is well tolerated. She continues with CPAP at home, with resolution of her symptoms.

> **Case 16.3** **Uvulopalatopharyngoplasty in the Treatment of Sleep Apnea**
>
> A man 43 years of age complains of snoring and frequently awakening at night with shortness of breath. His wife says that he seems to be struggling for air at these times. The patient frequently travels for work and complains of sleepiness during business meetings.
>
> Physical examination shows enlarged tonsils and an elongated soft palate that, on fiberoptic exam, collapses against the posterior pharyngeal wall. Occlusion is normal. A sleep study shows and RDI of 32 and desaturations to 78%.
>
> The symptoms are reduced with CPAP, but the patient cannot tolerate a variety of masks and has difficulty taking the equipment with him on business trips. He undergoes uvulopalatopharyngoplasty, and his symptoms are eliminated.

midification; and a more moderate pressure "ramp," or build-up, from zero (Fig. 16.5). A higher patient education level and a greater sense of improvement when using CPAP are associated with better long-term compliance.

Nasal obstruction can cause or aggravate OSAS. The **treatment of nasal obstruction** may involve treatment of rhinitis with topical or systemic medications (*see* Chapter 8). If there is alar collapse, then external nasal dilator adhesive strips (Fig. 16.6) or internal nasal dilator devices may be helpful. Sometimes, surgery of the nasal skeleton is required before a patient is able to use CPAP.

Over the years, mechanical devices have been used for the treatment of snoring and OSAS. Many antisnoring devices have been patented in the United States during the past century, including oral prostheses and body harnesses. An old remedy is the "snore ball"—one or more tennis balls inserted into an ath-

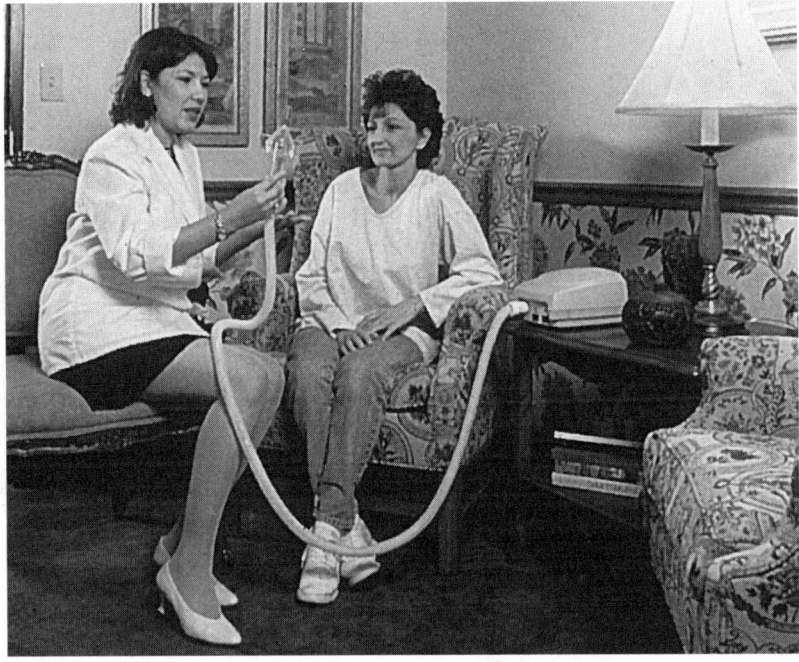

Figure 16.4 Model of nasal continuous positive airway pressure. (Courtesy of Dr. Samuel Kuna.)

letic sock that has been sewn to the central back of the patient's pajama top (with a Velcro closing so the balls can be removed easily). Ideally, this contraption prevents the snorer from sleeping in a supine position; however, most often it fails because of noncompliance and the fact that the aging process can lead to a loosening of pharyngeal tissue.

Tongue-retaining devices and other oral appliances have been developed as well (Fig. 16.7). An example of these involves the use of a mouthpiece into which the tongue is inserted and held throughout the night. Because the tongue is advanced, the air space widens, resulting in less snoring and apnea. Again, this device is difficult to wear, and compliance is a problem.

Surgical Management

The surgical management of the patient with obstructive sleep apnea involves the use of a number of procedures. Tracheostomy is the "gold standard" by which all treatments are judged; it effectively bypasses the upper airway obstruction and is curative in most cases. Unfortunately, patients rarely accept it as a treatment. A great deal of controversy exists about the timing, effectiveness, and the proper procedure in treating the OSAS patient surgically, because sleep-

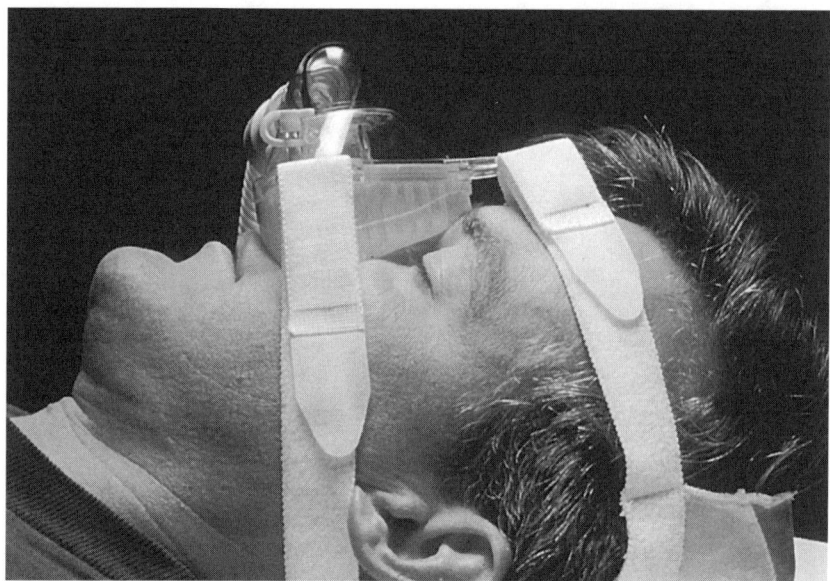

Figure 16.5 Nasal mask for nasal continuous positive airway pressure secured in place with soft Velcro straps. (Courtesy of Dr. Samuel Kuna.)

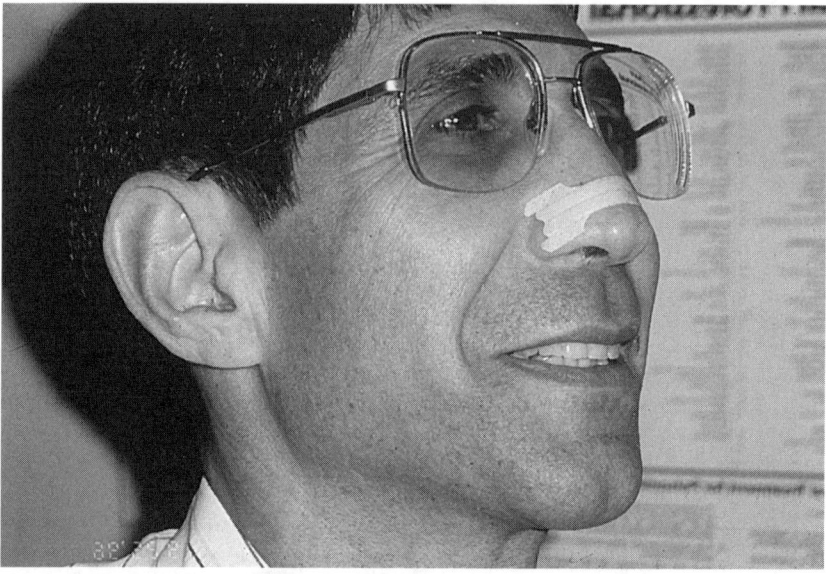

Figure 16.6 External nasal dilator adhesive strips properly positioned on the nose. (Courtesy of Dr. Samuel Kuna.)

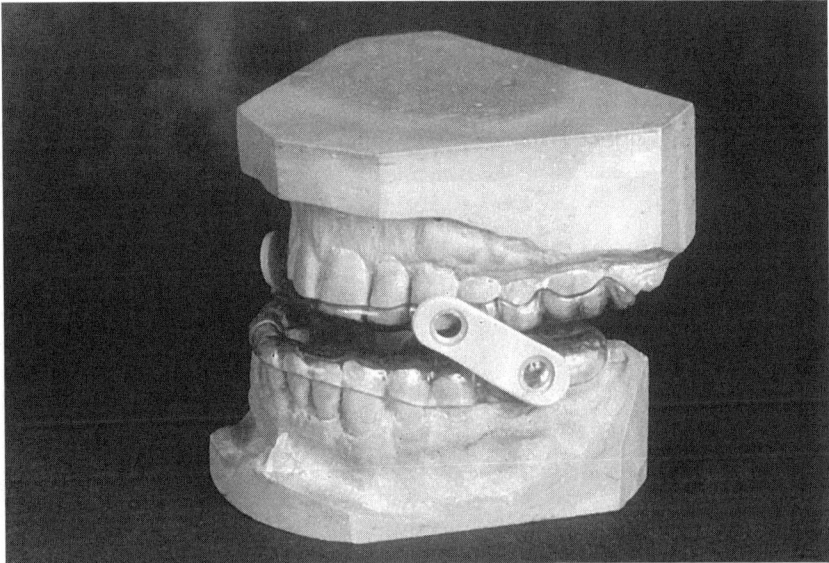

Figure 16.7 One of many available oral devices used to pull the mandible and the attached genioglossus muscle anteriorly, which opens up the retroglossal airway.

related airway collapse usually involves the retropalatal airway, the retroglossal airway, or both. The value of the RDI can help direct which level or levels need to be addressed. An RDI of less than 20 usually indicates palatal involvement, an RDI of greater than 20 means that multiple levels need to be addressed, and an RDI of greater than 60 usually requires a tracheostomy.

Since 1981, **uvulopalatopharyngoplasty (UPPP)** has been used to treat retropalatal collapse (Fig. 16.8). A significant improvement in the severity of symptoms is achieved in approximately 50% to 60% of patients undergoing UPPP and tonsillectomy (5). However, a dilemma occurs when determining which patients will benefit from this procedure. Patients with an RDI of less than 20 often respond favorably, whereas those with a higher RDI usually have significant improvement but are not cured. UPPP involves trimming the soft tissue of the soft palate and pharynx. The tonsils are removed, if present, and the anterior and posterior pillars are sutured together. The underlying muscle is left intact to avoid the complication of velopharyngeal incompetence. Other surgical procedures that address collapse of the retropalatal airway include **laser-assisted uvulopalatoplasty**, radiofrequency fibrosis, and palatal advancement.

Surgical procedures that are designed to improve the upper airway behind the base of tongue (retroglossal) include **genioglossal advancement, hyoid advancement, midline glossectomy**, and **bimaxillary advancement**. These are

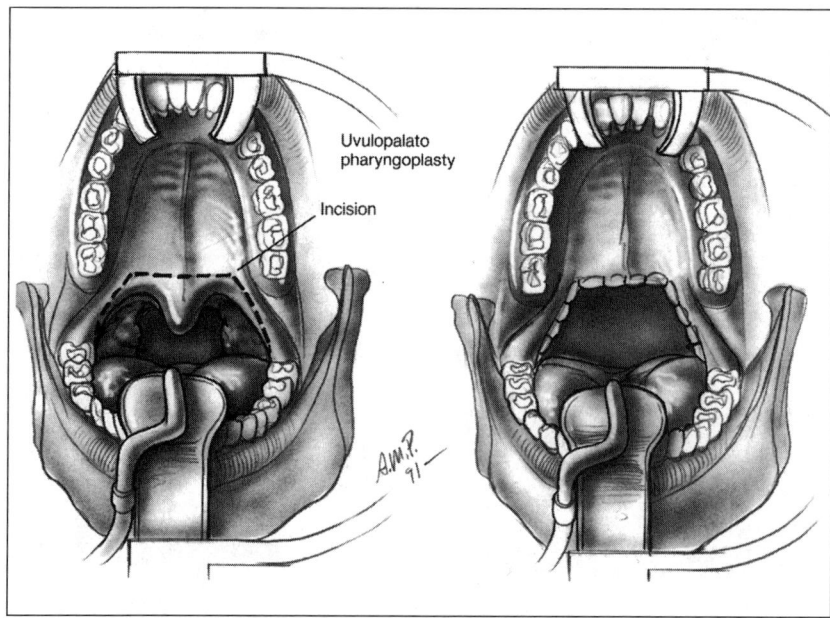

Figure 16.8 Anatomical changes made during the uvulopalatopharyngoplasty procedure. (Republished with permission from Bailey BJ (ed). *Head and Neck Surgery–Otolaryngology*, 1st ed. Philadelphia: Lippincott;1993.)

used in patients with narrow retroglossal airways in whom palatal surgery has failed or in patients with airway narrowing in both the retropalatal and retroglossal airways (Fig. 16.9). Most of these patients have been found to have small retroglossal airways with inferiorly located hyoid bones.

Two procedures that are performed simultaneously to improve the airway are the **inferior sagittal mandibular osteotomy** for genioglossus advancement and the **hyoid suspension**. Both have been found to be effective in reducing the average number of respiratory events and improving the average oxygen saturations significantly. Riley reported a series of 42 patients with OSAS who could not tolerate CPAP. These patients underwent simultaneous UPPP, sagittal mandibular osteotomy, and hyoid suspension and were found to have a 67% success rate in reducing the respiratory disturbance index by 50% (6).

Tonsillectomy and **adenoidectomy** have been shown to be effective in curing selected patients with OSAS (more commonly in the pediatric age group). Adenoidectomy should be performed with an inspection of the nasopharynx via an angulated mirror to ensure the opening of posterior choanae. Patients with craniofacial abnormalities may continue to have OSAS symptoms because of a tendency toward airway collapse. Some patients (especially children) may require a tracheostomy to obtain relief.

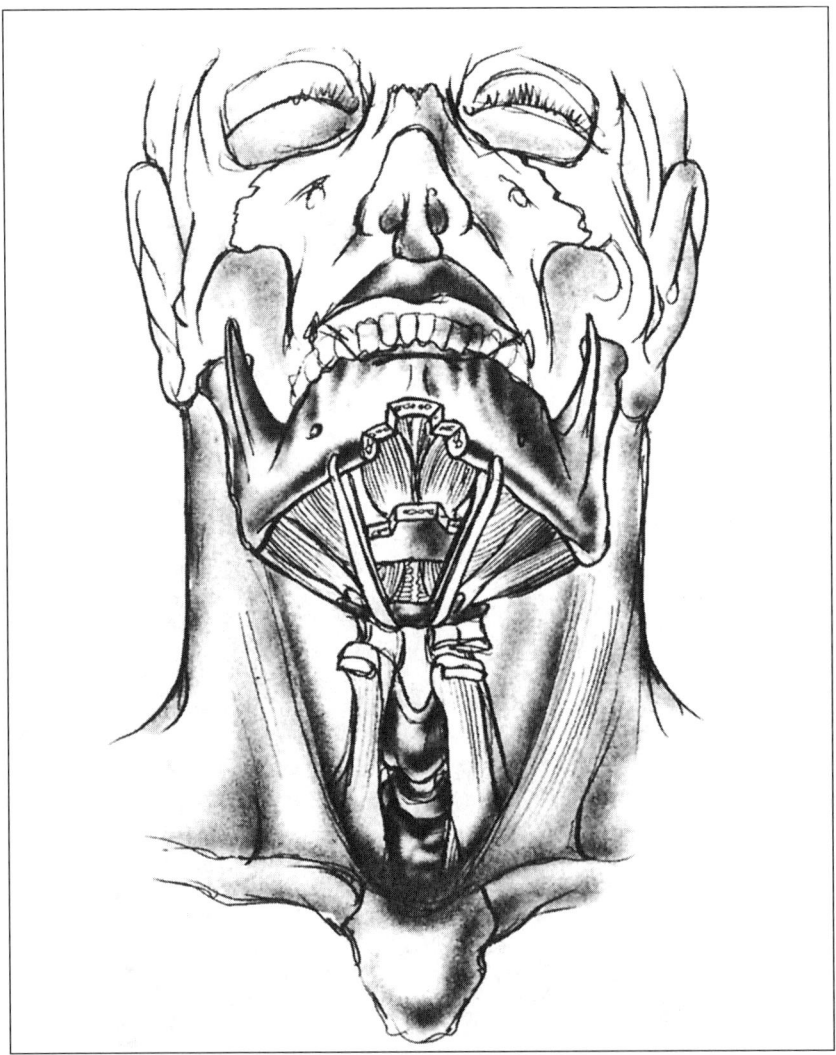

Figure 16.9 The anatomical changes made by advancement genioplasty and hyoid suspension, which enlarges the retroglossal airway. (Republished with permission from Bailey BJ (ed). *Head and Neck Surgery–Otolaryngology*, 1st ed. Philadelphia: Lippincott;1993.)

Danger Signs

The worst immediate danger for sleep apnea patients is falling asleep in inappropriate settings (e.g., while driving or operating critical machinery), resulting in injury to them and others. The long-term dangers of sleep apnea are the systemic medical problems (e.g., hypertension, arrhythmias, cor pulmonale) that increase with both the severity and duration of untreated sleep apnea.

Summary

A great deal of work is being done to define more clearly the anatomic and physiologic differences in patients with OSAS. With this information, we may be able to delineate further which patients will benefit from surgical versus other treatments. It may be possible in the future to predict which patients will have resolution of their symptoms with a simple surgical procedure compared with those who will need CPAP regardless of other treatments. More work also needs to be done regarding the specific role that OSAS has in associated medical problems, particularly hypertension and the disability of daytime somnolence.

REFERENCES

1. **Lugaresi E, Cirignotta F, Coccagna G.** Some epidemiological data on snoring and cardiocirculatory disturbances. *Sleep.* 1980;2:221-4.
2. **Koskenvus M, Daprio J, Telakiri T, et al.** Snoring as a risk factor for ischemic heart disease and stroke in man. *BMJ.* 1987;294:16-9.
3. **Kales A, Bixler ED, Cadieux RJ, et al.** Sleep apnea in a hypertensive population. *Lancet.* 1984;2:1005-8.
4. **Walsh RE, Michailson ED, Harkleroad LE, et al.** Upper airway obstruction in obese patients with sleep disturbance and somnolence. *Ann Intern Med.* 1972;76:185-92.
5. **McGuirt WF Jr, Johnson JT, Sanders MH.** Previous tonsillectomy as prognostic indicator for success of uvulopalatopharyngoplasty. *Laryngoscope.* 1995;105:1253-5.
6. **Riley RW, Powell NB Guilleminault C.** Maxillofacial surgery and obstructive sleep apnea: a review of 80 patients. *Otolaryngol Head Neck Surg.* 1989;101:353-61.

SUGGESTED READINGS

American Sleep Disorders Association. Practice parameters for the indications for polysomnography and related procedures. *Sleep.* 1997;20:406-22.
This is an excellent and up-to-date review of clinical guidelines for the use of sleep-study testing.

American Sleep Disorders Association. Practice parameters for the treatment of obstructive sleep apnea in adults: the efficacy of surgical modifications of the upper airway. *Sleep.* 1996;19:152-5.
This is an overview of the outcomes of various types of surgical treatment of OSAS.

Ancoli-Israel S. Sleep problems in older adults: putting myths to bed. *Geriatrics.* 1997;52:20-30.
This article discusses not only sleep apnea but also other sleep problems, including periodic limb-movement disorder, poor sleep habits, effects of medical illnesses, chronic medication use, and circadian rhythm changes that decrease the sleep an older person gets during the night, resulting in daytime sleepiness.

Cemons WW, Tsai W. Quality-of-life consequences of sleep-disordered breathing. *J Allergy Clin Immunol.* 1997;99:S750-6.

This article discusses the disturbances of daily life that result from breathing problems during sleep as well as the improvements that occur with treatment.

Fischer J, Raschke F. Economic and medical significance of sleep-related breathing disorders. *Respiration.* 1997;64(Suppl 1):39–44.

This article details the economic impact in Germany of treating sleep-related breathing problems. Even taking into account the costs of medical care and follow-up, there is a large mean annual monetary net benefit from such treatment.

Guilleminault C, Clerk AA, Dement WC. Nasal obstruction and obstructive sleep apnea: a review. *Allergy Asthma Proc.* 1997;18:69–71.

This reviews the contribution of nasal obstruction to sleep-related breathing problems as well as how treatment affects patient outcome.

Hudgel DW. Treatment of obstructive sleep apnea. *Chest.* 1996;109:1346–58.

Another excellent overview of treatment outcomes for obstructive sleep apnea.

Johnson NT, Chinn J. Uvulopalatopharyngoplasty and inferior sagittal mandibular osteotomy with genioglossus advancement for treatment of obstructive sleep apnea. *Chest.* 1994;105:278–83.

SECTION IV

Laryngeal Disorders

17

Hoarseness and Other Voice Disorders

Clark A. Rosen, MD
Thomas Murry, PhD
David E. Eibling, MD

Hoarseness is a common presenting symptom to the internist. There are many causes of hoarseness—from simple upper respiratory infections to serious pathologies such as head and neck cancer. Because hoarseness is frequently the only symptom and can be an early feature of head and neck cancer, patients with hoarseness require prompt and thorough evaluation. This chapter discusses voice changes that may be described by patients as hoarseness, the most important causes of which are listed in Table 17.1. The physiology of voice production, diagnostic techniques for laryngeal evaluation, and recommendations for prevention of a voice disorder also are discussed.

Hoarseness, or dysphonia, is defined as abnormal voice quality. Because the patient's and the clinician's perceptions of hoarseness are frequently different, it is important to clarify exactly what the patient means by his or her complaint. (Questions to ask the patient for the determination of hoarseness are listed in Table 17.2). Voice quality may be described as breathy, strained, rough, tremulous, or weak. On questioning, hoarseness may actually be increased vocal effort, vocal fatigue, or cough. Changes in pitch or abnormal pitch range, particularly in singers, may be primary complaints. These specific disturbances often help to focus on the various diagnoses. Often, voice change may not be recognized by the patient and his or her family because of preexisting voice disorders or a gradual onset. In these instances, voice abnormalities noted by the clinician should be pursued and should not be assumed to be long-standing or of little significance.

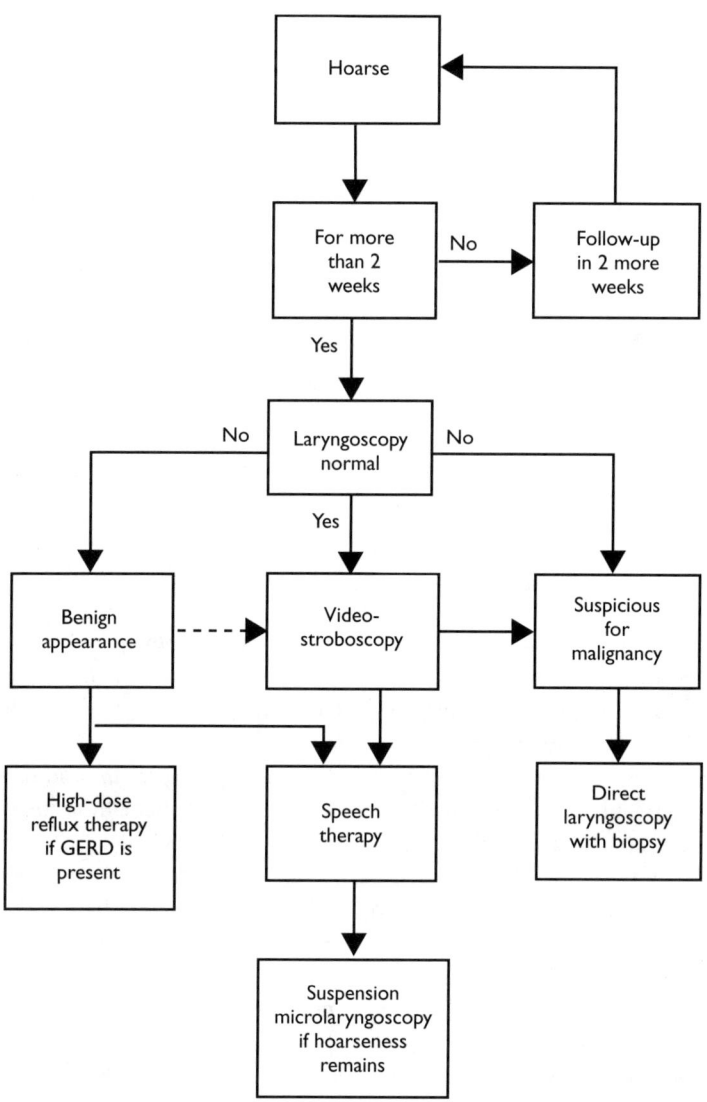

Algorithm Management of hoarseness. GERD = gastroesophageal reflux disease.

History

In the absence of an upper respiratory infection, any patient with hoarseness that persists for more than 2 weeks requires evaluation. The history can yield important information that can focus the differential diagnosis in these patients

Table 17.1 Definitions of the Common Causes of Hoarseness

Hoarseness Cause	Definition
Vocal fold nodules	Callus formations on the vocal folds, commonly referred to as nodes
Vocal fold paralysis	A weakness or immobility of the vocal folds, commonly referred to as the vocal "cords"
Reinke's edema	An accumulation of fluid in the vocal folds; this condition is seen in patients who smoke, are vocally abusive, and have reflux laryngitis
Laryngeal papilloma	Growths on the larynx caused by infection with human papillomavirus
Spasmodic dysphonia	A condition that results in irregular voice breaks and interruptions of phonation; this is a focal dystonia of the laryngeal muscles similar to blepharospasm and torticollis
Reflux laryngitis	An inflammation of the larynx caused by gastric acid reflux into the larynx and pharynx
Muscle tension dysphonia	A voice disorder that results from excessive or unequal tension of the laryngeal muscles while speaking; this condition results from improper use of the laryngeal muscles and occurs commonly with reflux laryngitis or after a severe upper respiratory infection
Functional dysphonia	An abnormal use of the vocal mechanism despite normal anatomy; this condition can be related to stress, psychological disturbance, or habituation of compensatory techniques developed during an upper respiratory infection

Table 17.2 Important Questions To Define Hoarseness

How does your voice sound different to you?
Does your voice consistently sound normal?
Is your voice worse at different times of the day?
Does your voice fatigue with use?

(Table 17.3). In a patient with hoarseness and a history of tobacco use, head and neck cancer is the primary diagnosis to exclude. Hoarseness is often the only presenting symptom of a laryngeal malignancy, and early detection significantly improves the patient's prognosis, for both cure and voice preservation.

An essential part of a thorough history is elucidating the patient's pattern of voice use, including an evaluation of the patient's "vocal personality" type with the amount and style of voice use. An inquiry about recent vocal use (e.g., screaming at a football game) and environment (e.g., noisy workplace) should be made. A history of hearing loss in the patient or a family member may contribute to shouting and subsequent voice changes. (The patient's entire family may speak loudly and have abnormal voices; it is often surprising

Table 17.3 Characteristics of Hoarseness

Voice Quality	Diagnosis
Low-pitched	Reinke's edema, vocal abuse, reflux laryngitis, vocal fold paralysis
Breathy	Vocal fold paralysis, abductor spasmodic dysphonia, functional dysphonia, vocal fold lesion (e.g., nodule, cyst, polyp)
Fatigued	Muscle tension dysphonia, vocal fold atrophy, vocal fold paralysis, reflux laryngitis, vocal abuse, vocal fold lesion (e.g., nodule, cyst, polyp)
Strained	Adductor spasmodic dysphonia, muscle tension dysphonia, reflux laryngitis
Tremulous	Parkinson's disease, essential tremor of the head and neck, spasmodic dysphonia, muscle tension dysphonia
Hoarse	Vocal fold lesion (e.g., nodule, cyst, polyp), muscle-tension dysphonia, reflux laryngitis

how much alike a family can sound.) Vocal abuse is a common, often preventable cause of dysphonia and may be underestimated by the patient; thus, it is important to question him or her as well as family members about specific patterns of voice use.

Special consideration should be given to the patient who is a professional voice user, i.e., anyone whose occupation or livelihood depends on the normal use of his or her voice—from teachers to professional singers (Table 17.4). These individuals need earlier and more aggressive intervention because of the high demands and the their livelihood's reliance on the voice. These patients also often require more specialized care and early referral to a formal "voice center."

Other aspects of the patient history include discovering the nature and occurrence of the dysphonia. Specific questioning should be used to explore 1) associated symptoms (e.g., pain, dysphagia, cough, shortness of breath), 2) symptoms of gastroesophageal reflux disease (GERD), 3) associated sinonasal diseases, 4) asthma, and 5) the use of medications that may dry the upper airway mucosa. Tobacco and ethanol use must be noted as well as exposure airborne irritants (e.g., chemicals in the workplace). The patient should be asked about previous surgery of the neck or chest or other procedures that require intubation or manipulation of the upper airway.

Physical Examination

A thorough head and neck examination, particularly of the larynx, is essential for any patient with a voice disorder. Assessing hearing acuity, upper airway mucosa, tongue mobility, and cranial nerve function are often required in a complete evaluation of the dysphonic patient. **Visualizing the larynx is central to the evaluation**. The larynx must be examined for the presence of mucosal lesions,

Table 17.4 Occupations in Which People Rely on Their Voices

Actor	Physician
Broadcaster	Receptionist
Clergy (e.g., priest, minister, rabbi)	Salesperson
Coach	Singer
Lawyer	Teacher
Nurse	Telephone operator

erythema, or edema. **Assessing vocal fold motion is crucial.** Laryngeal examination methods include **mirror or telescopic indirect laryngoscopy** or **flexible fiberoptic nasopharyngoscopy**. It is essential to visualize the entire larynx and pharynx. Assessing laryngeal abnormalities and vocal fold mobility can be challenging, often requiring a repeat examination (Fig. 17.1). The patient also should be examined for signs of associated systemic disease, such as hypothyroidism or neurological dysfunction (e.g., tremor, Parkinson's disease) (Table 17.5).

Video Laryngostroboscopy

During phonation, the vocal folds vibrate 80 to 400 times per second, too fast for the unaided eye. (Viewing the vocal folds during phonation is like trying to see a hummingbird's wings during flight.) Subtle abnormalities in motion, therefore, cannot be seen by standard laryngoscopic methods. However, video laryngostroboscopy uses a rapidly flashing strobe light that is synchronized with vocal fold vibrations to evaluate vocal fold mucosal motion. This examination allows the examiner to view the vocal folds in "slow motion," identifying subtle changes in the mucosa or tension of the vocal fold that can result in hoarseness (Fig. 17.2). Video laryngostroboscopy is especially important in evaluating subtle lesions that affect the vibration of the folds (e.g., vocal fold scar, hemorrhage, or cyst)

Diagnosis and Management

The management of hoarseness is summarized in the Algorithm.

Exposure of the larynx to gastric contents often causes pharyngeal symptoms (e.g., globus sensation, frequent throat clearing, cough) and often is not associated with the classic symptoms of GERD (e.g., "heartburn") (Case 17.1). This condition is highly prevalent, with a previously unrecognized effect on the larynx and pharynx.

Treatment for reflux laryngitis should be more aggressive than for GERD, with high-dose H_2-blockers or proton-pump inhibitors in combination with

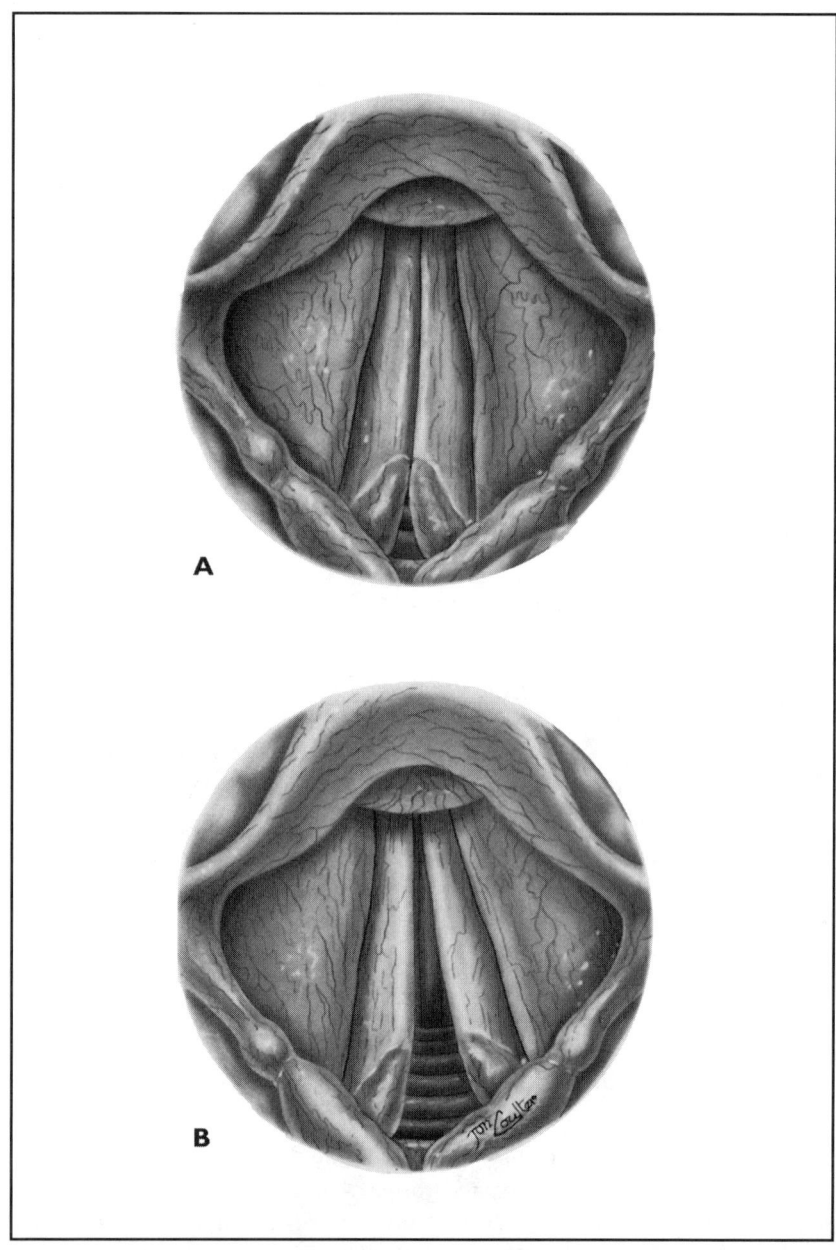

Figure 17.1 A, Normal vocal cords in the midline position during phonation. **B,** Right vocal cord paralysis during phonation, with the normal-moving left cord at the midline and the paralyzed right cord in a more lateral position. Because the cords are unable to come together during phonation, the voice has a breathy quality to it. (Reprinted with permission from Johns ME, Rood SR. *Vocal Cord Paralysis: Diagnosis and Management SiPac.* Washington, DC: American Academy of Otolaryngology Head and Neck Surgery; 1987.)

Table 17.5 Differential Diagnosis of Hoarseness

Neoplastic	Neurological
Vocal fold polyp	Vocal fold paralysis (unilateral)*
Vocal fold nodule*	Spasmodic dysphonia*
Vocal fold granuloma	Movement disorder (e.g., Parkinson's disease)
Vocal fold cyst	Essential tremor
Laryngeal papilloma*	Cerebral vascular accident
Squamous cell cancer of the larynx	
	Miscellaneous
Inflammatory	Vocal abuse
Gastroesophageal reflux laryngitis*	Vocal fold atrophy
Viral laryngitis	Vocal fold scarring
Bacterial laryngitis	Hypothyroidism (myxedematous laryngitis)
Tuberculosis or fungal laryngitis	Psychogenic dysphonia*
Allergic laryngitis	Muscle tension dysphonia*
	Reinke's edema*
	Medications

* See Table 17.1 for definition

behavioral modification. It is important to consider the diagnosis of reflux laryngitis in patients with hoarseness or pharyngeal symptoms even when heartburn symptoms are absent. Occasionally, dual-probe pH monitoring for 24 hours is necessary for diagnosis (1).

Vocal fold nodules are common in children and in female adults. These nodules are areas of epithelial thickening, similar to "calluses," on the medial surface of each vocal fold (Case 17.2). A history of vocal abuse or misuse usually can be elucidated. Voice therapy, a special form of speech therapy, is the cornerstone of treatment; if ineffective, then typically either the patient has been noncompliant or the speech therapy is not being administered properly. These patients rarely require surgery to remove the nodules; optimal results can be obtained by nonsurgical treatments (2).

Unilateral vocal fold paralysis typically presents with a breathy, weak voice due to incomplete vocal fold closure. The paralysis causes the vocal fold to be flaccid and immobile, preventing the vocal fold from moving to the midline to oppose the contralateral vocal fold during phonation. Unilateral vocal fold paralysis can be caused by a lesion anywhere along the path of the vagus or recurrent laryngeal nerve (i.e., from the base of skull to the left mediastinum) (Case 17.3). Patients also may have difficulty swallowing (typically the aspiration of liquids because of an inability to close the glottis). Discovering the site of the lesion requires imaging from the base of the skull to the level of the aortic arch for left vocal cord paralysis and to the subclavian artery for right vocal cord paralysis.

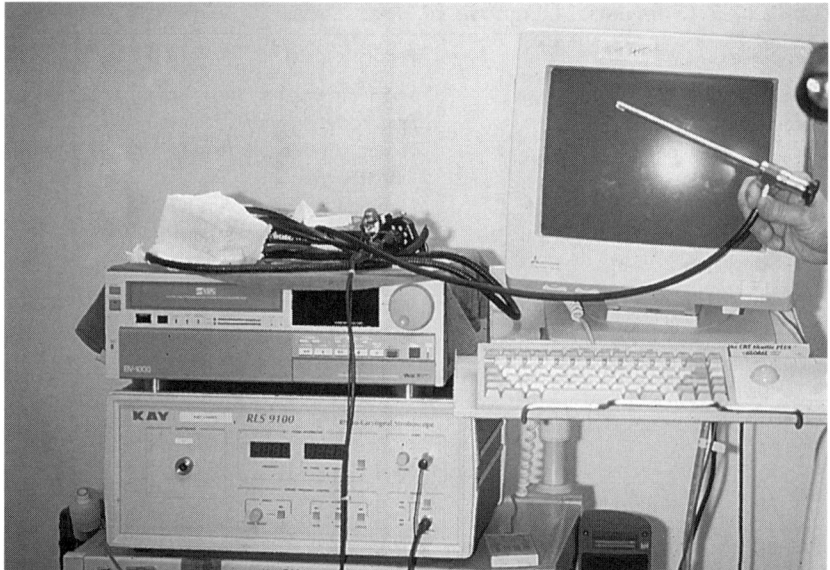

Figure 17.2 The typical setup for performing a video laryngostroboscopy. (Courtesy Dr. Karen H. Calhoun).

> ### Case 17.1 Man with Reflux Laryngitis
>
> An overweight college professor 49 years of age presents with a 6-month history of hoarseness, which he states is worse in the morning. He also reports a "dry throat" with excessive mucus and frequent throat clearing. He denies heartburn or any classic symptoms of GERD. He is a nonsmoker and denies dysphagia or other pharyngeal symptoms.
>
> Laryngeal visualization reveals subtle edema and erythema of a posterior commissure and generalized swelling of his vocal folds. The patient has normal vocal fold motion without mucosal lesions. He is diagnosed with suspected reflux laryngitis
>
> Treatment is begun with behavior modification omeprazole 20 mg/d to reduce reflux. Within 2 weeks, the patient notices a significant improvement of his hoarseness; by 6 weeks, his symptoms have resolved completely. He is switched to an H_2-blocker, and he continues behavioral modification on a long-term basis.

Injury to the recurrent laryngeal nerve also can occur during thyroid surgery, carotid endarterectomy, cervical trauma, thoracic surgery, or anterior cervical disc surgery. Medialization laryngoplasty (thyroplasty or arytenoid adduction) is the primary treatment option for permanent vocal fold paralysis (Fig. 17.5) (3).

Case 17.2   Woman with Hoarseness Caused by Vocal Fold Nodules

A woman 34 years of age complains of hoarseness for more than a year. She sings in the church choir and has two young children. She does not smoke or drink alcohol.

Physical examination reveals a mass at the junction of the anterior third and posterior two thirds of each vocal fold (Fig. 17.3).

The patient is treated with voice therapy (a total of 10 sessions in 6 weeks) that includes avoidance of voice abuse at home and in her church choir. Reevaluation after voice therapy finds complete resolution of the patient's hoarseness and vocal nodules.

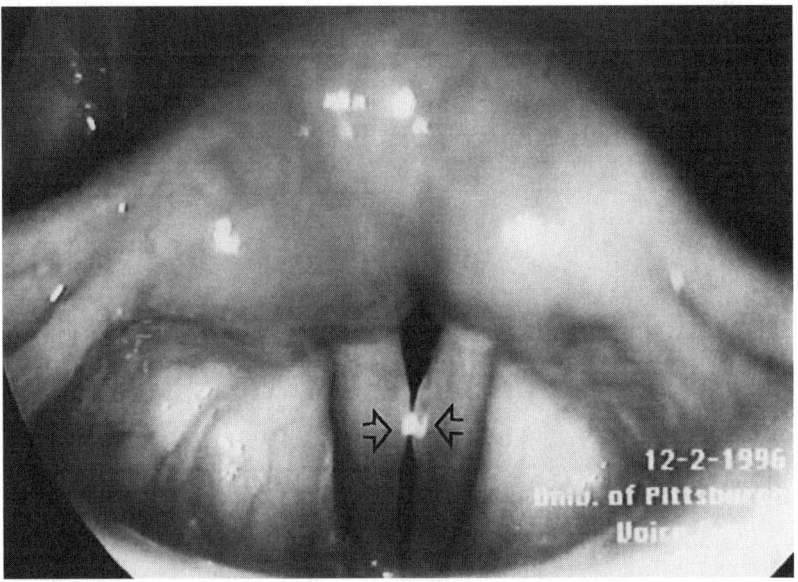

Figure 17.3 Vocal nodules can be seen on each fold as focal protuberances on the medial margin of the vocal folds (*arrows*).

Hoarseness can be caused by **inappropriate laryngeal muscle tension** that affects the vibratory characteristics of the vocal folds (Case 17.4). Called *muscular tension dysphonia*, it occurs primarily in individuals who use their voice extensively (either socially or professionally). Vocal fatigue and discomfort are common presenting symptoms (in addition to hoarseness) seen in patients with muscle tension dysphonia (4). Voice therapy is appropriate in such patients.

Any adult patient with hoarseness and a history of tobacco use may have a **laryngeal malignancy**, and the vocal folds are the most common site for la-

> **Case 17.3** **Smoker with Vocal Fold Paralysis Secondary to Mediastinal Adenopathy**
>
> A male smoker 67 years of age reports the recent onset of hoarseness and easy fatigability of his voice. He also states that he has difficulty being heard in a crowd and complains of the recent onset of coughing that is most noticeable when drinking liquids.
>
> Physical examination reveals paralysis of the left vocal fold (Fig. 17.4). Chest radiography reveals a solitary lesion in the left lung field with mediastinal adenopathy. Computed tomography–directed needle biopsy reveals large cell carcinoma of the lung. Left recurrent laryngeal nerve paralysis is secondary to mediastinal adenopathy that is invading the left recurrent laryngeal nerve in the mediastinum.
>
> Medialization laryngoplasty is performed under local anesthesia to enhance the patient's ability to speak and swallow. After surgery, he experiences a significant improvement in his swallowing and a near normal return of his vocal quality.

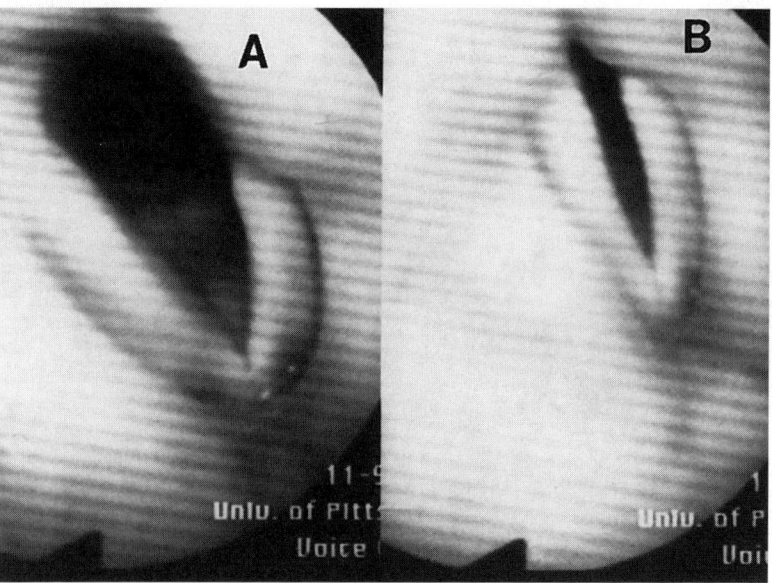

Figure 17.4 Unilateral vocal fold paralysis during abduction (*part A*) and phonation (*part B*). Note incomplete closure of the glottis with a short and flaccid left vocal fold.

ryngeal cancers (Cases 17.5 and 17.6). Patients with laryngeal cancer often present early with hoarseness and usually can be cured with minimal sequelae if detected early. Sore throat, hemoptysis, dysphagia, referred otalgia, or neck mass can develop after the hoarseness. Radiation therapy or surgery are

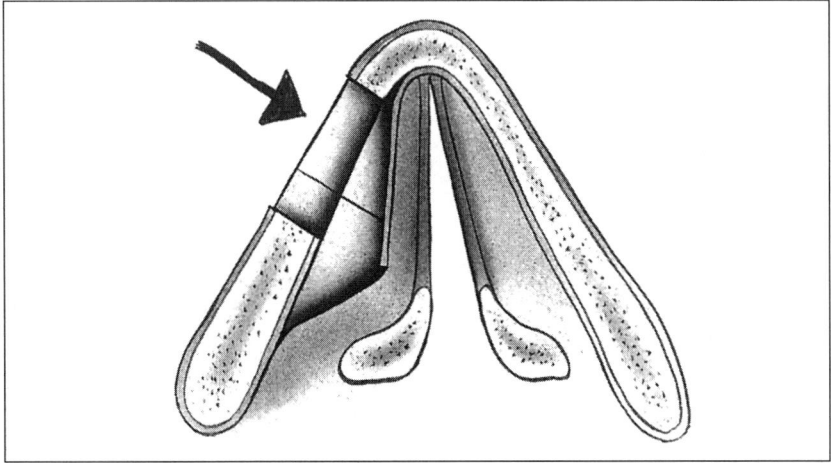

Figure 17.5 Medialization laryngoplasty involves the placement of a custom-designed implant (*arrow*) to medialize a paralyzed vocal fold. (Reprinted with permission from Wanamaker JR, Netterville JL, Ossoff RH. Phonosurgery: Silastic medialization for unilateral vocal fold paralysis. In *Operative Techniques in Otolaryngology–Head and Neck Surgery*. 1993;4:215.)

Case 17.4 Clergyman with Hoarseness Caused by Laryngeal Muscle Tension

A minister 45 years of age complains of hoarseness and pain in his throat and neck at the end of the day or after preaching on Sundays. He is a nonsmoker and is concerned that his voice is beginning to affect his ability to function in his profession.

Palpation of his neck reveals muscle tension in his strap muscles (especially at their insertion on the hyoid bone). Laryngeal examination finds inappropriate adduction of his false vocal folds and a "squeezing" of the supraglottis. There are no vocal cord abnormalities. The patient is diagnosed with muscle tension dysphonia.

Voice therapy with emphasis on abdominal breath support and laryngeal relaxation techniques results in vocal quality improvement and in discomfort resolution.

---

equally effective for early cancer, whereas a combination of both usually is required for more advanced cancers. Laryngeal cancer has a 90% to 95% cure rate when detected early and treated promptly (5). (*See* Chapter 31 for a more detailed discussion of the management of laryngeal cancer.)

Other causes of hoarseness, such as vocal cord granuloma (Case 17.7), and their treatment are described in Table 17.6.

> **Case 17.5** **Clergyman with Hoarseness Caused by Laryngeal Cancer**
>
> A man 35 years of age with a long history of smoking one pack of cigarettes per day and drinking two to three beers per week reports a 1-month history of hoarseness. He denies a recent upper respiratory infection, symptoms of airway compromise, dysphagia, and throat pain.
>
> Laryngeal examination reveals an irregular exophytic lesion of the mid-portion of his right true vocal fold (Fig. 17.6). His vocal folds demonstrate normal mobility, and a neck examination reveals no masses. The patient undergoes direct laryngoscopy and biopsy. On the basis of these findings (and a negative chest radiograph), a diagnosis of squamous cell carcinoma (stage T1) is made.
>
> The patient undergoes surgical excision of the lesion and has remained free for cancer for 5 years.

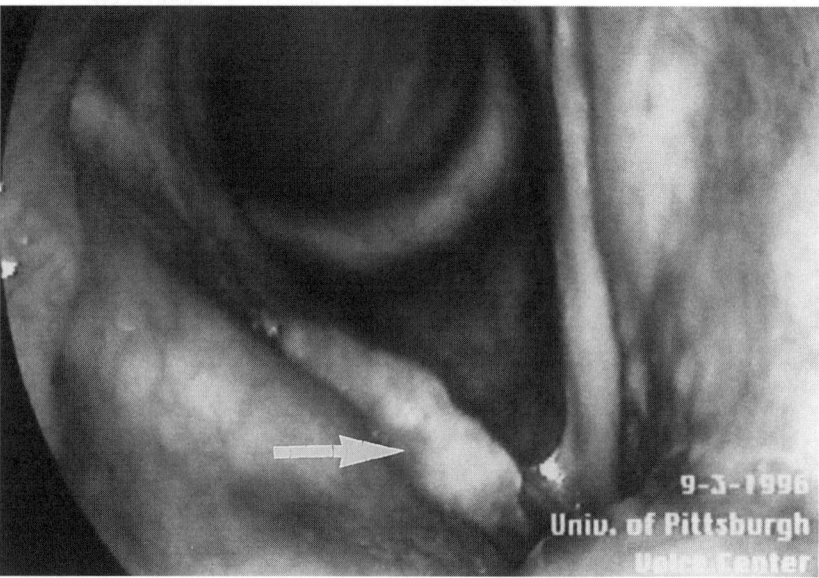

Figure 17.6 Laryngeal cancer (T1) arising from the right vocal fold (*arrow*).

Prevention

An integral aspect of hoarseness prevention is good vocal hygiene. Patients should avoid shouting, whispering, or attempting to talk extensively over excessive background noise. The importance of hydration should be empha-

> **Case 17.6** **Smoker with Hoarseness Caused by Glottic Cancer**
>
> A woman 64 years of age with a history of abusing alcohol (2 alcoholic beverages per day) and tobacco (50 pack-years, and she continues to smoke) is evaluated because she has been hoarse for the past 4 months. She relays a history of right-sided sore throat that is not alleviated with a 10-day course of antibiotics. Three weeks ago, she noted right ear pain and dyspnea on exertion. She denies fevers, chills, dysphagia, and weight loss. Her past medical history is positive for hypertension that has been well controlled by medication.
>
> Physical examination reveals severe hoarseness in a thin woman who appears older than her stated age. Flexible fiberoptic examination shows an erythematous, ulcerative lesion of the entire superior and medial surface of the right vocal fold that extends superiorly onto the false vocal fold anteriorly and crosses the midline at the anterior commissure. The right hemilarynx does not move with phonation or respiration. The nasopharynx and hypopharynx appear normal. Palpation of the neck reveals a 2.0-cm right jugulodigastric mass that is mobile and well delineated. Fine-needle aspiration of the right neck mass shows moderately differentiated squamous cell carcinoma. A metastatic work-up to rule out second primary and metastatic lesions includes liver function studies, chest radiogram and barium swallow, all of which are negative. On the basis of physical findings, the patient is diagnosed with T3N1M0 squamous cell carcinoma of the glottis.
>
> The recommendation of the multi-disciplinary head and neck tumor board is primary chemoradiation for possible preservation of the larynx. Salvage laryngectomy and right modified neck dissection are reserved for persistent or recurrent disease.

sized. Certain medications, such as antihistamines and drugs that have anticholinergic side effects (e.g., tricyclic antidepressants), may create unfavorable drying of the laryngeal mucosa; hence, these drugs should be avoided if possible. Irritants (e.g., tobacco, alcohol, marijuana, industrial chemicals) also should be avoided. Smoking cessation alone is associated with a significantly decreased risk of laryngeal cancer after 5 to 6 years, returning to near the risk of a nonsmoker after 10 to 15 years (Table 17.7 provides more guidelines on vocal hygiene). **Patients with the following symptoms should be advised to consult a physician: hoarseness that lasts more than 2 weeks, pain that occurs with speech or swallowing, or a foreign body sensation in the throat.**

Voice Therapy

Many causes of hoarseness can be treated promptly and effectively with voice therapy, a behavioral-based process in which maladaptive vocal habits and tech-

> **Case 17.7** **Young Woman with Hoarseness Caused by Postintubation Granulation Polyp**
>
> A female college student 24 years of age presents with hoarseness. She reports that her voice had been normal until 3 months ago when she underwent general anesthesia for an emergency appendectomy. She denies voice overuse or abuse, tobacco use, dysphagia, choking, dyspnea on exertion, pain, and weight loss. Past medical and surgical histories are negative. Social history is remarkable for moderate alcohol use.
>
> Flexible fiberoptic laryngoscopy reveals an erythematous polypoid lesion on the posterior medial edge of the left true vocal cord. The lesion occupies approximately half of the posterior air space and moves in and out of the glottis with respiration. Both arytenoids and vocal folds have normal range of motion. Videostroboscopy confirms the appearance of the lesion and shows a normal right vocal fold. The patient is diagnosed with granulation polyp (postintubation) as opposed to other neoplastic processes.
>
> Treatment begins with preoperative antacids and reflux precautions. Microscopic direct laryngoscopy and excisional biopsy of the lesion is performed. Pathologic specimens show a granulation polyp, and the patient is continued on reflux treatment postoperatively. Two months after surgery, a videostroboscopic examination of the larynx is normal.

Table 17.6 Management of Disorders Associated with Hoarseness

Condition	Cause	Treatment
Vocal cord polyp	Vocal abuse, sudden acute episode of vocal trauma	Surgical removal of the polyp, voice therapy
Reinke's edema	Vocal abuse, smoking, drinking alcohol	Voice therapy, abstinence from tobacco and alcohol, surgical removal
Laryngeal papilloma	Human papillomavirus	Surgical removal
Spasmodic dysphonia	Spasm of the laryngeal muscles	Botulism toxin injections
Vocal cord cyst	Congenital disorder, acute trauma	Surgical removal
Vocal cord granulomas	Trauma, GERD	Antireflux medication
Functional dysphonia	Psychiatric disturbance	Reassurance, psychiatric referral

GERD = gastroesophageal reflux disease.

niques are replaced with appropriate use of the vocal mechanism. Voice therapy is a specialized form of speech therapy that has four major components:

1. **Vocal hygiene:** the maintenance of healthy attitudes, use, and treatment of the voice mechanism; it is similar to a dental hygiene program

Table 17.7 Do's and Don'ts of Vocal Abuse

Don't...

Smoke tobacco or marijuana
Use drugs
Drink alcohol or coffee
Shout at sporting events
Attempt to be heard in noisy places like bars or airports
Phonate while yawning
Clear your throat continually
Try to talk over a cold or laryngitis
Whisper loudly or for long periods
Try to change your natural speaking voice

Do...

Get plenty of rest
Avoid places with foul air
Drink plenty of water (eight glasses per day)

Chemicals That Can Cause Problems in the Larynx

Antihistamines
Aspirin
Cigarette smoke (marijuana or tobacco)
Steroids
Tricyclic antidepressants
Any substance that blunts perception (e.g., alcohol, sleeping pills)

---

2. **Vocal production:** includes the analysis and alteration of speaking pitch, loudness, and voice quality using auditory, visual, and kinesthetic feedback techniques and proper alignment
3. **Muscle relaxation and respiratory support:** involve posture, timing, and coordination of respiration and phonation and respiratory effort
4. **Vocal mechanism education:** provides a basis for understanding the goals of treatment

The treatment process of voice therapy incorporates auditory biofeedback through visual and proprioceptive channels to produce a healthy and efficient voice. Voice therapy typically is administered in six to 14 sessions (30-40 minutes each) over a 6- to 8-week period (voice therapy rarely requires prolonged treatment). Preoperative voice therapy can prepare the patient for the rehabilitation period after surgery. An examination of the larynx, documenting any improvement, is done routinely after the completion of therapy.

Danger Signs

Hoarseness is a ubiquitous symptom. If it does not resolve with conservative medical treatment (e.g., voice rest, antireflux measures, humidity) after 2 weeks, then referral or evaluation of the vocal cords by direct or indirect laryngoscopy is warranted. In a smoker or an abuser of alcohol, the vocal cords should be visualized sooner (1–2 weeks). Chronic hoarseness requires evaluation of the vocal cords in any patient.

Summary

A thorough evaluation of dysphonia requires a detailed history (including vocal environment and social history) and a complete head and neck examination, with thorough visualization of the vocal folds. The differential diagnosis includes structural and neurological lesions that interfere with the production of voice from the lungs to the lips. **Head and neck cancer is the most important diagnosis to consider in any patient with hoarseness.** Vocal abuse is one of the most common causes of hoarseness and can be avoided by maintaining good vocal hygiene. Voice therapy is an integral part of the management of many voice problems (e.g., vocal fold nodules).

REFERENCES

1. **Koufman JA.** The otolaryngologic manifestations of gastroesophageal reflux disease. *Laryngoscope.* 1991;101(Suppl 53):1–78.
   This artcile is a comprehensive review of the otolaryngologic manifestations of GERD, including animal studies and results of a large clinical series.
2. **Murry T, Woodson GE.** A comparison of three methods for the management of vocal fold nodules. *J Voice.* 1992;6:271–6.
   This article details the study of three different methods for the treating vocal fold nodules, demonstrating a high degree of efficacy using voice therapy.
3. **Benninger MS, Crumley RL, Ford CN, et al.** Evaluation and treatment of the unilateral paralyzed vocal fold. *Otolaryngol Head Neck Surg.* 1994;111:497–508.
   This article is a thorough review of the causes, work-up, and treatment options for unilateral vocal fold paralysis.
4. **Morrison MD, Rammage LA.** Muscle misuse voice disorders: description and classification. *Acta Otolaryngol.* 1993;113:428–34.
   This article discusses the anatomy, pathophysiology, and treatment for muscle tension dysphonia.
5. **Johnson JT.** Review of early laryngeal carcinoma [Editorial]. *Am J Otolaryngol.* 1994;15:241.
   This article is an overview of the treatment modalities and their success for early laryngeal carcinoma, with extensive references for both surgery and radiation therapy of this condition.

SUGGESTED READINGS

Brown WS, Vinson BP, Crary MA (eds). *Organic Voice Disorders: Assessment and Treatment.* San Diego: Singular Publishing Group; 1996.

This text provides an excellent introduction to the types of voice disorders that exist and also a framework for understanding the diagnosis and management of these disorders.

Colton R, Casper JK (eds). *Understanding Voice Problems: A Physiological Perspective for Diagnosis and Treatment,* 2nd ed. Baltimore: Williams & Wilkins; 1996.

This text gives detailed information about the anatomy and physiology of changes in the sound of the human voice, facilitating an understanding of the functional relationship between anatomical form and sound production.

Sataloff RT. The human voice. *Sci Am.* 1992;Dec:110–1.

A superb review of the vocal fold anatomy and physiology required for voice production.

18

Upper Airway Obstruction

Randall L. Plant, MD

Upper airway obstruction can present with life-threatening hypoxemia and hypercapnia. During the initial assessment of patients with these diseases, the first priority is always to establish a stable patent airway. Sometimes an airway must be established immediately by intubation or other intervention. Upper airway distress is often due to mechanical obstruction (by tumor or foreign body), and oral intubation may not be possible. In these cases, an airway must be created surgically, by either cricothyrotomy or tracheostomy. Treat all patients who have airway obstruction with extreme caution, and use minimal manipulation before confirming that the airway is secure and stable. Sudden catastrophic obstruction can be precipitated by something as seemingly insignificant as placing a tongue blade in the mouth.

Signs of Upper Airway Obstruction

Patients with upper airway obstruction usually have inspiratory stridor. The intraluminal pressure in the upper (extrathoracic) airway drops below atmospheric pressure during inspiration. The airway collapses, and air flow becomes turbulent, producing inspiratory stridor. During expiration, the intraluminal pressure exceeds that of the surrounding tissue, dilating the airway and improving airflow. The configuration of the glottis also may contribute to its propensity to collapse during inspiration but not expiration (Fig.

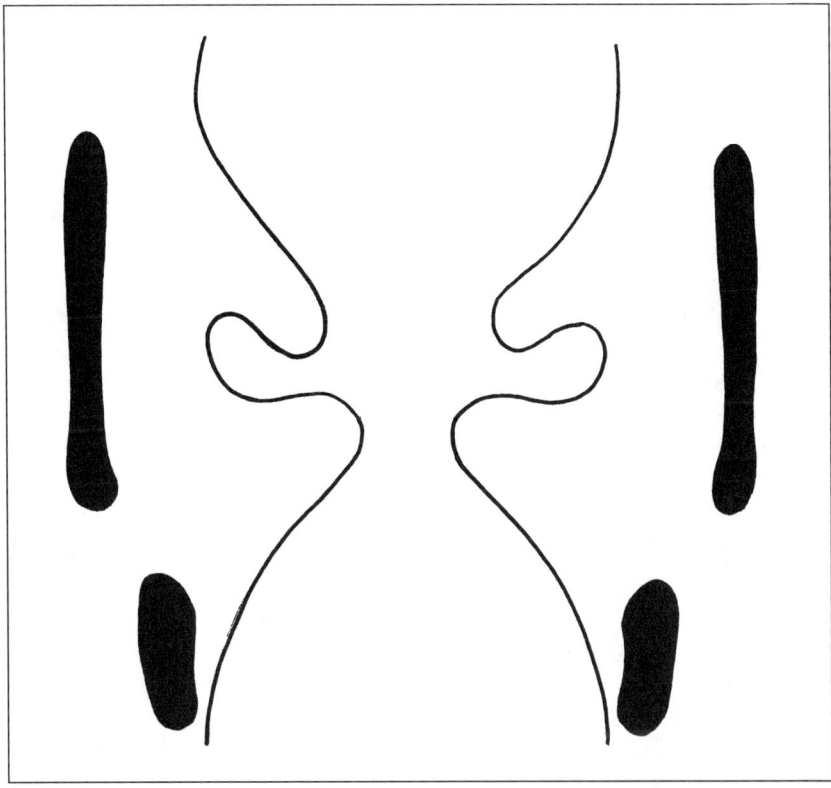

Figure 18.1 Glottic airway configuration. The glottis is the region of the airway that has the smallest cross-sectional area; thus, it is the most critically affected by narrowing. Inspiratory stridor occurs as a result of the Bernoulli effect as air moves rapidly through the small lumen. Becaues the tapered, funnel-shaped subglottis may help expand the glottic airway during expiration, expiratory wheezing at the level of the glottis is unusual.

18.1). Large lesions or critically narrowed portions of the airway produce turbulent flow on both inspiration and expiration, resulting in biphasic stridor.

In intrathoracic obstruction, the situation is reversed. During inspiration, the expansion of the chest wall decreases the intrapleural pressure compared with the intraluminal pressure. The trachea dilates, and the obstruction is reduced. During forced expiration, the intrapleural pressure exceeds the intraluminal pressure, compressing the lumen and increasing resistance to expiratory air flow. Expiratory wheezing, a classic sign of asthma, is caused by the collapse of small airways during expiration. Careful auscultation with attention to the timing of the wheezing can help differentiate between upper and lower airway obstruction.

Diagnostic Evaluation: An Overview

Physical Examination

The most important step in the initial evaluation is determining whether an airway needs to be established immediately. Other supportive measures, such as steroids or antibiotics, often need to be instituted while the diagnostic evaluation is in progress.

Pulse oximetry is monitored in patients with upper airway obstruction. **Blood oxygenation can remain normal until the moment of respiratory arrest; hence, normal pulse oximetry does not mean that obstruction is insignificant.** Hypercapnia and acidosis are early abnormalities that result from hypoventilation. The clinician should assess overall status, such as agitation and cyanosis. The patient's respiratory effort also should be assessed. The lungs are examined for wheezing and symmetry of breath sounds. Placing a hand on the patient's chest or abdomen during auscultation can help verify whether airway noises are occurring during inspiration or expiration. Retractions in the neck or abdomen during inspiration are a sign that accessory muscles are necessary to maintain airflow and suggest that fatigue is imminent. Airway intervention and respiratory support should be considered. **These patients must not be sedated** because a reduction in voluntary breathing can precipitate hypercapnia, acidosis, and respiratory arrest.

If the rapid assessment indicates that the patient is stable, a careful head and neck examination should be performed. The nasal cavity should be examined for crusting or septal abnormalities that would suggest a systemic autoimmune disorder. Severe septal deviation obstructs airflow, compelling patients to be mouth-breathers, but does not cause catastrophic airway obstruction. The oral cavity should be inspected for signs of cellulitis, abscess, and dental problems. Swelling of the anterior floor of the mouth suggests Ludwig's angina, and finger palpation of the anterior floor of the mouth demonstrates firm, woody induration. Angioedema can present with massive tongue and uvula swelling, or the swelling may be confined to the supraglottic region out of direct view. The posterior pharynx is inspected to assess the size of the tonsils and any unilateral palatal swelling that may suggest peritonsillar abscess. Large amounts of adherent debris on the posterior pharyngeal wall suggests that other debris may be occluding the laryngeal inlet, which is not an uncommon condition in elderly, debilitated, dehydrated individuals in chronic care facilities.

The neck should be inspected for obvious masses or goiter and then palpated for adenopathy that may indicate malignancy. The presence of a supraclavicular mass suggests pulmonary malignancy with associated vocal cord paralysis. Auscultation of the neck for stridor can help determine the level of obstruction.

Examination of the larynx is required in all cases of upper airway obstruction. Urgent flexible fiberoptic examination of the larynx is the "gold standard" in the diagnosis of airway obstruction and should be readily available in emergency and urgent care settings. If the obstruction is severe or progressive, then this examination must be performed as soon as possible to best direct the treatment algorithm.

History

Certain features in the patient history can be useful in the differential diagnosis (Table 18.1). A history of heavy alcohol or tobacco use raises suspicion for squamous cell carcinoma. Use of angiotensin-converting–enzyme (ACE) inhibitors or a family history of airway problems or sudden death suggests angioedema. In these cases, the patient should be asked if any minor episodes of oral or pharyngeal swelling have preceded the presenting complaint.

A history of throat pain or fever suggests an infectious cause. The throat pain of supraglottitis may seem out of proportion to a usual sore throat. Previous dental pain and poor dentition typically are associated with Ludwig's angina.

Previous endotracheal intubation and tracheostomy are clues to possible subglottic stenosis. These symptoms can develop slowly over many years. The patient also should be asked about any previous history of laryngeal or chest trauma.

If the patient's voice has changed, the time course of the change should be noted. Similarly, the duration of the breathing disorder must be ascertained.

Table 18.1 Key History or Symptom Features and Their Diagnostic Implications

History or Symptom Features	Considerations
Severity of symptoms (pending airway collapse)	May need to establish airway immediately (either by intubation or surgical airway)
History of heavy tobacco or alcohol use	Increases likelihood of squamous cell cancer in upper airway
Presence of fevers, chills, or pain	Consider infectious cause; site of infection is most often apparent on examination
Recent neck or chest surgery	Possible injury to recurrent nerve, leading to vocal fold paralysis
History of previous intubation	Intubation can produce posterior glottic or subglottic scar tissue and obstruction
History of hypertension or family history of airway obstruction	Angioedema, either from ACE inhibitors or inherited
Severe hoarseness	Obstruction at the glottic level (e.g., neoplasm, polyp, papilloma)

ACE = angiotensin-converting enzyme

Symptoms that have developed over a span of hours may result in respiratory collapse in a period of minutes.

The presence or absence of other systemic disorders should be determined. In some unusual cases, the initial presentation of a systemic disorder may be its laryngeal manifestation.

An historical clue of imminent respiratory failure is a patient's inability to sleep. Before presentation, patients with impending respiratory failure often have had to sit up for one or more nights.

Radiologic Studies

Lateral neck soft tissue films are occasionally useful in establishing a diagnosis. However, it is imprudent to send patients to the radiology department for these films because this would delay treatment of an airway emergency. Although these radiographs may assist in determining the presence of epiglottic edema or a retropharyngeal abscess, they cannot replace direct visualization of the pharyngeal and subglottic structures.

Computed tomography and magnetic resonance imaging are useful in diagnosing subglottic narrowing and compression from mediastinal masses and in identifying possible causes of recurrent laryngeal nerve (RLN) paralysis. Sagittal or coronal reconstructions allow accurate, noninvasive measurement of the stenotic region's length and diameter, and they assist in the differential diagnosis of infectious or neoplastic masses throughout the airway.

Pulmonary Function Tests

Flow volume loops are useful in distinguishing upper from lower airway obstruction. They are seldom used in the acute setting but may be valuable in the study of slowly progressive obstructions.

Management of Airway Obstruction: An Overview

As mentioned previously, **airway support** (if required) is the first treatment priority (**A**irway, **B**reathing, **C**irculation). If airway collapse occurs, direct laryngoscopy with **intubation** is attempted. Occasionally, a bag mask can be used to ventilate a patient with an obstruction that has been caused by vocal cord paralysis. More commonly, however, ventilation by this means is impossible, and intubation or tracheostomy may be required. Although fiberoptic intubation is rarely useful in an emergent situation, it may be of value in a controlled environment when an obstruction is developing slowly. If laryngoscopy is not feasible because of a neoplasm, foreign body obstruction, or infection of the tongue, pharynx, or larynx, then an urgent **cricothyrotomy** (or **tracheostomy**) is usually the best option.

A tracheostomy is performed most optimally in the operating room by experienced personnel. If this is not possible, a **cricothyrotomy** can be performed safely and expediently by any physician with knowledge of anatomy, a sharp knife, and some courage. It is wise to remember that the cricothyroid membrane and overlying tissues are not bloodless, and the "surgeon" must not be deterred by bleeding encountered en route to the airway. Once the airway is opened and a tube is inserted (an endotracheal tube is appropriate), hemostasis can be obtained at leisure.

Because airflow resistance is highly dependent on the lumen radius, even small increases in the airway diameter can improve symptoms significantly. High-dose steroids are used frequently in the acute setting to decrease swelling. For adults, intravenous dexamethasone (10–12 mg every 6 hours for 24 hours) is administered and then rapidly tapered. Oxygen is given if blood oxygenation is low. Cool, misted air reduces crusting along the lumen wall and may have a dramatic effect. A helium–oxygen mixture ("Heli-Ox") may provide significant short-term relief by reducing the resistance of gas flow across the obstruction. If an infectious process is suspected, intravenous **antibiotics** should be administered.

Patients with any airway difficulty should be admitted to a hospital's intensive care unit where they can receive continuous cardiac and respiratory monitoring, with a tracheostomy tray placed at the bedside.

Diagnosis and Management of Specific Pathologic Processes Associated with Upper Airway Obstruction

Upper airway obstruction may result from a variety of pathologic processes; its major causes are summarized in Table 18.2.

Subglottic Airway Obstruction

Subglottic airway obstruction occurs below the true vocal cords at the level of the cricoid cartilage (Fig. 18.2). Infectious subglottic swelling (croup) is common in children but rare in adults. In adults, the common causes of subglottic obstruction are endotracheal intubation or other airway trauma. Prolonged intubation, gastroesophageal and pharyngeal reflux, infection, tube movement, and hypotension all contribute to the risk of edema, injury, and subsequent permanent subglottic stenosis.

Subglottic stenosis can occur with some autoimmune disorders (e.g., Wegener's granulomatosis) and can produce a diffuse tracheitis that eventually

Table 18.2 Major Causes of Upper Airway Obstruction

Tumors of the Upper Airway

Malignant Tumors
  Squamous cell cancer of the larynx, tongue base, hypopharynx, and trachea
  Adenoid cystic carcinoma of the trachea
  Thyroid carcinoma, producing compression, and invasion of the trachea

Benign Tumors
  Recurrent respiratory papillomas (most common)
  Chondromas, lipomas, and fibromas

Infections
  Epiglottis
  Supraglottis
  Tracheitis
  Cellulitis of floor of mouth (Ludwig's angina)
  Retropharyngeal abscesses

Inflammatory Processes
  Gastroesophageal reflux disease associated with layrngospasm
  Angioedema (hereditary or acquired)

Subglottic Stenosis

Vocal Fold Paralysis
  Recurrent nerve injury (traumatic or tumor compression)
  Systemic neurological disorder
  Idiopathic

Other Vocal Fold Mobility Disorder
  Cricoarytenoid joint fixation (inflammatory, tumor invasion)
  Inspiratory adduction ("functional laryngospasm")
  Scar tissue formation in the interarytenoid region

Other Vocal Fold Lesions
  Vocal fold polyps
  Glottic webs

---

causes subglottic scarring. Subglottic stenosis also has occurred spontaneously in some patients with no previous history of intubation or known systemic disorders. Gastroesophageal reflux disease (GERD) is known to exacerbate intubation-induced subglottic stenosis in infants and probably plays a role in "spontaneous" cases.

Obstructive subglottic lesions, such as granulomas or thin webs, often can be managed with an endoscope. Laser ablation may be useful in some circum-

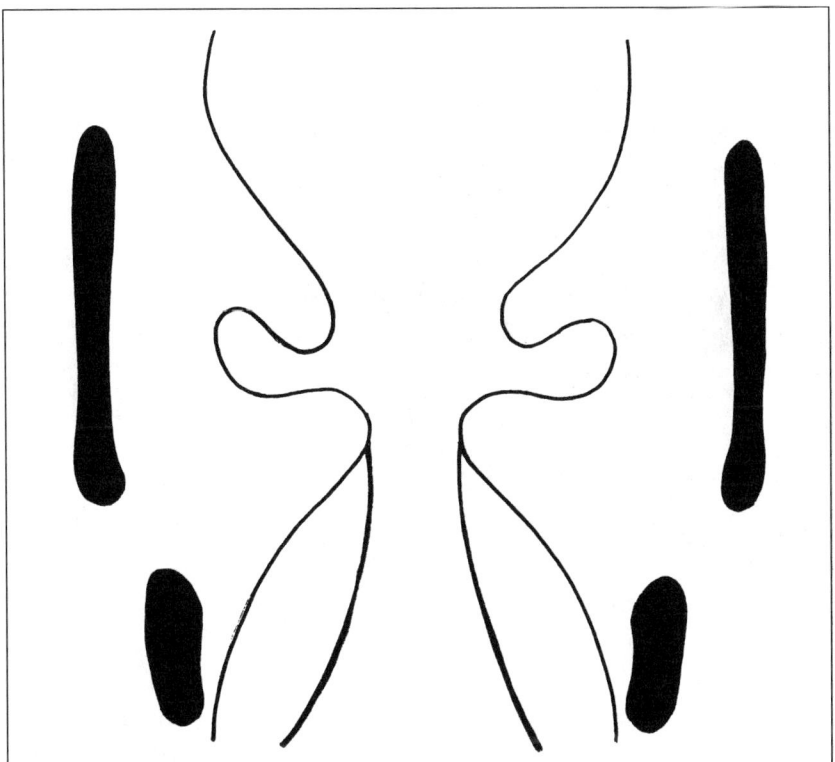

Figure 18.2 Croup. This diagram illustrates edema in subglottic soft tissue within the cricoid ring. Very small reductions in lumen diameter lead to dramatic changes in airstream velocity and airway collapse due to the Bernoulli effect.

stances. Longer stenotic segments usually require an open surgical procedure. Tracheal segments of up to 5 cm in length can be removed as a sleeve resection with immediate end-to-end anastomosis. Bone or cartilage also can be used to stent the anterior and posterior airway, increasing lumen diameter.

Tracheal mucosal injury can occur if the pressure of an endotracheal tube cuff against the tracheal wall exceeds the capillary perfusion pressure of the mucosa. Prolonged, high cuff pressure causes vascular compromise, leading to inflammation, fibrosis, and the formation of a circumferential stenosis. Mediastinal and cervical tumors (e.g., adenoid cystic carcinoma) can compress the subglottic lumen directly. Large benign goiters also can shift or compress the trachea (Fig. 18.3).

Tracheostomy Stomal Granulation Tissue

Chronic inflammation at a tracheostomy site can induce exuberant granulation tissue. If the granulation tissue is intraluminal but superior to the tra-

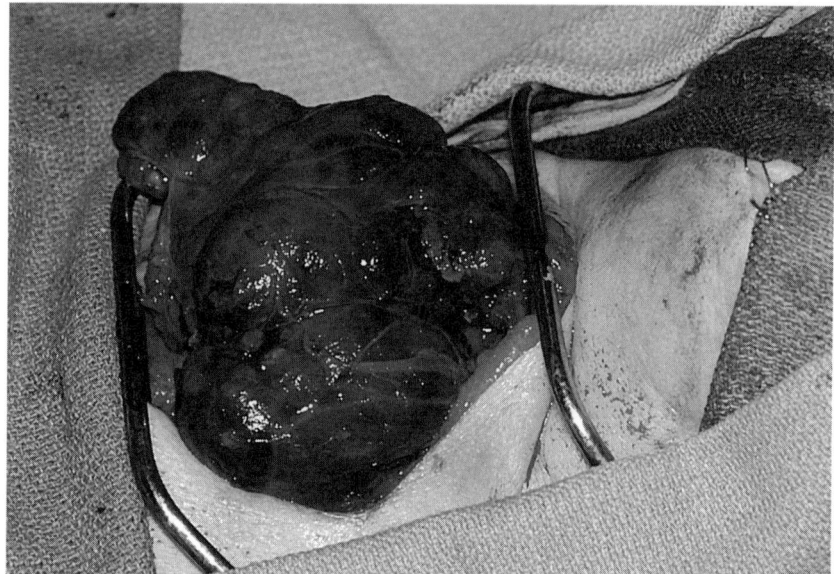

Figure 18.3 Massive thyroid tumor causing airway obstruction.

cheostomy tube, it causes no symptoms as long as the tube is in place (because the tube bypasses this area). When the tube is removed, the granulation tissue can obstruct the airway. Any patient who develops a breathing difficulty after decannulation (removal of a tracheostomy tube) should be examined for the presence of subglottic granulation tissue below the vocal cords but above the tracheostomy site. This can be visualized easily with a fiberoptic endoscope introduced through the stoma in the neck and directed upward.

Glottic Obstruction

Glottic obstruction is caused either by failure of the vocal folds to open or by an obstructive lesion at the level of the vocal folds. Failure of the vocal folds to open (i.e., vocal fold immobility or paralysis) can be caused by **abductor muscle paralysis**, **cricoarytenoid joint fixation** (Case 18.1), central neurological disorder, or **soft tissue scarring** (e.g., a web formation that impairs vocal cord motion).

Glottic stenosis due to soft tissue scarring in the interarytenoid region is difficult to treat. The scar tissue can be removed easily through the laryngoscope with a carbon dioxide laser, but there is a high rate of recurrence. Various open-neck surgical procedures with bone or cartilage stenting of the posterior cricoid cartilage have been used with better results but at greater surgical risk.

> **Case 18.1** **Elderly Woman with Cricoarytenoid Joint Fixation**
>
> A woman 76 years of age with long-standing rheumatoid arthritis presents with 3 weeks of gradually increasing inspiratory stridor and exercise intolerance. Past medical history is significant for multiple, successful joint replacements and chronic pharmacologic management of her rheumatoid disease.
>
> Physical examination reveals a short, elderly, alert, dyspneic woman with severe kyphoscoliosis, inspiratory stridor, and characteristic features of long-standing rheumatoid disease. Despite her stridor, her voice is normal. Indirect laryngoscopy cannot be performed due to the kyphoscoliosis, but flexible fiberoptic laryngoscopy reveals bilateral vocal cord immobility and erythema of the arytenoid mucosa. A diagnosis of rheumatoid fixation of the cricoarytenoid joints is suspected; however, due to impending airway collapse, immediate intervention is required.
>
> Her kyphoscoliosis precluded oral intubation, so a tracheotomy is performed. The procedure is technically difficult due to her short stature and neck rigidity. After her airway is secured, she is anesthetized, and direct operative laryngoscopy is attempted. Again, due to her severe spine disease, the larynx cannot be visualized, nor the arytenoids palpated. After the procedure, transcutaneous electromyography of the thyroarytenoid muscles is performed, revealing normal action potentials. She is treated with high-dose steroids and empirical antireflux medication.
>
> Although there is improvement, adequate vocal cord mobility does not return. Laser cordotomy to improve her airway is considered but is not performed because of anticipated technical difficulties and a fear of exacerbating her already-compromised swallowing function and voice (the latter of which she uses actively in various activities). After her tracheostomy stoma matures, her tube is replaced with a small uncuffed tube, and an expiratory speaking valve is inserted to permit communication. Although she thinks the tracheostomy is "a nuisance," she is able to care for it easily (with the help of her elderly sister with whom she lives) and to resume her active lifestyle.
>
> **Discussion**
>
> This case illustrates the successful management of a potentially difficult situation. Early suspicion of the diagnosis precluded inappropriate attempts to treat other causes of dyspnea, and early tracheotomy precluded emergent attempted oral intubation that undoubtedly would have resulted in catastrophe. A long-term tracheostomy is "a nuisance," but with appropriate support can be managed by most cognitively intact individuals.

Vocal Cord Paralysis
A singe pair of muscles—the posterior cricoarytenoid muscles—are responsible for abducting (opening) the vocal folds. These muscles, and most muscles responsible for adducting (closing) the vocal folds, are innervated by the RLNs.

The RLN follows a circuitous route through the lower neck on the right side, and around the aorta on the left side, before reaching the larynx. As a result, the nerve is exposed to injury by numerous pathologic processes and by surgery anywhere along its track from the skull base to the mediastinum.

Glottic obstruction and airway difficulty typically do *not* occur with unilateral vocal fold immobility. The voice may be quite hoarse or breathy (*see* Chapter 17), but the contralateral functioning vocal fold usually abducts sufficiently to provide an adequate airway. Shortness of breath with unilateral vocal fold immobility usually suggests that an additional process (e.g., asthma, congestive heart failure, emphysema) is playing a role.

In contrast, bilateral vocal fold immobility frequently produces breathing difficulty and often requires tracheostomy or other intervention. If the folds are immobilized near the midline, the voice may be normal but airway obstruction is severe. Bilateral vocal fold paralysis may resolve spontaneously; however, recovery may require 12 months or more. Tracheostomy is often necessary for immediate treatment. The airway can be improved by transection of the vocal fold (cordotomy) or by partial resection of the arytenoid and the vocal fold. The goal of this treatment is to resect enough of the glottis to allow air flow without significantly deteriorating voice quality. Nevertheless, neither the voice nor the airway is normal after this procedure.

Causes of Vocal Cord Paralysis

The most frequent cause of bilateral vocal fold paralysis is surgery. Thyroid surgery, especially total thyroidectomy, can place both of the RLNs at risk. In most cases, the symptoms are apparent immediately after surgery, occasionally necessitating reintubation in the recovery room. Carotid endarterectomies and cervical spine surgery can cause unilateral nerve paralysis, but airway obstruction is unusual and encountered only if performed bilaterally (or if there is a preexisting immobility on the opposite side). If the nerves have not been transected, some degree of recovery can be expected. However, until vocal fold movement returns (in up to 12 months), the patient may have airway obstruction that requires a temporary tracheostomy.

Neoplasms or other pathology in the neck and upper chest can present with bilateral vocal fold paralysis, although unilateral paralysis is more common. The left side is affected more often because the left RLN travels through the chest as well as the neck. Thyroid cancer can compress both RLNs. Upper mediastinal masses that cause vocal cord paralysis usually arise from a primary lung tumor. Lymphoma, esophageal cancer, or metastatic tumors from infradiaphragmatic sites also commonly cause paralysis.

Neurological disorders can produce bilateral vocal fold paralysis; sarcoidosis and Lyme disease rarely cause it. Bilateral vocal fold paralysis can be acquired from congenital anomalies, such as myelomeningocele, hydrocephalus, and Arnold–Chiari malformation. These anomalies almost always present in childhood but may be diagnosed rarely at older ages. In adults, bilateral vocal fold paralysis has been seen with a postpolio syndrome, cerebral vascular accidents, myasthenia gravis, Guillain–Barré syndrome, and Parkinson's disease. A variant of Parkinson's disease known as the Shy–Drager syndrome presents with Parkinson-like symptoms, autonomic nervous system failure, and bilateral vocal fold paralysis.

Endotracheal intubation alone can produce vocal fold immobility due to nerve, joint, or soft tissue injury. Short-term intubation (e.g., during a surgical procedure) is suspected to cause muscle paralysis due to the pressure placed on the RLN by the endotracheal tube cuff. Others have suggested that RLN stretching during intubation may be the cause of this paralysis.

Vocal Cord Fixation

The **cricoarytenoid joint**, like other synovial joints elsewhere in the body, can be damaged by systemic or local inflammatory disorders. Rheumatoid arthritis can cause cricoarytenoid joint fixation and airway obstruction. This condition is frequently associated with advanced systemic disease, and patients usually exhibit serologic abnormalities such as elevated rheumatoid factor. Oral endotracheal intubation may be difficult or impossible because of kyphoscoliosis and cervical spine changes associated with the advanced age of these patients. Thus, tracheostomy may need to be performed under local anesthesia. The joints also can be invaded and immobilized by hypopharyngeal or vocal fold cancer (Fig. 18.4).

Prolonged intubation can result in vocal cord fixation. Pressure of the endotracheal tube on the posterior cricoid cartilage in the interarytenoid area can lead to inflammation of the joint capsule and fixation of the vocal folds. The soft tissue between the arytenoids also can become scarred, preventing full abduction of the vocal folds even if joint mobility returns. This posterior glottic scar can be difficult to diagnose and manage and frequently requires operative endoscopy with arytenoid manipulation for diagnosis.

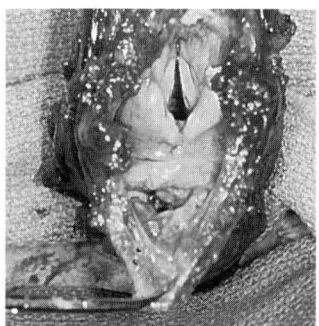

Figure 18.4 Tumor of hypopharynx that has invaded both posterior cricoarytenoid muscles, leading to bilateral vocal cord fixation.

In the sedentary individual, bilateral vocal fold immobility may be surprisingly well tolerated and, therefore, remain undiagnosed. However, because the airway is already compromised, very small decreases in the remaining glottic opening can lead to obstruction. A minor upper respiratory infection, allergic irritation, or mild viral laryngitis may rapidly produce respiratory distress in this situation. Fortunately, because the anatomy is typically normal, endotracheal intubation usually is feasible and provides time for further investigation.

Episodic Laryngospasm

Paroxysmal episodes of shortness of breath can be caused by laryngeal irritation from refluxed gastric contents (i.e., GERD). The highly acidic contents produce laryngospasm when they come in contact with the arytenoids or the vocal folds. Typically, the patient is awakened at night with significant shortness of breath; however, episodes may occur at any time. The condition can be mistaken for the paroxysmal nocturnal dyspnea of heart failure or obstructive sleep apnea. Pharyngeal reflux often occurs without heartburn symptoms. If laryngeal examination is normal or suggestive of GERD (i.e., inflamed mucosa in the posterior larynx, especially over the arytenoids), empirical therapy for GERD is appropriate.

Aggressive management of GERD includes changes in diet, head-of-bed elevation, avoidance of food within 2 hours of bedtime, and drug therapy with either H_2-blockers or proton-pump inhibitors. If heartburn is present, it may resolve immediately; however, the resolution of voice and throat symptoms (e.g., hoarseness) may require 4 to 6 weeks of treatment. Episodic laryngospasm usually responds within this period as well. The use of 24-hour dual-probe pH-metry may be required to confirm or exclude the diagnosis if symptoms persist.

Paradoxical Vocal Fold Motion

Inappropriate vocal fold adduction can sometimes occur during inspiration. The condition can mimic asthma, but wheezing is inspiratory. It is often treated as asthma but is refractory to steroids or bronchodilators. Patients frequently have a history of multiple trips to the emergency room. Certain smells or emotional events may trigger obstructive episodes. The condition is occasionally called **functional laryngospasm**, although this may be misleading because the larynx is not in true spasm. Even during episodes of distress, the vocal folds often fully abduct when the patient is relaxed or distracted. The exact cause of this is unknown, but it is thought to have a psychological component. However, it does not seem to be a focal laryngeal dystonia such as adductor spasmodic dysphonia, because spasmodic dysphonia is seldom associated with breathing problems. Diagnosis can be exceptionally difficult, requiring carefully performed flexible laryngoscopy. Asking the patient to either sniff or swallow can often "break" an episode. Accurate diagnosis with explanation and reassurance obviates the need for airway intervention.

Functional inspiratory adduction is treated primarily by speech pathologists who use various speech and breathing techniques to help reduce laryngeal muscle tension. Relaxation therapy and psychological counseling is often useful. GERD may exacerbate the muscle-tension disorder, so antireflux precautions and medications (e.g., proton-pump inhibitors, H_2-blockers) are warranted. Tracheostomy should be avoided if possible. Although botulinum toxin (Botox, a long-acting muscle relaxant) has been used in cases of true adductor laryngeal dystonia, its effectiveness in functional adduction has not been reported.

Laryngeal Neoplasms

Neoplasms of the larynx can present with airway obstruction, and the most common malignant vocal cord tumor is **squamous cell carcinoma**. Heavy tobacco and alcohol use are major risk factors; however, such tumors occasionally occur without such a history. Carcinomas arising on the vocal fold produce hoarseness as an early symptom, which is sometimes ignored by the patient and his or her family (Case 18.2). Recognizing this important warning sign leads to early diagnosis and an excellent chance of cure. Advanced tumors may be accompanied by airway distress and respiratory stridor, which may be misdiagnosed as asthma. As opposed to tumors on the vocal folds, tumors of the supraglottic larynx do not cause hoarseness and may become quite large before airway obstruction symptoms occur (Fig. 18.5). Treatment of airway obstruction due to neoplasm is directed toward eliminating the neoplasm. Surgery, radiation therapy, or chemotherapy is used for malignant tumors, depending on the extent and histology (*see* Chapter 31).

The most common benign vocal fold neoplasm is recurrent respiratory papillomatosis. This occurs frequently in children but also can present for the first time in adults. Involvement in adults is usually less aggressive and extensive than in younger patients. The voice is hoarse and obstruction is usually progressive over a prolonged period. Recurrent respiratory papillomatosis is treated with endoscopic removal using forceps or a carbon dioxide laser. Success also has been achieved with interferon therapy, although the side effects of this treatment may be worse than the disease.

Benign vocal fold polyps can enlarge but do not usually result in airway obstruction. Polyps are seen most often in smokers and begin as a thickened fluid collection (Reinke's edema) in the superficial lamina propria of the vocal folds. Hoarseness is common but, if diagnosed early, may resolve with smoking cessation. With continued smoking, however, this edema can develop into true polyps. Once polyps are present, they seldom resolve spontaneously and must be removed surgically.

Case 18.2   Man with Airway Obstruction Caused by Squamous Cell Carcinoma

A male smoker 67 years of age with known chronic obstructive pulmonary disease presents to the emergency department with a 3-day history of increasing inspiratory stridor. He has been hoarse for a few years but recently has experienced a worsening of his voice and an increase in his "asthma." Over the past 8 hours, his symptoms have become so severe that he cannot lie flat, and he has not slept or eaten for more than 12 hours.

Physical examination reveals a thin man sitting on the stretcher in obvious distress. There is loud inspiratory wheezing (stridor) and suprasternal, subxiphoid, and intercostal retractions. There are no visible or palpable neck masses noted, and the oral cavity examination is normal. Oxygen via nasal cannula was begun at the time of his arrival, and pulse oximetry reveals a saturation of 100. Urgent transnasal flexible fiberoptic laryngoscopy reveals an ulcerated mass that involves his entire left hemilarynx, with fixation of the vocal cord and a severely compromised airway.

The patient is placed on a monitor, an intravenous line is inserted, and he is transported emergently to the operating room where he undergoes a tracheotomy under local anesthesia. The procedure is made difficult because of the patient's sitting position and because of the caudal motion of the larynx during forced inspiration. Immediately after an opening into the trachea is created, his stridor and agitation resolves, and he becomes relaxed and breathes quietly. After general anesthesia is induced, the patient undergoes laryngoscopy and biopsy of his tumor. Esophagoscopy and bronchoscopy also are performed to rule out second primary cancers.

Three days later, after the histologic diagnosis of squamous cell carcinoma is confirmed and the treatment options with the patient and his family have been discussed, he undergoes total laryngectomy. Pathologic examination reveals negative margins, but the tumor extends into the trachea, 2 cm below the level of the vocal cords. He is treated with external-beam radiation to the upper mediastinum and stoma. During several years of follow-up, he remains free of disease.

Discussion

Acute upper airway obstruction may be the initial presentation of patients with cancer of the larynx. Typically, tumors of the supraglottic structures (e.g., arytenoids, epiglottis) present with a "hot potato" voice, whereas glottic cancer is associated with a long history of hoarseness. Airway obstruction is characterized as inspiratory stridor and often may be confused by the patient as progression of asthma rather than an indication of new disease. Symptoms may become quite dramatic before the patient presents, necessitating emergency intervention. Generally, the patient is able to maintain near-normal oxygen saturations until he fatigues; hence, the history that he had not slept for some time was quite worrisome, despite normal oxygen saturation. In most instances, tracheotomy is required; however, occasionally, the airway can be controlled with intubation and the tumor debulked sufficiently to permit leisurely treatment planning.

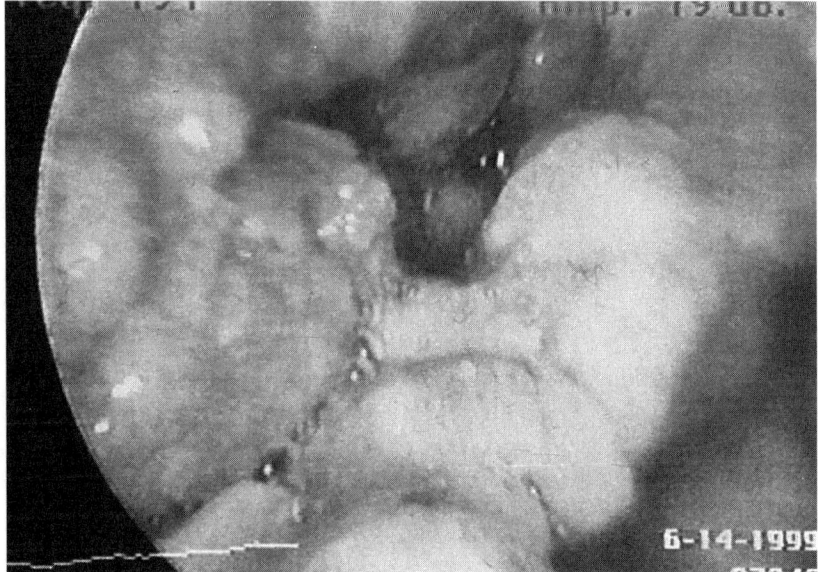

Figure 18.5 Large, obstructing supraglottic cancer. The *arrow* notes the only visible airway. Hoarseness is a late sign in supraglottic tumors, and they can reach very large size with relatively minimal symptoms.

Supraglottic Obstruction

Supraglottic obstruction usually presents with dysphagia and the muffled voice change sometimes called "hot potato" voice, but it rarely causes hoarseness. Supraglottic obstruction usually is caused by edema or neoplasm. Edema most often occurs as a result of either infection or angioedema. The typical presentation is **epiglottitis** in children; however, its incidence has decreased dramatically since the introduction of the *Haemophilus influenza* vaccine.

Infectious Supraglottitis

Infection of the supraglottis in adults that is similar to epiglottitis in children is called **supraglottitis** and usually involves not only the epiglottis but also the arytenoids, aryepiglottic folds, and pharyngeal walls. Supraglottitis presents with severe sore throat, fever, muffled voice, and dysphagia—a sore throat that is out of proportion to other complaints is an important clue to this disease. Supraglottitis can progress rapidly, with sudden airway blockage. This infection in adults is caused by *H. influenza, Streptococcus pneumoniae, Streptococcus viridans,* and *Staphylococcus aureus.* The risk of airway obstruction is less in adults (because of their larger airways) than in children. These patients require extremely close monitoring. When airway support is required, the infection often has distorted the anatomy so much that endotracheal intubation is impossible. Emergent cricothyrotomy or tracheostomy may be necessary.

Supraglottitis in adults is treated most optimally with broad-spectrum antibiotics that are effective against *H. influenza* (usually resistant to ampicillin), gram-positive streptococci, and anaerobes. Subglottic stenosis often can be associated with mild tracheitis, which also responds well to antibiotics. Parenteral steroids are useful in reducing inflammation and swelling even in the presence of infection; however, their empirical use probably should be limited to 24 hours or less.

Angioedema

Angioedema produces a boggy, painless edema that can involve the supraglottic larynx, the palate, tongue, lips, and face. Four types of angioedema have been described: hereditary angioedema, hereditary allergic angioedema, nonhereditary allergic angioedema, and idiopathic edema (Fig. 18.6). Angioedema is treated most effectively with a combination of airway support, steroids, and antihistamines.

Angioedema Associated with the Use of Angiotensin-Converting–Enzyme Inhibitors

The idiopathic variant of angioedema is most often associated with ACE inhibitors and also can be associated with nonsteroidal anti-inflammatory drugs

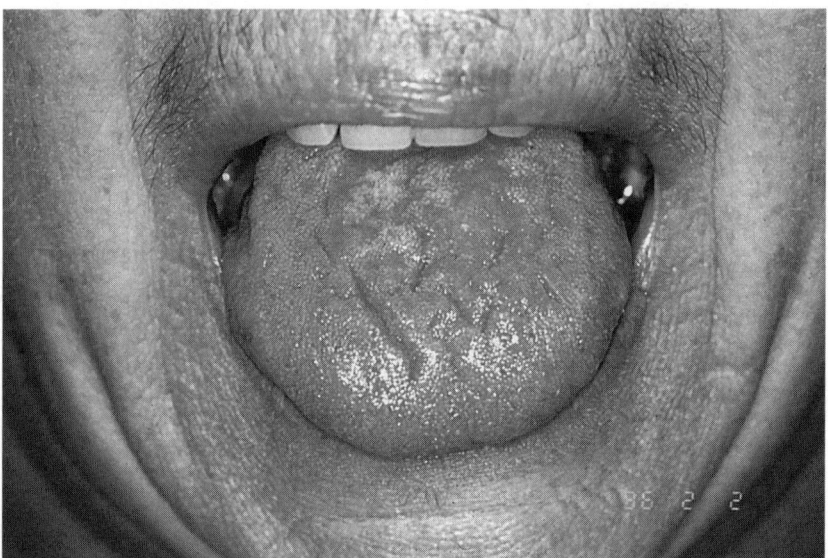

Figure 18.6 Angioneurotic edema of the tongue can develop extremely rapidly (this patient required a tracheotomy). The differential diagnosis includes allergic edema or edema due to use of angiotensin-converting–enzyme inhibitors.

> **Case 18.3** **Man with Life-Threatening Angioedema Caused by Angiotensin-Converting–Enzyme Inhibitor Use**
>
> A black man 55 years of age with essential hypertension presents to the emergency department with acute swelling of his tongue and difficulty breathing and swallowing. Three weeks ago, he had a mild episode of cheek and lip swelling, but it resolved rapidly after treatment with an injection of subcutaneous epinephrine. His hypertension is well controlled on Vasotec, an angiotensin-converting–enzyme (ACE) inhibitor. The current episode began 30 minutes before his presentation and is progressing rapidly. Epinephrine is administered urgently after his arrival.
>
> Physical examination reveals an uncomfortable, moderately obese man sitting upright with massive edema of his tongue, which is protruding from his mouth. During the course of the history, examination, and consultation, the size of the tongue is enlarging. The patient develops dysphagia and dyspnea. By the time the otolaryngology resident has completed documenting his findings, the swelling has progressed to the point that airway intervention is urgently required, despite treatment with intravenous steroids, epinephrine, and Benadryl.
>
> Intubation is not feasible via either oral or nasal route due to the massive edema, which now involves his supraglottis as well. An urgent cricothyrotomy is performed with some difficulty due to the patient's thick, short neck and because he could not lie flat or extend his neck. He is admitted to the intensive care unit, his Vasotec is withheld, and intravenous steroids are administered.
>
> Over the next 3 days, his tongue swelling resolves. One week after the event, his tracheotomy tube is removed.
>
> **Discussion**
>
> Life-threatening angioneurotic edema is a rare complication of ACE-inhibitor therapy for essential hypertension. About two thirds of cases occur within a week of drug initiation, but angioneurotic edema can occur at any time. Hence, just because a patient has been treated with long-term ACE inhibitors does not preclude the disorder. There is a predilection for those of African ancestry to be at higher risk. Occasionally, the patient experiences minimal transitory mucosal edema that resolves spontaneously before an episode of massive edema; therefore, the occurrence of mild edema should suggest the possible diagnosis.

(e.g., aspirin, morphine, codeine). Angioedema occurs in 0.1% to 0.2% of those taking ACE inhibitors. Although the reactions can occur several days to many months after starting the medications, two thirds of patients have reactions that occur within a week. The effect is not dose related and is thought to arise from a reduction in the normal degradation of bradykinin by ACE inhibitors. An initial mild reaction may be followed in several months by a severe life-threatening obstruction (Case 18.3). Early symptoms may include only a globus sensation. Because of the airway risk of this condition, pharyngeal symptoms that occur in patients being treated with ACE inhibitors require prompt investigation.

Steroids may not be effective in this ACE-inhibitor induced syndrome. Instead, subcutaneously injected epinephrine (0.5 mL of 1:1000) can be used. Many of these patients have hypertension, and the additional epinephrine may elevate their blood pressure further. Swelling typically resolves within 24 to 48 hours.

Hereditary Angioedema

The hereditary form of angioedema is an autosomal-dominant trait that affects C1-esterase inhibitors. Approximately 85% of affected patients have decreased levels of normally functioning inhibitors; most others have normal levels of a defective C1-esterase inhibitor. A family history may be present but vague; nonspecific early death in affected family members may be the only history. The absence of a history is not always helpful, because previous episodes of swelling may have been mild and, therefore, ignored. For the hereditary variant, prophylaxis with ε-aminocaproic acid and fresh-frozen plasma occasionally is recommended.

Other Causes of Supraglottic Obstruction

Other systemic diseases can have supraglottic laryngeal manifestations. Sarcoidosis of the larynx presents with swelling in the epiglottis, aryepiglottic

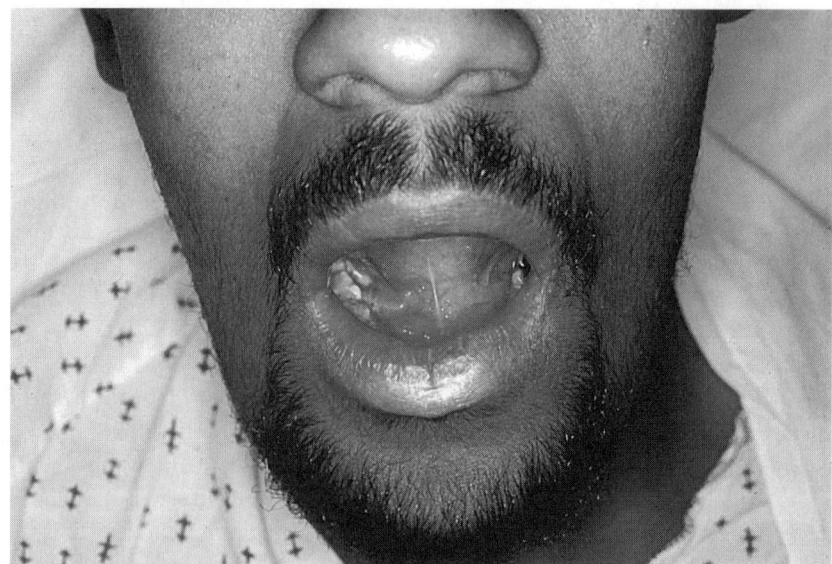

Figure 18.7 Edema of the floor of the mouth in a patient with Ludwig's angina.

folds, and arytenoids. As in other parts of the body, histologic examination of biopsied lesions demonstrates noncaseating granulomas. Long-standing involvement can lead to soft tissue scarring that limits vocal fold abduction and reduces the diameter of the airway.

Amyloidosis of the larynx is a pink granular lesion that can grow to become obstructive. Thick, adherent secretions in dehydrated, dysphagic, or debilitated individuals may accumulate and obstruct the airway.

Infections of the Oral Cavity

Ludwig's angina is an infection of the floor of the mouth, often seen in individuals with poor dentition. The muscular sling formed by the mylohyoid muscle beneath the mouth floor limits the inferior spread of the infection, resulting in woody edema on the floor of the mouth (Fig. 18.7). Rapid expansion of the cellulitis can displace the tongue base posteriorly into the pharynx, causing precipitous airway obstruction. In rare instances, Ludwig's angina can be controlled with antibiotics alone; usually it requires surgical drainage. Severe infections necessitate the establishment of a secure airway. Because intubation usually is not possible, an airway must be created surgically (cricothyrotomy or tracheostomy) is required. A tracheostomy is performed under local anesthetic (i.e., an "awake tracheostomy"). Abscesses in other parts of the airway, especially the **retropharyngeal region**, require drainage as well.

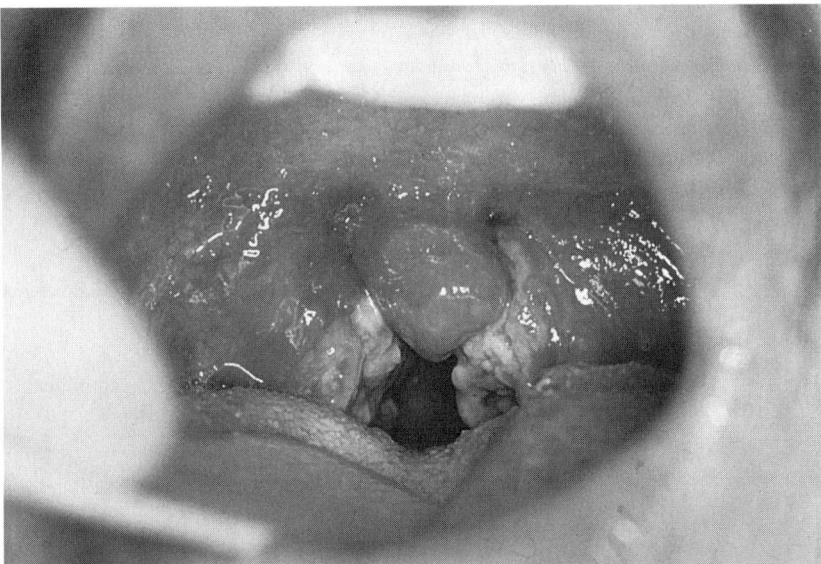

Figure 18.8 Massive tonsillar enlargement with the typical shaggy exudate of mononucleosis.

Infectious mononucleosis can present with massive tonsillar swelling that causes upper airway obstruction (Fig. 18.8). Other systemic symptoms of mononucleosis are present, and the obstruction usually responds rapidly to intravenous steroids and antibiotics. Occasionally, urgent tonsillectomy is required. Peritonsillar abscesses are common but do not result in airway obstruction unless they are bilateral (an extremely rare occurrence).

Summary

Upper airway obstruction can arise from a variety of pathologic processes. The common denominator is reduced airflow. The obstruction can progress rapidly to respiratory arrest, and the clinician must be prepared to establish an airway. Intubation often is not possible due to the obstruction, and it may be necessary to create an airway surgically. Initial medical treatment is usually a combination of antibiotics, steroids, antihistamines, oxygen, and closely monitored observation. Early examination of the larynx, usually with a flexible fiberoptic instrument, is required.

SUGGESTED READINGS

Aboussounan LS, Stoller JK. Diagnosis and management of upper airway obstruction. *Clin Chest Med.* 1994;15:35–53.
   An excellent review of the pathophysiology and etiology of upper airway obstruction.
Christopher KL, Wood RP, Eckert RC, et al. Vocal cord dysfunction presenting as asthma. *N Engl J Med.* 1983;308:1566–70.
   A detailed description of findings in five patients with inspiratory vocal fold adduction.
Heffner JE. Medical indications for tracheostomy. *Chest.* 1989;96:186–90.
   Geared primarily toward the critically ill patient, but still a good review of the decision making and consequences pertaining to tracheostomy.
Lauretano AM, Cardonna DS, Michel JL, Weinstein L. Laryngeal infections. In Fried MP. *The Larynx: A Multidisciplinary Approach.* St. Louis: Mosby-Year Book; 1996.
   A thorough chapter covering viral, bacterial, and fungal infections of the larynx.
Roberts JR, Wuerz RC. Clinical characteristics of ACE inhibitor–induced angioedema. *Ann Emerg Med.* 1991;20:556–8.
   A case study and literature review of this common complication.
Weymuller EA, Bishop MJ, Santos PM. Problems associated with prolonged intubation in the geriatric patient. *Otol Clin N Am.* 1990;23:1057–74.
   A description of the various injuries leading up to and including laryngeal stenosis.

19

Aspiration

David E. Eibling, MD

The classic presentation of a patient with aspiration of food or gastric contents is a single dramatic event that is recognized easily (Table 19.1). Massive aspiration usually occurs with serious life-threatening illness and requires immediate and aggressive management. The less-obvious aspiration that occurs with many chronic illnesses is not recognized as easily but also can lead to significant morbidity and even death.

Many patients with symptomatic or occult dysphagia (especially after stroke, head injury, or other neurological disease) develop chronic aspiration, often with significant pulmonary sequelae. Reactive airway disease that is triggered by microaspiration can cause significant alterations in pulmonary function. Surgery of the oral cavity, larynx, or hypopharynx disrupts normal swallowing, putting patients at high risk for aspiration-related pulmonary complications.

Patients with a wide variety of illnesses may aspirate, but the aspiration may not be readily apparent. (*See* Chapter 15 for a review of the physiology of normal swallowing and the pathophysiology of dysphagia and aspiration.)

Identifying Aspiration

Massive aspiration typically occurs after an acute change in a patient's level of consciousness after neurological injury, myocardial infarction–related hypoxia, or intoxication with drugs, alcohol, or anesthetic agents. Aspiration

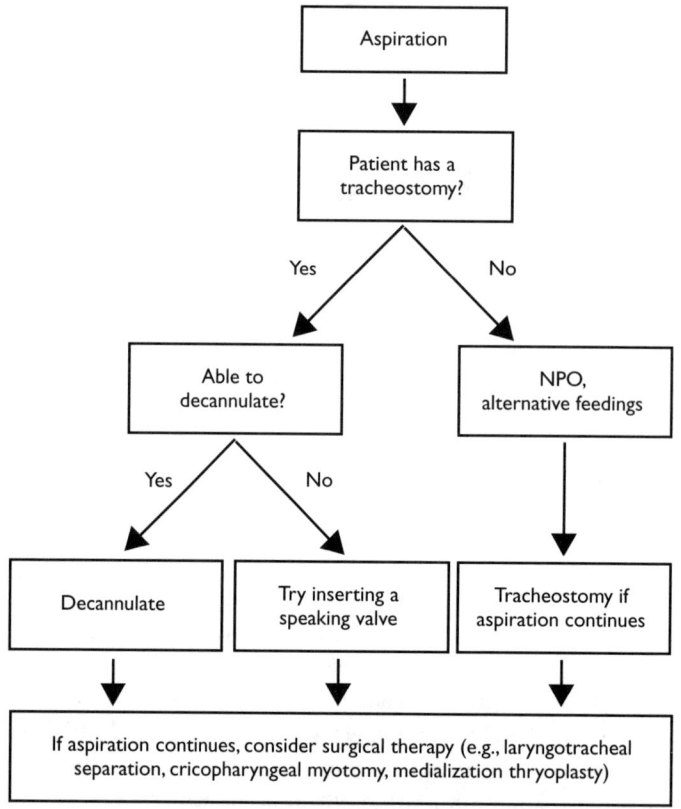

Algorithm Management of aspiration. NPO = nothing by mouth.

prevention during anesthetic induction is critical because protective reflexes are suppressed by drug-related loss of consciousness. Preventive measures include ensuring that the patient has an empty stomach and using drugs to reduce acid production or to promote gastric emptying. When an emergency requires anesthetic induction in a patient with a full stomach, specific anesthetic techniques that minimize aspiration of gastric contents include conscious intubation using a flexible fiberoptic endoscope and so-called "rapid-sequence induction" (i.e., anesthetizing, paralyzing, and intubating the patient within 15 to 30 seconds, with no attempt to ventilate the patient by mask because it may precipitate vomiting).

Chronic aspiration is more common than massive aspiration and more difficult to recognize (Table 19.2).

Table 19.1 Signs of Massive Aspiration

Gastric contents in endotracheal tube after respiratory arrest and resuscitation
Hypoxia after CNS injury or sudden change in level of consciousness
Chest radiograph with evidence of aspiration after an acute respiratory "event"
Lung abscess in patient who is predisposed to massive aspiration (e.g., alcohol abuser)
Hypoxia and decreased breath sounds after endotracheal intubation
Patient who has had obvious tube feedings or gastric contents suctioned from trachea after intubation

CNS = central nervous system.

Table 19.2 Signs of Chronic Aspiration

Weight loss and sarcopenia	Recurrent fevers
Choking with meals, especially liquids	Chronic or recurrent pneumonitis
Poor oral intake	"Bronchorrhea" after tracheostomy
"Wet" cough	Drainage from around tracheostomy tube
Weak voice	Unexplained hypoxia

Causes and Complications of Aspiration

Aspiration Due to Stroke and Other Neurological Diseases

Neurological and neuromuscular diseases associated with aspiration are listed in Table 19.3. The most common underlying cause of chronic aspiration is neurological disease (Table 19.4). Aspiration and dysphagia are common in patients with loss of central nervous system function after a vascular event or head injury. This problem is also common in patients with chronic progressive neurological disease, such as multiple sclerosis and amyotrophic lateral sclerosis. At the University of Pittsburgh, nearly all patients who required laryngotracheal separation for severe aspiration had suffered some major neurological insult.

The economic effect of aspiration-induced pulmonary complications in stroke patients is high. Up to 90% of these patients have swallowing problems, and many aspirate. Stroke patients in rehabilitation units frequently develop aspiration pneumonia secondary to either food aspiration during feeding or oropharyngeal secretion aspiration (Case 19.1).

Table 19.3 Neurological and Neuromuscular Disease Associated with Aspiration

Cerebrovascular accident	Huntington's chorea
Intracranial tumors	Dystonia or tardive dyskinesia
Amyotrophic lateral sclerosis	Myoclonus
Parkinson's disease	Elevated intracranial pressure
Myasthenia gravis	Vocal cord paralysis (laryngeal or vagal nerve injury)
Myotomic dystrophy	
Polymyositis or dermatomyositis	Progressive muscular dystrophy
Guillain–Barré syndrome	Pseudobulbar or bulbar palsy
Bulbar poliomyelitis	Stroke

Table 19.4 Pathologic States Associated with Chronic Aspiration

Altered level of consciousness	Gastrointestinal disease
Neurological disease	Head and neck surgery
Neuromuscular disease	Tracheostomy
Cranial nerve deficits	

Aspiration Pneumonia

Aspiration pneumonia causes approximately 40,000 deaths per year in the United States. The cumulative cost of treating aspiration pneumonia in these patients is estimated to be more than $3 billion dollars per year.

Chronic aspiration in the ill, **hospitalized patient** is a common cause of pneumonia. Broad-spectrum antibiotics for the treatment of recurrent aspiration-induced nosocomial pneumonia are costly (because of patient isolation, prolonged hospitalization, and intensive nursing care) and enhance the development of resistant organisms. Early recognition and management of aspiration could reduce both morbidity and cost.

Recognition of potential aspiration is critical to reducing the risk and cost of pulmonary morbidity. The symptoms are often poorly defined, without an obvious association with aspiration (*see* Table 19.2). In many centers, the speech–language pathologist plays an active role in management of the dysphagic patient and is key to the early identification of aspiration. A dysphagia (multispecialty) team can help identify patients who are at risk for aspiration. An overview of this evaluation process can be found in Chapter 15.

> **Case 19.1** **Elderly Woman with Aspiration After a Stroke**
>
> A woman 74 years of age who has suffered two strokes (one recently) and has developed significant dysarthria with a "wet" voice. On admission, she is evaluated by the multidisciplinary dysphagia team, and it is determined that she is not to be given anything by mouth (NPO). Nasogastric feedings are instituted. Because she seems to have improved during the first 3 days, a modified barium swallow is performed, revealing significant delay in swallowing and silent aspiration of both thick and thin liquids.
>
> She was advanced to, and did well on, a pureed diet with nonpourable liquids. Two weeks later, the modified barium swallow was repeated, demonstrating significant improvement; she was tolerating solid food and had only minimal aspiration of thick liquids and moderate difficulties with thin liquids. Moreover, she was noted to cough with aspiration. Her nasogastric tube was removed, and she was begun on a mechanical soft diet with thickened liquids.
>
> One month after discharge, a repeat examination demonstrated further improvement, and she was permitted to ingest thin liquids without restriction.
>
> **Discussion**
>
> This is a common scenario for patients who have suffered stroke. Silent aspiration is essentially a radiographic (or endoscopic) diagnosis; hence, decisions about feeding have to be made on the basis of objective studies (repeated modified barium swallows in this case). Similar information could have been obtained via flexible endoscopic examination of swallowing (FEES) during test feeding.

Aspiration Associated with Head and Neck Cancer

Patients with head and neck cancer often aspirate after surgery, both acutely and chronically. Surgical defects in the palate, tongue, larynx, or pharynx disrupt normal swallowing with timing errors, poor bolus control, decreased pharyngeal sensation, glottic closure defects, or nonpassage of the bolus into the esophagus. Successful management of postoperative aspiration begins with the anticipation that all of these patients will aspirate, especially after surgery of the tongue base, pharyngeal wall, or supraglottic larynx. Surgical reconstruction to minimize aspiration and postoperative instruction for "relearning" how to swallow are vital.

Dysphagia and aspiration also occur after other surgery, such as esophageal and cervical spine surgery. **The key to early recognition and successful management is to remember that copious secretions or pneumonia that develops after head and neck surgery is most likely due to aspiration.**

Aspiration Due to Vocal Cord Paralysis

Impaired glottic closure due to **vocal cord paralysis** can cause aspiration. Aspiration occurring with a high vagal lesion (by either surgical injury to the va-

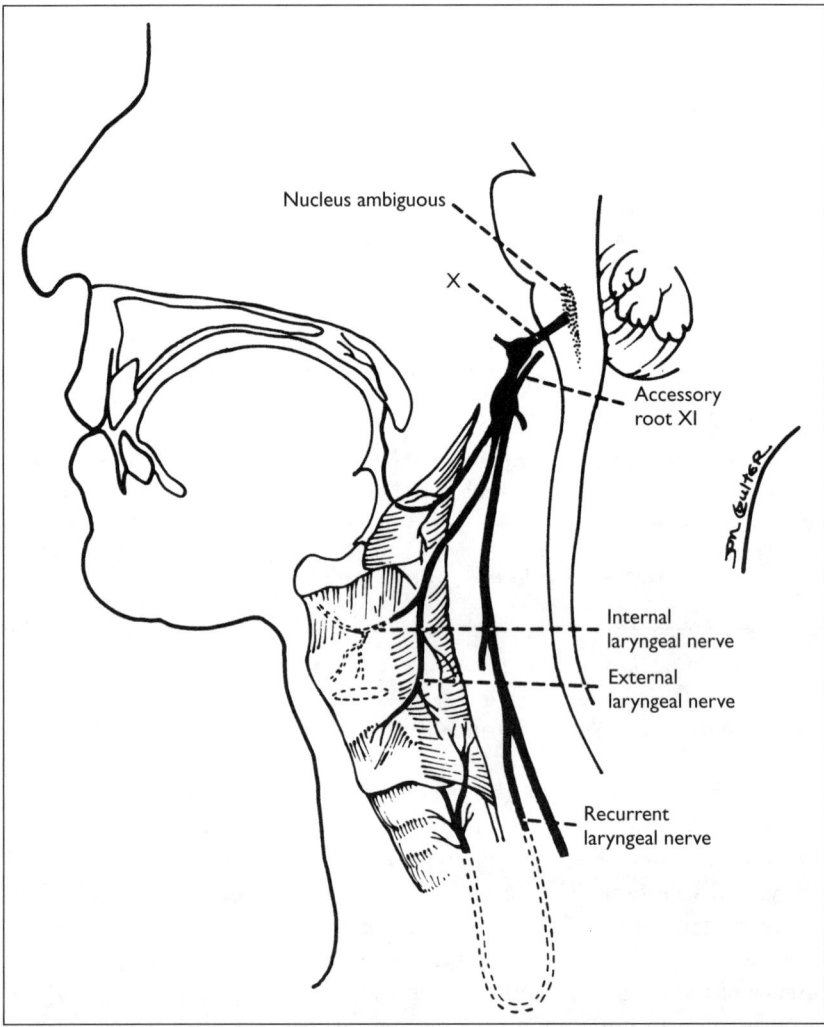

Figure 19.1 The path of the left vagus and recurrent laryngeal nerve. The site of a high vagal lesion that results in ipsilateral laryngeal anesthesia, pharyngeal paresis, and vocal cord paralysis is shown (X). Although rare, this lesion will result in aspiration. A more common condition is isolated recurrent laryngeal nerve injury (see Fig. 19.2), which results in voice change; however, aspiration is less common. (Republished with permission from Eibling DE, Johnson JT, Bacon G. *Understanding and Treating Aspiration SIPac*. Alexandria, VA: American Academy of Otolaryngology–Head and Neck Surgery; 1993.)

gus nerve by surgery or tumor at the skull base or high in the neck) is more likely to be severe than is isolated recurrent laryngeal nerve injury (Fig. 19.1). This causes both ipsilateral vocal cord paralysis and pharyngeal paresis, with sensory denervation of the hypopharynx and supraglottis. This sensory denervation impairs swallow timing, increasing aspiration risk. If the paralyzed vocal cord is positioned laterally, the widely patent glottic opening allows aspiration into the trachea (Fig. 19.2).

A high vagal interruption is not always diagnosed easily. Symptoms may be limited to hypoxia, an inability to decannulate or extubate the patient, or the poor handling of oral secretions. This clinical picture may not immediately suggest an open, insensate glottis. We routinely consider the possibility of a high vagal interruption in any patient with pulmonary difficulties, hoarseness, or aspiration after surgery of the posterior fossa, skull base, or neck (Case 19.2).

Aspiration Caused by Tracheostomy

Aspiration often occurs in patients with tracheotomies. Although the secretions suctioned from the tracheostomy are sometimes called "bronchorrhea," they usually consist of aspirated saliva. A cuffed tracheostomy tube does not guarantee protection of the lower airways from aspirated secretions. A cuff can decrease the quantity of material aspirated, especially with frequent tube

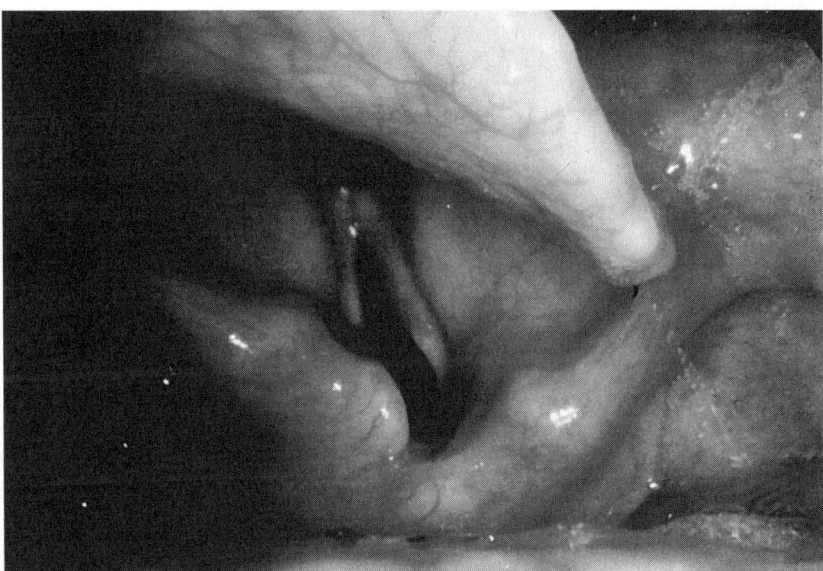

Figure 19.2 Larynx exhibiting paralysis of the left vocal cord. The aspiration risk depends on the degree of vocal cord closure that the patient can achieve.

> ### Case 19.2 Man with Aspiration Caused by a High Vagal Lesion
>
> A man 30 years of age is referred for evaluation of hoarseness. Past surgical history is remarkable for previous excision of a small right vagal paraganglioma at age 25. Postoperatively, Gelfoam injection of the right vocal fold was performed twice, but he was lost to follow-up thereafter. Over the past year, he has noted increased coughing associated with liquid intake and voice weakness. He denies weight loss, pneumonia, and bronchitis. He recently started working as a salesman and is interested in anything that could "strengthen" his voice. Past medical and surgical histories are otherwise unremarkable.
>
> Head and neck examination shows a well-healed transverse surgical scar on the right neck. There are no cervical masses. Fiberoptic examination of the larynx shows an immobile, lateralized, right true vocal cord. The left vocal fold crosses the midline on phonation but does not approximate the right completely. There is pooling of saliva in the right pyriform sinus. The mucosal surfaces of the larynx and hypopharynx appear normal. The remaining cranial nerves function normally. Videostroboscopy confirms an immobile right vocal fold without evidence of a mucosal wave. A modified barium swallow, with a speech therapist in attendance, shows microaspiration of thin liquids. Computed tomography of the neck shows postoperative changes without evidence of recurrent disease.
>
> The patient is diagnosed with a high vagal lesion after excision of a vagal paraganglioma, resulting in hoarseness and aspiration. He is offered vocal cord medialization (type I thyroplasty) to treat his symptoms.
>
> **Discussion**
>
> This patient's primary complaint was of voice problems, not aspiration. Nevertheless, questioning revealed that he had symptoms of aspiration that were also bothersome. Treatment with vocal cord medialization is expected to resolve both his voice and swallowing difficulties.

suctioning, but secretions pooled above the tube cuff inevitably leak into the distal trachea and lower airways. Some health care workers assume that aspirating patients can eat without aspiration so long as tracheostomy cuffs are inflated. Unfortunately, the tracheostomy tube disrupts swallowing function, leading to aspiration and allowing the accumulation of significant debris above the tracheostomy tube cuff. This debris is eventually aspirated, leading to pneumonitis. Testing with dyed food or liquid can identify such aspiration rapidly and should be performed routinely.

A tracheostomy tube facilitates the suctioning of aspirated secretions; thus, it is a reasonable first step in managing aspiration. Once the acute process (for which the tracheostomy was required) resolves, aspiration often is managed most optimally by decannulation or with the use of an expiratory speaking valve (described later in this chapter) to improve swallowing.

Diagnostic Evaluation

Aspiration cannot be diagnosed by physical examination alone. Neck auscultation during the swallowing of liquids can reveal gurgling sounds of aspirated material in the airway or residual liquid in the pharynx. Coughing or choking during eating suggests aspiration, but "silent aspiration" occurs without symptoms, especially in the neurologically impaired. Suctioning gastric contents, tube feeding, or oral feeding from a tracheostomy tube means the patient is aspirating. Giving dyed food orally, or dyeing the tube feeding, identifies whether suctioned material is aspirated secretion.

Examination with a flexible fiberoptic laryngoscope permits the identification of laryngopharyngeal abnormalities. Inadequate glottic closure can be discovered by asking the patient to phonate or by touching supraglottic mucosa with the tip of the endoscope to elicit reflex glottic closure (Case 19.3). Failure of glottic closure suggests aspiration risk, especially when decreased laryngopharyngeal sensation also exists. Estimating the sensation of the pharyngeal and supraglottic mucosa can be performed by touching the mucosa with the tip of the endoscope; newer instrumentation can help quantify sensory loss. Pooled secretions in the oral cavity or hypopharynx strongly suggest dysphagia and associated aspiration. A fiberoptic examination that is made difficult because of thick or pooled pharyngeal secretions strongly suggests severe pharyngeal dysfunction with a high risk of aspiration.

Modified Barium Swallow

Because a traditional barium esophogram uses a large volume of barium, patients may aspirate a large quantity of it. A modified barium swallow (or "cookie swallow") avoids this problem and is the preferred evaluation for dysphagia and aspiration. Performed jointly by a speech pathologist and a radiologist, this study is videotaped, which permits slow-motion replay to evaluate the individual phases of swallowing.

Barium is administered in small quantities and in varying consistencies (e.g., thin liquid, thick liquid, pudding-like) to identify maneuvers or consistencies that reduce aspiration. Gastrographin is not used, because it can cause significant chemical pneumonitis if aspirated. The degree of aspiration can be estimated radiographically, using guidelines to distinguish clinically significant from clinically insignificant aspiration.

Aspiration can be quantified by swallow scintigraphy. Technetium-99–la-

> ### Case 19.3   Elderly Man with Presbylarynx
>
> A man 84 years of age is referred for evaluation of a weak voice that he has had for the past 5 years. He also reports intermittent "coughing spells" when drinking fluids. He denies weight loss, chronic cough, pneumonia, dysphagia, otalgia, and dyspnea on exertion. Past medical and surgical histories are unremarkable. There is no history of stroke.
>
> Physical examination reveals a healthy-appearing elderly man with a weak and quavering voice. Flexible fiberoptic examination of the larynx reveals mobile and symmetric vocal cords that do not adduct completely in the midline. There is salivary pooling above the vocal folds and in the hypopharynx. The cranial nerves are normal. No cervical masses are noted, and the remainder of the head and neck examination is normal. Videostroboscopic examination of the larynx confirms equal mobility of the vocal folds bilaterally, with bilateral "bowing" and a reduced mucosal wave. Mild salivary pooling without gross aspiration is noted. A modified barium swallow shows microaspiration of thin liquids and no suggestion of a hypopharyngeal or cervical esophageal lesion. The esophogram shows no evidence of extrinsic compression or mucosal lesions. A chest radiograph and computed tomography scan of the neck are normal. On the basis of these findings, the patient is diagnosed with presbylarynx.
>
> **Discussion**
>
> It is important to rule out neoplasm as the cause of this man's symptoms. He tolerates microaspiration and is otherwise healthy; therefore, management is elective. His risk of pneumonia is minimal, and it probably would not be appropriate to alter his diet. The first line of therapy is speech and swallowing therapy, with particular emphasis on proper vocal technique to improve the quality of his voice. Surgical therapy is not indicated at this time.

beled food or liquid is administered, and scintigraphic imaging measures the radioactive count over the pharynx, lungs, and stomach. There is no precise correlation between the amount of material aspirated and the resultant morbidity for the patient, because the morbidity caused by aspiration varies from patient to patient. Clinical judgment is required to assess the risk to the patient in light of his or her underlying medical condition, particularly pulmonary reserve.

Endoscopic Examination of Swallowing

Endoscopic examination of the hypopharynx during swallowing provides excellent qualitative evaluation of swallowing. A nasopharyngoscope is passed to the level of the soft palate, and a variety of dyed liquids and foods of varying consistencies is administered. This examination permits the evaluation of glottic function; amount of secretion; degree of mucosal sensation; and the patient's ability to control oral material, to initiate a swallowing reflex, and to clear a bolus residue.

Patients who cannot control an oral bolus (usually because of neurological disease or oral surgery) often have bolus material that escapes into the pharynx before the swallow initiation. This "premature loss" is a significant aspiration risk and is identified easily by endoscopic examination or fluoroscopy. Failure of, or significant delay in, swallow initiation is also easily identifiable. In patients under 50 years of age, swallow initiation occurs so rapidly that the food material cannot be visualized endoscopically. In normal patients aged 50 years or over, swallow is initiated more slowly so the food can be visualized, but there is no aspiration. Neurologically impaired patients may have a much longer delay (several seconds) before swallow initiation, and the glottis is often incompetent, causing significant aspiration risk. Thickened liquids or pureed foods move more slowly than do thin liquids, allowing adequate time for reflex glottic closure and protecting the patient with a delayed response from aspiration. Feeding pureed and thickened liquids (i.e., a dysphagia diet) to patients who have had a cerebrovascular accident often can reduce the risk of aspiration.

After a cerebrovascular accident or other brain injury, a weak swallow cannot clear food or liquid residue from the hypopharynx. Food that is retained in the vallecula (between the epiglottis and the tongue base) spills passively into the hypopharynx and is aspirated during the next inspiration. A weak swallow also cannot move thick liquids or solids through the hypopharynx, so these patients must rely on liquids. Frequent liquid rinses and repeated swallows (two or three consecutive swallows before inspiration) can assist in clearing hypopharyngeal residue.

Patients with both delayed swallow and excessive residue almost always aspirate due to 1) food in the hypopharynx several seconds before the swallow begins, and 2) residue at the swallow's completion just before the next inspiration. Videostroboscopy uses a stroboscope with direct fiberoptic examination of the vocal cords, allowing accurate assessment of vocal cord motion and evaluation of normal vocal cord physiology.

Management

When potential aspiration is identified, **oral feeding is stopped (NPO)** and a nasogastric tube is placed (*see* Algorithm). If the cause of the aspiration (e.g., vocal cord paralysis) can be identified, correction (by medialization thyroplasty, which is described later in this chapter) may prove curative. Correction may be all that is necessary for a short-term disability (e.g., postoperative status, acute stroke, self-limiting disease process). If prolonged aspiration is anticipated (e.g., after subarachnoid hemorrhage, brainstem stroke, head injury, or skull base surgery), **gastrostomy** feedings may suffice for long-term management. Antibiotic therapy for recurrent aspiration pneumonia is ineffective in the long term, resulting in the colonization of resistant organisms. Early identification and control of aspiration with measures such as these decrease morbidity and cost.

Massive aspiration of gastric contents (e.g., vomiting during cardiac resuscitation) requires steroids, antibiotics, and often intubation with mechanical ventilation. Emergent therapeutic bronchoscopy to lavage aspirated vomitus or other irritating substances can reduce the incidence of acute pulmonary failure, saving lives.

Tracheostomy Tubes

As mentioned previously, aspiration is common even with a cuffed tracheostomy or endotracheal tube in place. It is important to remember that the tracheostomy tube assists in the management of aspiration but also may hinder it—the proverbial double-edged sword. Tracheostomy tube cuffs vary widely in their fit and their ability to serve as tracheal-occluding devices. Foam-filled cuffs often provide a better seal; however, motion, tracheal size, and inflammation all affect the degree of occlusion obtained.

Ventilator-dependent, tracheotomized patients may benefit from **continuous suction** of subglottic secretions from above the tracheostomy tube cuff. This can reduce the incidence of pneumonia in chronically ventilated patients. One way to do this is with a "speaking" tracheostomy tube, which has a small opening just above the cuff. Its intended use is to insufflate air above the cuff for speaking, but a small suction catheter can be attached for the continuous removal of accumulated secretions.

Decannulation

Removal of the tracheostomy tube (decannulation) can reduce aspiration in some patients and can reverse the impairments in glottic closure and swallowing that accompany open tracheostomy. Airway-protection reflexes, however, do not return to normal immediately after the tracheostomy tube is removed, so an orderly sequence of decannulation minimizes aspiration risk. The first step is cuff deflation. If increased coughing or choking occurs or if more material is suctioned from the trachea, the cuff is reinflated, and the tube removal is postponed. Patient tolerance of decannulation also can be evaluated by temporary tracheostomy tube removal, using a finger to plug the stoma. If no respiratory distress or increase in secretions occurs, decannulation is likely to be successful.

If the patient remains a candidate for decannulation, the cuffed tracheostomy tube is changed to a smaller cuffless tube, and oronasal breathing is begun with the smaller tracheostomy tube in place to prepare the patient for resuming normal breathing. The external end of the tracheostomy tube is intermittently closed, using a plug that cannot be aspirated through the tube. Alternately, a "speaking" valve (e.g., Passy–Muir valve) can be placed on the neck end of the tracheostomy tube, permitting inspiration. During expiration, air is forced upward between the vocal cords and out the normal oronasal route, allowing vocalization (Fig. 19.3). Both techniques are effective in preparing a patient for decannulation.

For either plugging or valving, there must be enough room between the tracheostomy tube and the tracheal wall to allow air to pass. This may require placing of a still smaller tracheostomy tube. A cuffed tube must be deflated; otherwise air would be forced out the tracheostomy tube, which is plugged. With the cuff deflated, air passes around the tube, up through the glottis and out the normal oronasal route. Most instances of a patient's failure to tolerate plugging or speaking-valve placement are caused by the tracheostomy tube being too large.

Once plugging is tolerated for 24 hours, the tracheostomy tube can be removed. An occlusive pressure dressing is placed over the neck opening, and

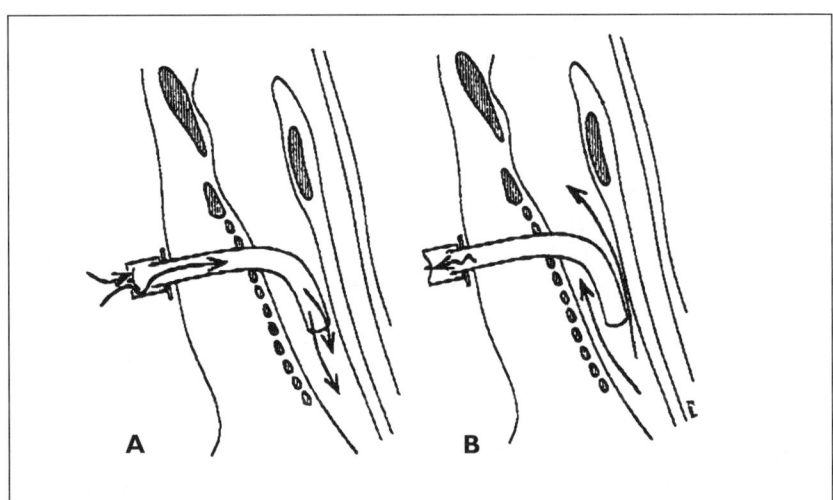

Figure 19.3 The function of an expiratory speaking valve, such as a Passy–Muir valve. **A**, Inspiratory flow. **B**, Note that the valve prevents expiratory air flow through the tracheostomy tube, forcing air around the tube and out through the larynx. (Republished with permission from Dettelbuch MA, Gross RD, Mahlmann J, Eibling DE. The effect of the Passy–Muir valve on aspiration in patients with tracheostomy. Head Neck. 1995; 17:277–302.)

the patient applies finger pressure over the stoma when speaking to decrease the amount of air escaping, enhancing rapid healing of the stoma. Stomal closure is usually complete within 48 to 72 hours.

Occasionally, the stoma does not close rapidly, especially in very thin patients or after prolonged cannulation. Because an open stoma hinders swallowing and speech, this tracheocutaneous fistula should be closed surgically if spontaneous closure does not occur within 1 to 2 weeks.

Swallowing Therapy

Swallowing therapy by a speech pathologist assists the patient in adopting specific therapeutic maneuvers to reduce aspiration risk (e.g., altering food consistency, using special head positions, using swallow and cough sequences during feeding). Patients with delayed swallow initiation use thickeners to slow bolus flow, permitting reflex glottic closure. Patients with poor clearance use a "supraglottic swallow"(i.e., coughing after swallowing) before inspiration, which clears saliva and food from the vocal cord surface and decreases aspiration.

Surgical Therapy

Some patients with chronic aspiration do not improve with conservative treatment. When tube feedings and frequent tracheal suctioning fail to protect the airway, surgery may be life saving. The goal of surgery for intractable aspiration can be either the reduction or elimination of aspiration.

Cricopharyngeal Myotomy

Cricopharyngeal achalasia can be identified on radiographic studies. Surgical division of the constricted cricopharyngeal sphincter can be effective, especially if a Zenker's diverticulum is also present (*see* Chapter 15). Nevertheless, cricopharyngeal opening failure can be caused by poor laryngeal elevation rather than true cricopharyngeal hypertonicity. Cricopharyngeal myotomy may not help such a patient, especially when pharyngeal muscle weakness (e.g., after a stroke) is also present.

Procedures That Enhance Glottic Closure

Swallowing difficulties and aspiration that accompanies vocal cord paralysis usually improve after surgical correction of glottic closure, because the problems resulted from too large an opening between the vocal cords (i.e., a "too open" glottis). The paralyzed vocal cord can be augmented by **Teflon injection**–a paste-like material that is injected directly into the cord, pushing its free edge medially and narrowing the glottic opening. Precise placement is difficult, however, and the injected cord is often stiff and poorly mobile, so alternative techniques are now used by many laryngologists.

Injecting an absorbable material such as **Gelfoam** into the vocal cord is a reversible procedure, ideal for short-term vocal cord paralysis. The material lasts approximately 6 weeks, after which the injection must be repeated unless another form of vocal cord medialization is selected.

Over the past decade, laryngeal framework surgery has become an alternative to Teflon injection. **Medialization thyroplasty** is the most common procedure. Under local anesthesia, a spacer (e.g., a carved silicone block) is placed through a window that has been cut in the thyroid cartilage just lateral to the paralyzed vocal cord (*see* Fig. 19.3), pressing against the paralyzed cord medially. The precise size and shape of the block is modified to obtain the best voice.

Another procedure (often performed simultaneously with medialization thyroplasty) is **arytenoid adduction**. A suture passed around the arytenoid cartilage pulls and anteriorly rotates the arytenoid medially, closing the posterior glottis. This also is performed under local anesthesia, and real-time "tuning" of the voice is done with incremental changes in vocal cord tension. Both procedures are theoretically reversible; however, in practice, they are used only in patients for whom return of function is thought to be unlikely. These procedures are highly effective in reducing aspiration in patients with paralyzed vocal cords.

Definitive Procedures

High-volume aspiration in patients with significant neurological impairment (e.g., brainstem stroke, progressive demyelinating diseases, bilateral vocal cord paralysis) may not respond to conservative measures or surgery. When more definitive therapy is required, a tracheostomy with the cuff inflated can be a temporizing first step. This can reduce aspiration enough to permit time for a definitive care plan to be developed.

Laryngotracheal Separation: The Definitive Procedure

Absolute long-term elimination of aspiration is best achieved by permanently separating the airway from the digestive tract. This can be performed by total laryngectomy or by sewing the vocal cords together, but laryngotracheal separation is the procedure that is performed most commonly. The trachea is divided, and the distal end is brought out to the neck (as is done after a laryngectomy). The larynx, although present, no longer communicates with the trachea, and the subglottic trachea ends in a blind pouch (Fig. 19.4). This technique is used mainly for chronically debilitated, aspirating patients. Home care becomes feasible because nursing care requirements are reduced, and pa-

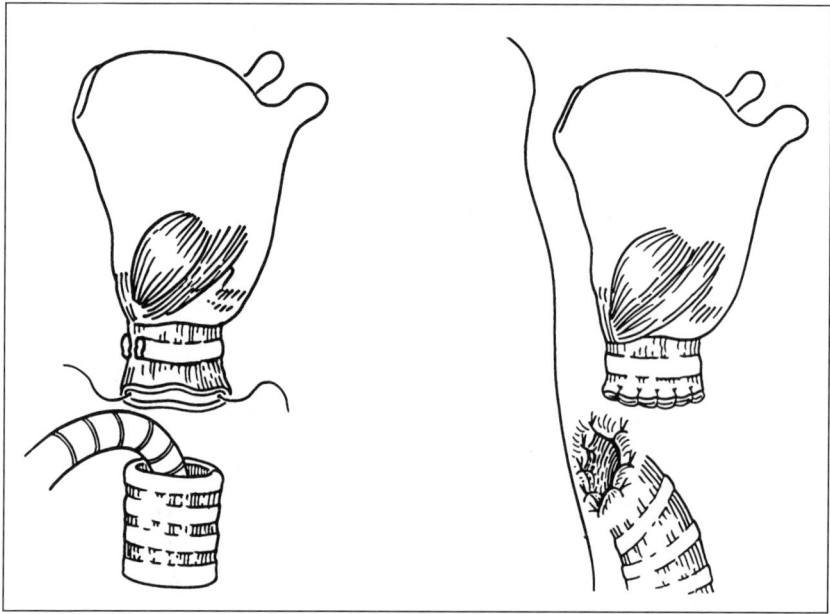

Figure 19.4 Laryngotracheal separation. Note that the trachea has been divided and that the proximal end has been closed. The result is a functional laryngectomy, with complete separation of the food and airway passages. This is an ideal means of eliminating morbid, intractable aspiration. (Republished with permission from Eibling DE, Johnson JT, Bacon G. *Understanding and Treating Aspiration SIPac*. Alexandria, VA: American Academy of Otolaryngology–Head and Neck Surgery; 1993.)

tients occasionally can resume an oral diet. Although normal speech is impossible after this procedure, most patients who undergo laryngotracheal separation have such severe neurological disease that loss of speech is not an issue. Aspiration pneumonia is the terminal event in many of these patients, so this procedure prolongs life, perhaps for years. The patient's prognosis and wishes, and the wishes of his or her family, must be considered thoroughly before undertaking such a major intervention. Case 19.4 illustrates the role of laryngotracheal separation when recovery would not occur otherwise.

Summary

A decision tree for selective management of patients with chronic aspiration includes initial nonsurgical therapy (e.g., alternative feeding routes, speech therapy evaluation and strategies) followed by the selection of adjunctive surgical procedures if required. If a tracheostomy tube is present, decannulation

> ### Case 19.4 Male Candidate for Laryngotracheal Separation After a Stroke
>
> A hypertensive man 45 years of age suffered a devastating brainstem stroke that left him unresponsive. Because he is unable to control his secretions, a tracheotomy is performed along with a gastrostomy for feedings. Two weeks after the stroke, he has demonstrated no evidence of recovery; however, transferring him to a long-term care facility was not feasible because of fevers, continuous radiographic evidence of pneumonia, and required frequent tracheal suctioning.
>
> Physical examination reveals an unresponsive man with copious tracheal secretions that have a foul odor. A team conference indicates that recovery is unlikely, and it was decided to proceed with a laryngotracheal separation. The procedure is performed uneventfully, and the patient rapidly demonstrates a decrease in tracheal secretions. His chest radiograph improves, and he no longer requires continuous antibiotics.
>
> **Discussion**
>
> Copious tracheal secretions nearly always represent aspirated saliva, and chronic pneumonia in these patients is usually due to continuous aspiration around the inflated tracheostomy tube cuff. One way to address this situation and reduce the episodes of pneumonia and the requirement for intensive nursing care is by performing a laryngotracheal separation. The procedure is well tolerated and, if acceptable to the patient and his family, can reduce care requirements dramatically.

is attempted. If decannulation is not possible, inserting an expiratory speaking valve may be efficacious. Gastrostomy feedings may diminish aspiration to nontroublesome levels. Patients with aspiration that is unresponsive to these measures can be considered for surgical therapy, such as laryngotracheal separation. These procedures may improve the quality of life in severely debilitated patients and may reduce health care costs.

SUGGESTED READINGS

Dettelbach MA, Gross RD, Mahlmann J, Eibling DE. The effect of the Passy–Muir valve on aspiration in patients with tracheostomy. *Head Neck.* 1995;17:297–302.

Eibling DE, Gross RD. Subglottic air pressure: a key component of swallowing efficiency. *Ann Otol Rhinol Laryngol.* 1996;105:253–8.

> *This paper reviews the evidence that restoration of subglottic air pressure is beneficial in preventing aspiration. The authors review previous basic science studies performed by Sasaki and coworkers and note improvements in swallowing as measured by transit time in patients with a Passy–Muir valve. This paper also provides a review of the effects of tracheostomy on swallowing.*

Eibling DE, Johnson JT, Bacon G. *Understanding and Treating Aspiration SIPac.* Alexandria, VA: American Academy of Otolaryngology–Head and Neck Surgery; 1993.

This publication is a self-instructional package published by the American Academy of Otolaryngology–Head and Neck Surgery Foundation for otolaryngologists and otolaryngology residents. The SiPac reviews normal swallowing function and addresses the cause, diagnosis, evaluation, and management of the aspirating patient. The surgical technique for laryngotracheal separation is also described.

Eibling DE, Snyderman CH, Eibling C. Laryngotracheal separation for intractable aspiration: a review of 34 patients. *Laryngoscope.* 1995;105:83–5.

This paper reviews the outcome in 34 patients who underwent laryngotracheal separation. Forty percent resumed an oral diet; however, the paper notes a complication rate of approximately 30% in patients undergoing the procedure.

Lindeman RC. Diverting the paralyzed larynx: a reversible procedure for intractable aspiration. *Laryngoscope.* 1975;85:157–80.

Lindeman RC, Yarington CT Jr, Sutton D. Clinical experience with the tracheoesophageal anastomosis for intractable aspiration. *Ann Otol Rhinol Laryngol.* 1976;85:609–12.

These two articles describe laryngotracheal diversion (1975) and then separation (1976), representing the landmark descriptions of this important surgical procedure. Subsequent to these procedures, many other authors have reported their experience with the use of laryngotracheal separation in the chronically aspirating patient.

Muz J, Mathog REH, Miller PR, et al. Detection and quantification of laryngotracheopulmonary aspiration with scintigraphy. *Laryngoscope.* 1987;94:1185–90.

This study illustrates with scintigraphy the value of plugging a tracheostomy tube in the reduction of aspiration.

Pou AM, Carrau RL, Eibling DE. Laryngeal framework surgery for the management of aspiration in high vagal lesions. *Am J Otolaryngol.* 1998;19:1–7.

This report notes a high degree of success in the management of aspiration in patients with paralyzed or weakened vocal cords by surgical medialization of the vocal cord with thyroplasty or arytenoid-adduction procedures.

Stackler RJ, Hamlet SL, Choi J, Fleming S. Scintigraphic quantification of aspiration reduction with the Passy–Muir valve. *Laryngoscope.* 1996; 106:231–4.

These two papers illustrate the effectiveness of an expiratory speaking valve in the management of the aspirating patient who has tracheostomy tube. Other authors have not been able to demonstrate similar findings, suggesting that the use of a valve does not benefit all patients.

SECTION V

THE NECK

20

Neck Masses

Karen M. Kost, MD

The correct diagnosis of neck masses can be established by using a systematic approach in which a careful history and physical examination lead to the selection of imaging and laboratory testing. This chapter guides the physician through the process of diagnosing neck masses in an orderly, stepwise fashion.

Anatomy

Neck masses are described by their location within a particular cervical triangle, along a specific lymphatic chain, or both. For example, congenital masses tend to occur in certain specific areas or triangles of the neck. Enlarged metastatic lymph nodes, by their location along a particular lymphatic chain, direct the physician to look for the cause in the part of the upper aerodigestive tract that those nodes drain.

The neck is divided into anatomical triangles (Fig. 20.1). The posterior triangle is bounded anteriorly by the sternocleidomastoid muscle, posteriorly by the anterior border of the trapezius muscle, and inferiorly by the middle third of the clavicle. Its contents include cutaneous branches of the cervical plexus, the spinal accessory nerve, two arterial branches of the thyrocervical trunk, and several lymph nodes.

The anterior triangle is defined posteriorly by the sternocleidomastoid muscle, anteriorly by the midline of the neck, and superiorly by the body of

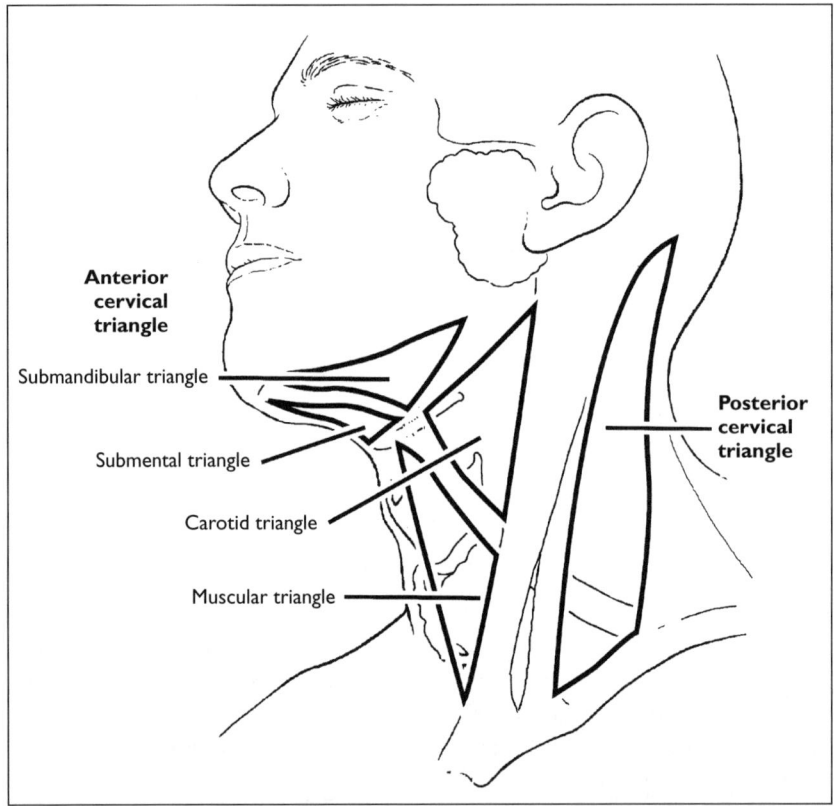

Figure 20.1 Major anatomic triangles of the neck.

the mandible. It is subdivided further into the submandibular, submental, carotid, and muscular triangles.

The submandibular triangle is bound by the anterior and posterior bellies of the digastric muscle and superiorly by the body of the mandible. It contains the submandibular gland and its accompanying lymph nodes and portions of the lingual and hypoglossal nerves.

The submental triangle is defined by the anterior bellies of the digastric muscles and inferiorly by the hyoid bone. It contains adipose tissue and lymph nodes.

The carotid triangle is bordered by the posterior belly of the digastric muscle, the superior belly of the omohyoid muscle, and posteriorly by the sternocleidomastoid muscle. Within this triangle are the common carotid artery (with its bifurcation into the internal and external branches), the internal jugular vein (with its associated lymph nodes), and cranial nerves IX, X,

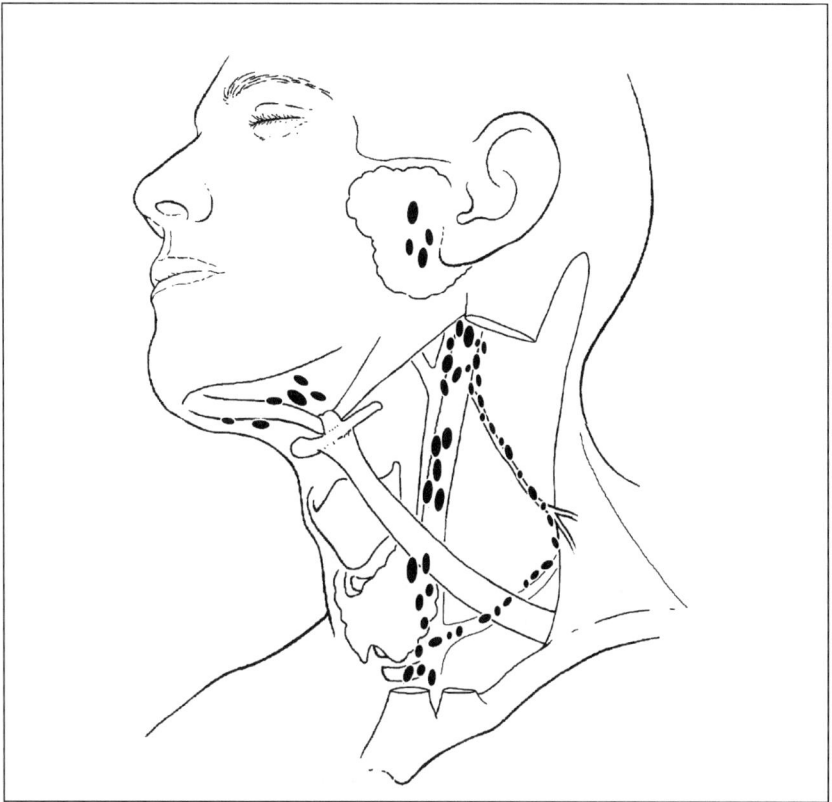

Figure 20.2 Major collections of lymph nodes in the neck.

XI, and XII (the glossopharyngeal, vagus, spinal accessory, and hypoglossal nerves, respectively).

The muscular triangle is bound by the superior belly of the omohyoid muscle, the sternocleidomastoid muscle, and the midline of the neck (*see* Fig. 20.1) (1).

The neck contains between 150 and 300 lymph nodes grouped according to their location (Figs. 20.2–20.4). The primary lymphatic drainage to the various nodal groups is summarized in Table 20.1.

Submental and Submandibular Groups (Level I)

The submental nodes drain the lower lip, tip of the tongue, and the anterior floor of the mouth. These nodes drain bilaterally into the submandibular nodes, except for one small lymphatic pedicle that leads to the middle jugular

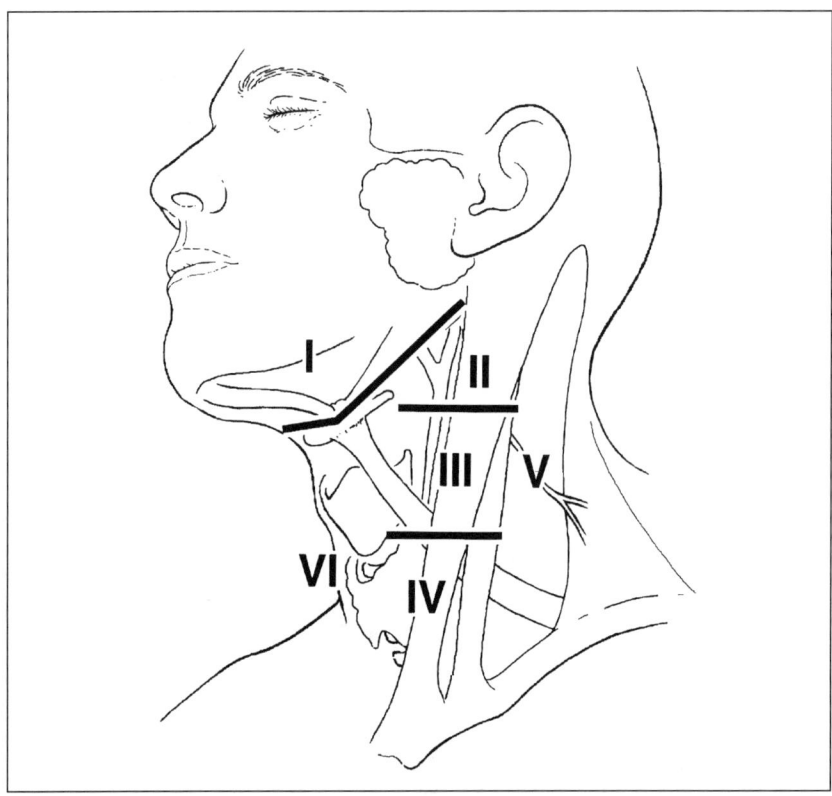

Figure 20.3 Levels of the neck. Specific anatomic areas drain to lymph nodes in each of these numbered areas. I = submental and submandibular areas; II = upper jugular; III = middle jugular; IV = lower jugular; V = posterior triangle; VI = anterior compartment.

nodes. The submandibular nodes drain the eyelids and conjunctiva, the skin and mucosa of the nose, the mucosa of the cheek, the upper lip and commissure, the anterior two thirds of the tongue, and the floor of the mouth. The submandibular nodes then drain into the upper jugular nodes, which are composed of three groups: upper (level II), middle (level III) and lower (level IV). The internal jugular nodes drain almost all of the head and neck.

Upper Jugular Nodes (Level II)

These are variably called the superior deep cervical, subdigastric, or jugulodigastric nodes. They drain the soft palate, palatine tonsils, lateral pharyngeal wall, posterior oral tongue, base of the tongue, pyriform sinuses, and supraglottic larynx. The upper jugular nodes receive lymph from the retropharyngeal, spinal accessory, parotid, and submandibular nodes. In general, the

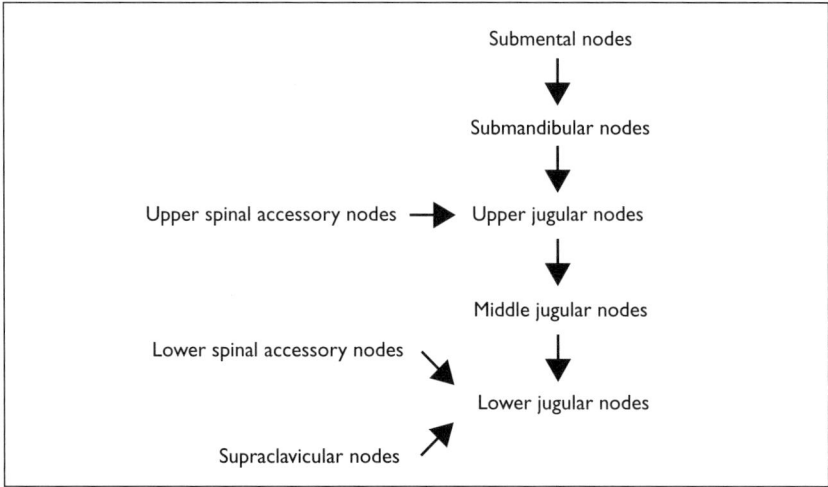

Figure 20.4 Relative lymphatic drainage routes to the various areas of lymph nodes in the neck.

upper jugular nodes receive efferent lymphatics from all head and neck nodes except the middle and lower jugular groups.

Middle Jugular Nodes (Level III)

These are called the middle deep cervical nodes; the jugulo-omohyoid node is included in this group, which drains the supraglottic larynx, lower pyriform sinus, the posterior cricoid area, and the upper jugular nodes.

Lower Jugular Nodes (Level IV)

These are the inferior deep cervical nodes. They drain the cervical esophagus, thyroid gland, and trachea and are connected to the supraclavicular nodes, which receive lymph from infraclavicular sites.

Posterior Triangle Nodes (Level V)

These cluster along the spinal accessory nerve and the transverse cervical artery and include the supraclavicular nodes (*see* Fig. 20.1). The spinal accessory nodes drain the nasopharynx and the paranasal sinuses via the retropharyngeal and parapharyngeal nodes. The upper spinal accessory nodes drain into the upper jugular nodes, whereas the lower spinal accessory nodes drain into the supraclavicular nodes.

Table 20.1 Primary Lymphatic Drainage to Nodal Groups of the Head and Neck*

Level	Lymph Node Location	Anatomical Areas Drained
1	Submental	Lower lip
		Tip of tongue
		Anterior floor of mouth
	Submandibular	Eyelids
		Conjunctiva
		Skin and mucosa of nose
		Mucosa of cheek
		Upper lip and commissure
		Anterior two thirds of tongue
		Floor of mouth
2	Upper jugular	Soft palate
		Palatine tonsils
		Lateral pharyngeal wall
		Posterior oral tongue
		Base of tongue
		Pyriform sinus
		Supraglottic larynx
3	Middle jugular	Supraglottic larynx
		Lower pyriform sinus
		Posterior cricoid
4	Lower jugular	Cervical esophagus
		Thyroid gland
		Trachea
5	Spinal accessory	Nasopharynx
		Paranasal sinuses
6	Anterior compartment	Trachea
		Thyroid gland
		Recurrent laryngeal nerve
		Cervical esophagus

* Levels I–VI correlate with those shown in Figure 20.3.

Anterior Compartment Nodes (Level VI)

These lymph nodes are located between the common carotid artery laterally, the hyoid bone superiorly, and the suprasternal notch inferiorly. These nodes lie around the trachea, thyroid gland, and the recurrent laryngeal nerves, draining these structures in addition to the cervical esophagus.

Table 20.2 Classification of Neck Masses*

Age	Diagnostic Groups (in order of decreasing frequency)
0–15 years	Inflammatory
	Congenital or developmental
	Neoplastic, malignant
	Neoplastic, benign
16–40 years	Inflammatory
	Congenital or developmental
	Neoplastic, benign
	Neoplastic, malignant
>40 years	Neoplastic, malignant
	Neoplastic, benign
	Inflammatory
	Congenital or developmental

* Patient age provides a clue as to the cause of the neck mass.

Important Considerations: Age and Location

Neck masses can be classified as congenital, inflammatory, and neoplastic, with the incidence of each varying with age (Table 20.2). In the pediatric age group (0–15 years), a neck mass is probably inflammatory, with congenital causes ranking a close second and malignant neoplasia third. Benign tumors are less common than are malignant tumors in children of this age group. In the young adult group (16–40 years), inflammatory causes also predominate, followed by congenital causes and neoplasia, with benign tumors predominating over malignant tumors. In adults over 40 years of age, new-onset neck masses are considered malignant until proven otherwise, because most neck masses are, in fact, malignant in this age group (3) (see Table 20.2).

Congenital neck masses tend to occur in predictable locations (Table 20.3 and Fig. 20.5). Dermoid cysts and thyroglossal duct cysts occur in the midline, whereas branchial cleft cysts are found along the anterior border of the sternocleidomastoid muscle. The location of the neck mass can suggest a focused search for the primary tumor (see Table 20.1). Inflammatory lesions follow similarly predictable patterns of lymphatic drainage (3).

History and Physical Examination

Family history can uncover genetically transmitted paragangliomas and neurofibromatosis. Past medical history can suggest recurrence of previous malig-

Table 20.3 Location of Congenital Neck Mass

Location	Type and/or Location of Mass
Lateral neck	Brachial cyst sinus
	Laryngocele
Midline	Thyroglossal duct cyst
	Thymic cyst
	Dermoid cyst
	Teratoma of the neck
Entire neck	Hemangioma
	Lymphangioma

nant tumor. One should look for a history of chronic granulomatous disease (e.g., sarcoidosis, systemic lupus erythematosus). Previous exposure to ionizing radiation in the head and neck area increases the likelihood of a thyroid mass being a carcinoma. Drugs (e.g., phenytoin, allopuranol, hydralazine) have been implicated in cervical lymph node enlargement. Nasopharyngeal carcinoma (Fig. 20.6) occurs frequently in Chinese and Inuit populations.

Patient age and event sequence help categorize the lesion as inflammatory, congenital, or neoplastic. A painful neck mass that enlarges over only a few days in a child suggests infection or an infected, previously unrecognized congenital lesion. Recent exposure to animals (cats in particular) may suggest cat-scratch disease. Other important details include a history of recent trauma, dental work, or travel abroad. A mildly tender neck mass that enlarges slowly over several weeks suggests atypical mycobacteria, particularly if the neck mass is in the submandibular area. A history of tuberculosis contact in a patient with a posterior cervical or supraclavicular neck mass raises the possibility of scrofula. A firm, slowly enlarging, painless neck mass in a young adult suggests the possibility of a lymphoma, particularly with associated fever, chills or weight loss.

A careful social and occupational history becomes increasingly important with age. The association between tobacco use (e.g., smoking cigarettes, cigars, or pipes; chewing tobacco) and squamous cell carcinoma of the upper aerodigestive tract is well known. Furthermore, alcohol interacts synergistically with tobacco to increase the risk of squamous cell carcinoma of the head and neck. Occupational exposure to asbestos, certain petroleum products, nickel, and wood dust are associated with an increased risk of head and neck carcinoma (4).

A complete head and neck examination is a necessity and includes meticulous inspection of the nasopharynx and larynx. In a child, large red tonsils

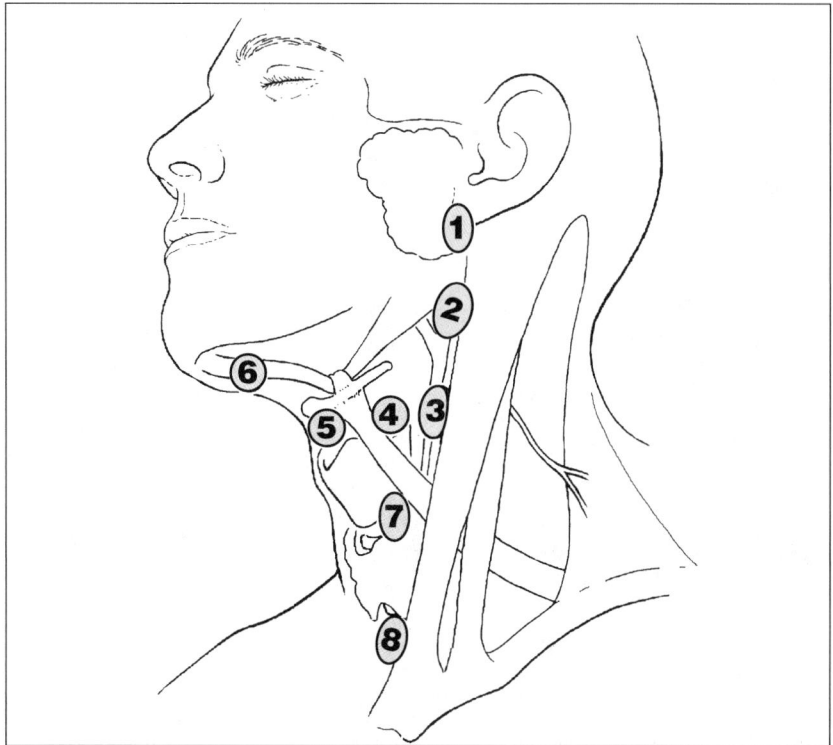

Figure 20.5 The location of a congenital neck mass often can be a clue to its origin. 1 = first branchial cleft cyst; 2 = second branchial cleft cyst; 3 = third branchial cleft cyst; 4 = laryngocele; 5 = thyroglossal duct cyst; 6 = dermoid cyst; 7 = teratoma; 8 = thymic cyst.

with exudate can indicate the presence of enlarged and tender jugulodigastric nodes. In a young adult, asymptomatic enlargement of a tonsil with an ipsilateral lymph node suggests lymphoma. In the older adult, the presence of an ulcerating or fungating lesion in the upper aerodigestive tract almost always determines a diagnosis of metastatic carcinoma.

The location, size, color, and consistency of any neck mass should be noted. Soft, compressible, poorly defined masses in newborns or young children suggest a congenital cause, such as a lymphangioma or hemangioma. A well-defined, fluctuant mass along the anterior border of the sternocleidomastoid muscle in a child or young adult likely represents a branchial cleft cyst. Firm, solid, nontender masses increase the probability of neoplasm. A pulsatile mass with an audible bruit suggests a vascular cause.

An appreciation of "normal" neck masses is also important. The presence of multiple small, nontender, mobile cervical lymph nodes in children under 10 years of age is considered normal. In older adults, the submandibular

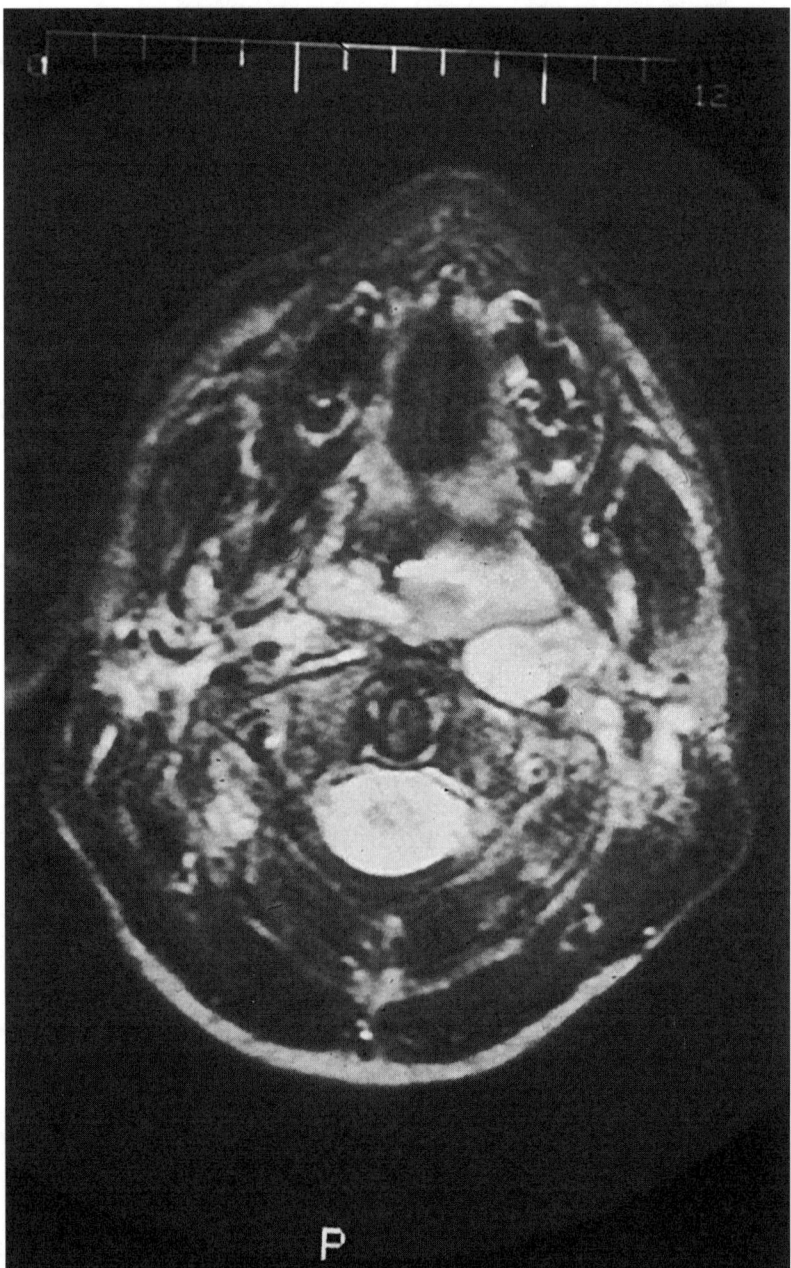

Figure 20.6 Magnetic resonance imaging scan showing nasopharyngeal carcinoma with retropharyngeal node involvement. (Republished with permission from McGirt WF, Johnson PE. *Evaluation and Treatment of the Patient with a Neck Mass*. Alexandria, VA: American Academy of Otolaryngology–Head and Neck Surgery; 1998.)

glands may be ptotic and thus easily palpable. The key to appreciating these findings as normal is the fact that the glands are symmetrical, soft, mobile, and nontender. In an individual with a long, thin neck, the transverse processes of the first cervical vertebra may be felt just above the jugulodigastric area; these are immobile and bone hard.

Differential Diagnosis

The differential diagnosis of neck masses is summarized in Table 20.4. A comprehensive history and physical examination, along with the age of the patient

Table 20.4 Differential Diagnosis of Neck Masses

Congenital
  Midline
    Thyroglossal duct cyst
    Dermoid cyst
    Teratoma
  Lateral
    Branchial cleft cyst, sinus, fistula
    Laryngocele
    Thymic cyst
    Congenital torticollis
  Variable Location
    Lymphangioma or cystic hygroma
    Hemangioma

Inflammatory
  Viral lymphadenopathy
  Bacterial lymphadenopathy
  Granulomatous lymphadenopathy
  Miscellaneous causes of lymphadenopathy
  Sialadenitis
  Sialolithiasis

Neoplastic
  Benign
    Neurogenic neck mass
    Paraganglioma
    Lipoma
    Salivary gland neoplasm
    Thyroid gland neoplasm
  Malignant
    Salivary gland neoplasm
    Thyroid gland neoplasm
    Rhabdomyosarcoma

Table 20.5 Major Diagnostic Categories of Common Neck Masses

Diagnostic Category	Type and/or Location of Mass
Congenital or developmental	Thyroglossal duct cyst
	Dermoid cyst
	Teratoma
	Branchial cleft cyst
	Laryngocele
	Thymic cyst
	Congenital torticollis
	Lymphangioma
	Cystic hygromas
	Hemangiomas
Inflammatory	Viral
	Bacterial
	Granulomatous
	Sialadenitis
	Sialolithiasis
Neoplastic	
Benign	Neurogenic
	Paragangliomas
	Lipomas
	Salivary gland
	Thyroid
	Metastases
Malignant	Lymphoma
	Salivary gland
	Thyroid
	Rhabdomyosarcoma

and the location of the mass, often reduce the differential diagnosis to a list of two or three possibilities (Table 20.5).

Diagnosis and Management

Congenital Neck Masses

Congenital masses are the most frequently encountered, noninflammatory neck masses in children and result from an aberration in normal embryonic development. Although most present between birth and young adulthood, they may be seen in all age groups (*see* Table 20.2 and Fig. 20.5).

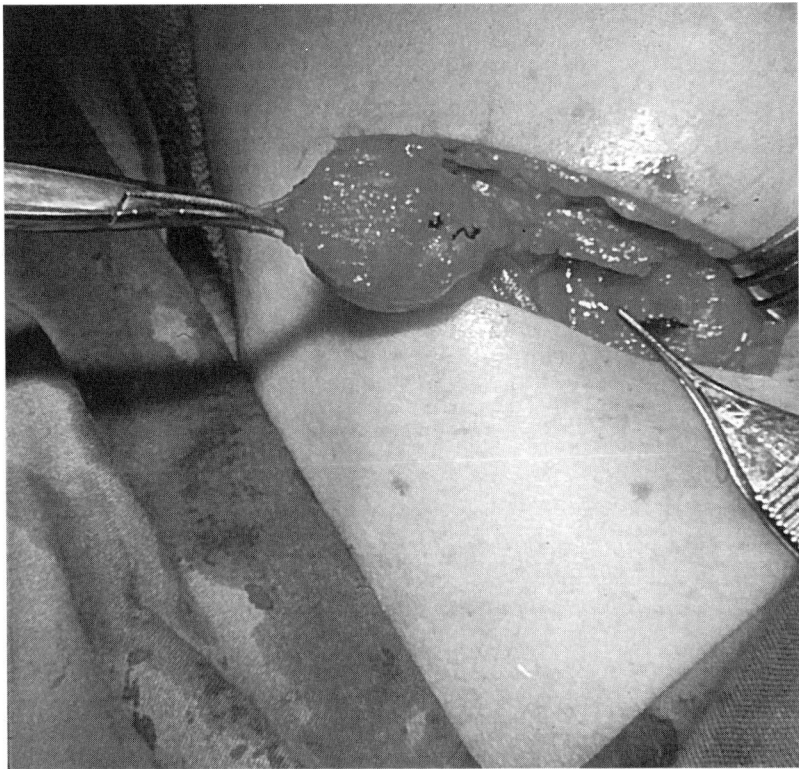

Figure 20.7 A distinct tract leading upward usually can be found during the removal of a thyroglossal duct cyst. (Courtesy of Dr. David E. Eibling.)

Midline Congenital Neck Masses

Thyroglossal Duct Cysts

Thyroglossal duct cysts are caused by incomplete involution of the thyroglossal duct after the thyroid gland descends from its origin at the foramen cecum to its final position in the neck. Although these cysts may occur anywhere along this path, most (85%) are located in the midline at or below the hyoid bone (Fig. 20.7).

Thyroglossal duct cysts account for approximately 70% of congenital neck masses and are the most common developmental abnormality in the neck. Although most appear in children between 2 and 10 years of age, they can occur at any age. Approximately two thirds appear as asymptomatic neck masses, with the remainder presenting as a tender, fluctuant mass after upper respiratory infection. Typically, these cysts are smooth and round and rise in the neck with swallowing or tongue protrusion. Fine-needle–aspiration biopsy

(FNAB) and ultrasonography reveal the cystic nature of the lesion; the latter test is also helpful in determining the presence of normal thyroid tissue in the cyst. Computed tomography (CT) is largely unnecessary, and the use of radionuclide scans should be reserved for those cases in which the presence of normal thyroid tissue is uncertain. Acute infections should be treated with antibiotics that are effective against both aerobic and anaerobic organisms; incision and drainage should be avoided if possible. Definitive treatment consists of surgical excision of the cyst, a portion of the hyoid bone, and any duct remnants up to the foramen cecum (5–10).

Dermoid Cysts

Dermoid cysts are composed of ectoderm and mesoderm and contain epidermal appendages such as hair follicles and sebaceous glands. Appearing as smooth, round, nontender masses that are usually situated at or above the hyoid bone, these cysts are often present at birth or shortly thereafter but may arise later in childhood or adolescence. Occasionally, they are found lower in the neck. Ultrasound demonstrates their cystic nature; thus, they may be confused clinically with thyroglossal duct cysts. Dermoid cysts do not elevate with tongue protrusion and, on FNAB, are found to contain sebaceous material (compared with the serous or mucoid material found in thyroglossal cysts). Treatment consists of complete excision.

Teratomas

Teratomas are true neoplasms that contain elements of ectoderm, mesoderm, and endoderm in various degrees of differentiation, ranging from teratoid cysts to true teratomas and epignathi that contain teeth, hair, or cartilaginous or osseous elements. They usually present at birth or within the first year of life as large midline or paramedian lesions with upper airway obstruction. Teratomas are firm, mobile, and well circumscribed, whereas lymphangiomas are poorly defined. Ultrasonography of teratomas shows mixed echogenicity compared with the multilocular pattern seen with cystic hygromas. Cartilaginous or osseous elements may be seen on plain radiographs or CT scan. In the presence of upper respiratory obstruction, endotracheal intubation (or tracheostomy) is followed by complete surgical excision.

Lateral Congenital Neck Masses

Branchial Cleft Cysts, Sinuses, and Fistulae

The branchial system appears during the fourth week of development as a series of four paired arches that are separated from each other externally by clefts of ectodermal origin and internally by pouches of endodermal origin. A thin epithelial plate separates each cleft and pouch. Each arch is supplied by an artery and nerve and consists of a condensation of mesoderm from which cartilage, muscle, and bone will form. Branchial cleft cysts, sinuses, and fistulae may develop from aberrations in the normal development of the first four arches. Cysts are the most common abnormality and represent trapped remnants of the clefts or pouches. Branchial sinuses represent vestigial clefts or pouches and, as such, may open externally through the skin or internally into the pharynx. By definition, branchial fistulae have both an internal and external opening and are presumed to be the result of persistent vestigial pouches and clefts with a loss of the interposed branchial plate. Generally, branchial cleft sinuses with openings to the skin are associated with the first and second arches, whereas branchial pouch sinuses with connections to the pharynx are associated with the third and fourth arches.

First branchial abnormalities may occur as sinuses, fistulae, or cysts and have two types. Type one abnormalities are ectodermal in origin and represent duplications of the membranous external auditory canal. They usually are located in the pre-auricular area parallel to the external canal, with the sinus opening being medial, inferior, or posterior to the pinna. Type two abnormalities are also duplications of the external auditory canal, with openings usually situated below the angle of the mandible. The sinus or fistula tract courses through the parotid gland with a variable relationship to the facial nerve and terminates at or near the bony cartilaginous junction of the external auditory canal. First branchial abnormalities are uncommon and usually present in early childhood with a mucoid discharge at the opening(s) situated below the angle of the mandible and/or within the external auditory canal. Treatment is complete surgical excision of the entire tract, cyst, or both. The location of first branchial abnormalities necessitates the identification and meticulous dissection of the facial nerve.

Second branchial abnormalities are the most common and account for approximately 90% of aberrations seen. Second branchial cleft cysts are encountered much more frequently than are sinuses or fistulae. These cysts present in the second or third decade of life (or even later) as slowly enlarging, painless, well-circumscribed, round, mobile masses that are located at the anterior border of the sternocleidomastoid muscle, just below the angle of the mandible (Fig. 20.8). Secondary infection is common, occurring in approximately 25% of cases. In contrast, second branchial sinuses or fistulae usually present at or shortly after birth. Their external openings are located along the anterior border of the sternocleidomastoid muscle and are associated with a persistent mucoid discharge. If a complete fistula is present, the tract courses between the carotid vessels and over the hypoglossal and glossopharyngeal nerves to enter the pharynx at the level of the tonsillar fossa.

Third branchial abnormalities, although very rare, have a similar clinical presentation to that of second branchial anomalies. The course of the associ-

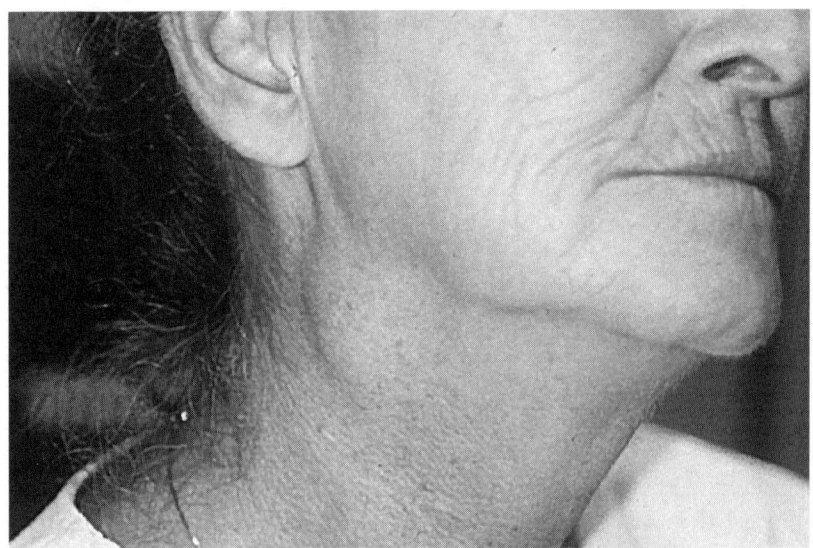

Figure 20.8 Second branchial cleft cyst presenting in an older adult. (Republished with permission from McGirt WF, Johnson PE. *Evaluation and Treatment of the Patient with a Neck Mass*. Alexandria, VA: American Academy of Otolaryngology–Head and Neck Surgery; 1998.)

ated tracts or fistulae differ in that they pass posterior to the carotid vessels and between the glossopharyngeal and hypoglossal nerves (i.e., above the former and below the latter), to enter the pharynx at the level of the pyriform sinus.

In most cases, the history and physical examination suggest the diagnosis of a branchial abnormality, particularly in the presence of a draining sinus or fistula. FNAB immediately identifies the lesion's cystic nature; ultrasound confirms it. CT is not necessary except when one suspects a sinus or fistula. A fistulogram is helpful when an external opening is present. Direct pharyngoscopy and laryngoscopy and a barium swallow may identify an internal opening. If these abnormalities become infected, treatment consists of antibiotic therapy with incision and drainage if necessary. Surgical therapy is best undertaken when acute inflammation has subsided.

Laryngoceles

The saccule is a blind pouch containing mucous glands that lubricate the vocal folds. It is vertically oriented on the inner surface of the thyroid cartilage and opens at the level of the laryngeal ventricles. Distension of this structure with air results in the formation of a laryngocele, which can be categorized as internal, external, or combined. Internal laryngoceles are confined to the interior of the larynx and extend posterosuperiorly into the false cord and the aryepiglottic fold. They can cause hoarseness and varying degrees of respiratory distress, or they may be asymptomatic. External laryngoceles appear laterally in the neck through the thyrohyoid membrane and are soft and compressible. Combined laryngoceles have both internal and external components and cause hoarseness, cough, dyspnea, and dysphagia. Infected laryngoceles (laryngopyoceles) may be firm, tender, and associated with systemic signs of inflammation (11). Treatment of infection precedes surgical excision.

Thymic Cysts
The bilateral thymic primordia arise from the third branchial pouch, descending caudally and medially from the pharynx and fusing before reaching the mediastinum. Connections with the pharynx remain as thymopharyngeal ducts. Rarely, cystic changes occur in ductal remnants, producing thymic cysts. These cysts occur in children and present as slowly enlarging, painless masses, usually in a left paramedian position. The presence of thymic tissue within the cyst wall distinguishes thymic cysts from branchial cleft cysts of third- or fourth-pouch origin, which share similarities in terms of location and histology. Treatment consists of surgical removal (5).

Congenital Torticollis
Congenital torticollis (fibromatosis colli) has uncertain etiology and affects infants at 2 to 4 weeks of age. Shortly after birth, the infant develops a hard fusiform mass, usually in the lower third of the sternocleidomastoid muscle. The infant may present with torticollis, a neck mass, or both. The mass initially tends to increase in size, followed by gradual resolution between 5 and 8 months of age. A fibrotic, noncontractile portion of the sternocleidomastoid muscle may remain, producing various degrees of contracture; the infant's head is pulled ipsilaterally and rotated to the opposite side. If left untreated, this contracture results in asymmetric growth of the skull and face. The diagnosis is based on history, physical examination, and selected investigations. FNAB is often diagnostic, revealing benign muscle fragments and fibroblasts. CT is useful in delineating the mass with respect to surrounding structures. Conservative therapy, consisting of stretching the sternocleidomastoid muscle, is effective within the first year of life. Surgical therapy to release of the contracture is reserved for children over 1 year of age who have failed physiotherapy (12).

Congenital Neck Masses of Variable Location
Lymphangiomas and Cystic Hygromas
Lymphangiomas, also known as cystic hygromas, represent developmental malformations of the jugular lymphatic sac and can be separated into three groups based on histologic characteristics: lymphangioma simplex, cavernous

lymphangioma, and cystic hygroma. This classification is somewhat academic because elements of all three types frequently coexist in the same lesion. With the possible exception of the cavernous lymphangioma, which may be more aggressive locally, the clinical behavior of all three types is similar. Local extension occurs by surrounding the normal structures in the neck, including blood vessels, nerves, and muscles.

Lymphangiomas are frequently present at birth, with 80% to 90% of them clinically apparent by 2 years of age; less than 10% occur in adults. Most lymphangiomas are found in the head and neck area, with the neck being the favored site. Characteristically, they are soft, painless, poorly defined masses in the anterior and/or posterior cervical triangles. Being cystic, multilocular lesions, they readily transilluminate and range in size from a few centimeters to large lesions that encroach on adjacent aerodigestive structures, with varying degrees of dysphagia and respiratory obstruction. Hemorrhage or infection within the lesion may result in rapid enlargement. The clinical course of these lesions is that of gradual enlargement. Spontaneous regression is rare.

History and physical examination establish the diagnosis. CT scanning or magnetic resonance imaging (MRI) demonstrates the cystic, multilocular nature of the lesion and its relationship to adjacent structures. Pharyngoscopy and laryngoscopy are useful in calibrating the airway.

Treatment consists of surgical excision, although the timing is somewhat controversial. In the absence of aerodigestive tract encroachment, excision may be delayed until 3 or 4 years of age. Complete removal can be extremely difficult and may require staged resections, particularly for suprahyoid lesions that extend into the floor of the mouth and tongue. In these cases, tracheostomy and the placement of a gastrostomy feeding tube may be necessary. Recurrences are expected in 5% to 10% of cases. Alternative therapies (e.g., irradiation, electrocautery, injection of sclerosing agents) have not been shown to be effective in treating lymphangiomas and may even increase the morbidity associated with these lesions.

Hemangiomas

Hemangiomas result from faulty vascular development and can be classified histologically as capillary, cavernous, mixed, juvenile (proliferative), or infiltrative. Most hemangiomas are noted shortly after birth, and 95% of them are evident by 6 months of age. Skin hemangiomas are clinically obvious but should prompt a search for hemangiomas elsewhere (e.g., in the subglottic region). **Subcutaneous hemangiomas** tend to be masses that are poorly defined, soft, cystic, and compressible. The diagnosis may be suggested by a bluish discoloration of the skin, the presence of a bruit, and an increase in size with crying or straining. Although they may be found anywhere in the head and neck, hemangiomas are the most common **congenital parotid masses.**

The diagnosis is based on the history and physical examination. Enhancement on contrast-aided CT is characteristic, highlighting the vascular nature of these lesions and defining their extent. Angiography (or magnetic resonance angiography [MRA] when available) demonstrates feeding vessels and lesion extent.

Treatment is best formulated by taking into account the natural history. In 90% of cases, there is a period of rapid growth during the first year, with complete spontaneous resolution over the next 4 to 5 years. When the initial period of rapid growth restricts aerodigestive passages or causes unacceptable facial deformity, systemic corticosteroid therapy is the treatment of choice. Systemic steroids have been shown to be helpful in arresting the growth of these lesions and frequently to promote or induce resolution. However, hemangiomas that appear in later life are less likely to involute spontaneously and often require surgical treatment. Resection (perhaps preceded by embolization) is indicated for hemangiomas that fail to involute or respond to systemic steroid therapy. Radiation therapy and sclerosing agents are of no use in the treatment of hemangiomas of the head and neck.

Inflammatory Neck Masses

Approximately 55% of normal children in all age groups have palpable lymph nodes that are not associated with infection or systemic illness (13). These vary in size from a few millimeters to 1 cm and are soft, mobile, and nontender. In contrast, palpable lymph nodes usually are not found in either young adults or adults over 40 years of age.

Most neck masses that are encountered in children and young adults are inflammatory in nature (*see* Table 20.5), with the source often found in the upper aerodigestive tract. Cervical lymphadenopathy may be viral, bacterial, or granulomatous. Causes include sialadenitis (parotid or submandibular) and odontogenic sepsis.

Viral Lymphadenopathy

Cervical lymphadenopathy from a viral upper inspiratory tract infection is a frequent cause of node enlargement. The illness is usually obvious, and the adenopathy tends to be diffuse and bilateral, involving the anterior and posterior triangles. Viruses that are responsible include the Epstein–Barr virus, cytomegalovirus, and HIV. Infectious mononucleosis (caused by the Epstein–Barr virus) occurs often in adolescents and young adults and is frequently associated with large confluent lymph nodes (>3 cm) in both the anterior and posterior triangles of the neck; cytomegalovirus produces a similar clinical picture. With the exception of HIV, these viral diseases are largely self-limiting. Treatment is supportive, and the nodes regress spontaneously. Investigations include screening hemogram and serology. Radiographic investigations are appropriate only if symptoms persist more than 3 weeks.

Cervical lymphadenopathy associated with HIV occurs in up to 70% of infected patients and is usually part of a diffuse, otherwise asymptomatic lymphadenopathy. Nodes are soft and symmetrically distributed and range from 1 to 5 cm in size. Both children and adults with this diagnosis are at risk for bacterial, fungal, and granulomatous (especially tuberculosis) infections as well as for malignant tumors (lymphomas).

Bacterial Lymphadenopathy

Bacterial lymphadenopathy appears as a unilateral tender node and usually is related to otitis media, pharyngitis, tonsillitis, or dental infection. Acute tonsillitis, for example, causes a tender, enlarged jugulodigastric or upper jugular node. Common pathogens include beta-hemolytic streptococci, *Staphylococcus aureus*, and gram-negative organisms. Although culture and sensitivity testing is useful, initial treatment is empirical and consists of a 10- to 14-day course of antibiotics known to be effective against the presumptive pathogens. Occasionally, the affected nodes become fluctuant and suppurate, which can be confirmed by ultrasound imaging and FNAB. Aspiration may be both diagnostic and therapeutic; however, incisional drainage may be necessary.

Odontogenic infections deserve special mention because of their sometimes-fulminant clinical course. Dental infections that affect the incisors, premolars, and first molars may involve not only the sublingual space but also the submental nodes and space. Infections of the second and third molars spread to the submandibular nodes and space. There is frequently a history of toothache, fever, and a progressive, poorly defined, tender swelling in the lateral neck. Clinically, the patient looks ill and there is an obvious, but poorly demarcated, tender neck mass involving the submandibular and submental areas. The floor of the mouth is swollen, sometimes superiorly displacing the tongue and posteriorly threatening the airway. Early assessment of the airway is essential, and patency is secured with either fiberoptic endotracheal intubation or a tracheostomy when necessary. If the airway is not in danger, the patient may be hospitalized and given high-dose intravenous antimicrobial agents that are known to be effective against both aerobic and anaerobic organisms (e.g., clindamycin), because these infections are almost always polymicrobial. Failure to improve within 24 hours or a progression of signs and symptoms is an indication to perform open surgical drainage of the affected spaces and to remove the offending tooth.

Granulomatous Lymphadenopathy

Nontuberculous or **atypical mycobacteria (ATM)** (*Mycobacterium avium-intracellulare* and *M. scrofulaceum* in particular) may cause unilateral cervical lymphadenopathy, usually affecting the submandibular or pre-auricular nodes. Although it is most common in children between 1 and 6 years of age, adults are affected occasionally; these infections are more prevalent in immunocompromised individuals. The route of transmission is from soil to mouth or eye. The clinical presentation is that of a firm, unilateral neck mass that over several weeks may become fluctuant with overlying skin changes and eventual skin breakdown. Culture and sensitivity testing of a FNAB specimen usually confirms the diagnosis. Acid-fast staining can provide a presumptive diagnosis during the 2 to 4 weeks necessary for identification by culture. Half of patients with these infections are negative on purified protein derivative (PPD) skin testing, and the other half are weakly positive (10–12 mm). Therapy with antimicrobial or antituberculous medications is unsuccessful. Definitive treatment consists of surgically excising the affected node(s) (14).

The most common form of head and neck involvement by **M. tuberculosis** is **cervical lymphadenopathy**. Also referred to as scrofula, this infection is less frequent than atypical mycobacterial infection, yet the incidence has been rising in North America because of the increased number of patients with AIDS and the increased number of immigrants from countries where classical tuberculosis is widespread (Case 20.1). In contrast to ATM infection, adults are affected more frequently than are children. Involved nodes tend to be multiple, matted, bilateral, firm, and nontender and are typically found in the posterior triangles or supraclavicular areas. In suspected cases, PPD testing is usually positive (>10 mm) and a chest radiograph should be requested. Excisional biopsy may be necessary for diagnosis, but incisional biopsy is not recommended because it can lead to a chronically draining fistula. Submitted tissue may reveal caseating granulomas and acid-fast bacilli on Ziehl–Neelsen staining. Obtaining positive cultures may take up to 6 weeks. Distinguishing scrofula caused by *M. tuberculosis* from ATM infection is important because ATM treatment is primarily surgical, whereas prolonged antituberculous therapy is necessary for the successful treatment of tuberculosis.

Cat-scratch disease is caused by the gram-negative bacillus *Bartonella (Rochalimaea) henselae* and occurs more frequently in children than adults. Arising in over half of patients after a still-visible cat scratch, this disease is characterized by a mild fever and tender, unilateral, regional adenopathy that usually involves the pre-auricular or submandibular areas. Diagnosis is based on a history of cat exposure, evidence of primary inoculation, regional lymphadenopathy, typical histologic features on FNAB or excisional biopsy (i.e., pleomorphic intracellular bacilli demonstrated with Warthin–Starry silver stain), and the absence of other causative agents. Treatment is supportive, with resolution expected within several weeks. Antibiotics, including erythromycin and doxycycline, are effective but are reserved for severe, persistent, or complicated cases (e.g., neurological involvement) (14,15).

> **Case 20.1** **Immigrant with Tuberculosis That Is Initially Diagnosed as Carcinoma**
>
> A woman 44 years of age presents with a 1-month history of an open, draining wound in the left supraclavicular area following a surgical procedure. She originally presented to a surgeon with a 3-month history of left cervical adenopathy that involved the posterior triangle and supraclavicular areas. At that time, the presumptive diagnosis was carcinoma, and an incisional biopsy was performed. The biopsy site never healed, and pathology showed granulomata. She was then referred to an otolaryngologist.
>
> Further inquiry reveals that she had emigrated from India to North America 1 year ago. There is no history of tobacco or alcohol use.
>
> Complete examination of the upper aerodigestive tract is negative. Examination of the neck reveals multiple matted nodes in the left posterior triangle and supraclavicular areas. In addition, there is a 2-cm, open, draining wound in the right supraclavicular area. Aspiration of purulent material from the site shows acid-fast bacilli, and her reaction to purified protein derivative (PPD) of tuberculin was strongly positive at 20 mm.
>
> Long-term antituberculous therapy is begun.
>
> **Discussion**
>
> This case illustrates the importance of a thorough history and physical examination. The history of immigration, absence of alcohol and tobacco use, and the location of the neck nodes all strongly suggest a diagnosis of tuberculosis. Progressing to an incisional biopsy without a proper history, physical examination, and work-up is inappropriate and potentially harmful to the patient. Useful tests in this situation include chest radiography, PPD, and FNAB aspirate for special staining and culture. These investigations, along with the history and physical examination, are more than enough to determine a diagnosis.

Actinomycosis is caused by *Actinomyces* species, and infection frequently follows dental manipulation or trauma. The submandibular and upper jugular nodes are affected most commonly, with occasional discoloration of the overlying skin. Positive cultures may be obtained after 1 to 2 weeks, and histologic examination reveals the presence of typical sulfur granules. Treatment consists of intravenous penicillin for 4 to 6 weeks, and surgical debridement is sometimes necessary (14).

Sarcoidosis is a multisystem, granulomatous disease of unknown etiology that affects primarily black women between 20 and 40 years of age. Head and neck manifestations may include bilateral cervical adenopathy and salivary gland involvement. In many cases, the disease is asymptomatic and found incidentally on chest radiograph. Diagnosis is based on the history, physical examination, and chest radiograph and on the presence of hypergammaglobulinemia, elevated erythrocyte sedimentation rate, hypercalcemia, and elevated levels of angiotensin-converting enzyme. Treatment (prednisone) is reserved for symptomatic patients.

Sjögren's syndrome (SS) is a systemic autoimmune disorder of the exocrine glands that frequently occurs with one or more connective tissue diseases. It affects women between 40 and 60 years of age and is characterized by xerostomia and keratoconjunctivitis sicca. There is intermittent, sometimes persistent, tender swelling of the major salivary glands. Diagnosis is based on the history, physical examination, positive SS-A and SS-B autoantibody tests, positive Schirmer's test, and characteristic histopathology on parotid or minor salivary gland biopsy. Treatment is primarily symptomatic, although systemic steroids occasionally are used for tender salivary gland enlargement. Long-term follow-up is required because of the increased incidence of non-Hodgkin's lymphoma and anaplastic carcinoma in this patient population. Measures to increase salivary flow (e.g., massage, sialogues) may help.

Toxoplasmosis is caused by the protozoan *Toxoplasma gondii* and is acquired by ingesting poorly cooked lamb or pork. Most patients are asymptomatic, although cervical lymphadenopathy occasionally is observed. Diagnosis is based on history and serologic testing. Treatment consists of pyrimethamine and trisulfapyrimidines.

Histoplasmosis is a fungal infection caused by *Histoplasma capsulatum*, which is spread by airborne transmission. Although clinical manifestations are related primarily to pulmonary infection or disseminated disease, cervical lymphadenopathy may be seen. Diagnosis is by culture on Sabouraud's medium. Treatment consists of amphotericin B.

Miscellaneous Causes of Lymphadenopathy

Kawasaki disease is a disorder of unknown etiology, affecting children under 9 years of age with cervical lymphadenopathy, fever, stomatitis, and conjunctivitis. The diagnosis is based entirely on clinical features, and antibiotic treatment is ineffective. High-dose acetylsalicylic acid is the mainstay of therapy along with intravenous gamma-globulins.

Sialadenitis

Acute suppurative sialadenitis primarily involves the parotid gland and is related to obstruction or the decreased production of saliva. Predisposing factors include calculi or strictures along the duct. Up to 40% of cases occur in postoperative patients, probably as a result of dehydration. Characteristically, the condition presents with fever and the rapid, diffuse enlargement of the involved gland. Induration and tenderness are noted on physical examination. Purulent saliva can be expressed from the duct orifice by massaging the affected gland. This material may be sent for Gram stain, culture, and sensitivity tests. The most frequently involved organism is coagulase-positive *S.*

aureus, although other aerobic and anaerobic organisms also may be found. Treatment consists of aggressive hydration, repeated massage of the gland, and intravenous antistaphylococcal antibiotics such as cloxacillin or clindamycin. Progression of symptoms or failure to improve within 48 hours is an indication for incision and drainage, which may be performed surgically or with needle aspiration under CT or ultrasound guidance.

Chronic sialadenitis is characterized by recurrent, mildly tender parotid enlargement that is exacerbated by eating. In contrast to acute sialadenitis, massaging the gland produces only scant amounts of saliva. When identified, calculi or ductal strictures should be treated. Massage, hydration, the use of sialagogues (e.g., lemonade, chewing gum) and antibiotics are helpful for acute exacerbations. Persistent symptoms are treated by surgically excising the affected gland.

Sialolithiasis

Approximately 80% of calculi occur in the submandibular gland, with the remaining 20% occurring in the parotid gland. Chronic sialadenitis and gout are predisposing factors. The submandibular gland and duct seem to be more susceptible to calculus formation for the following reasons: 1) the duct is oriented against gravity, which leads to salivary stasis; and 2) the saliva is more alkaline, with higher concentrations of calcium and phosphate. The calculi are composed largely of calcium phosphate. For reasons that are not entirely clear, 90% of submandibular calculi and only 10% of parotid calculi are radiopaque. The presenting history consists of recurrent pain and swelling in the involved gland that is provoked or exacerbated by eating. The obstruction produced by the calculus leads to salivary stasis and acute suppurative sialadenitis. The gland is enlarged and mildly tender; bimanual palpation often reveals the offending calculus. Massaging the gland produces very small quantities of saliva.

When the condition has progressed to sialadenitis, there is marked tenderness of the gland and a purulent discharge from the duct orifice. Diagnosis is by history and physical examination. Plain radiographs often reveal the calculus when the submandibular gland is involved. If the diagnosis is uncertain, ultrasound or CT is helpful in demonstrating the calculus. Treatment consists of antibiotics, gland massage, and removal of accessible intraoral calculi. Any calculi situated at the hilum of the gland necessitate removal of the entire gland, which is best undertaken after the acute infection has resolved.

Benign Neoplastic Neck Masses

Neurogenic Neck Masses

Neurogenic tumors that present as neck masses are rare and usually involve cranial nerves IX, X, XI, and XII or the cervical plexus. Although a consensus on terminology is lacking, in this chapter both neurofibromas and schwannomas are considered individually because clear histologic and clinical differences distinguish them.

Neurofibromas are usually numerous and are often associated with von Recklinghausen's disease. In approximately 10% of these patients, malignant transformation to a sarcoma eventually occurs in one neurofibroma. Unlike schwannomas, neurofibromas are not encapsulated; the involved nerves pass right through the tumor. Cystic and degenerative changes are uncommon. Cutaneous and subcutaneous neurofibromas do not involve major nerves, may be found anywhere in the head and neck, and are often cosmetically deforming. On CT and MRI, the lesions are poorly defined, may show evidence of fatty degeneration, and can be confused with lipomas. Complete surgical excision is the treatment of choice. When this is not possible, debulking may improve the patient's appearance (16).

Schwannomas are well-encapsulated, solitary lesions that rarely are associated with von Recklinghausen's disease. Although cystic degeneration and necrosis occur frequently in these tumors, malignant changes are rare. The vagus nerve is most often involved and usually is draped over the lesion, often in the parapharyngeal space. There is a single, firm, lateral neck mass that may vary in size from 2 to 20 cm. Dysfunction of the affected nerve is uncommon. In contrast to neurofibromas, however, pain and/or paresthesias are features of schwannomas. CT with contrast reveals a hypovascular mass. MRI with gadolinium demonstrates a well-defined ovoid lesion that paradoxically shows significant enhancement. This finding may suggest incorrectly the presence of a vascular tumor. Further testing with MRA reveals the true hypovascular nature of schwannomas. Of note, neurogenic and salivary gland lesions that occupy the parapharyngeal space share identical magnetic resonance findings. The only difference is that schwannomas displace the internal carotid artery anteriorly, whereas salivary tumors displace it posteriorly. Traumatic neuromas result from faulty regeneration of a previously injured or transected nerve. They are usually less than 2 cm in size and are frequently found in a previous surgical site. Symptoms include paresthesias and tingling. Excision may be necessary for control of symptoms.

Paragangliomas

Historically, these tumors have been assigned a number of other names, including **glomus tumors**, **chemodectomas**, and **nonchromaffin paragangliomas**. Of these terms, *paragangliomas* is the most appropriate. They arise from paraganglionic tissue, which originates embryologically from neural crest cells. This tissue contains catecholamines and has been identified in many locations, including the vagus nerve, the carotid bifurcation, and the adrenal medulla. Paragangliomas may secrete catecholamine, although most of these lesions are nonfunctioning. Tumors that present in the neck arise from either the vagus nerve or the carotid bifurcation. Approximately 10% of sporadic paragangliomas are multicentric. In patients with a positive family history of these neoplasms, the incidence of multicentricity rises to 30%. Paragangliomas present as slow growing, painless lateral cervical masses, and their malignant potential is low (established not by histologic findings but by the presence of metastases).

Vagal paragangliomas usually arise from the nodose ganglion and displace the carotid artery anteriorly and laterally. Small lesions present as slow-growing, painless, lateral cervical masses. Further growth results in hoarseness or a breathy voice, with possible aspiration from paralysis of the vagus nerve. Expansion into the jugular foramen results in tinnitus and may produce jugular foramen syndrome with additional involvement of cranial nerves IX and XI, with symptoms of dysphagia, nasal regurgitation, and shoulder drop. Eventually, the hypoglossal nerve is affected with paralysis of the ipsilateral tongue. Pain is a late symptom. Physical examination reveals a lateral neck mass that is sagittally but not axially mobile and signs of cranial nerve dysfunction. The presence of pulsations and bruits is unusual.

Carotid paragangliomas arise from the carotid body that is situated at the bifurcation of the common carotid artery. They usually present as painless lateral neck masses that occupy a lower position in the neck relative to their vagal counterparts. Symptoms of pressure, dysphagia, cough, and hoarseness are encountered with larger lesions that may even produce paralysis of the tenth nerve. Physical examination reveals a neck mass that is only sagittally mobile. Unlike vagal paragangliomas, the mass is pulsatile with a bruit in more than 50% of patients.

Diagnosis is based on the history, physical examination, a high index of suspicion, and appropriate imaging studies. The differential diagnosis includes aneurysms, metastases (e.g., papillary thyroid carcinoma), and rare primary vascular malignancies (e.g., angiosarcomas, hemangiopericytomas, extramedullary plasmacytomas). Fine-needle–aspiration cytology and incisional biopsy are not helpful in establishing the diagnosis, and the latter procedure may result in hemorrhage. CT with contrast shows marked enhancement consistent with a vascular lesion. MRI demonstrates a smoothly contoured mass with vascular flow voids and frequently a "salt and pepper" appearance on T_2-weighted images. Vagal paragangliomas have an oval shape if they are exclusively within the neck and a dumbbell shape with jugular foramen involvement; the internal carotid artery is displaced anteriorly. Typically, carotid paragangliomas are oval and displace both the internal and external carotid arteries anteriorly while splaying them at the bifurcation (16). MRA may show an apparently nonvascular mass because small-caliber, slow-flow vessels are beyond its resolution capabilities. For this reason, conventional angiography remains the "gold standard" for determining the true vascular nature of these tumors. Because of the high incidence of bilateral and multicentric lesions, routine study of both the left and right carotid arteries is advised.

Treatment consists primarily of surgical excision with or without preoperative embolization of the main feeding vessels. Radiotherapy is helpful postoperatively for incompletely resected lesions or as primary therapy in elderly patients or in those who are not fit to withstand surgery.

Lipomas

Lipomas are benign, encapsulated, subcutaneous collections of adipose tissue and may occur anywhere in the neck. The presenting complaint is usually of an asymptomatic mass that is easily mobile and has a doughy consistency on palpation (Fig. 20.9). Simple enucleation constitutes definitive treatment, and recurrence is rare. Infiltrating lipomas are nonencapsulated and more deeply situated in the neck. As their name suggests, they infiltrate surrounding tissue and may be difficult to remove completely. Liposarcomas are rare and require complete surgical removal.

Benign Salivary Gland Neoplasms

Benign salivary gland neoplasms, which arise from the parotid or submandibular glands, may present as neck masses. (*See* Chapter 21 for a discus-

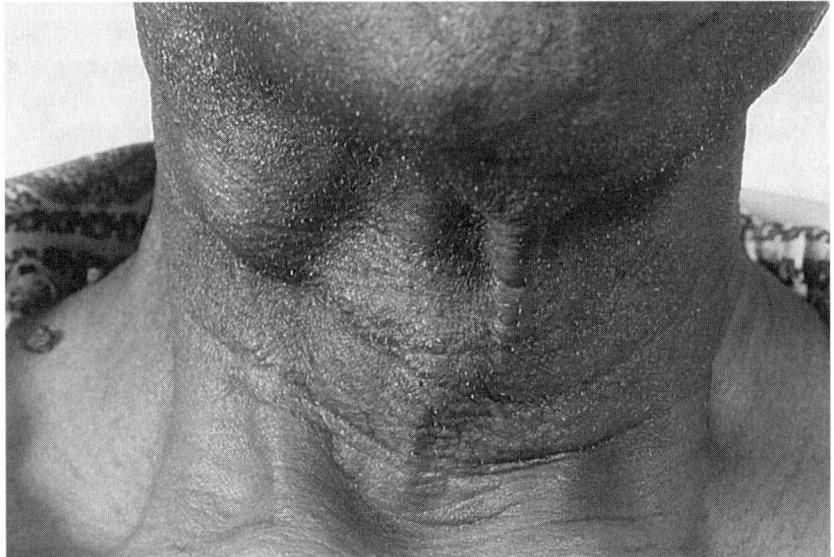

Figure 20.9 Lipomas are usually soft and doughy on palpation. (Republished with permission from McGirt WF, Johnson PE. *Evaluation and Treatment of the Patient with a Neck Mass*. Alexandria, VA: American Academy of Otolaryngology–Head and Neck Surgery; 1998.)

sion of these and other salivary gland disorders). Approximately 80% of all salivary gland neoplasms occur in the parotid gland; 80% of these are benign. They present as painless masses in the pre-auricular area or, more commonly, in the tail of the gland (just below the lobule of the ear). In the latter location, they can be confused with a jugulodigastric lymph node. Neoplasms that are located in the deep lobe of the parotid often extend into the parapharyngeal space and may present with a poorly defined neck mass and medial displacement of the tonsil on intraoral examination. In the submandibular gland, the incidence of benign salivary tumors drops to 50% to 60%. Presentation is also of an asymptomatic mass located in the submandibular triangle. The presence of facial nerve paresis or paralysis, fixation to overlying skin or adjacent structures, regional adenopathy, and possibly pain are all indicators of malignancy. In the hands of an experienced cytopathologist, FNAB is reliable in establishing the diagnosis of both benign and malignant salivary gland neoplasms. Incisional biopsy generally is contraindicated because of the risk for facial nerve injury and tumor seeding. Incisional biopsy may be considered when FNAB is not diagnostic in the presence of a massive tumor and when the probability of lymphoma exists. Otherwise, when the diagnosis is questionable, excisional biopsy with a cuff of normal tissue is preferable. CT and MRI are useful in delineating tumor size, margins, and relationship to adjacent structures.

By far the most common benign salivary gland neoplasm of the parotid and submandibular glands in both children and adults is the **benign mixed tumor (or pleomorphic adenoma)**. It occurs more frequently in women between 40 and 50 years of age, and most patients present with a history of a painless mass growing slowly over months to years. A history of recent rapid enlargement suggests the possibility of malignant change to a carcinoma ex-pleomorphic adenoma, which occurs in approximately 10% of cases. Physical examination reveals a nontender, mobile mass. FNAB often establishes the diagnosis and should be repeated if the first specimen is inadequate. The histologic hallmark of these tumors is the presence of both epithelial and mesenchymal elements. CT or MRI establishes the limits of the lesion. Treatment consists of surgical excision with a cuff of normal tissue while preserving the facial nerve (usually referred to as a superficial parotidectomy). Simple enucleation should be avoided because it results in a high recurrence rate resulting from frequent tumor extension beyond the borders of the apparent capsule. Long-term follow-up is required because recurrences may occur several years later, even after adequate removal.

Warthin's tumor (or papillary cystadenoma lymphomatosum) accounts for 6% of all salivary gland tumors. It occurs almost exclusively in the parotid gland and is the second most common benign neoplasm involving this gland. It has been reported to occur rarely as an isolated lateral neck mass. Older men (>40 years) are affected far more frequently than are women. Of note, these tumors are frequently bilateral as well as being multicentric within the same gland. Typically, they are soft and freely mobile on examination and have one or more cystic cavities demonstrable on CT or MRI. Warthin's tumors and oncocytomas share the unique feature of showing strong uptake on technetium pertechnetate scanning. FNAB may reveal the mucinous material within the cystic cavity or may show the classic findings of a papillary glandular epithelium in a lymphoid stroma. Surgical excision with preservation of the facial nerve is curative.

Other benign neoplasms that may affect the salivary glands include oncocytomas and a variety of adenomas. In most cases, FNAB confirms the benign nature of the lesion. Excision is the treatment of choice.

Lymphoepithelial cysts of the parotid gland are associated with HIV infection and are often bilateral. Patients usually present with several months of progressive parotid swelling with minimal tenderness. Generalized cervical adenopathy may be noted even though other manifestations of HIV may be absent. Both CT and MRI demonstrate multiple, thin-walled, cystic masses within the gland. FNAB may be diagnostic and typically shows fluid-containing benign lymphocytes and squamous epithelial cells. The clinical course of these lesions is benign. Treatment is not required except in cases in which the cysts are large when recurrent aspiration or parotidectomy may be helpful (18).

Benign Thyroid Gland Neoplasms

Follicular adenomas are solitary, nonfunctioning, benign, encapsulated neoplasms found most frequently in young and middle-aged adults. (*See* Chapter 22 for a discussion of these and other thyroid and parathyroid disorders.) Most of these lesions are solid, but they can undergo degenerative changes such as hemorrhage, fibrosis, and cyst formation. Several microscopic patterns have been identified, including **embryonal adenomas, microfollicular adenomas, follicular adenomas, colloid adenomas, atypical adenomas**, and **trabecular adenomas**. These patterns have no clinical significance and many of them often coexist within a single lesion. The presenting complaint is usually of a painless round or oval mass within the thyroid gland, either in the midline of the neck or slightly to the right or left. On physical examination, the mass is delineated sharply from the surrounding thyroid gland and moves with swallowing. Thyroid function tests are expected to be normal, and ultrasound demonstrates the solid nature of the lesion. Follicular carcinoma is characterized histologically by blood vessel and capsular invasion, features that cannot be demonstrated on FNAB. Excision and histologic examination are required to distinguish benign from malignant follicular neoplasm. In patients with a clinically benign lesion that is at low risk for malignancy, treatment may consist of thyroid suppression and follow-up; otherwise, the lesion should be removed surgically to rule out malignancy.

Purely cystic lesions of the thyroid gland are usually benign and present as painless thyroid masses. The cyst is demonstrated on ultrasound and FNAB.

Simple aspiration performed once or twice may be curative; otherwise, excision is indicated.

Malignant Neoplastic Neck Masses

An asymmetric neck mass in a patient over 40 years of age should be considered malignant until proven otherwise (Fig. 20.10). Approximately 50% of these masses are found to be malignant, with most of them representing cervical metastasis from a primary upper aerodigestive tract lesion. Up to 80% of head and neck malignancies are squamous cell carcinoma, which is strongly linked to the use of alcohol and tobacco. This point must be emphasized and understood, because simple excisional biopsy of the node can disseminate tumor cells and should be avoided. **Non-squamous cervical metastasis** is far less common but may originate from mesenchymal tumors or other head and neck sites such as the thyroid and salivary glands. Rarely, malignancies from distant sites such as the kidney or breast metastasize to cervical lymph nodes. Primary lymph node malignancies include Hodgkin's lymphoma as well as the non-Hodgkin's lymphomas (Fig. 20.11). (For a discussion of head and neck cancer in general, *see* Chapter 31.)

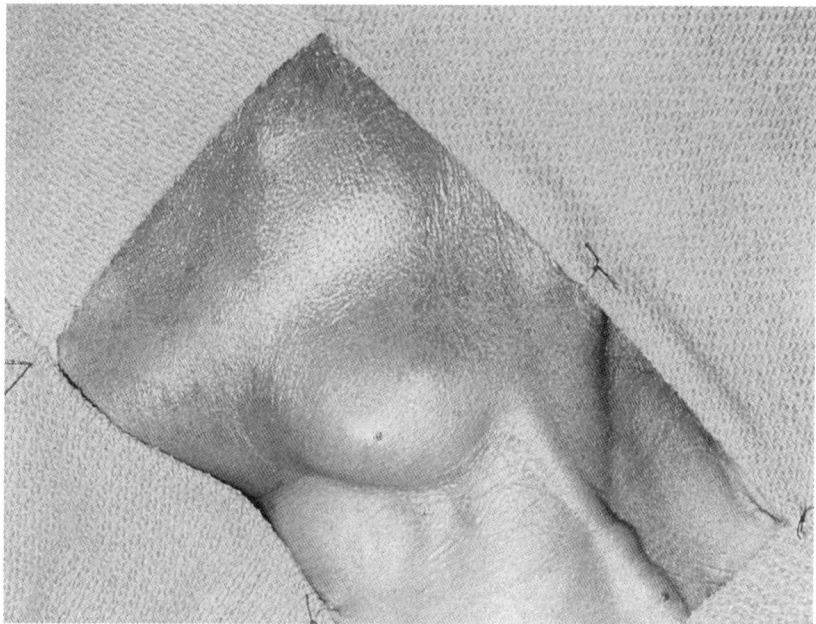

Figure 20.10 Mass in the upper neck, highly suspicious for squamous cell carcinoma. (Courtesy of Dr. Gary Clayman.)

Cervical Metastasis and Lymph Node Malignancies

Cervical metastasis from a primary upper aerodigestive tract lesion usually presents with progressive, painless enlargement of one or more cervical lymph nodes. If present, symptoms from the upper aerodigestive tract often help identify the site of primary involvement. Dysphagia and otalgia indicate a possible lesion in the base of the tongue, tonsil, or pharynx, whereas hoarseness may signify a laryngeal neoplasm.

Physical examination reveals one or more unilateral, but sometimes bilateral, firm to hard, round or oval masses that vary in size from 1 cm to several centimeters. When small, these nodes are freely mobile; unchecked growth results in gradual fixation to adjacent structures such as the mandible, carotid artery, skin, and the muscles underlying the deep cervical fascia. The jugulodigastric area often is involved because of its importance as a primary or ultimate drainage site for the head and neck. Because specific areas of the upper aerodigestive tract are known to have predictable lymphatic drainage patterns to specific nodal groups, the location of the involved lymphatic group often indicates the primary site of the head neck carcinoma (*see* Table 20.1 and Figs. 20.3 and 20.4). Thus, a thorough head and neck examination is essential. All mucosal surfaces, including the nasopharynx, oropharynx, hypopharynx, larynx, and oral cavity, are inspected using a mirror or a fiberoptic endoscope. Digital palpation is equally important because of the possibility of a submucosal lesion. This is particularly true in the base of the tongue and tonsil

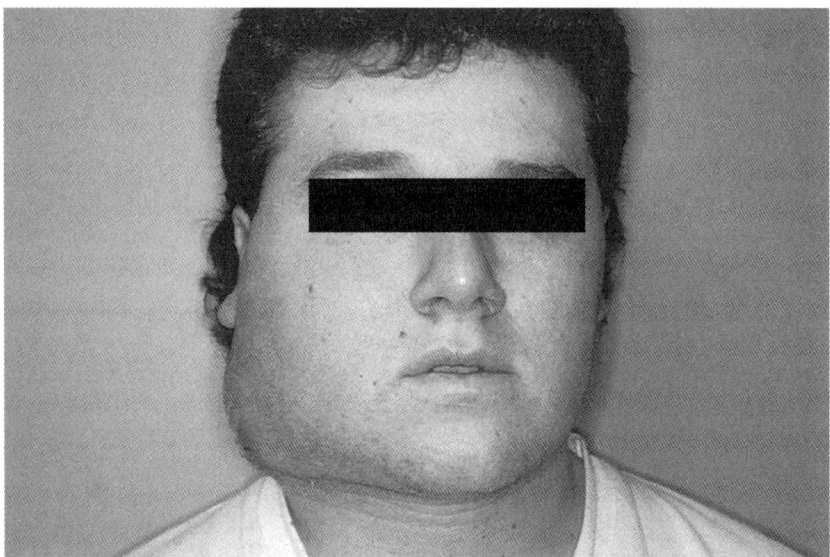

Figure 20.11 Young man with Burkitt's lymphoma. (Courtesy of Dr. David E. Eibling.)

where visual inspection may be unremarkable but when palpation reveals an area of induration signifying a submucosal lesion. Lymphadenopathy that involves the supraclavicular area usually indicates an infraclavicular primary site—primarily the gastrointestinal tract, tracheobronchial tree, and breast—at which identification efforts should be directed.

If the initial history and physical examination fail to reveal the cause of the neck mass, a thorough physical examination should be repeated. Then nasopharyngoscopy, laryngoscopy, esophagoscopy, and bronchoscopy should be performed under general anesthesia, which is necessary to allow for biopsies of obvious or probable sites and to facilitate the search for a second synchronous carcinoma (identified in up to 15% of patients.) Obvious lesions should be biopsied; when none have been found, guided biopsies should be obtained from the most suspicious sites based on known lymphatic drainage patterns. In the presence of an enlarged jugulodigastric node, special attention should be directed toward the oropharynx; an adequate sampling of this area includes tonsillectomy and deep biopsies from the base of the tongue (Case 20.2). Adenopathy that involves the posterior triangle suggests a primary site

---

Case 20.2   Smoker with an Enlarged Jugulodiagastric Node

A man 51 years of age presents with a 4-month history of a right neck mass that is increasing in size. He has a 50-pack-year history of smoking and admits moderate alcohol intake.

A thorough examination of all mucosal surfaces reveals a small indurated area in the right tongue base. The examination of the neck is significant for the presence of a firm, mobile right jugulodigastric node 4 cm in diameter. FNAB shows an acellular specimen. Repeat FNAB is positive for squamous cell carcinoma. Panendoscopy under general anesthesia confirms the presence of an indurated area in the right tongue base. Biopsy specimens taken from this area reveal squamous cell carcinoma.

Treatment consists of surgery and radiotherapy.

Discussion

The patient's age and history of tobacco and alcohol use strongly suggest that his neck mass is metastatic squamous cell carcinoma from a primary head and neck tumor. The location of the mass in the jugulodigastric area provides an important clue to the primary site. The search in this case should be directed toward the tonsil, pharynx, and base of the tongue. An inadequate FNAB is not an indication for open biopsy; however, it is an indication for repeat FNAB. Because the procedure is quick, easy, and safe, it may be repeated several times if necessary.

in the nasopharynx, whereas enlarged submandibular lymph nodes indicate a possible tumor of the oral tongue or mouth floor. If the primary site is identified, the tumor is staged with the help of CT or MRI. Treatment consists of surgery, radiotherapy, or both.

In some cases, a search fails to reveal the primary source of the suspected cervical metastasis. The next step is to perform FNAB of the neck mass, which is extremely useful in diagnosing **metastatic squamous cell carcinoma** (Fig. 20.12) and is reliable in identifying nonsquamous metastasis from distant sites as well as from thyroid and salivary gland malignancies. FNAB is usually not helpful in the diagnosis of lymphoma and actually may be misleading by describing sheets of benign-appearing lymphocytes. Such a report should arouse suspicion of a possible lymphoma and is an indication for excisional biopsy.

If FNAB confirms a diagnosis of metastatic squamous cell carcinoma and the primary site remains unknown, treatment may be planned based on the staging of the neck metastases. This usually consists of surgery or radiotherapy alone for N1 neck cancer and combined therapy for more advanced disease. Long-term follow-up with repeated examinations is necessary for several reasons: 1) the possibility of local recurrence, 2) some of the primary sites declare themselves months to years later, and 3) the increased risk of developing squamous cell carcinoma at another head and neck site.

Excisional biopsy in patients over 40 years of age with suspected cervical metastasis should be considered only if the above steps have failed to establish

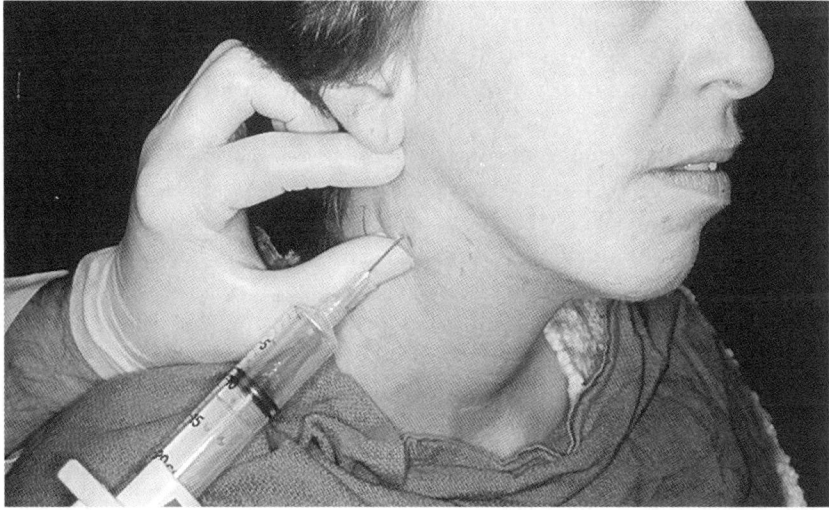

Figure 20.12 Fine-needle–aspiration biopsy being performed. (Courtesy of Dr. David E. Eibling.

a diagnosis. Furthermore, this procedure should be performed only by a surgeon who is prepared to proceed with a therapeutic neck dissection if the intraoperative frozen section reveals metastatic squamous cell carcinoma. There are ample data to show that an excisional biopsy performed before definitive therapy adversely affects long-term survival by increasing the risk of both local recurrence and distant metastasis. If the frozen section indicates a nonsquamous metastasis (e.g., from the salivary or thyroid glands) or the possibility of lymphoma, the wound should be closed and definitive therapy should be undertaken after appropriate staging.

Hodgkin's disease, **non-Hodgkin's lymphomas**, and **lymphosarcomas** are seen most frequently in children and young adults. Together, they account for up to 55% of all pediatric malignancies. Most have at least one neck mass at the time of diagnosis. The presenting complaint is the progressive enlargement of a painless lateral neck mass with possible constitutional symptoms, such as fevers and night sweats. Physical examination reveals a well-circumscribed, painless mass with a rubbery texture. A full head and neck examination is indicated, paying particular attention to Waldeyer's ring (which should be biopsied if any abnormalities are detected). Other findings on physical examination that support a diagnosis of malignancy include hepatomegaly, splenomegaly, and inguinal or axillary adenopathy. A high index of suspicion should be maintained in this patient population and should prompt the appropriate investigations with blood smears and a chest radiograph. The diagnosis is made rarely with FNAB, which is more likely to demonstrate benign-appearing lymphocytes. The physician should not be reassured by such a report and should proceed with an open biopsy. Excisional biopsy of the mass in this setting is acceptable and, in fact, indicated because of the low probability of a primary mucosal squamous cell carcinoma. With the diagnosis established, appropriate staging procedures are followed and treatment can be instituted.

Malignant Salivary Gland Neoplasms

Approximately 20% of **parotid neoplasms** are malignant, with the incidence rising to 50% to 60% in the **submandibular gland**. The presenting complaint is usually of an asymptomatic mass. In the parotid gland, it may be located in the pre-auricular area or more commonly in the tail of the gland just below the earlobe. Deep lobe tumors, which occupy the parapharyngeal space, usually are seen intraorally as a medial displacement of the ipsilateral tonsil. Submandibular neoplasms are situated below the mandible in the submandibular triangle. Small masses are usually well-circumscribed, whereas larger masses tend to be firm or hard. Establishing the diagnosis on the findings of the history and physical examination alone is difficult unless there are clear signs of malignancy, including facial nerve paralysis, fixation to skin or adjacent structures, and regional adenopathy. The significance of pain is controversial and thought by some to be an additional indicator of malignancy. FNAB is an excellent diagnostic tool that can differentiate benign from malignant lesions. Imaging studies such as CT or MRI cannot distinguish between benign and malignant neoplasms; thus, they need not be used routinely in small lesions that are primarily managed surgically. However, CT is useful in evaluating tumor extent and invasion with respect to adjacent structures in large lesions, and MRI is particularly helpful in assessing neoplasms that occupy the parapharyngeal space.

Mucoepidermoid carcinoma is the most common malignant tumor of the parotid gland and the second most common malignancy of the submandibular gland. Microscopically, these lesions are characterized by the presence of epidermoid and mucous cells in varying proportions. Tumors are divided into low-grade and high-grade categories based on the relative epidermoid-to-mucus ratio of cells—the higher the proportion of epidermoid cells, the higher the grade and the poorer the prognosis. FNAB is useful in establishing the diagnosis. Malignant and benign neoplasms can be distinguished, and often the precise histologic type of tumor can be determined—information that is important for preoperative planning and counseling. Imaging studies are helpful in delineating tumor extent for surgical planning. Treatment consists of complete surgical excision with preservation of the facial nerve unless the nerve is directly involved with tumor. Neck dissection is indicated for high-grade tumors or in the presence of regional adenopathy. Postoperative radiotherapy improves locoregional control in large (T3 or T4) or high-grade lesions. Long-term follow-up is necessary to detect locoregional recurrence or distant metastasis.

Adenoid cystic carcinoma is the most common malignancy of the submandibular gland and the second most common malignancy of the parotid gland. It usually appears as a slow-growing, asymptomatic mass and facial paralysis and pain are occasionally the only presenting symptoms. Microscopically, small basaloid cells surround an eosinophilic hyaline stroma and are often arranged in cylindrical shapes. Attempts to correlate the histologic appearance of these tumors with ultimate prognosis have provided conflicting results. The hallmark of this tumor is perineural invasion. FNAB may establish the diagnosis preoperatively. Treatment consists of radical surgery with preservation of the facial nerve, if possible, and neck dissection for locally advanced disease or palpable lymph nodes. Because of the propensity for perineural invasion, complete removal is difficult and adjuvant radiotherapy generally is recommended. Patients may remain free of disease for several years, only to present with recurrent disease or pulmonary metastases; however, even with this complication, survival for many years is not unusual.

Carcinoma ex-pleomorphic adenoma represents malignant transformation of a previously benign but long-standing mixed tumor. Typically, the patient has had a parotid or submandibular mass for many years with a recent, sudden increase in growth. Diagnosis may be difficult if the carcinoma is present in only a small portion of the tumor and occasionally is made on histologic examination of the entire surgical specimen. In general, prognosis is poor with frequent locoregional and distant metastasis. Adjuvant radiotherapy usually is recommended.

Other malignant tumors of the salivary glands are much less common. Acinous (or acinic cell) carcinoma occurs mainly in the parotid gland and is the second most common salivary gland malignancy in children (mucoepidermoid carcinoma is most common). The tumor is bilateral in 3% of cases, and treatment consists of surgical removal with facial nerve preservation. Adenocarcinoma, squamous cell carcinoma, and undifferentiated carcinoma are all rare but aggressive tumors that require a combination of surgery and radiotherapy for treatment. Rarely, lymphomas arise within the salivary glands and usually are diagnosed at the time of surgery. Malignant tumors from distant sites, such as the kidney or breast, occasionally metastasize to the parotid gland.

Malignant Thyroid Gland Neoplasms

Thyroid malignancies present in much the same way as benign thyroid neoplasms, namely as neck masses in the lower anterior compartment of the neck in all age groups. The incidence of malignancy in children who present with a solitary nodule is approximately 50%. Factors from the history that are associated with an increased risk of malignancy include age less than 20 years or greater than 50 years, history of ionizing radiation to the head and neck, male gender, family history of medullary thyroid carcinoma, rapid growth, and hoarseness.

Findings on physical examination that suggest malignancy include a firm to hard, nontender nodule, regional lymphadenopathy, fixation to adjacent structures, and vocal cord paralysis (19). Most patients present with an asymptomatic firm to hard, nontender mass in the region of the thyroid gland that moves with swallowing. Thyroid function tests are usually normal. In autonomously functioning nodules, however, the level of serum thyrotropin (thyroid-stimulating hormone) is low, as is the risk of malignancy. The level of serum calcitonin is a reliable marker for medullary thyroid carcinoma and should be measured in patients with a family history of medullary cancer or multiple endocrine neoplasia syndrome type 2.

Although imaging is helpful in evaluating masses that involve the thyroid gland, the ideal choice of studies is controversial and varies greatly from one physician to the next. Radioisotope scans are used primarily to determine the functional status of a nodule and are less useful as indicators of malignancy. The incidence of malignancy is 2% in hyperfunctioning (or "hot") nodules, 5% in normally functioning nodules, and 5% to 25% in nonfunctioning (or "cold") nodules. Ultrasound has been used to determine whether a nodule is solid or cystic, because pure cysts, although unusual, are rarely malignant. This test is probably most useful in assessing lesions that are difficult to palpate and in guiding FNAB when previous attempts have yielded insufficient material. Ultrasound also may be helpful in identifying small contralateral nodules in patients with carcinoma, thus facilitating the decision between total thyroidectomy and hemithyroidectomy. FNAB has become the mainstay in the evaluation of thyroid masses—its sensitivity and specificity in determining thyroid cancer are 83% and 92%, respectively. Limitations of FNAB include its inability to determine whether follicular and Hürthle cell neoplasms are benign or malignant. This is because capsular and vascular invasion are necessary for the diagnosis of malignancy and can be demonstrated only histologically. CT and MRI are useful in assessing tumor extent and lymph node involvement in cases in which malignancy has been proven or is suspected.

To a large extent, indications for surgical removal of a thyroid nodule are guided by risk factors elicited in the history and on physical examination as well as by the results obtained from FNAB.

Papillary carcinoma is the most common thyroid malignancy, accounting for 70% of all thyroid carcinomas. It occurs more frequently in women and is characterized by an excellent prognosis. A history of radiation is a well-known risk factor for this type of malignancy. Papillary carcinoma arises from the follicular cells and is frequently multifocal. Lymph node metastases are common, with frequencies ranging from 46% to 90%. The diagnosis is confirmed easily with FNAB. Treatment is surgical and may involve hemithyroidectomy or total thyroidectomy (*see* Chapter 22).

Follicular carcinoma is the second most common malignancy of the thyroid and is more common in women. Presentation is usually of an asymptomatic nodule that measures 2 to 4 cm. Regional lymphadenopathy is relatively uncommon, occurring in approximately 10% of patients. The cell of origin is the follicular cell. Surgery is required to make the diagnosis because neither FNAB nor frozen section is reliable. Treatment is surgical excision by hemithyroidectomy, subtotal thyroidectomy, or total thyroidectomy. Prognosis is generally good; however, factors that adversely affect the outcome include age greater than 40 years, tumor size greater than 4 cm, male gender, poor histologic grade, and the presence of distant metastasis.

Hürthle cell neoplasm is believed to be a variant of the follicular neoplasm and is defined as an encapsulated group of follicular cells with at least a 75% Hürthle cell component. Demonstration of capsular or vascular invasion is necessary for the diagnosis of malignancy; thus, the presence of Hürthle cells on FNAB is an indication for surgery. Because this tumor behaves in a more aggressive manner than does papillary or follicular carcinoma, total thyroidectomy is indicated.

Medullary thyroid carcinoma accounts for only 5% to 10% of thyroid neoplasms. Eighty percent of these carcinomas are sporadic, whereas 20% are familial and occur as part of a multiple endocrine neoplasia syndrome in which multicentricity and bilaterality are the rule. The tumor arises from the parafollicular cells (or C cells) of the thyroid, which produce calcitonin, a calcium-lowering hormone. Diagnosis can be made on FNAB, with the demonstration of amyloid and positive staining for calcitonin. Serum calcitonin levels are elevated and can be used in the postoperative period to detect recurrence or metastases. Treatment consists of total thyroidectomy and dissection of the paratracheal lymph nodes. Postoperative radiation is indicated in the presence of soft tissue invasion and multiple positive lymph nodes.

Anaplastic thyroid carcinoma occurs principally in elderly individuals and is characterized by rapid growth and invasion of adjacent structures (e.g., esophagus, trachea, carotid artery, recurrent laryngeal nerve.) Up to 20% of patients have a previous history of follicular carcinoma. The diagnosis often can be made with FNAB. Because the nature of this cancer is extremely aggressive, it is rarely cured. Treatment is usually palliative and is directed at securing an airway with tracheostomy, if necessary, and improving local control. Surgery alone is rarely effective. Current treatment includes doxorubicin (Adriamycin) and cisplatin with concomitant radiotherapy.

Thyroid lymphomas are uncommon and occur more frequently in women in the sixth decade of life. There is often a history of a rapidly enlarging thyroid mass with possible symptoms of encroachment onto adjacent structures, producing symptoms of hoarseness, dysphagia, and pain. Non-Hodgkin's B-cell lymphomas are the most common type of lesion, and a diagnosis is often suggested on FNAB. Open biopsy is occasionally necessary for complete characterization of the tumor. The principal treatment modality is chemotherapy with or without radiotherapy.

Rhabdomyosarcomas

Rhabdomyosarcomas are the most common malignant soft tissue tumor in children, involving the head and neck in 40% of cases. FNAB may be helpful in establishing the diagnosis, although open biopsy may be necessary. Imaging studies are required to delineate the extent of the lesion, and a full metastatic work-up is necessary to rule out distant metastasis. Treatment consists of wide surgical excision of the primary site, when possible, followed by radiation and chemotherapy because of the high propensity for local recurrence and distant metastasis.

Work-Up: An Overview

The initial work-up of a neck mass consists of a thorough history and physical examination as described previously in this chapter. This essential step should, at the very least, allow classification of the neck mass into one of the major groupings: inflammatory, congenital, or neoplastic.

Inflammatory neck masses in children and young adults are usually viral or bacterial in origin, with an obvious source in the upper aerodigestive tract. An uncomplicated viral upper respiratory tract infection associated with a few small mobile neck nodes does not require any investigations and may be treated expectantly, with a follow-up in 3 to 4 weeks. **Culture and sensitivity studies** are useful in tonsillitis and pharyngitis to rule out beta-hemolytic *Streptococcus* group A. In the presence of cervical lymphadenopathy and marked enlargement of the tonsils, it may be useful to distinguish between a viral and a bacterial cause. A positive heterophil antibody test for mononucleosis or cytomegalovirus titers confirms a viral infection but does not preclude the presence of a superimposed bacterial infection. If such an overlapping of infections is suspected, a culture and sensitivity test of the tonsils and a complete blood count with differential should be obtained.

Inflammatory neck masses of a granulomatous nature tend to have more of a subacute presentation. The location of the mass and unsuccessful antibiotic treatment are often clues to the cause. Culture and sensitivity testing are useful but take several weeks. More immediate results may be obtained from **PPD skin tests** and by using special stains to identify acid-fast bacilli on aspirated material. Clinical clues, such as the age of the patient and the location of the neck mass, are useful distinguishing features between ATM infection and tuberculosis.

Culture and sensitivity studies are useful in the identification of bacterial infections from acute tonsillitis (beta-hemolytic *Streptococcus* group A) or after dental manipulation (*Actinomyces* species). Cultures using special media are also helpful in the diagnosis of fungal infections such as histoplasmosis and mycobacterial diseases caused by ATM and *M. tuberculosis*. Positive cultures require several weeks and an adequate specimen, which often can be obtained with FNAB. Obtaining an adequate tissue sample for culture sometimes requires excisional biopsy.

Serologic studies may be obtained for the diagnosis of toxoplasmosis and histoplasmosis. Viral infections can be identified using cytomegalovirus titers and the heterophil antibody test for mononucleosis.

Although nonspecific, a complete blood count with differential may be useful in certain inflammatory or malignant processes. The erythrocyte sedimentation rate may be elevated in inflammatory, autoimmune, or connective tissue disorders. In connective tissue diseases, rheumatoid factor is positive and antinuclear antibodies are elevated. Measurement of SS-A and SS-B autoantibodies are useful in the diagnosis of Sjögren's syndrome. Angiotensin-converting–enzyme levels are elevated in sarcoidosis.

Skin tests may be useful in the diagnosis of mycobacterial disorders. Special stains on material obtained from FNAB may demonstrate acid-fast bacilli in mycobacterial infections or pleomorphic intracellular bacilli in cat-scratch disease.

Chest radiographs are indicated in all cases of malignancy, including lymphoma, and may be abnormal in sarcoidosis, toxoplasmosis, and suspected cases of tuberculosis. In sialolithiasis that involves the submandibular or parotid glands, plain radiographs may demonstrate the presence and location of calculi. However, aside from these specific indications, plain radiographs are of limited value in the assessment of head and neck masses.

Fine-needle-aspiration biopsy has become one of the most useful techniques in the evaluation of head and neck masses. Because the information obtained from this simple test is so valuable, it should precede imaging studies in most cases. The diagnosis provided by FNAB often obviates the need for an open surgical procedure and serves to direct further investigation and treatment of the presenting mass. It can be used in children and adults and is simple, accurate, safe, and inexpensive. However, FNAB is sensitive to technique and requires an experienced cytopathologist. It is of proven value in the diagnosis of both benign and malignant neoplasms. Cellular material may be subjected to all the ancillary studies currently available for surgically excised tissue, including morphometry, molecular hybridization reactions, lymphocyte surface-marker studies, flow cytometry for DNA ploidy analysis, immunohistochemistry, and electron microscopy. FNAB is also extremely useful in the diagnosis of congenital and inflammatory lesions. Aspirated material may be sent for culture or subjected to special stains. When submitted material is insufficient or inadequate for diagnosis, the technique can and should be repeated at least once, even twice. Limitations of the technique are well recognized. Because the demonstration of malignancy requires histologic evidence of capsular or vascular invasion, benign and malignant follicular cell neoplasms of the thyroid gland cannot be distinguished on FNAB. It is also unreliable in the diagnosis of lymphoma, and a negative report in an otherwise suspicious mass is an indication for excisional biopsy. FNAB complications are few but include bleeding (easily controlled with local pressure) when performed on a vascular lesion. Tumor seeding along the needle tract has never been documented (20,21).

Ultrasonography can distinguish between solid and cystic lesions; thus, it is particularly helpful in distinguishing congenital cystic masses from solid masses. Ultrasound-guided FNAB may be used to obtain material for cytology or culture when previous attempts at conventional aspiration have been unsuccessful. In addition, ultrasound is useful in evaluating the thyroid gland in specific clinical situations, including patients with suspected lesions that are difficult to palpate and those in whom a nonpalpable lesion has been detected by a radioisotope scan.

Computed tomography is one of the most useful imaging modalities in the assessment of neck masses, playing a particularly important role in the evaluation and staging of cervical metastases from a head and neck primary site. Clinically occult nodes may be detected, particularly in short thick necks, which are difficult to examine. CT may be helpful in localizing the site of an occult primary carcinoma, but by no means is it intended to supplant the need for repeated, thorough head and neck examinations. CT also may be of value in the imaging of congenital lesions such as thyroglossal duct cysts, branchial cleft cysts, and cystic hygromas. In infectious or inflammatory processes, CT can help guide therapy by differentiating between cellulitis, edema, and abscess formation.

Information obtained by **MRI** is often complementary to that provided by CT. MRI is superior in evaluating submucosal lesions of the upper aerodigestive tract and in demonstrating tumor extension into the laryngotracheal complex and esophagus. In the neck, it also can detect the invasion of adjacent neurovascular structures and the deep cervical musculature. MRI is the imaging modality of choice for the assessment of parapharyngeal space lesions.

Occasionally, a definitive diagnosis cannot be reached by using FNAB and other appropriate studies. In these instances, excisional biopsy of the mass is appropriate and indicated. A frozen section may be obtained, and the surgeon should be prepared to tailor the procedure on the basis of the results. If there is doubt as to whether the lesion is inflammatory or neoplastic, tissue should be sent for cultures and special stains as well.

Management and Follow-Up: An Overview

The diagnosis of congenital neck masses is usually straightforward based on age, location, and the aspiration of fluid in the case of cystic lesions. The treatment of choice for congenital midline lesions and branchial cleft cysts or sinuses is surgical excision. Recurrence is infrequent and usually results from a failure to excise associated ducts or sinuses. Hemangiomas and lymphangiomas must be distinguished clinically because the treatments differ. After a period of initial growth during the first year, 90% of hemangiomas undergo spontaneous resolution by 5 or 6 years. Systemic steroids are used when involution is incomplete or when rapid growth results in facial deformity or airway compromise. Lymphangiomas rarely undergo spontaneous regression, and most require one or more surgical procedures after 3 or 4 years of age. In massive lesions, the priority is to secure the airway, usually with a tracheostomy.

As mentioned previously, inflammatory neck masses in children and young adults are often viral or bacterial in origin, with an obvious source in the upper aerodigestive tract. An uncomplicated viral upper respiratory tract infection with a few small mobile cervical nodes requires no investigation and can be treated expectantly. When a bacterial infection is suspected, cultures should be taken and appropriate antibiotics should be begun. Failure of the nodes to regress as expected is an indication for reevaluation and possible FNAB. Special mention should be made of odontogenic neck infections, which must be treated aggressively because of their potentially fulminant course. Treatment must consist, first and foremost, of securing the airway, followed by intravenous antibiotics and incision and drainage if necessary.

Granulomatous neck masses generally have a more subacute presentation over weeks to months and may be suspected after an unsuccessful course of antibiotics. Differentiating between the various causes is important because the treatment of each entity is different. Occasionally, despite every effort (including a repeat FNAB), a precise diagnosis cannot be reached. In this instance, excisional biopsy of the mass may be indicated, provided that metastatic squamous cell carcinoma and tuberculosis have been excluded in the diagnosis.

It may be difficult to distinguish between **ATM** infection and tuberculosis. ATM infection usually occurs in children with the pre-auricular and submandibular nodes affected; treatment consists of surgical excision of the affected nodes. Tuberculosis is more common in adults, and involved nodes are found in the posterior triangle; appropriate treatment consists of antituberculous drugs. In this setting, incisional biopsy may well result in an open, draining wound and should be avoided. The diagnosis of cat-scratch disease is largely one of exclusion, requiring only supportive therapy, with antibiotics reserved for persistent or complicated cases. A high index of suspicion is required in identifying sarcoidosis, which predominantly affects young black women. Treatment is mainly supportive, with systemic steroids reserved for exacerbations. Long-term follow-up is required because of the disease's chronic nature, multisystem involvement, and potential complications. Sjögren's disease is a chronic autoimmune disorder that requires principally symptomatic therapy, although steroids may be used for marked enlargement of the salivary glands. Prolonged follow-up is necessary because of potential dental and ocular complications, association with other autoimmune disorders, and the well-known risk of developing non-Hodgkin's lymphoma. Histoplasmosis is treated with amphotericin B, whereas toxoplasmosis is treated with pyrimethamine and trisulfapyrimidines.

The diagnosis of **sialadenitis** is usually obvious. Empirical antistaphylococcal antibiotics are begun while awaiting final culture and sensitivity test results. Repeated massage and the use of sialagogues as salivary stimulants help "flush out" the gland. Predisposing factors, such as dehydration or the presence of calculi, must be identified and addressed. If possible, calculi are removed intraorally; otherwise, removal of the gland may be necessary after the infection resolves. If the infection progresses to abscess formation, surgical incision and drainage is required. When operating on the parotid gland, care must be taken not to injure the facial nerve.

As a general rule, most **neoplastic neck masses** require some form of surgical intervention, ranging from simple excision to radical removal of a primary malignancy to neck dissection. The key is to use FNAB preoperatively to discover whether the neoplasm is benign or malignant and, if possible, the histologic type.

For vascular lesions in adults (e.g., **paragangliomas**), planning includes determining the blood supply of the lesion for possible embolization and ruling out the presence of additional lesions. In the latter circumstance, surgical treatment may carry a risk of unacceptable morbidity, and radiotherapy is preferable.

In patients over 40 years of age (when the risk of metastatic squamous cell carcinoma from a head and neck primary is high), every effort must be made to establish the diagnosis by means of a thorough examination of the upper aerodigestive tract under general anesthesia and with guided biopsies. FNAB of the mass may be repeated if necessary.

In the few instances in which these diagnostic steps fail and a mucosal primary lesion is not found, open biopsy is to be undertaken by a surgeon who is prepared to proceed with a therapeutic neck dissection if the frozen section is positive. It has been demonstrated clearly that excisional biopsy of a neck node that contains squamous cell carcinoma results in a poor prognosis, even when appropriate treatment (e.g., neck dissection and/or radiotherapy) is instituted at a later time. To clarify, N1 disease may be treated with surgery or radiotherapy alone; more advanced disease (N2 or N3) is treated with combined surgery and radiotherapy. Long-term follow-up is mandatory as part of an ongoing search to detect the primary carcinoma and also because 15% to 20% of these patients develop a second head and neck squamous cell carcinoma. Yearly chest radiographs are necessary because of the risk of developing a primary lung cancer or metastasis.

In patients under 40 years of age (when the risk of metastatic squamous cell carcinoma is low), neck mass management is different. If no diagnosis is established initially, it is reasonable to proceed with a 2-week trial of antibiotic therapy. If the mass has not regressed or has increased in size during this period, FNAB is indicated (Case 20.3). A report documenting the presence of benign-appearing lymphocytes should prompt an excisional biopsy to rule out lymphoma.

Establishing an exact diagnosis may be difficult in follicular neoplasms of the thyroid. FNAB can establish the presence of follicular cells but cannot distinguish between benign and malignant characteristics. This is a limitation that must be interpreted in light of the clinical situation, so that a decision can be made about whether to proceed with medical or surgical treatment. If the mass is small, clinically benign, and in a low-risk individual, initial treatment consists of observation and thyroid-suppression therapy. Continued growth of

> **Case 20.3** **Young Man with a Neck Mass and No History of Recent Infection**
>
> An otherwise healthy man 24 years of age presents with a left neck mass that he recently discovered while shaving. The mass is nontender and has grown only slightly. There is no history of recent upper respiratory tract infection.
>
> A complete head and neck examination reveals only a 3-cm, rubbery, nontender, mobile left neck mass situated below the angle of the mandible. FNAB indicates that the mass is solid.
>
> The patient is sent home on a 2-week course of antibiotics. At the time of follow-up 3 weeks later, there is no change in the mass. The FNAB report indicates that an adequate specimen was taken, showing only benign-appearing lymphocytes. An excisional biopsy of the mass is performed, revealing Hodgkin's lymphoma.
>
> **Discussion**
>
> Although inflammatory and congenital masses are most common in this age group, there is no history of infection in this particular case, and the mass is solid as demonstrated by FNAB. Nonetheless, a 2-week trial of antibiotics is reasonable. The absence of response to antibiotic therapy heightens the index of suspicion for a neoplastic process. Because the incidence of squamous cell carcinoma in this age group is extremely low, an excisional biopsy is reasonable and indicated. The FNAB results must be interpreted in the context of the clinical situation. There is no history of infection and no response to antibiotics, but there is the presence of lymphocytes on cytology. These lymphocytes could represent reactive hyperplasia or lymphoma. FNAB cannot differentiate these two entities and therefore an open biopsy is necessary.

the lesion is an indication for excisional biopsy. Firm or hard thyroid masses in high-risk patients should be removed with hemithyroidectomy as the minimum procedure. Long-term follow-up of patients with thyroid malignancies is necessary to detect recurrence or metastasis.

Summary

An organized approach to the patient who presents with a neck mass begins with a detailed history and thorough physical examination. Integrating this information with the age of the patient and the location of the neck mass starts the process of narrowing the list of diagnostic possibilities by categorizing the lesion as inflammatory, congenital, or neoplastic. In many instances, the list can be reduced to just a few serious choices. At this point, carefully selected investigations may be requested (e.g., cultures in inflammatory conditions, imaging studies in congenital and neoplastic conditions).

An invaluable diagnostic aid is FNAB; it is safe, rapid, and can be repeated if necessary. Its usefulness extends beyond the cytologic diagnosis of neoplasms; aspirated material can be sent for culture and sensitivity and special staining, thereby confirming the diagnosis in inflammatory conditions as well. However, FNAB is limited in the diagnosis of lymphomas and follicular thyroid neoplasms. A clear understanding of these limitations and an ability to interpret the results are essential in proceeding to diagnosis and treatment.

Ultimately, in carefully selected cases, excisional biopsy may be the final diagnostic and therapeutic (sometimes) step. This is especially true in children and young adults in whom removal is indicated for congenital lesions and certain inflammatory granulomatous conditions (e.g., ATM infection). The diagnosis of lymphoma usually depends on sufficient material obtained from excision of the neck mass. Understanding when open biopsy is or is not appropriate is essential, because the inappropriate use of this option may adversely affect prognosis. As we have seen, long-term survival is compromised when an excisional biopsy is performed on a cervical metastatic node that contains squamous cell carcinoma.

REFERENCES

1. **Graney DO.** Anatomy. In Cummings CW, Fredrickson JM, Harker LA, et al. (eds). *Otolaryngology Head Neck Surg.* St. Louis: CV Mosby; 1986.
2. **Alvi A, Johnson JT.** The neck mass: a challenging differential diagnosis. *Postgrad Med.* 1995;97:87–97.
3. **McGuirt WF.** Diagnosis and management of masses in the neck with special emphasis on metastatic malignant disease. *Oncology.* 1990;4:85–97.
4. **Cann CI, Fried MP, Rothman KJ.** Epidemiology of squamous cell cancer of the head and neck. *Otolaryngol Clin North Am.* 1985;18:367–88.
5. **Cunningham MJ.** The management of congenital neck massses. *Am J Otolarygol.* 1992;13:78–92.
6. **Guarisco JL.** Congenital head and neck masses in infants and children: Part I. *Ear Nose Throat J.* 1991;70:40–7.
7. **Guarisco JL.** Congenital head and neck masses in infants and children: Part II. *Ear Nose Throat J.* 1991;75–82.
8. **Pincus RL.** Congenital neck masses and cysts. In Bailey BJ (ed). *Head and Neck Surgery–Otolaryngology.* Philadelphia: JB Lippincott; 1993.
9. **Burton DM, Pransky SM.** Practical aspects of managing nonmalignant lumps of the neck. *J Otolaryngol.* 1992;21:398–403.
10. **Ward R, Selfe RL, Bowling D.** Computed tomography and the thyroglossal duct cyst. *Otolaryngol Head Neck Surg.* 1986;95:93–8.
11. **DeSanto LW.** Laryngocele, laryngeal mucocele, large saccules, and laryngeal saccular cysts: a developmental spectrum. *Laryngoscope.* 1974;84:1291.
12. **Gonzales J, Ljung B-M, Guerry T, Schoenrock L.** Congenital torticolis: evaluation by fine-needle–aspiration biopsy. *Laryngoscope.* 1989;99:651–4.

13. **Park Y.** Evaluation of neck masses in children. *Am Fam Phys.* 1995;51:1904–12.
14. **Littlejohn MC, Bailey BJ.** Granulomatous diseases of the head and neck. In Bailey BJ (ed). *Head and Neck Surgery–Otolaryngology.* Philadelphia: JB Lippincott;1993.
15. **Smith DL.** Cat-scratch disease and related syndromes. *Am Fam Phys.* 1997;55: 1783–94.
16. **Som PM, Curtin HD.** Lesions of the paralaryngeal space: role of MR imaging. *Otolarygol Clin North Am.* 1995;28:515–42.
17. **Toriumi DM, Atiyah RA, Murad T, Sisson GA.** Extracranial neurogenic tumors of the head and neck. *Otolaryngol Clin North Am.* 1986;19:609–17.
18. **Lee KC, Cheung SW.** Evaluation of the neck mass in the human immunodeficiency virus-infected patients. *Otolaryngol Clin North Am.* 1992;25:1287–1305.
19. **Singer PA.** Evaluation and management of the solitary thyroid nodule. *Otolaryngol Clin North Am.* 1996;29:577–91.
20. **Patt BS, Schaefer SD, Vuitch F.** Role of fine-needle aspiration in the evaluation of neck masses. *Med Clin North Am.* 1993;77:611–22.
21. **Mobley D, Wakely P, Frable M.** Fine-needle–aspiration biopsy: application to pediatric head and neck masses. *Laryngoscope.* 1991;101:469–72.

SUGGESTED READINGS

Guarisco JL. Congenital head and neck masses in infants and children (Parts I & II). *Ear Nose Throat J.* 1991;70:40–7, 75–82.
This article provides a detailed account of the embryology and management of congenital neck masses. Of particular interest is the large number of beautiful illustrations and photographs.
McGuirt WF. Diagnosis and management of masses in the neck with special emphasis on metastatic malignant disease. *Oncology.* 1990;4:85–97.
This is an excellent general review of the appropriate approach to neck masses. Dr. McGuirt places particular emphasis on metastatic cervical lymphadenopathy from an unknown primary lesion in the head and neck. The points are stated clearly, and the information is well organized.

21

Salivary Gland Disorders

David E. Eibling, MD

Swelling of a major salivary gland is the most common presenting complaint in a patient with salivary gland disease. Painless, slow-growing masses generally are assumed to be benign neoplasms; however, these growth characteristics do not rule out malignancy in tumors of salivary origin (Fig. 21.1). An asymptomatic mass that suddenly becomes tender or increases in size usually indicates infection or hemorrhage into the mass but also may indicate malignant change. A fixed, firm mass may signify malignancy, inflammation, or fibrosis. Patients with acute infection or obstruction of a major duct complain of a tender, enlarged salivary gland that often fluctuates in size, especially at mealtime. A foul-tasting discharge in the mouth is another sign of infection, but this is usually a minor complaint compared with the pain and swelling of the gland.

Anatomy and Physiology

There are three pairs of major salivary glands: the parotid, submandibular, and sublingual glands. Hundreds of minor salivary glands are distributed throughout the mucosa of the oral cavity, pharynx, and sinuses. The largest of the salivary glands, the parotid gland, lies just anterior to the ear between the ascending ramus of the mandible and the mastoid process, extending up to the level of the tragus. The tail of the parotid gland curves posteroinferiorly

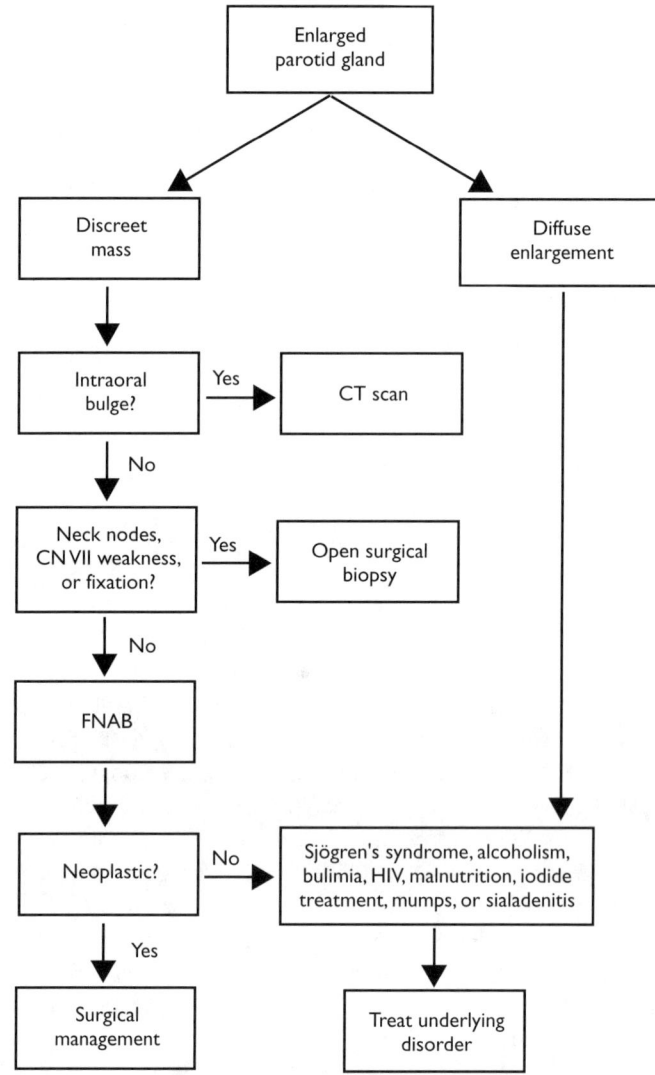

Algorithm Diagnosis and management of salivary gland disorders. CN = cranial nerve; CT = computed tomography; FNAB = fine-needle–aspiration biopsy.

to just below the ear lobe. The parotid gland drains via Stensen's duct to an orifice on the buccal mucosa opposite the second maxillary molar.

The secretomotor innervation of the salivary glands is parasympathetic, and the path taken by the preganglionic fibers is tortuous and fascinating. The secretomotor innervation of the parotid gland arises in the inferior salivatory

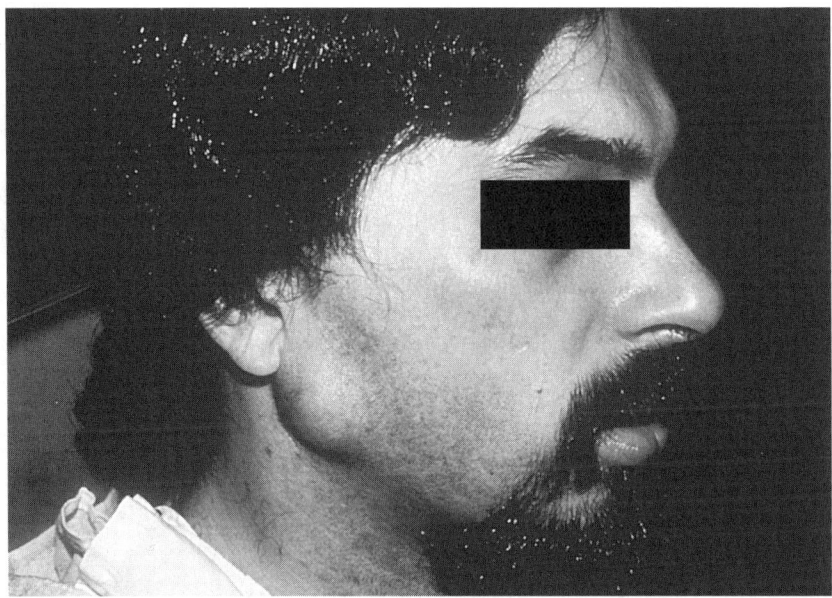

Figure 21.1 Young man with a mass in his upper neck. The location of the mass, just behind and below the angle of the mandible, is typical of a mass in the tail (inferolateral part) of the parotid gland. (Republished with permission from McGuirt WF, Johnson PE. *Evaluation and Treatment of the Patient with a Neck Mass*. Alexandria, VA: American Academy of Otolaryngology Head and Neck Surgery; 1998.)

nucleus of the brainstem and travels with cranial nerve (CN) IX. After passing through the jugular foramen, a branch turns superiorly to enter the middle ear. The nerve crosses the middle ear cleft and enters the middle cranial fossa. The secretomotor fibers course along the floor of the middle cranial fossa as the lesser superficial petrosal nerve and then exit the skull via the foramen ovale along with CN V3. The preganglionic parasympathetic fibers synapse in the otic ganglion, and the postganglionic fibers course along the auriculotemporal nerve to innervate the parotid gland.

The submandibular (or submaxillary) gland lies deep to the posterior floor of the mouth in the triangle formed by the mandible and the two bellies of the digastric muscle. Most of the gland rests on the mylohyoid muscle, but a portion wraps around the mylohyoid to rest between the mylohyoid and the hyoglossus. The gland drains via Wharton's duct, which opens through the sublingual caruncle adjacent to the lingual frenulum.

The sublingual gland is oblong in shape and lies next to the submandibular duct just deep to the mucosa of the anterior floor of the mouth. There is no specific duct for the sublingual gland, because it drains through several small ductules in the floor of the mouth as well as into the submandibular duct.

Secretomotor innervation of both the submandibular and sublingual glands begins in the superior salivatory nucleus of the brainstem. The fibers exit the brainstem in the cerebellopontile angle on the intermediary nerve, which joins CN VII in the internal acoustic meatus. The fibers leave CN VII via the chorda tympani and course through the middle ear. Occasionally, this nerve can be visualized just behind the tympanic membrane adjacent to the posterosuperior annulus. After traversing the petrotympanic fissure, the fibers join the lingual nerve. In the floor of the mouth, the fibers synapse in the submandibular ganglion. The postganglionic fibers then innervate the submandibular and sublingual glands.

Histologically, all salivary glands are made up of acini, which contain mucus and serous-producing cells. This acinus fluid empties into a ductal system that actively modifies water content and electrolyte composition before secretion. Saliva composition is gland specific. Parotid saliva is primarily serous, whereas minor salivary gland saliva is mainly mucinous. Submandibular and sublingual saliva is mixed.

History

The presenting symptoms, their onset, and their rate of development are critical. The symptoms may be acute or chronic, intermittent or relentlessly progressive, associated with time of day or activity, or associated with palliative or provocative events. It is important to know whether the symptoms are located in one or more glands; systemic symptoms are also important. The relationship of any swelling or pain with meals, recent regional trauma, and recent dental extraction may be important clues to the diagnosis. The growth rate, mobility, and pain associated with any mass should be explored and described. Facial nerve weakness or previous skin cancers on the ipsilateral side of the head (including the scalp), upper lip, or pinna suggest malignant neoplasm (either primary or metastatic).

Physical Examination

When the contralateral gland is normal, it may serve as a reference. The size, shape, and consistency of the gland should be noted with regard to induration, masses, or tenderness.

The parotid gland is generally not palpable as a distinct entity. The submandibular glands often become progressively ptotic with age and may mimic an enlarged submandibular gland or lymph node. **Bimanual examination** easily differentiates these entities and should be routine in the examination.

The tail of the parotid gland lies immediately inferior to the earlobe; a mass in this location can be confused with a cervical lymph node. The transverse process of the first cervical vertebra is also in this region and can mimic a parotid mass, especially in thin individuals.

Intraoral examination of the salivary ducts and ductal orifices may disclose erythema, edema, or discharge. The affected gland should be massaged while observing the respective duct orifice to determine salivary character. This maneuver may be uncomfortable for the patient who has an acute infection, so gentleness is important. It is helpful to dry the duct orifice area first with clean gauze to facilitate visualization of the saliva.

The oropharynx and mouth floor should be examined for masses or stones. A mass in the deep portion of the parotid gland may extend into the parapharyngeal space and cause medial displacement of the palate and tonsillar pillar, with little external swelling of the parotid gland itself. These and other parapharyngeal space masses are often asymptomatic and identified only by routine intraoral examination. Salivary stones are often visible as hard yellow objects at the orifice of Wharton's duct. Bimanual palpation of both Wharton's and Stensen's ducts should be performed to localize occult stones and to detect inflammation.

Facial nerve function should be evaluated in all patients with parotid lesions. The **House–Brackman** rating system is standard and should be used (*see* Chapter 24). Lingual and hypoglossal nerve function should be examined in patients with submandibular or sublingual gland processes.

Differential Diagnosis

The differential diagnosis of salivary gland diseases is listed in Table 21.1. Disorders can be divided broadly into three categories: inflammatory, metabolic, and neoplastic. Although the histology of most neoplastic disorders of the head and neck is straightforward, tumors of the salivary glands comprise a wide range of histologic types, with an equally wide range of biological behavior. Diagnosis and management are a challenge for the clinician and pathologist alike.

Additional Diagnostic Evaluation

The history and physical examination are important in the evaluation of salivary gland disorders. However, in nearly all cases of salivary gland masses, the need to make a histologic diagnosis is even more critical. One technique that can be performed in the office is fine-needle–aspiration biopsy (FNAB),

Table 21.1 Differential Diagnosis of Salivary Gland Diseases

Inflammatory Diseases
  Acute
    Acute suppurative sialadenitis
    Mumps
  Chronic
    Sialolithiasis
    Benign lymphoproliferative lesions
    Granulomatous diseases
    Sialadenitis
    Stricture
    HIV
    Mycobacterial infection
    Actinomycosis
    Sarcoidosis
    Heerfordt's disease

Neoplastic Diseases
  Benign
    Pleomorphic adenoma
    Warthin's tumor
    Oncocytoma
    Monomorphic adenoma
    Sebaceous adenoma
  Malignant
    Mucoepidermoid carcinoma
    Adenoid cystic carcinoma
    Malignant mixed tumor
    Acinic cell carcinoma
    Adenocarcinoma
    Carcinoma ex pleomorphic
    Oncocytic carcinoma
    Primary squamous cell carcinoma
    Undifferentiated carcinoma
    Metastatic

Metabolic and Endocrine Diseases
  Diabetes
  Menopause
  Malnutrition
  Gouty parotitis

Cysts
  Congenital
  Acquired

Trauma

Radiation-Induced Xerostomia

Hypersalivation
  Medications
  Oral dyskinesia

which is helpful in suggesting a cytologic diagnosis. However, because FNAB is not 100% accurate, its results must be interpreted carefully.

Conventional radiography provides little useful information. In experienced hands, **contrast sialography** (i.e., instillation of contrast material through the oral opening of a salivary duct) can demonstrate evidence of chronic inflammation, sialectasis, and intraglandular obstructions. It is usually performed with **computed tomography (CT)** but is rarely used because other imaging techniques provide equally useful information with less discomfort.

Nuclear scans using **technetium-99m pertechnetate** demonstrate a "hot spot" in a patient with Warthin's tumor or oncocytoma. FNAB provides even more information. CT and **magnetic resonance imaging (MRI)** are helpful in identifying the location and anatomical relationship of salivary neoplasms and are useful in planning surgical excision (Fig 21.2). These scans cannot differentiate between benign and malignant lesions. Radiographic characteristics, such as tumor margins and the presence of nodal disease, can help predict malignancy, but a biopsy is always needed to confirm this determination. The ultimate biopsy required in most instances is a complete excision of the submandibular gland and, in the case of the parotid salivary gland, a superficial parotidectomy.

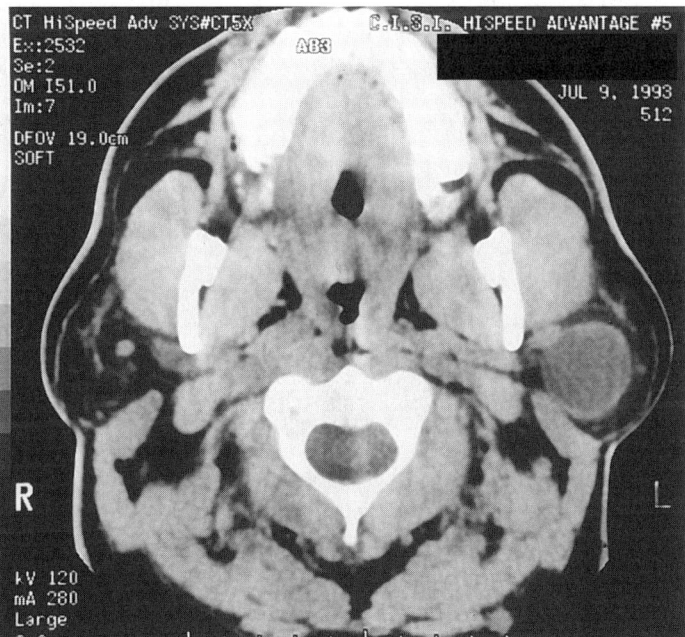

Figure 21.2 Computed tomography scan showing the typical appearance of a well-encapsulated pleomorphic adenoma (benign mixed tumor) of the parotid gland. (Courtesy of Dr. Gary Clayman.)

Diagnosis and Management of Specific Salivary Gland Disorders

The diagnosis and management of salivary gland disorders are summarized in the Algorithm.

Acute Inflammatory Diseases

Acute suppurative sialadenitis typically presents with a unilateral, swollen, tender gland associated with fever. Eating may worsen pain and swelling (Case 21.1). Leukocytosis is common, and sepsis can develop (especially in elderly and debilitated patients who become dehydrated). Massaging the gland while watching the intraoral opening of the gland's duct often demonstrates frank pus. Bimanual palpation (i.e., with one hand on the skin and the other in the mouth) is used to detect obstructing calculi. Radiologic studies, including plain films of the floor of the mouth and CT scans, are often helpful in identifying obstructing stones (Fig. 21.3).

Treatment consists of hydration; antibiotics; warm, moist compresses; and sialagogues (i.e., activities or substances that increase saliva flow [e.g., lemon drops, chewing gum]). The common bacterial pathogens are *Staphylococcus* in the parotid gland and *Streptococcus* in the submandibular gland. Cultures of expressed pus can be obtained easily before instituting antibiotic therapy. Antibiotic coverage is directed against these bacteria by using appropriate drugs for resistant organisms; they are continued for 10 days. Warm, moist compresses to the area may provide some symptomatic if not therapeutic assistance, and sialagogues promote physiologic irrigation. Vigorous oral care in debilitated, dehydrated elderly patients with **acute parotitis** is necessary and may help

---

Case 21.1 **Man with Acute Suppurative Sialadenitis**

A man 65 years of age is just recovering from an episode of gastroenteritis. He says only during the past 24 hours has he been able to "keep anything down." Approximately 2 days ago he noticed some pain under his left jaw. Now, whenever he gets ready to eat anything, his jaw hurts more and begins to swell up. With this history of probable dehydration and intermittent swelling associated with eating, submaxillary sialadenitis is high on the differential diagnosis list. Intraoral examination reveals scant clear saliva from the left Wharton's duct.

The patient is given 2 L intravenous rehydration fluids in the office and is begun on oral antibiotics. He maintains good hydration at home and sucks on lemon drops to stimulate saliva flow. Two days later, his symptoms have resolved completely.

enhance the flow of saliva. Patients with dentures should leave their dentures out, especially their lower denture, which may contribute to inflammation that obstructs Wharton's duct. The removal of obstructing stones is critical, and frequent reexaminations should be performed to ensure that additional stones have not become impacted at the duct orifice. Follow-up is necessary to assess treatment response; complete resolution of induration may take several weeks. Failure to respond to treatment may signify abscess formation or an obstruction that requires surgical drainage. In some cases, urgent excision of the submandibular gland may become necessary. Urgent parotidectomy for infection is performed rarely due to the risk to the facial nerve. As a result, parotitis that is unresponsive to antibiotics and hydration is treated occasionally with low-dose radiotherapy as palliation to decrease salivation. Chronic acute parotitis may require total parotidectomy, which is usually associated with temporary facial nerve weakness that resolves with time.

Mumps is an acute, febrile, viral disease that usually involves the salivary glands and occasionally affects the gonads, meninges, and pancreas. The peak age of onset is between 4 and 6 years, and 95% of adults have antibodies to the virus, indicating that infection is essentially universal. As many as 25 of every 1000 people have some meningeal involvement. Labyrinthitis and hearing loss may occur, with the latter usually being unilateral and total. One or all of the major salivary glands may become swollen and tender. The associ-

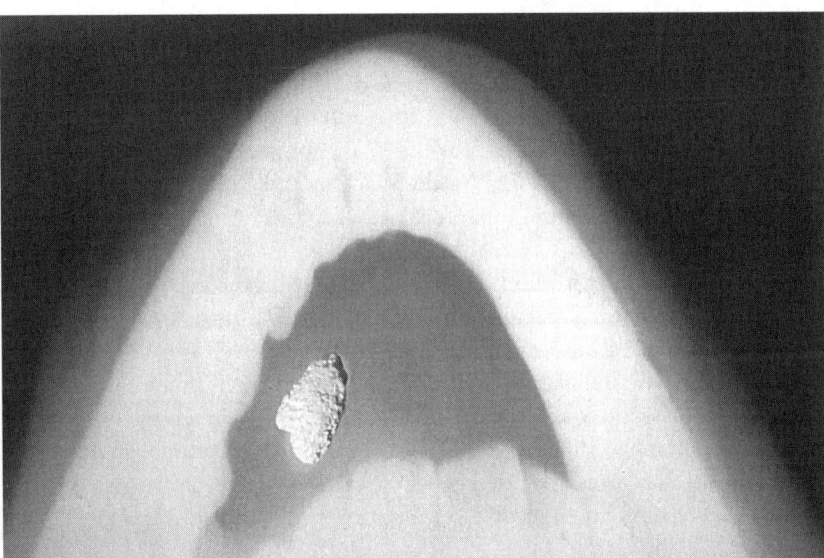

Figure 21.3 Submandibular duct stone superimposed on a submentovertex radiograph. (Courtesy of Dr. David E. Eibling.)

ated duct orifice is erythematous and swollen, but clear saliva is expressed. The diagnosis is made by the demonstration of virus in the urine up to 6 days before and 11 days after the acute symptoms. Temperature may range from 100° to 103°F and patients have significant lethargy, headache, and discomfort. White blood cell count is often normal. Treatment is symptomatic, and recovery is usually complete; however, sequelae can include sensorineural hearing loss and diabetes. Mumps that occurs in adults may be associated with orchitis, with the possible sequela of sterility. The introduction of the mumps vaccine 30 years ago has reduced the incidence of the acute disease dramatically.

Chronic Inflammatory Diseases

Chronic sialolithiasis affects the submandibular gland 90% of the time, with only approximately 10% of salivary stones occurring in the parotid gland. The sublingual gland rarely is affected. Stones can arise anywhere within the gland or duct, with intermittent symptoms of swelling and pain that are made worse by eating. The extent of symptoms is highly dependent on size and location of the calculus and, specifically, on the degree of salivary obstruction. The swelling generally subsides slowly between episodes. The stones often can be noted in the duct by bimanual palpation, and occasionally a white or yellow stone can be seen at the papilla.

Small stones sometimes can be expressed by gently milking the gland, whereas others may require a small incision to open the duct. Because approximately 20% of submandibular stones and 80% of parotid stones are radiolucent, the presence of a stone cannot be ruled out by radiography alone.

Therapy consists of removing the stone and treating any acute suppurative sialadenitis with antibiotics, warm moist compresses and sialagogues. Repeated episodes and glands with stones that cannot be removed require surgical removal of the offending gland (Case 21.2). Prevention is facilitated by adequate hydration and sialagogues.

Benign lymphoepithelial lesions include **Sjögren's syndrome (SS)**, **Mikulicz's syndrome**, **sicca complex**, and **chronic punctate sialadenitis**. SS is the complex of **keratoconjunctivitis sicca and xerostomia** due to glandular lymphocytic infiltration and is the second most common autoimmune disease (after rheumatoid arthritis). The term *Mikulicz's syndrome* suggests idiopathic asymptomatic enlargement of the salivary and/or lacrimal glands and is rarely used. *Sicca complex* is used to describe SS-like symptoms without evidence of a collagen vascular disease. *Chronic punctate sialadenitis* is a term based on the sialographic appearance in these patients.

Although SS presents most often in middle-aged women, it can occur in either sex at any age. It is a multiglandular disease in which one or all salivary

> **Case 21.2** **Man with Chronic Sialolithiasis**
>
> A man 34 years of age is referred for the evaluation of recurrent episodes of swelling and tenderness in the left floor of the mouth and the submental region. He states that a painless swelling, brought on by eating, occurs several times per month. However, approximately four times per year, the swelling is associated with redness, pain, and a foul, gritty taste. These episodes resolve with outpatient antibiotics, warm compresses, and sialagogues. He denies dry eyes, dry mouth, and constitutional symptoms. Past medical and surgical histories are negative.
>
> Physical examination of head and neck is normal, except for left submandibular fullness on neck palpation. Bimanual palpation of left floor of the mouth and submandibular area are remarkable for firmness and ropy texture in the left proximal Wharton's duct. Clear saliva is expressed from bilateral Stensen's and right Wharton's duct; a scant mucoid discharge is expressed from the left Wharton's papilla. No cervical adenopathy is appreciated. Further studies include a submental vertex radiograph, which suggests calcification in the left floor of the mouth. A FNAB shows chronic inflammation.
>
> A submandibular stone is suspected and the treatment options are presented, including continued medical management, transoral excision of suspected salivary stone, or submandibular gland excision. The patient opts for left submandibular excision to relieve symptoms and to rule out a neoplastic process. The pathology report shows chronic inflammation, multiple stones in the proximal duct, and no evidence of neoplasm.

glands may be involved at any time and in any combination. The presentation is usually with asymptomatic, diffuse glandular swelling; however, occasionally, there may be mild pain. The disease can be divided into two categories: primary (with glandular involvement only) and secondary (with other associated collagen vascular diseases [rheumatoid arthritis is most common]). Parotid gland swelling, which can be unilateral, occurs in 80% of primary cases and in approximately one third of secondary cases (Fig. 21.4). Diagnosis can be confirmed by detecting SS-A and SS-B antibodies in the serum. A high percentage of patients demonstrate other serologic evidence of autoimmune disease, with rheumatoid factor and antinuclear antibodies present in their serum. Xerostomia generally is caused by the involvement of the minor salivary glands; however, occasionally, thickened saliva can be visualized extruding from the parotid duct orifices. Biopsy of the minor salivary glands can also help in the diagnosis. Histologic examination shows periductal infiltration of lymphocytes and atrophy of acini. Over time, myoepithelial cells become more prominent.

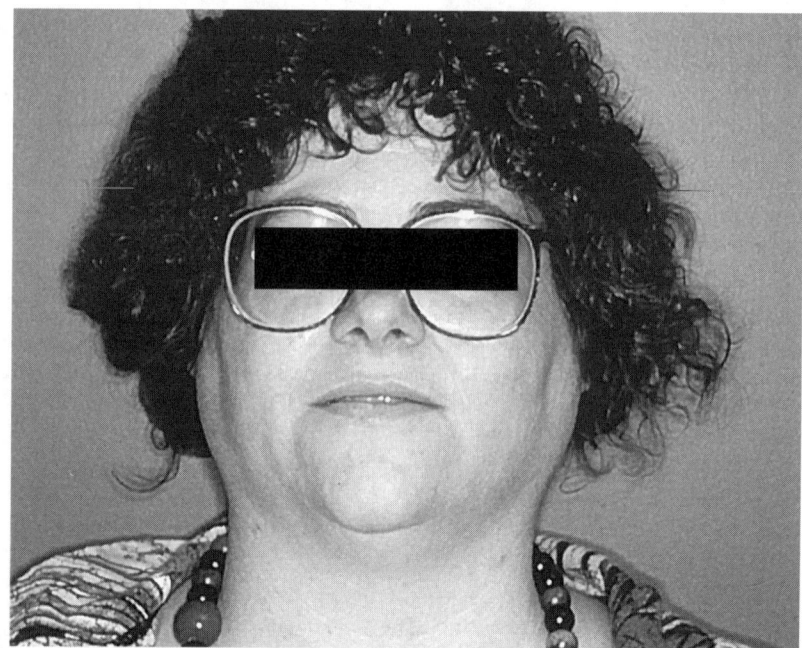

Figure 21.4 Patient with bilateral parotid swelling from Sjögren's disease. (Courtesy of Dr. Stephen Cass.)

Treatment is aimed at increasing salivary flow and at preventing inspissation of secretions, which eventually leads to infection. Increasing oral fluid intake, sialagogues, and gland massage is helpful. Antibiotics are indicated for secondary infection. Rarely, surgical excision of the glands is required for chronic infection or for cosmesis. There are recent reports that the use of oral pilocarpine can assist in symptomatic relief (*see* Radiation-Induced Xerostomia section below). A number of conditions are associated with SS, including Raynaud's phenomenon, myositis, diffuse interstitial lung disease, and renal abnormalities. These patients are also at increased risk for lymphoma and anaplastic carcinoma.

Granulomatous diseases are relatively uncommon processes that can affect the salivary glands, but they rarely exist in isolation. Salivary involvement generally is associated with signs of systemic disease. Salivary flow is usually normal, and pain is uncommon. Examples of granulomatous processes that may involve the salivary glands are tuberculosis, actinomycosis, and sarcoidosis. Treatment is directed toward the systemic disease.

Mycobacterial infection may involve the periparotid lymph nodes, rarely affecting the gland directly. **Actinomycosis** also may involve the periparotid nodes and usually is associated with recent dental work or trauma. "Sulfur granules" in the pus is pathognomonic, and culture requires specific media and growing conditions. Treatment of choice is penicillin and surgical drainage. **Sarcoidosis** may present as bilateral parotid enlargement in which the lacrimal glands are frequently involved. **Heerfordt's disease (uveoparotid fever)** is a variant that includes fever, lacrimal and parotid swelling, multiple CN palsies, and chorioretinitis. These symptoms usually resolve spontaneously; thus, treatment is necessary only for complications.

HIV disease can cause xerostomia, and histologic findings are similar to that of SS. Salivary gland masses can arise from Kaposi's sarcoma, non-Hodgkin's lymphoma, and lymphoepithelial cysts. FNAB helps to make a diagnosis. **Lymphoepithelial cysts in the parotid salivary gland** are often bilateral and massive, with a multilocular radiographic appearance. Treatment for these cysts remains controversial because excision usually results in recurrence. Aspiration provides temporary relief, and many find that repeated aspiration on an as-needed basis is the best therapy.

Chronic sialadenitis is thought to occur after repeated episodes of acute suppurative sialadenitis. It arises from scarring and fibrous replacement of the gland during acute episodes, eventually leading to obstruction and salivary stasis. Asymptomatic periods vary in length from weeks to months. Cure is obtained only through surgical excision of the affected gland, although total parotidectomy is required, and there is a significant risk of temporary facial nerve paresis.

Stricture of a salivary duct is a rare disorder that usually results from trauma. Symptoms are similar to those of calculi. Dilatation may be helpful, but surgical repair is often necessary.

Neoplastic Diseases

Approximately 80% of all salivary gland neoplasms occur in the parotid gland, 15% occur in the submandibular gland, and 5% occur in the minor and sublingual glands. Malignancy rates tend to increase as the gland size decreases. A rough estimate of malignancy rates provides an easy-to-remember rule of thumb for salivary gland malignancy: 80% of parotid masses are benign, and 20% are malignant; 50% of submandibular gland tumors are benign, and 50% are malignant; and 20% of minor salivary gland growths are benign, and 80% are malignant.

Benign neoplasms usually present as slow-growing asymptomatic masses. Rapid growth, a hard or fixed mass, overlying skin or mucosal ulceration, and facial nerve weakness suggest malignancy; however, malignant tumors also may grow slowly and be asymptomatic. Because a FNAB that suggests malignancy also indicates further evaluation, surgical excision (or incisional biopsy in select cases) makes the diagnosis. Incisional biopsy, if performed, must be done carefully to avoid risking facial nerve injury.

Although the differential diagnosis for both benign and malignant neoplasms of the salivary glands is extensive, each list is dominated by one type: **pleomorphic adenomas (benign mixed tumors)**, which account for approximately 65% of the benign tumors (Fig. 21.5). **Warthin's tumors** and monomorphic adenomas also occur with relative frequency. Malignant lesions are most often mucoepidermoid carcinoma, but adenoid cystic carcinoma and occasional malignant mixed tumors also are seen. Other neoplasms occur with much less frequency.

Factors that influence survival in patients with malignant lesions include histopathologic diagnosis, stage at presentation, presence of lymph node metastasis, and whether the tumor represents a recurrence. In contrast with mucosal malignancy, tumor grade may affect prognosis dramatically in salivary gland malignancy. Facial nerve weakness and spontaneous pain suggest an unfavorable prognosis. Patients with salivary gland malignancies must be followed for periods of up to 15 or 20 years after initial treatment, because delayed recurrence is common, especially with adenoid cystic carcinoma (Fig. 21.6).

Treatment of both benign and malignant neoplasms is surgical. The most common parotid neoplasm is pleomorphic adenoma, for which the risk of recurrence and iatrogenic facial nerve injury is increased considerably if the tu-

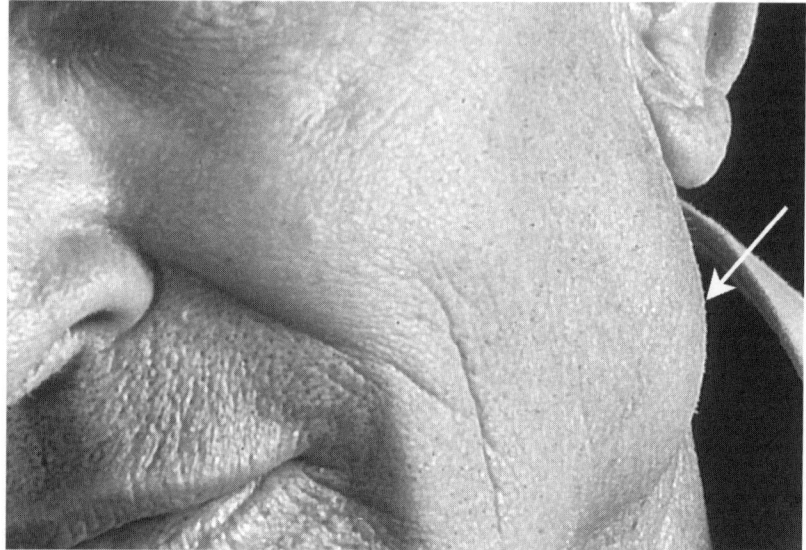

Figure 21.5 Patient with a pleomorphic adenoma in the tail of his parotid gland (*arrow*). (Courtesy of Dr. Jonas T. Johnson.)

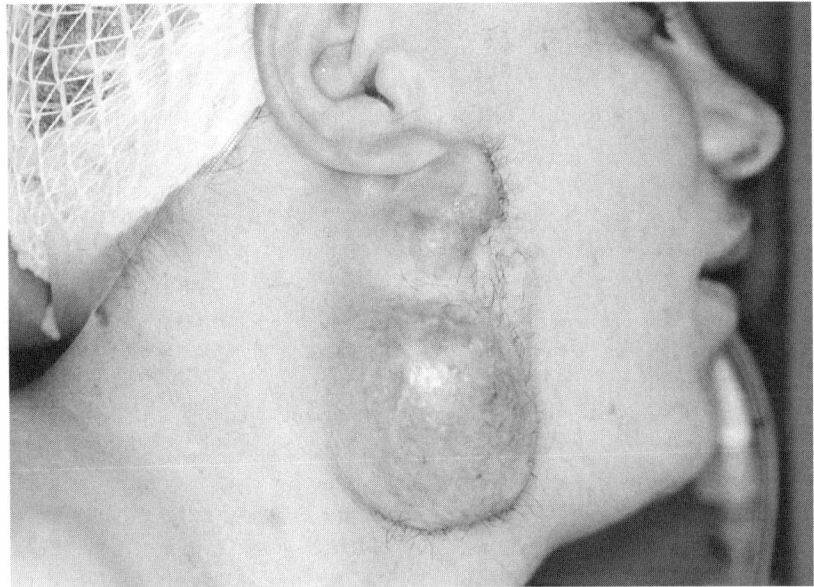

Figure 21.6 Young man about to undergo surgery for an adenoid cystic carcinoma of his parotid gland. (Courtesy Dr. Gary Clayman.)

mor is simply enucleated. Therefore, the minimal surgical excision for parotid tumors is considered to be superficial parotidectomy. In this technique, the facial nerve is identified first and that portion of the parotid gland superficial to the nerve (not an actual "lobe") is removed completely, usually excising the entire tumor with a cuff of surrounding normal gland (Fig. 21.7). Facial nerve weakness is uncommon and, if present, is temporary. Cutting into a tumor should be avoided because recurrences are problematic and usually multiple. The surgical management of recurrent pleomorphic adenoma is technically challenging and is associated with a high risk of permanent facial nerve injury. Hence, any mass in the region of the parotid gland must be dealt with appropriately, or else the patient may be burdened with the lifelong sequelae of enucleation with tumor spillage and facial nerve injury.

Deep lobe and parapharyngeal parotid gland tumors also are removed surgically after identification of the facial nerve and its branches by superficial parotidectomy. Temporary nerve paresis occurs because the nerve filaments have to be displaced to remove the tumor below them; both the stretching and the disruption of their blood supply contribute to the paresis. Submandibular gland tumors are removed by gland excision, and minor salivary tumors are treated as necessary to ensure complete tumor excision. Malignant tumors are treated according to the stage and histologic type and grade, with extended resection, facial nerve sacrifice, and neck dissection when indicated. Postoperative radiotherapy has been demonstrated to reduce the incidence of recurrence in some higher-grade tumors and is used routinely in these cases (Case 21.3). There are insufficient data to support the routine use of adjuvant chemotherapy, although it is used in selected cases of advanced or recurrent disease.

Management of the sequelae and complications of parotidectomy consists primarily of managing **facial nerve paralysis** (especially its related eye complications) and **Frey's syndrome**. (*See* Chapter 24 for more details on the management of facial paralysis.) Frey's syndrome is gustatory sweating that the affected patient feels as drainage at the surgical site during meals after parotidectomy (Case 21.4). The condition can be problematic, causing embarrassment and soaked collars, coats, etc. The patient usually believes that the drainage is from a fistula or other leak, when in fact the moisture is simply sweat that has been triggered by a postganglionic parasympathetic cross-innervation of the sweat glands in the skin after the removal of the physiologic target organ. The syndrome can be treated by interrupting 1) the preganglionic parasympathetic fibers as they cross the middle ear (tympanic neurectomy), or 2) the postganglionic fibers by elevating the skin flap off the nerves and interposing a layer of fascia. Both options carry some risk; hence, most physicians elect to treat the syndrome with liberal applications of roll-on an-

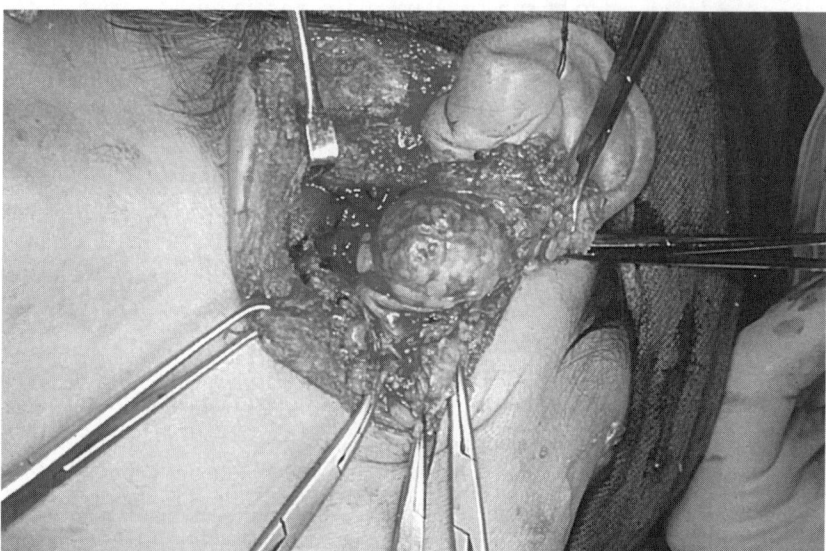

Figure 21.7 Intraoperative photograph showing the facial nerve freed from the surrounding tissue. (Courtesy of Dr. Jonas T. Johnson.)

Case 21.3 — Young Woman with a Malignant Neoplasm

A woman 21 years of age presents with a 2-month history of fullness in the right submandibular region. There is no pain, fluctuance, foul or gritty taste, fever, or weight loss. Past medical and surgical histories and a review of systems are unremarkable.

Physical examination shows a healthy-appearing young woman. The head and neck examination is normal except for a discretely enlarged right submandibular gland that is mobile and nontender and measures 5 cm x 6 cm. A 1.5 cm right jugulodigastric mass also is noted. Examination of the cranial nerves is normal. A computed tomography scan of the neck shows a heterogeneous neoplasm within the parenchyma of the right submandibular gland that measures 2 cm x 3 cm. FNAB is not diagnostic, and a repeat study suggests malignant cells. Excisional biopsy of the right submandibular gland shows high-grade mucoepidermoid carcinoma; frozen section examination of the jugulodigastric mass shows reactive adenopathy. The margins of excision were clear.

The multidisciplinary tumor board recommends postoperative radiation therapy for this case.

Case 21.4 — Woman with Frey's Syndrome That Developed After Parotidectomy for Pleomorphic Adenoma

A woman 35 years of age who is recovering from an upper respiratory infection notices a small lump just behind her right jawbone near her ear. It is not tender and does not really bother her. Approximately 6 months later, she becomes concerned that the lump seems bigger. Her physician performs a fine-needle–aspiration biopsy, which yields salivary tissue consistent with a pleomorphic adenoma.

After discussing treatment options, the patient decides on surgical treatment. Several weeks later, she undergoes a superficial parotidectomy, with an uneventful recovery. Four months after her surgery, at a Fourth of July picnic, the patient notices a lot of sweating on her face while eating her meal. At first, she ascribed it to the hot weather, but the sweating over her right cheek continued and now occurs every time she eats.

Seeking advice from her physician, the patient is diagnosed with Frey's syndrome (or gustatory sweating). Topical roll-on antiperspirant helps, but she still experiences some sweating, which is bothersome to her in more formal dining settings. Trial injection with Botox provides complete symptom relief. She understands that periodic reinjection will be needed but is satisfied with the results.

tiperspirant. Recent use of Botox for suppression of gustatory sweating has been promising.

Metabolic and Endocrine Diseases

Metabolic and endocrine diseases are rare causes of salivary gland disorders and are most often seen in postmenopausal women, diabetes patients, and alcoholic individuals. The presentation is usually of asymptomatic, diffuse enlargement of the parotid glands. Biopsy specimens generally reveal fatty degeneration of glandular elements; fatty infiltration also can be visualized on CT and MRI scans. This condition may occur in malnourished patients. Gout may cause a rare form of parotitis diagnosed by uric acid crystals in the saliva. Treatment is directed at any symptoms referable to the systemic disease and is the same as that for the underlying disease.

Cysts

Salivary gland cysts may be congenital or acquired. Congenital cysts of the parotid gland generally originate from the first branchial cleft. Although present from birth, these cysts may not develop until adulthood, usually in association with an infection. Treatment is surgical excision, and may be challenging due to the proximity of the facial nerve and the disordered anatomy. Uncommonly, aspiration is diagnostic and leads to cyst resolution. Acquired cysts are often obstructive pseudocysts resulting from surgery or trauma, or associated with HIV disease (Case 21.5).

Obstruction of sublingual gland ducts may result in a cyst appearing in the floor of the mouth called a **ranula**–a word derived from Latin for "little frog"–because these types of cysts resemble the round protrusion of a frog's neck as it croaks (Fig. 21.8). These may extend inferiorly through the mylo-

---

Case 21.5 **Man with Salivary Gland Cysts Associated with AIDS**

A male AIDS patient 29 years of age is bothered by the facial distortion caused by his parotid cysts. For the past 2 years, his physician has aspirated the cysts before important social events but now offers the patient a trial of sclerosis.

The next time the cysts are aspirated, a sclerosing substance is injected into the cyst immediately after aspiration. Although the cysts never get any smaller than their usual size just after aspiration, they do not enlarge again. The patient is pleased with the results.

hyoid muscle to present as a swelling in the submental region (plunging ranula). Treatment is surgical excision in continuity with the entire sublingual gland. Recurrences are difficult to manage due to scarring and the disordered anatomical relationships with the adjacent submandibular gland duct and lingual nerve.

Hypersalivation

Disorders of increased salivation are unusual but particularly problematic for the clinician. Many cases of perceived hypersalivation are, in fact, a manifestation of **oral dysphagia**, with decreased oral control, reduced spontaneous swallowing frequency, and an accumulation of saliva in the oral cavity. Oral dyskinesias associated with neurological dysfunction or drug use also can enhance salivation while reducing salivary clearance. In severe cases, the patient may be incapacitated due to constant drooling or having to spit continuously into a container or towel. Certain drugs and toxins (e.g., mercury, lithium) also can induce hypersalivation. Discontinuation and avoidance of the implicated chemical may provide relief. In rare cases, surgical excision of the major salivary glands or even radiotherapy may be warranted. In severely neurologically impaired patients, rerouting the salivary ducts posteriorly can reduce the drooling associated with this condition.

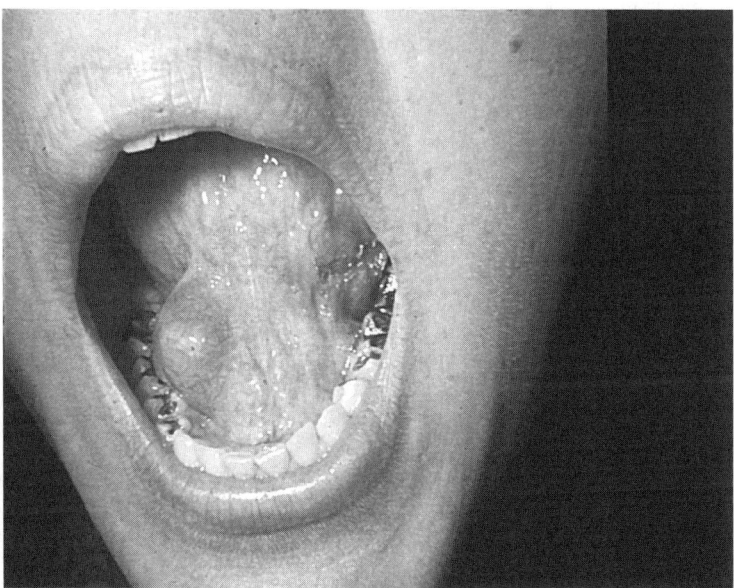

Figure 21.8 This mass on the right floor of the mouth represents a ranula and is filled with thick mucous secretions. (Courtesy of Dr. David E. Eibling.)

Radiation-Induced Xerostomia

Treating head and neck malignancies with radiotherapy that encompasses the salivary glands inevitably results in a rapid reduction of salivary flow. Although radiation-induced stomatitis may resolve several weeks to months after completion of therapy, the reduction in quantity and increase in viscosity of salivary flow is irreversible. This effect leads to secondary xerostomia, dysphagia, increased dental caries, and generalized oral discomfort. For many patients, it is the most significant sequela of their malignancy. The use of topical solutions, artificial saliva, and increased hydration can provide some symptomatic relief. Most patients carry a water bottle with them at all times and must make other lifestyle changes to accommodate to the condition.

The use of oral pilocarpine as a parasympathomimetic agent to increase salivation both during and after radiotherapy has been demonstrated to increase salivary flow, decrease viscosity, and greatly enhance patient comfort. The drug is available in 5-mg tablets (Salogen) administered at a dosage of 5 mg three times daily. Current recommendations call for consultation with an ophthalmologist to rule out glaucoma and, for patients with a history of cardiac disease, a cardiac physician before initiating therapy. Some radiotherapists begin therapy with this medication at the beginning of radiotherapy if the salivary glands are in the radiation field. Recently, there has been evidence that some patients with SS also may experience symptomatic improvement with pilocarpine.

Trauma

Although the salivary glands are protected by surrounding bone and soft tissue, they are often injured in knife or gunshot wounds or, more commonly, in automobile or industrial accidents. The wounds are categorized as blunt, sharp, or penetrating, and there is usually trauma to the surrounding bony or soft tissue as well. Parotid gland injuries in particular can lead to significant long-term morbidity and require immediate surgical management. During the initial examination, it is important to note facial nerve function and to question paramedical personnel who were at the scene, because delayed-onset, traumatic facial nerve paralysis has a markedly different prognosis and treatment from immediate-onset facial nerve paralysis. Early repair of severed facial nerve branches and Stensen's duct is important to ensure an optimal outcome.

Danger Signs

Signs and symptoms that require immediate treatment or specialist consultation include the following:
- Parotid mass with decreased or absent ipsilateral facial nerve function
- Infection that worsens despite antibiotic treatment
- Palpable or visible ductal stones with acute infection
- Sublingual or mouth floor swelling with woody induration (Ludwig's angina)
- Positive FNAB for malignancy
- Mass associated with mucosal or skin erosion
- Trauma with decreased nerve function, fractures, or significant soft tissue injury

Summary

Salivary gland disorders are common and may present as anatomical or functional abnormalities. Swelling or masses may represent tumor, either benign or malignant, and require evaluation and treatment. Surgical excision usually is required for both diagnosis and treatment. Functional disorders represent clinical challenges, although symptomatic relief may enhance patient comfort significantly. Identifying the underlying systemic disease may provide an opportunity for early intervention and a reduction of long-term complications.

SUGGESTED READINGS

Ottaviani F, Capaccio P, Rivolta R, et al. Salivary gland stones: ultrasound evaluation in shock-wave lithotripsy. *Radiology.* 1977;204:437–41.
   This article describes the use of ultrasound with extracorporeal electromagnetic shock-wave lithotripsy for the treatment of parotid gland or submandibular duct stones. This may be a reasonable alternative to surgery in patients who are poor surgical candidates.

Ron E, Saftlas AF. Head and neck radiation carcinogenesis: epidemiologic evidence. *Otolaryngol Head Neck Surg.* 1996;115:403–8.
   This article reviews the effects of medical radiation exposure on the head and neck tissues. The authors make an estimate of relative risk and support a connection between radiation exposure and salivary tumors.

Spiro RH. Changing trends in the management of salivary tumors. *Semin Surg Oncol.* 1995;11:240–5.

Kamal SA, Othman EO. Diagnosis and treatment of parotid tumors. *J Laryngol Otol.* 1977;111:316–21.
   These two articles review the situations in which the use of FNAB, CT, and MRI is and is not helpful in evaluating salivary gland masses. They contain a nice review of diagnostic points on history and physical examination and a concise summary of treatment recommendations.

22

Surgical Treatment of Thyroid and Parathyroid Gland Disease

Gregory W. Randolph, MD
Jon K. Thiringer, DO
Peter J. Martin, MD

Thyroid nodular disease is common. Approximately 5% of the adult population has a palpable thyroid nodule, and between 30% and 50% of the older adult population have thyroid nodules that are evident on sonography (1). Thyroid cancer occurs in approximately 5% of thyroid nodules (2,3). Approximately 13,900 new cases of thyroid cancer are diagnosed annually in the United States, comprising 1% of all new thyroid cases (4). Despite a generally good prognosis, almost 1200 patients per year die of this disease. Surgical intervention is indicated for 1) proven carcinoma or lesions that are judged suspicious for carcinoma, 2) substernal or cervical goiter that affects adjacent cervical viscera, and 3) patients with Graves' disease and toxic nodules who are not candidates for antithyroid medications or radioactive iodine ablation.

Anatomy

The thyroid isthmus overlies the second, third, and fourth tracheal rings and is fixed to the trachea through the anterior and posterior (Berry's) suspensory ligaments. These attachments allow the thyroid to move superiorly with the larynx during deglutition, permitting the examiner to distinguish between a thyroid nodule (which moves up with the larynx) and an adjacent nonfixed cervical node (which does not). Thyroid lobes are bordered laterally by the carotid artery and medially by the trachea and esophagus. The vascular supply to the thyroid is via the superior thyroid artery, a branch of the external carotid artery, and the inferior thyroid artery that arises from the thyrocervical trunk of the subclavian artery. The recurrent laryngeal nerves branch from the vagus in the upper chest and return into the neck by traveling deep to the thyroid lobes and close to the tracheoesophageal groove. Exact recurrent laryngeal nerve position varies, especially with goitrous thyroid enlargement; these nerves provide motor function to the larynx, entering the larynx on either side at the level of the cricothyroid joint. Injury to a recurrent laryngeal nerve results in vocal cord paralysis, which is typically manifested by a weak and breathy voice (rather than a hoarse voice) and by dysphagia or aspiration. The external branch of the superior laryngeal nerve arises from the vagus in the neck and travels to the cricothyroid muscle, running close to the thyroid superior pole. Injury to this nerve results in more subtle vocal cord dysfunction, a reduction in vocal cord tensing, and a loss of high vocal registers.

Embryologically the thyroid derives from a base-of-the-tongue midline diverticulum and descends in the midline neck along the thyroglossal duct tract to assume its normal adult position in the base of the neck. If embryologic migration has been arrested completely, a lingual thyroid results, without normal tissue in the orthotopic site. If only the most inferior portion of the thyroglossal duct tract is maintained, a pyramidal lobe is formed. If remnant tissue persists higher in the neck, it may manifest clinically in the adult as a midline upper neck cyst (thyroglossal duct cyst).

Thyroid Function Tests

Thyroid hormone (TH) production and secretion is regulated by the anterior pituitary gland's thyroid-stimulating hormone (TSH). Ninety percent of circulating TH is thyroxine (T_4); 10% is triiodothyronine (T_3), the more physiologically active form of TH. Eighty percent of T_3 is made through peripheral conversion of T_4. Anterior pituitary thyrotrophs with appropriate hypothalamic thyroid-releasing hormone monitor the plasma levels of T_3 and T_4 and elaborate TSH. Exogenous T_4 taken for "suppression" results in decreases in TSH level. The decreased TSH level during suppressive therapy leads to a reduction in thyroid gland size and vascularity, which can be associated with the reduction of thyroid nodule size during suppressive therapy. Circulating T_3 and T_4 are predominantly protein bound (mainly to thyroid-binding globulin [TBG]), with only 1% representing free active hormone. Therefore, total T_3 and T_4 laboratory measures (the total of free and protein-bound hormone) can fluctuate with changes in the TBG level; however, pituitary thyroid axis maintains free TH within strict physiologic ranges. Pregnancy can increase the TBG level; hypoproteinemic states can decrease it. T_3 resin uptake and its related TH-binding ratio are measures that allow for correction of total T_4 levels for TBG fluctuation.

When obtained as a third-generation ultrasensitive assay capable of detecting 0.01 mU/L, TSH levels allow definitive diagnosis of thyroid functional status (hypothyroidism, euthyroidism, or hyperthyroidism) and thus represents an excellent screening test to exclude thyroid functional disease during work-up of the thyroid nodule. Other thyroid function tests should be obtained only if TSH level is abnormal. If TSH level is high, the patient is hypothyroid. If TSH level is low, the patient is hyperthyroid. In patients with multinodular goiter, multiple nodules grade toward autonomous function slowly over time. In such patients, the TSH can be in the low-to-normal range with normal T_3 and T_4 measures, representing a state of prehyperthyroidism called subclinical hyperthyroidism. Iodine loads, such as computed tomography (CT) scan dye, actually can cause subclinical hyperthyroidism to become frank hyperthyroidism and therefore should be avoided until thyroid function test results are obtained. TSH level also is used to monitor the adequacy of replacement and suppressive therapies.

Thyroid Nodular Disease

A thorough history, physical examination, and fine-needle–aspiration biopsy (FNAB) should be performed in euthyroid patients who present with a palpable thyroid abnormality (Fig. 22.1).

History

Patients under 20 years of age have an increased risk of thyroid carcinoma (5); patients over 50 years of age have a significantly worse prognosis if a thyroid malignancy is diagnosed. A history of exposure to low-dose ionizing radiation therapy increases the risk of thyroid carcinoma in patients who present with a palpable thyroid abnormality (6). A family history of medullary carcinoma dramatically increases the risk of this relatively rare form of thyroid cancer. A rapid increase in nodule size often indicates hemorrhage into a benign nodule but may represent malignancy. Pain is associated commonly with the rapid enlargement of a nodule through hemorrhage or subacute granulomatous thyroiditis, but it also can be present in advanced thyroid malignancies. Similarly, symptoms of respiratory distress, hoarseness, cough, and dysphagia may occur with both benign goiter and advanced thyroid malignancies. In general, thyroid malignancy is not associated with functional thyroid disorders; therefore, historical evidence of hypo- or hyperthyroidism reduces the risk of malignancy (7).

Surgical Treatment of Thyroid and Parathyroid Gland Disease   453

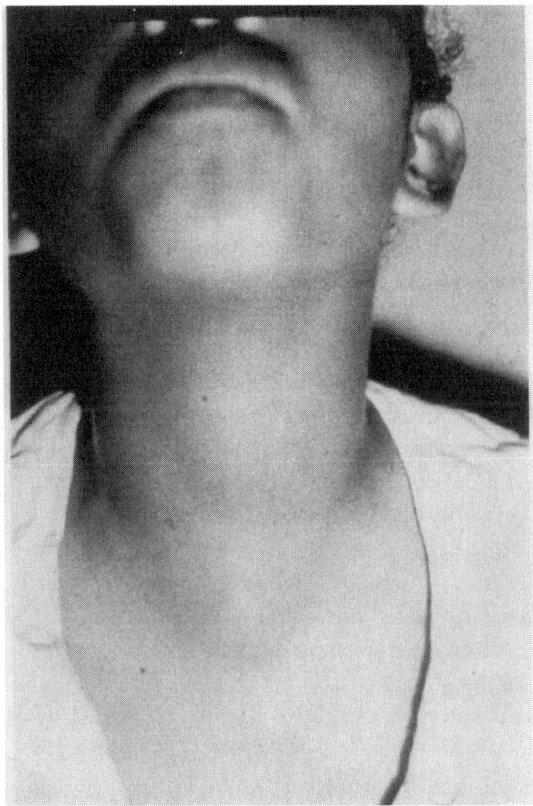

Figure 22.1 A large right-sided thyroid mass. (Republished with permission from McGuirt WF, Johnson PE. *Evaluation and Treatment of the Patient with a Neck Mass*. Alexandria, VA: American Academy of Otolaryngology–Head and Neck Surgery; 1998.)

Physical Examination of the Thyroid

During the physical examination of the thyroid, it is essential to orient the gland to its normal position adjacent to the laryngeal cartilage. Locating the midline thyroid cartilage notch (Adam's apple) allows identification of the thyroid cartilage lamina. Directly below the thyroid cartilage is the anterior arch of the cricoid, which is palpated easily. The anterior arch of the cricoid can be identified as a thick, hard, ring-like prominence below the thyroid cartilage in the midline neck. One finger's breadth below the anterior cricoid ring is the thyroid isthmus, which can be palpated as a tubular prominence overlying the upper cervical trachea. Laterally, the thyroid lobes are palpable in the cleft between the trachea medially and the sternocleidomastoid muscle and carotid sheath structures laterally. A helpful maneuver is to have the patient swallow, which allows the isthmus and thyroid lobes to move up and roll under the examining finger. With this maneuver, one can identify thyroid nodules 1 cm and greater in size. During the physical examination of large or inferiorly situated goiters, extension of the goiter's lower edge to the clavicle may indicate substernal extension and thus the need for CT. Pemburton's sign also should be assessed (*see* Evaluation in the section on Goiter below).

The presence of more than one nodule in the thyroid should not deter the examiner from performing **FNAB of the dominant nodule**, because the risk of malignancy in a multinodular gland with a dominant nodule is equivalent to that in a solitary nodule (2,8). The concern for malignancy increases in larger firm nodules and in those affixed to the laryngotracheal complex. **Malignancy is also more likely if the examination reveals coexistent cervical lymphadenopathy or vocal cord paralysis**. All patients with thyroid lesions should have their vocal cord mobility assessed. The classic symptoms of unilateral vocal cord paralysis are a weak and breathy voice (as opposed to true hoarseness) and cough while swallowing liquids. However, vocal cord paralysis may be present with normal voice and swallowing due to contralateral vocal cord compensation. Vocal cord paralysis rarely occurs in benign disease. Malignant infiltration of the nerve is also rare.

The history and physical examination are relatively insensitive in the detection of thyroid malignancy; however they do provide a clinical setting in which one can then interpret the FNAB results (Table 22.1).

Work-Up

Assessment of TSH is recommended in the work-up of the thyroid nodule to exclude a functional thyroid disorder. Almost all patients with thyroid nodules and thyroid cancer are euthyroid (7,9). In general, an abnormal TSH level diverts the evaluation from a work-up directed at ruling out malignancy with FNAB toward diagnosing the underlying thyroid functional disorder (e.g., Hashimoto's thyroiditis, toxic nodule), which usually does not involve FNAB. Such a work-up includes full thyroid function tests and perhaps I^{123} scanning. Thyroglobulin level, although helpful in follow-up after thyroid surgery and radioiodine-remnant ablation in patients with well-differentiated thyroid cancer (papillary and follicular carcinoma), has no role in the work-up of the thyroid nodule. **Calcitonin** is a marker for medullary carcinoma; however, because of the rarity of these tumors, calcitonin level also has no place in the work-up of a routine thyroid nodule. In patients with medullary carcinoma of the thyroid, calcitonin testing (basal and provocatively stimulated calcitonin levels with **calcium or pentagastrin infusion**), **pheochromocytoma urine studies**, and an assessment of parathyroid function should be performed. Patients who are diagnosed with medullary carcinoma of the thyroid

Table 22.1 Degree of Clinical Concern for Carcinoma in a Thyroid Nodule Based on History and Physical Examination

Findings of Less Concern

Chronic stable examination
Evidence of a functional disorder (e.g., Hashimoto's thyroiditis, toxic nodule)
Multinodular gland without dominant nodule

Findings of More Concern

Age <20 years and >60 years
Male gender
Rapid growth, pain
History of radiation therapy
Family history of thyroid carcinoma
Hard, fixed lesion
Lymphadenopathy
Vocal cord paralysis
Size >4 cm
Aerodigestive tract compromise (e.g., stridor, dysphagia)
Recurrent cyst formation after aspiration

Adapted from Lopresti J. Laboratory tests for thyroid disorders. *Otolaryngol Clin North Am.* 1996;29:557–73.

also should undergo *ret* **oncogene analysis** and should have family members screened for the *ret* oncogene mutation that is present in familial forms of this disease (10).

If there is a question about the physical examination, one can obtain a **thyroid ultrasound**—the most sensitive modality available for assessing thyroid gland architecture. Ultrasound does not allow differentiation between benign and malignant lesions. Solid lesions are not necessarily malignant, and cystic lesions are not necessarily benign. Chest radiographs can be obtained in patients with proven malignancy to assess for metastasis or for tracheal deviation in patients with goiter (Fig. 22.2). However, because chest radiographs can underrepresent the degree of tracheal compression in patients with laryngotracheal deviation, CT should be performed (Figs. 22.3 and 22.4).

Currently, **iodine or technetium scanning** (which, in the past, often had been obtained in the work-up of the thyroid nodule) is now thought to provide little useful information; approximately 95% of all nodules scanned are found to be "cold" (11,12) (Fig. 22.5). Although this group of patients (i.e., those with "cold" nodules) includes those with thyroid malignancy, the group is so large that the scan finding is not helpful in deciding a course of treatment.

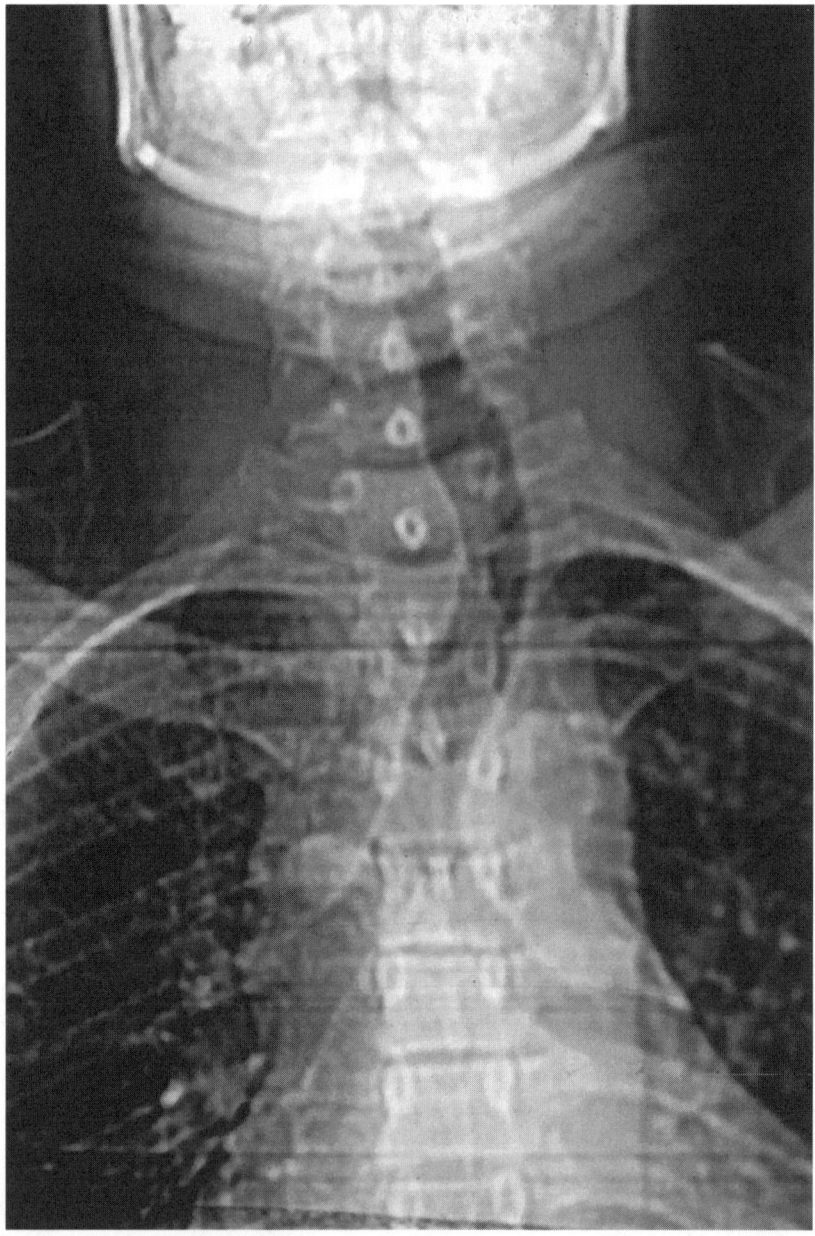

Figure 22.2 Radiograph showing tracheal deviation secondary to a large thyroid mass. (Courtesy of Dr. Faustino Guinto.)

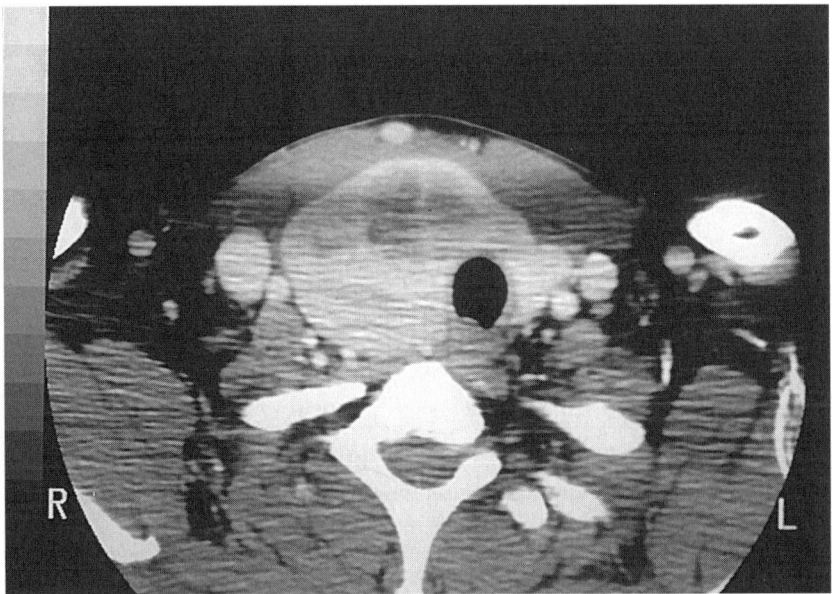

Figure 22.3 Computed tomography scan showing tracheal deviation resulting from a large thyroid mass. (Courtesy of Dr. Faustino Guinto.)

Fine-Needle–Aspiration Biopsy

Management of thyroid nodular disease is based primarily on FNAB, which has decreased the number of patients going to surgery, increased the incidence of carcinoma in patients treated surgically, and resulted in cost savings. FNAB is accurate and reliable, with high sensitivity and specificity (13–15). All palpable nodules in euthyroid patients require FNAB. In patients with thyroid nodules, approximately 70% of FNAB specimens are read as benign. Such aspiration reports typically describe nodules as being colloid, adenomatous, or macrofollicular in nature. False-negative rates range from 1% to 10% with experienced cytopathologists. Patients with benign thyroid FNAB specimens can be assured that, without other historical or physical examination correlates of malignancy, their disease can be managed nonsurgically. False-negative rates can be higher in lesions smaller than 1 cm (which can be missed because of their size) or in lesions greater than 3 cm (which may not be able to be sampled adequately with aspiration techniques). False-negative rates are also higher in patients with cystic lesions in which the cellular component of the smear is low.

Approximately 4% of thyroid-nodule FNAB specimens are read as malignant. The false-positive rate for these aspirates is approximately 1% (14).

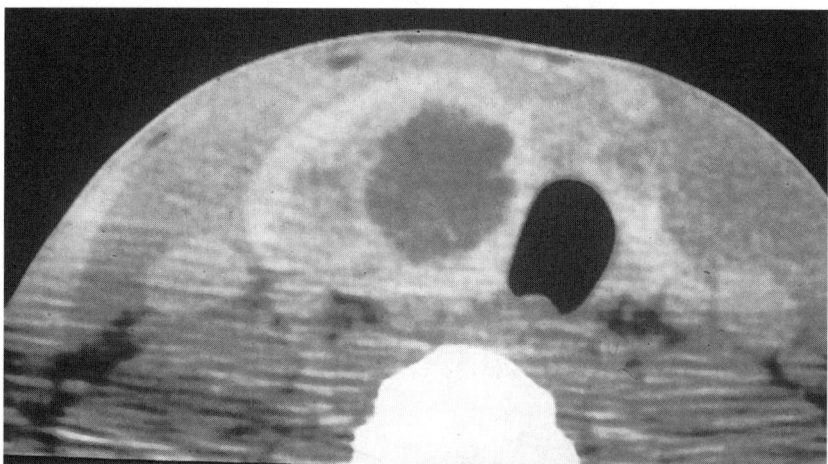

Figure 22.4 Computed tomography scan showing a large cystic mass in the right thyroid lobe. (Courtesy of Dr. Faustino Guinto.)

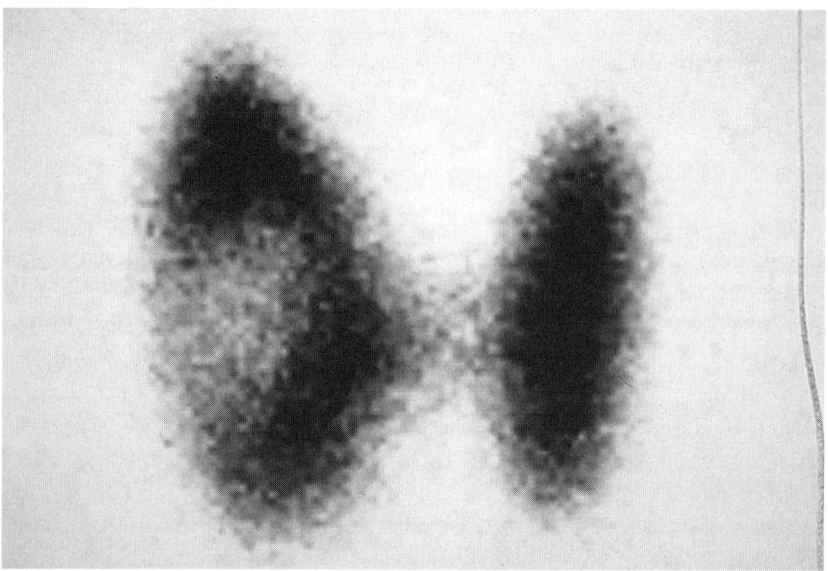

Figure 22.5 Thyroid scan (technetium) showing a nodule (4 cm x 4 cm) in the right lobe; the left lobe is normal. (Courtesy of Dr. Faustino Guinto.)

False-positive readings usually result from the aspiration of lesions that should not be probed (e.g., toxic nodules, Graves' disease, or Hashimoto's thyroiditis). Medullary, papillary, and anaplastic carcinomas usually can be diagnosed on FNAB.

In expert series, approximately 15% of smears are nondiagnostic. It is important not to describe such aspirates to patients by telling them "no malignancy was seen." In nondiagnostic smears, there is really no usable information. Such aspirations should be repeated and turn out to be diagnostic approximately 50% of the time. It is reasonable to consider sonogram-guided aspiration for this second attempt. Nondiagnostic FNAB rates correlate partly with the skill of the aspirator.

One major problem with thyroid-nodule FNAB is that it is impossible to differentiate follicular adenoma from follicular carcinoma on the basis of cytology. The distinction between these two lesions is based on **histopathologic identification of vascular invasion** at the level of the nodule capsule, a goal that cannot be obtained cytologically with FNAB. When smears are significantly hypercellular with microfollicular profiles in cell clusters with reduced colloid, cytologists describe the aspiration with the words "follicular neoplasm, can't rule out follicular carcinoma" and categorize it as suspicious or indeterminate. Aspirates that are described in this manner have an approximate 10% to 20% risk of follicular carcinoma and thus should be removed. The risk of carcinoma in such an aspirate increases with the size of the nodule. Similarly, **Hürthle cell adenomas cannot be distinguished from Hürthle cell carcinomas on the basis of FNAB**. Therefore, the finding of predominant Hürthle cells on thyroid FNAB also is regarded as suspicious.

Thyroid cysts account for approximately 20% of all thyroid nodules. Drainage of the cyst by FNAB may be the definitive treatment of cysts smaller than 3 cm; larger cysts typically recur. The risk of malignancy increases if a cyst persists or recurs after FNAB; such cysts should be removed (8).

Patients with benign FNAB specimens can be followed nonsurgically. Some patients may not be reassured by the low false-negative rate and may request surgery. This should be considered after a full discussion. In patients managed nonsurgically, baseline ultrasonography can be considered. Such patients should have repeat clinical examination in approximately 3 months. **Ultrasonography** can be repeated in the future as needed and compared with the initial baseline ultrasound. Repeat FNAB can be considered every 1 to 2 years. The nodule should be reevaluated promptly if there is any enlargement or significant change during follow-up.

The differential diagnosis of thyroid nodules is summarized in Table 22.2.

Suppressive Therapy

Suppression of T_4 is based on the assumption that exogenous T_4 administration induces TSH suppression, which effectively withdraws a trophic factor for the thyroid gland and the nodules within it. Nonrandomized uncontrolled studies have shown that suppressive therapy reduces nodule size in approxi-

Table 22.2 Differential Diagnosis of the Thyroid Nodule

Benign Nodule

Colloid or adenomatous nodule
Follicular adenoma
Thyroid cyst (cystification of colloid nodule or follicular adenoma)
Focal thyroiditis

Malignant Nodule

Papillary carcinoma
Follicular carcinoma
Hürthle cell carcinoma
Medullary carcinoma
Anaplastic carcinoma
Lymphoma
Metastasis to the thyroid (e.g., breast, renal, melanoma)

---

mately 30% of patients (16). However, out of five randomized prospective trials of T_4 therapy that was sufficient to suppress TSH levels in euthyroid patients with benign clinically solitary thyroid nodules, only one study showed a statistically significant decrease in nodule size by 50% (3). A meta-analysis of controlled studies on the effect of TSH suppression on bone-mineral density showed **substantial decreases in bone-mineral density in postmenopausal women. Suppressive treatment also increases the risk of cardiac arrhythmia**, especially in patients over 60 years of age (17,18). Given the questionable efficacy and the potential side effects of suppressive therapy, some clinicians question its appropriateness. There is also a problematic lack of consensus on the length of suppressive trials, the degree of TSH suppression, and even the exact goal of suppressive therapy itself. Should it stabilize or shrink the thyroid nodule? Should these changes be based on palpation or sonographic criteria? Furthermore, **malignant nodules can shrink with suppressive therapy**, and only a small percentage of nodules that grow on suppressive therapy are malignant (8).

Clearly, patients with enlarging nodules on suppression should undergo surgery. Suppressive therapy should not be offered to hyperthyroid patients or those with subclinical hyperthyroidism; also, it is generally not performed in patients with a TSH level below 1 mU/L. Similarly, elderly patients or those with cardiac disease are not good candidates for suppressive therapy. It seems most appropriate to treat only those patients who have a TSH level greater than 1 mU/L and solid, small, nonautonomous nodules for limited periods of time (~4 months) and then reevaluate. TSH level should not be suppressed below 0.3 mU/L.

Occasionally, surgery may be indicated on the basis of history and physical examination alone. In such cases, FNAB still can be obtained and may help in surgical planning. The work-up continues with TSH assessment and then FNAB in all patients who are euthyroid. Management of the lesion is determined by the FNAB results (2).

Goiter

Goiter may be diffuse or multinodular, involve both lobes symmetrically, or be strikingly asymmetric. Goiter may be associated with abnormal thyroid function tests or may occur in the euthyroid patient. Through an effect on adjacent cervical viscera or an extension into the chest, large goiters can present several clinical problems that are usually treated surgically. These problems include tracheal, esophageal (Fig. 22.6), or venous compression; extension through the thoracic inlet into the upper mediastinum; local positional discomfort; and cosmetic deformity (Fig. 22.7). The airway may be impacted because of laryngeal and tracheal deviation or compression, recurrent laryngeal nerve stretching, or vocal cord paralysis. The esophageal compression may result in dysphagia or a globus sensation (*see* Fig. 22.6). A massive goiter that extends to the root of the neck and thoracic inlet can compress head and neck venous outflow, resulting in the proliferation of subcutaneous venous collaterals and a positive Pemburton's sign. With goitrous enlargement of the thy-

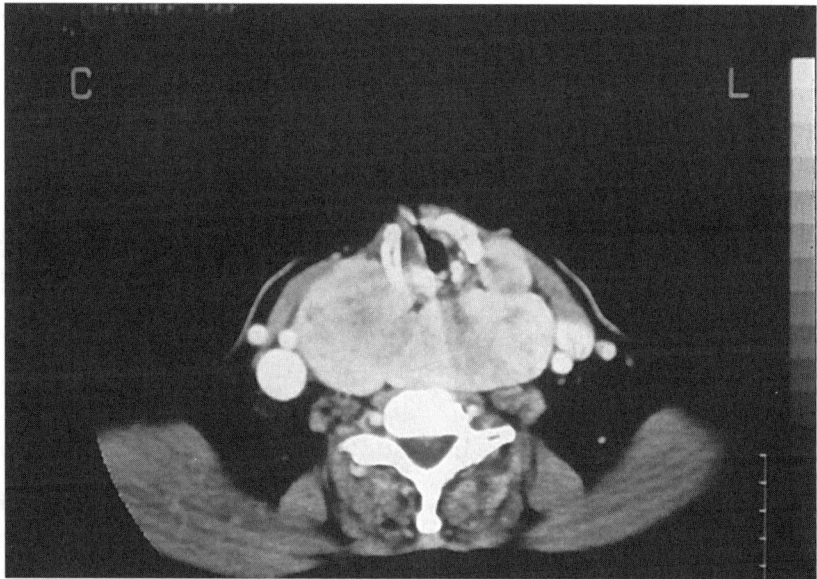

Figure 22.6 Computed tomography scan demonstrating massively enlarged thyroid gland. The retroesophageal component was responsible for the dysphagia in this patient.

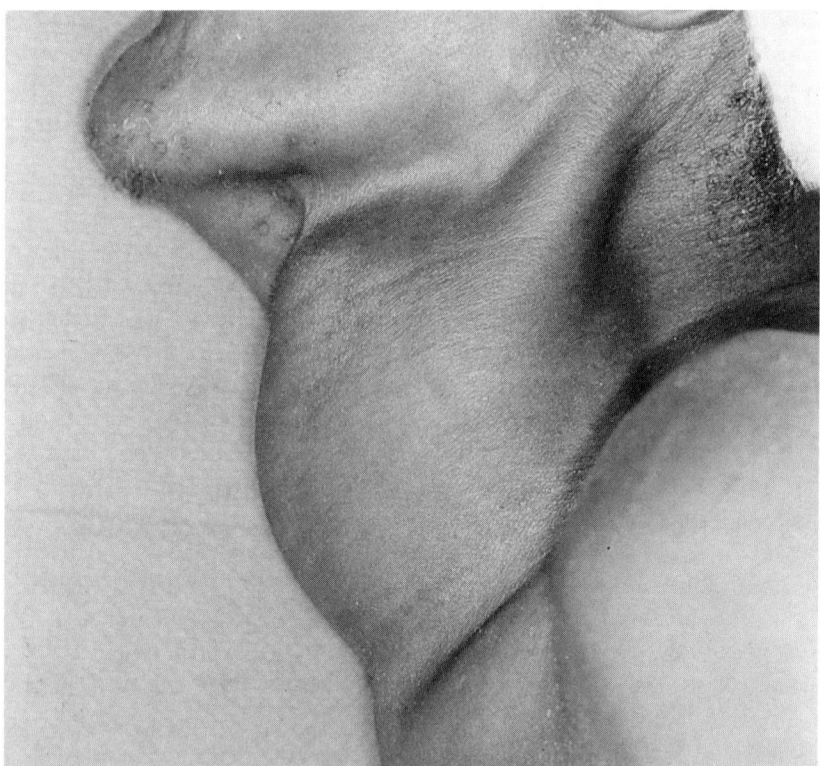

Figure 22.7 Long-standing neck mass in a patient from a third-world country where iodine deficiency is endemic.

roid, extension into the upper chest can occur. Most clinicians believe that surgically removing the goiter with significant substernal extension is reasonable, because the segment extending into the chest cannot be followed on serial physical examinations or studied with FNAB. Additionally, if hemorrhagic enlargement of the substernal segment of the goiter occurs, the airway can be compressed at the mediastinal level (20). Goiter also may cause regional discomfort (especially with rapid enlargement and capsule stretching from intrathyroidal hemorrhage) or may present with a cosmetic issue.

Evaluation

Goiter size may be stable over many years or may slowly increase. An acute increase in size can occur despite many years of stability and may occur from hemorrhage into a preexisting nodule or cyst, leading precipitously to profound airway symptoms. Patients may have up to 50% airway obstruction and be asymptomatic with a long history of stable goiter size (21). Such patients may present with positionally triggered dyspnea and chronic cough and may be diagnosed erroneously with asthma or obstructive sleep apnea. Patients with esophageal compression may present with a sensation of fullness, globus, or frank solid-food dysphagia (*see* Fig. 22.6).

The physical examination of patients with goiter includes an assessment of respiratory status, a determination of laryngotracheal deviation, and an estimate of substernal extension. The development of venous engorgement or subjective respiratory discomfort when the arms are lifted over the head (a positive Pemburton's sign) implies thoracic inlet obstruction from a large or substernal goiter. Vocal cord mobility should be assessed during the evaluation of a patient with goiter. Vocal cord stretch may occur secondary to goiter, yet voice may be normal because of contralateral vocal cord compensation.

Chest radiography provides a good assessment of tracheal deviation, but tracheal compression can be underrepresented (*see* Fig. 22.2). In such cases, noncontrast CT fully assesses the degree of airway compression and substernal extension. CT scans should be obtained in all symptomatic patients and in all patients in whom the physical examination suggests retrosternal extension; CT should be considered in all patients with massive goiter. Although ultrasonography is helpful when viewing intrathyroidal architecture, CT is the best study to help judge retrosternal extension and the relationship of the goiter to the adjacent cervical viscera (*see* Fig. 22.3) **It is important to avoid iodinated contrast agents until thyroid function tests are obtained, which prevents patients with multinodular goiter and subclinical hyperthyroidism from developing frank hyperthyroidism through the exogenous iodine load** that CT scan from the contrast represents (referred to as the **Jod–Basedow phenomenon**). Flow volume loops, although a good dynamic assessment of airway adequacy, are not as directly helpful as is CT in deciding a course of treatment.

Management

Surgery is successful in alleviating symptoms, is well tolerated, and can prevent acute airway emergencies. All symptomatic patients with goiter and all asymptomatic patients with significant radiographic airway deviation and compression (or retrosternal extension) should undergo surgery (Case 22.1). Surgery for nontoxic multinodular goiter usually involves resection of the more affected side via lobectomy and isthmectomy. If the goiter is bilateral, then bilateral subtotal thyroidectomy is a safe and effective procedure. Although they extend into the chest, retrosternal goiters are cervical in origin; thus, nearly all of these goiters can be extracted through the neck without sternotomy or thoracotomy.

> **Case 22.1** **Man with Substernal Goiter and Thyroid Nodular Disease**
>
> A man 40 years of age is referred for evaluation of an anterior neck mass and tracheal deviation. He presented to his primary care provider with symptoms of an upper respiratory infection and recent onset of dyspnea on exertion. A chest radiograph obtained for evaluation of these symptoms showed marked tracheal deviation to the right. Ten years ago, he was evaluated for an enlarged thyroid and was told that he had a benign goiter. He received no follow-up and has not been taking Synthroid. He denies dysphagia, hoarseness, aspiration, and a recent change in his voice. There is no history of childhood irradiation or family history of thyroid carcinoma. Past medical and surgical treatments have been unremarkable. He takes no medications and does not use alcohol or tobacco.
>
> Physical examination reveals a healthy-appearing man who is in no acute distress. The pertinent finding on head and neck examination is that the patient's laryngeal cartilage and trachea are deviated markedly to the right. The left lobe of the thyroid is diffusely enlarged and there is a dominant nodule in the midline that measures 5 cm x 6 cm. The right lobe of the thyroid is enlarged slightly, and the inferior extent of the left lobe is not appreciated on palpation. The gland moves normally with swallowing, and the gross appearance of the larynx and mobility of the vocal cords are normal on flexible fiberoptic examination. The upper airway structures are also normal. TSH and free T_4 levels are normal. CT scan of the neck without contrast shows substernal extension of the left thyroid lobe and a dominant nodule. A smaller 1.5-cm nodule is noted in the right lobe. There is no evidence of invasion of the trachea, larynx, or surrounding soft tissue or of tracheal compression. In this case, FNAB will not change the treatment plan. The site, location, and sex of the patient all require surgical resection. A diagnosis of substernal goiter with a dominant nodule is made.
>
> The patient meets two criteria for surgical excision of the thyroid: a substernal goiter and a thyroid nodule larger than 4 cm. The patient has consented for a total thyroidectomy. The left lobe and isthmus are excised first, and no complications are encountered. A right thyroid lobectomy is performed to biopsy the right thyroid nodule, preventing recurrence of substernal extension in the right lobe.

Small goiters without retrosternal extension and airway compression (especially if diffuse [i.e., anodular]), may be managed with TH suppression and rarely I^{131} ablation. TH can be offered if the patient is not hyperthyroid or subclinically hyperthyroid. Goiter size frequently increases when TH is stopped. Additionally, TH treatment usually results in only a modest decrease in goiter size. **There is no evidence that long-term TH treatment alters ultimate progressive enlargement in patients with multinodular goiter** (3). Although it is effective in some forms of hyperthyroidism (e.g., Graves' disease; *see* the section on Hyperthyroidism below), radioactive iodine treatment (I^{131}) is less effective in the treatment of euthyroid goiter, because thyroid uptake may be too low to concentrate the radioactive isotope sufficiently. Transient radiation-induced thyroiditis results from this treatment, which may initially worsen airway symptomatology. Furthermore, radioactive iodine ablation causes only a gradual decrease in goiter size and often results in the development of hypothyroidism after treatment. Approximately 5% of patients treated with radioactive iodine for goiter may ultimately develop **autoimmune hyperthyroidism (Graves' disease)** secondary to radiation-induced antigen exposure (3). Although the risk of radiation-induced thyroid malignancy is low, and the risk of carcinoma development elsewhere in the body is only marginally increased by radioactive iodine treatment, such treatment is best avoided in young patients (22). Surgery allows rapid and safe symptomatic relief and provides pathologic data. Radioactive iodine ablation should be considered only in patients who are not surgical candidates.

Hyperthyroidism

Hyperthyroidism is caused most commonly by Graves' disease or toxic nodules. Graves' disease usually is treated initially with antithyroid medicines (e.g., propylthiouracil, methimazole) then ultimately with radioactive iodine unless remission occurs. Radioactive iodine ablation with I^{131} may be less effective in Graves' disease patients who have large goiters. Additionally, radioactive iodine treatment for Graves' disease may result in a worsening of its associated ophthalmopathy and is generally **avoided in children** because of empirical teratogenic concerns. This treatment also is associated with a high rate of radioactive iodine–induced hypothyroidism (in ~80% of Graves' disease patients) (23). Surgery (usually bilateral subtotal thyroidectomy) is an excellent treatment option for the following patient groups: Graves' disease patients with large goiters who wish to avoid radioactive iodine, young patients, patients with severe eye disease, and patients who require a rapid return to euthyroid status.

Toxic nodules are treated initially by antithyroid medicines to induce euthyroidism. Hyperthyroidism is likely to recur with the cessation of antithyroid medicine treatment, so definitive ablative treatment (either surgery or radioactive iodine) is typically necessary for these nodules. I^{131} ablation can be used; however, reports vary about the dose and the number of treatments necessary; there is an approximate 50% rate of radiation-induced hypothyroidism (24). Because thyroid nodules represent a focal discrete abnormality within the thyroid gland, a surgical approach that preserves the normal remaining thyroid gland always should be considered.

Thyroid Cancer

Approximately 80% of all thyroid cancers (**papillary carcinoma** [70%] and **follicular carcinoma** [10%–15%]) are well differentiated. Both papillary and follicular cancers arise from the thyroid follicular epithelium and most cases have a favorable prognosis. Patients with well-differentiated thyroid carcinoma can be separated into one of two divergent prognostic groups based on age, sex, size of lesion, degree of invasiveness, and presence of metastatic disease (25,26). Papillary carcinoma is strongly lymphotrophic, often presenting with intrathyroidal lymphatic spread (which, in the past, has been misinterpreted as multifocal disease) to the cervical lymphatic beds. Approximately 30% of patients who present with papillary carcinoma show gross nodal disease on their initial physical examination (19). Follicular carcinoma occurs as a single lesion, spreading through direct extension and hematogenously, usually without nodal metastasis. Papillary carcinoma can be induced through exposure to low-dose radiation therapy. Follicular carcinoma can occur with endemic goiter in the setting of chronic TSH-level elevations.

Medullary carcinoma accounts for approximately 5% of thyroid cancers and is derived from the parafollicular C cells. These lesions secrete calcitonin and occur in both sporadic (75%) and familial (25%) autosomal-dominant forms. Inherited medullary thyroid carcinoma can be associated with multiple endocrine neoplasia (MEN) types IIa (with pheochromocytoma and hyperparathyroidism) and IIb (with pheochromocytoma and marfanoid habitus). Anaplastic carcinoma, an undifferentiated carcinoma, arises from thyroid parenchyma, usually in an elderly population (Case 22.2). Because patients usually present with advanced disease, prognosis is poor and survival is often measured in months. Thyroid lymphoma often arises in a setting of autoimmune Hashimoto's thyroiditis and usually represents a B-cell malignancy (Table 22.3).

Management

Although there is disagreement among the surgical oncology literature, patients with papillary carcinoma in low-risk prognostic groups can be offered **unilateral thyroid surgery** with good results. In patients with follicular carcinoma or high-risk papillary carcinoma, **bilateral thyroid surgery** (total or nearly total thyroidectomy) should be offered. Patients with a preoperative FNAB that indicates follicular neoplasm should undergo **hemithyroidectomy with frozen section**. If the frozen section is negative, the procedure should be terminated. If final pathology reveals a follicular carcinoma, most clinicians believe that **whole-body scanning** is warranted. To perform this study, the remaining lobe needs to be removed through either completion thyroidectomy or radioactive iodine ablation. Medullary carcinoma requires a to-

Case 22.2 Woman with Anaplastic Thyroid Carcinoma That Presents as an Enlarging Neck Mass

A woman 60 years of age is referred for an evaluation of a rapidly enlarging anterior neck mass. She was in her usual state of health until 3 weeks ago when she noticed a painless mass to the right of the trachea. She denies dysphagia, aspiration, shortness of breath, and hoarseness. Past medical and surgical histories are noncontributory, and there is no history of alcohol or tobacco abuse or of childhood neck irradiation.

The pertinent findings on head and neck examination are a diffuse right thyroid mass that measures 6 cm along its greatest extent. Fixation to the trachea is suggested on palpation and observation during swallowing. Flexible fiberoptic examination shows decreased mobility of the right vocal fold and normal appearance of the subglottis. The differential diagnosis of a rapidly enlarging thyroid mass includes hemorrhage into a nodule, lymphomatous degeneration of Hashimoto's thyroiditis, and anaplastic thyroid carcinoma. FNAB suggests anaplastic thyroid carcinoma. An open biopsy confirms the diagnosis.

Palliative chemoradiation is recommended.

Table 22.3 Occurrence, Survival, and Characteristics of Thyroid Cancer

Cell Type	Percent of Thyroid Malignancy	5-Year Survival	10-Year Survival	Comments
Well-differentiated thyroid carcinoma	Papillary: 70% Follicular: 15%	—	~90%	High- and low-incidence groups depend on age, sex, size, invasiveness, and presence of metastasis
Medullary thyroid carcinoma	~5%	~85%	~65%	Sporadic or inherited forms with *ret* oncogene mutation
Anaplastic thyroid carcinoma	~5%	0%–8%	—	Presents in an older age group with advanced disease
Lymphoma	<5%	50%	—	Typically associated with Hashimoto's thyroiditis

Adapted from Lopresti J. Laboratory tests for thyroid disorders. *Otolaryngol Clin North Am.* 1996;29:557–73.

tal thyroidectomy in all cases, because preoperative discrimination of familial multifocal disease from sporadic unifocal disease is imprecise. **Neck dissection** is offered for patients with well-differentiated thyroid carcinoma if gross

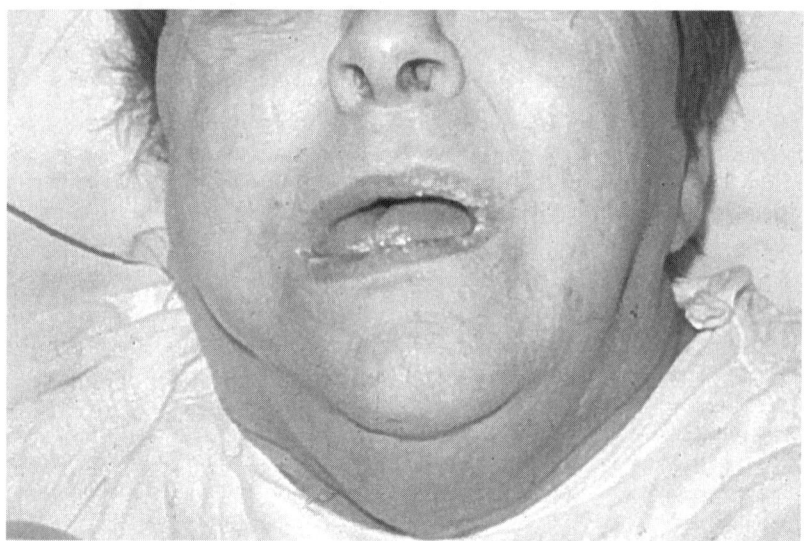

Figure 22.8 Classic myxedema in a woman who had undergone a total thyroidectomy and had stopped taking her thyroid replacement medication.

nodal disease is present and also is considered for patients with medullary carcinoma because of its high incidence of microscopic cervical nodal disease. Surgery for anaplastic carcinoma and thyroid lymphoma usually is restricted to biopsy for diagnosis.

Permanent recurrent laryngeal nerve paralysis occurs in expert series in approximately 1% to 2% of patients; however, many series have reported higher rates. **Rates of postoperative vocal cord paralysis** are higher in the following instances: 1) when the recurrent laryngeal nerve is not identified during surgery, 2) in cases of surgery performed for thyroid malignancy and retrosternal goiter, 3) in revision surgery, and 4) in patients reoperated for hemorrhage (19). Hypoparathyroidism occurs after bilateral thyroid surgery in expert series in approximately 6% of patients, but higher rates have been reported in many series. The rate of postoperative hypoparathyroidism is higher in surgery performed for malignancy, during which thyroidectomy is combined with nodal dissection, and correlates with the experience of the surgeon (Fig. 22.8) (19).

Hyperparathyroidism

Over the past decade, with more widespread use of laboratory screening, the detection rate of hypercalcemia has risen to 100 cases per 100,000 population

Table 22.4 Causes of Hypercalcemia

Primary Hyperparathyroidism	Metabolic and Drug-Related Disorders
Parathyroid adenoma	Milk alkali syndrome
Parathyroid hyperplasia	Lithium
Double adenoma	Thiazides
Parathyroid carcinoma	Vitamin A or D intoxication
	Immobilization
Secondary Hyperparathyroidism	
	Endocrinopathy
Tertiary Hyperparathyroidism	Addison's disease
Malignancies	Hyperthyroidism
PTH-like tumor factors (pseudohyperparathyroidism)	Acromegaly
Bony metastasis	**Benign Familial Hypocalcinuric Hypercalcemia**
Granulomatous Disorders	
Sarcoidosis	
Tuberculosis	
Coccidioidomycosis	

PTH = parathyroid hormone.

in men and twice that rate in women, increasing with advancing age (27). Most patients are now diagnosed through incidentally detected calcium elevation on routine lab screening. In the past, patients would present with advanced symptomatic disease with one or more of the classic symptoms of hypercalcemia (i.e., "painful bones, kidney stones, abdominal groans [pancreatitis, ulcer disease], psychic moans, and fatigue overtones"). The most common cause of hypercalcemia in the outpatient setting is primary hyperparathyroidism. Among hospitalized patients, malignancy is the leading cause of hypercalcemia attributed to calcium mobilization from bony metastatic disease. Multiple causes of hypercalcemia are listed in Table 22.4.

The four parathyroid glands are normally located adjacent to the thyroid gland near the tracheoesophageal groove (Fig. 22.9). In approximately 5% of patients, there are five (or more) glands. The parathyroid glands produce parathormone (PTH), which raises serum calcium by increasing bone-calcium mobilization, increasing calcium absorption from the gut and decreasing renal calcium excretion and stimulation of renal hydroxylase to maintain vitamin D levels (28).

Primary hyperparathyroidism is a disorder of calcium metabolism caused by the excess PTH produced by the hyperfunctioning of one or more parathyroid glands. Approximately 80% of primary hyperparathyroidism is

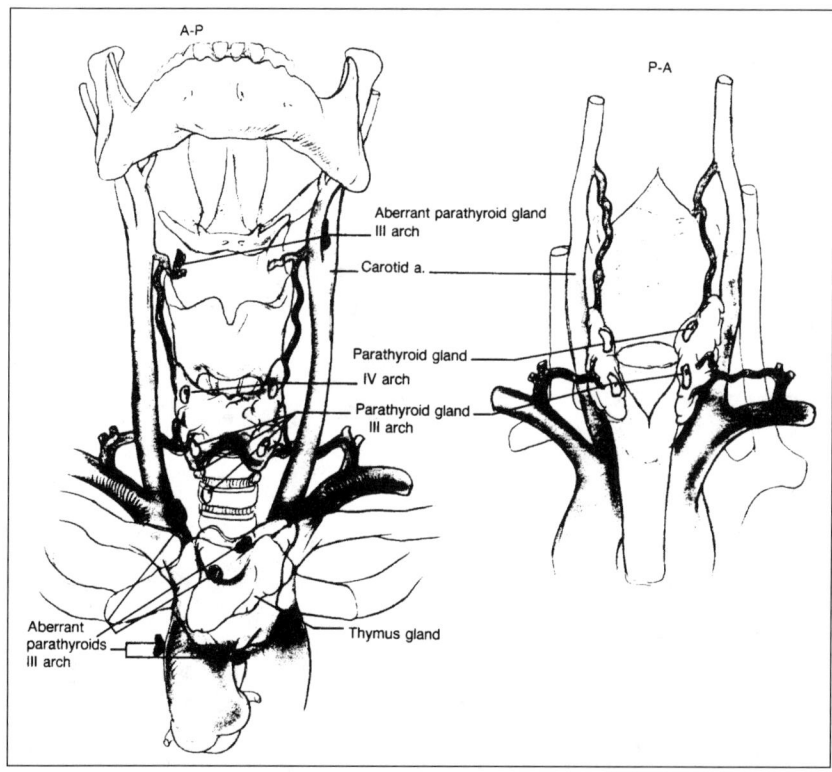

Figure 22.9 Location of the parathyroid glands. (Republished with permission from Bailey BJ. *Head and Neck Surgery–Otolaryngology*. Philadelphia: Lippincott; 1993.)

due to the hyperfunctioning of a single gland (single adenoma). Approximately 10% to 15% of primary hyperparathyroidism results from diffuse four-gland hyperplasia. Double adenoma occurs in approximately 2% to 3% of patients, whereas parathyroid carcinoma occurs in approximately 1%. Primary hyperparathyroidism is usually sporadic but can occur in familial forms or in MEN I or IIa syndromes. **Secondary hyperparathyroidism** typically represents a hyperplastic parathyroid response to renal failure. When this hyperplastic function fails to correct with treatment of the underlying renal disease, it is called **tertiary hyperparathyroidism.**

Patients who present with primary hyperparathyroidism generally have few physical findings. Patients with long-standing disease have multiple systems that are affected (29) (Table 22.5). Some mild constitutional symptoms (e.g., fatigue, joint pain, change in memory) may be present and difficult to elicit until successful surgery makes them apparent in retrospect (30).

Table 22.5 Manifestations of Chronic Hypercalcemia

Musculoskeletal and Dermatologic Disorders	Cardiovascular Disorders
Muscle weakness	Hypertension
Muscle fatigue	
Bone and joint pain or arthritis	**Genitourinary Disorders**
Osteoporosis	Polyuria
Pruritus	Renal stones
	Nephrocalcinosis
Neurological Disorders	**Ophthalmologic Disorders**
Depression or memory impairment	Band keratitis
Confusion, lethargy, or coma	Palpebral fissure calcium deposition
Decreased deep-tendon reflexes	
Gastrointestinal Disorders	
Polydipsia	
Constipation	
Nausea and vomiting	
Peptic or duodenal ulcer or pancreatitis	

Evaluation

Laboratory diagnosis of primary hyperparathyroidism is based on the finding of elevated serum calcium and elevated serum intact PTH level. These findings are associated with a decreased phosphorous level and strongly suggest primary hyperparathyroidism. Several assays are available for **PTH assessment**, including N terminal, C terminal, and intact. Intact PTH assay is the most sensitive measure for actual PTH level elevation. During initial laboratory evaluation, **benign familial hypocalciuric hypercalcemia (BFHH)** can be confused easily with primary hyperparathyroidism. BFHH can be associated with elevated calcium and PTH levels and indicates an inherited defect in renal calcium sensing. Such patients have a lifelong history of high calcium level and a low urine calcium level with a positive family history (autosomal dominance). Therefore, the initial laboratory evaluation for primary hyperparathyroidism should include a 24-hour urine test to exclude BFHH (calcium level < 100 mg suggests BFHH).

Many imaging techniques are available to localize enlarged hyperplastic parathyroid glands. Commonly used modalities include **sestamibi scanning** (Fig. 22.10), ultrasonography, magnetic resonance imaging, and technetium-thallium scanning. Sestamibi scanning has proven to be highly sensitive in the detection of **adenoma location** (31). The inclusion of such localization tests preoperatively depends on the surgeon's experience and philosophy. How-

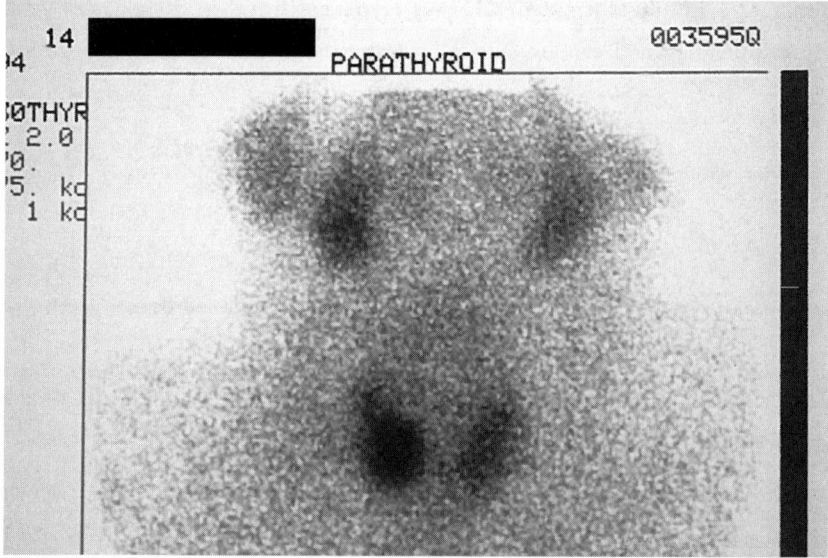

Figure 22.10 This sestamibi scan shows a parathyroid adenoma located near the right inferior lobe of the thyroid gland. (Courtesy of Dr. Faustino Guinto.)

ever, it is important to note that localization tests are intended to assist with intraoperative parathyroid gland localization; they are not meant to confirm the diagnosis of hyperparathyroidism. If localization tests are negative, one should not question a diagnosis that has been made on valid chemical grounds. Importantly, if a patient is judged to be a surgical candidate, referral should not be aborted if a given localization study is negative.

Surgical Treatment

All agree that symptomatic patients with primary hyperparathyroidism (e.g., those with renal disease secondary to hypercalcemia, bone disease, or significant gastrointestinal complaints [e.g. gastric ulcer]) require surgical exploration. Treating asymptomatic patients with primary hyperparathyroidism remains controversial. **Growing evidence suggests that the natural history of asymptomatic primary hyperparathyroidism may be clinically benign. Long-term medical surveillance may be appropriate in selected cases.** Other researchers, however, continue to believe that virtually all patients with primary hyperparathyroidism are treated most optimally with parathyroid exploration (30). Several studies show that asymptomatic patients who are not treated surgically have an **increased risk of cardiovascular dis-**

ease and that approximately 25% of these patients ultimately develop symptoms during long-term follow-up. It is not possible to determine which patients will develop symptoms (32,33). These points should be interpreted in the context of a surgical cure rate that is over 95% and a lack of other effective alternate forms of treatment. Therefore, the National Institutes of Health consensus opinion suggests that **surgery should be offered all patients under 50 years of age**. For patients over 50 years of age who are asymptomatic, surgery is suggested if there is evidence of 1) significant hypercalcemia with a calcium level greater than 11.5 mg/dL, 2) a history of a life-threatening episode of hypercalcemia, 3) biochemical evidence of significant bone loss (bone density > 2 SD below the mean, adjusted for age, race, and gender), or 4) biochemical evidence of significant renal disease with creatinine clearance of less than 30% (adjusted for age) or urinary calcium level above 400 mg/dL (34). Advances in operative technique and postoperative care have reduced hospitalization to 24 to 48 hours in most instances (30). An exciting new development in the surgery for hyperparathyroidism is the intraoperative PTH assay; if there is a drop in the PTH level within 15 minutes after an adenoma is removed, surgical success is confirmed.

Danger Signs

A more serious thyroid disorder in a patient with a thyroid mass is suggested by a history of ionizing radiation or a family history of medullary carcinoma. Potentially ominous physical findings include pain, vocal cord paralysis (recurrent laryngeal nerve paralysis), tracheal deviation or compression, tracheal invasion, a rapid increase in nodule size, and cervical adenopathy.

Signs of hypercalcemia, including the classic "painful bones, kidney stones, abdominal groans (pancreatitis or ulcer disease), psychic moans, fatigue overtones" should prompt a search for the cause of the hypercalcemia, particularly to rule out bony metastases from a malignancy.

Acknowledgements

We wish to acknowledge the contributions of members of the American Academy of Otolaryngology–Head and Neck Surgery Endocrine Subcommittee in the development of this chapter: James Denneny, MD; David Eisele, MD; Helmuth Goepfert, MD; W. Jarrard Goodwin, MD; David Myssiorek, MD; Frederic Ogren, MD; Lisa Orloff, MD; Robert Ossoff, MD; Mark Persky, MD; Nestor Rigual, MD; and Maisie Shindo, MD.

REFERENCES

1. **Mazzaferri E.** Thyroid cancer in thyroid nodules: finding a needle in a haystack. *Am J Med.* 1992;93:359.
2. **Hermus AR, Hysmans DA.** Treatment of benign nodular thyroid disease. *N Engl J Med.* 1998;338:1438–47.
3. **Wingo A, Tong T, Bolden S.** Cancer statistics, 1995. *CA Cancer J Clin.* 1995;45:8–30.
4. **McHenry C, Smith L, Lawrence A, et al.** Nodular disease in children and adolescents: a higher incidence of carcinoma. *Am Surg.* 1998;54:444–7.
5. **Simpson WJ, McKinney SE, Carruthers JS, et al.** Papillary and follicular thyroid cancer: prognostic factors in 1578 patients. *Am J Med.* 1987;104:940.
6. **Schlumberger MJ.** Papillary and follicular carcinoma of the thyroid. *N Engl J Med.* 1998;338: 297–306.
7. **Rojeski M, Gharib H.** Nodular thyroid disease. *N Engl J Med.* 1985;313:418–36.
8. **Randolph GW.** Thyroid and parathyroid glands. In Lee KJ (ed). *Essential Otolaryngology,* ed 7. Stamford, CT: Appleton & Lange; 1998:573–643.
9. **Randolph GW.** Medullary carcinoma of the thyroid. *Curr Opin Otolaryngol Head Neck Surg.* 1997;5:55–66.
10. **Ashcraft M, van Herle A.** Management of the thyroid nodule: Part 1. *Head Neck Surg.* 1981;Jan/Feb:216–27.
11. **Ashcraft M, van Herle A.** Management of the thyroid nodule: Part 2. *Head Neck Surg.* 1981;Mar/Apr:297–322.
12. **Hamburger JI.** Diagnosis of thyroid nodules by fine-needle biopsy: use and abuse. *J Clin Endocrinol Metabol.* 1994;79:335–9.
13. **Gharib H.** Fine-needle–aspiration biopsy of thyroid nodules: advantages, limitations, and effects. *Mayo Clinic Proc.* 1994;69:44–9.
14. **Gharib H, Goelner J, Johnson D.** Fine-needle–aspiration cytology of the thyroid: a 12-year experience with 11,000 biopsies. *Clin Lab Med.* 1993;13:699–709.
15. **Molitch ME, Beck JR, Dreisman M, et al.** Cold thyroid nodule: an analysis of diagnostic and therapeutic options. *Endocrine Rev.* 1984;5:185–99.
16. **Uzzan B, Campus T, Cucherat M, et al.** Effects on bone mass of long-term treatment with thyroid hormone: a meta-analysis. *J Clin Endocrinol Metabol.* 1996;81:4278–89.
17. **Sawin CT, Geller A, Wolf PA, et al.** Low serum thyrotropin concentration as a risk factor for atrial fibrillation in older persons. *N Engl J Med.* 1994;331:1249–52.
18. **Allo MD, Thompson NW.** Rationale for operative management of substernal goiter. *Surgery.* 1983;94:967–77.
19. **Lopresti J.** Laboratory tests for thyroid disorders. *Otolaryngol Clin North Am.* 1996;29:557–73.
20. **Melliere B, Saada F, Etienne G, et al.** Goiter with severe respiratory compromise: evaluation and treatment. *Surgery.* 1987;103:367–73.
21. **Holm LE, Hall P, Wiklund K, et al.** Cancer risk after iodine-131 therapy for hyperthyroidism. *J Natl Cancer Inst.* 1991;83:1072–7.
22. **Wise PH, Ahmad A, Burnet R, et al.** Intentional radioiodine ablation in Graves' disease. *Lancet* 1975;20:1231.

23. **Toft AD, Irvine WJ, Seth J.** Thyroid function in long-term follow-up of patients treated with I[131]. *Lancet.* 1975;2:576.
24. **Hay ID, Grant CS, Taylor WP, et al.** Ipsilateral lobectomy versus bilateral lobar resection of papillary carcinoma of the thyroid: a retrospective analysis of surgical outcome using a novel prognostic scoring system. *Surgery.* 1987;102:1088–95.
25. **Cady B, Rossi R.** An expanded view of risk group definition in differentiated thyroid cancer. *J Surg.* 1998;104:947–53.
26. **Clark O.** Diagnosis of primary hyperparathyroidism. In Clark O, Duh Q (ed). *Textbook of Endocrine Surgery.* Philadelphia: WB Saunders; 1997.
27. **Fukayama S, Bosma T, Goad D, et al.** Human parathyroid hormone related protein and human PTH: comparative biological activities on human bone cells and bone resorption. *Endocrinology.* 1988;123:2841.
28. **Stock J, Marcus R.** Medical management of primary hyperparathyroidism. In Bilezidian JP (ed). *The Parathyroids: Basic and Clinical Concepts.* New York: Raven Press; 1994.
29. **Clark O.** Presidential address: "Asymptomatic" primary hyperparathyroidism: Is parathyroidectomy indicated? *Surgery.* 1994;116:947–53.
30. **Sofferman RA, Nathan MH, Fairbank J, et al.** Preoperative technetium sestamibi imaging. *Arch Otolaryngol Head Neck Surg.* 1996;122:369–74.
31. **Palmer A, Adami HO, Bergstrom R, et al.** Survival and renal function in persons with untreated hypercalcemia: a population-based cohort study with 14-year follow-up. *Lancet.* 1987;1:59.
32. **Scholz DA, Pernell DL.** Asymptomatic primary hyperparathyroidism. *Mayo Clin Proc.* 1981;56:473.
33. **Consensus Development Conference Panel.** Diagnosis and management of asymptomatic primary hyperparathyroidism. *Ann Intern Med.* 1991;114:539.
34. **Boggs JE, Irvin GC, Molinari AS, et al.** Intraoperative parathyroid hormone monitoring as an adjunct to parathyroidectomy. *J Surg.* 1996;120:954–8.

SUGGESTED READINGS

Hermus AR, Hysmans DA. Treatment of benign nodular thyroid disease. *N Engl J Med.* 1998;338:1438–47.

The authors of this population-based study found palpable nodules in 1.5% of men and 6.4% of women in the general population. The authors review the current treatment concepts, including suppression, observation, radio-iodine, and surgery.

Mazzaferri E. Management of a solitary thyroid nodule. *N Engl J Med.* 1993;328:553–9.

This article reviews various aspects of the solitary thyroid nodule, including prevalence, differential diagnosis, laboratory and imaging studies, natural history, and treatment. The authors recommend fine-needle–aspiration biopsy as the first line diagnostic study in euthyroid patients with a solitary nodule.

Palmer A, Adami HO, Bergstrom R, et al. Survival and renal function in persons with untreated hypercalcemia: a population-based cohort study with 14-year follow-up. *Lancet.* 1987;1:59.

This study of 172 people with hypercalcemia found that those who were under 70 years of age when the diagnosis of hypercalcemia was made had a lower survival rate. This lowered survival rate correlated to the degree of hypercalcemia and seemed to be mainly from disorders of the circulatory organs. Patients over 70 years of age at the time of diagnosis of hypercalcemia had no decreased survival rate.

Schlumberger MJ. Papillary and follicular carcinoma of the thyroid. *N Engl J Med.* 1998;338:297–306.

Papillary and follicular carcinomas of the thyroid are generally curable cancers. This article reviews the epidemiology, pathogenesis, histopathology, diagnosis, treatment, and follow-up.

Uzzan B, Campus T, Cucherat M, et al. Effects on bone mass of long-term treatment with thyroid hormone: a meta-analysis. *J Clin Endocrinol Metabol.* 1996;81:4278–89.

This is a meta-analysis of the effects of long-term TH treatment on bone mass. The authors found that suppressive therapy was correlated with significant bone loss in the lumbar spine and hip in post-menopausal women, whereas replacement therapy was correlated with significant spine and hip bone loss in premenopausal women.

SECTION VI

THE FACE

23

Atypical Facial Pain and Related Entities

Steven M. Houser, MD
Diana N. Traquina, MD

A diagnosis of atypical facial pain is made only after the following common causes of head and neck pain have been excluded: sinusitis, common headache forms (e.g., migraine, musculoskeletal tension, cluster headache), dental infection, cervical arthritis, and temporomandibular joint (TMJ) disease. Diagnosing pain syndromes that have no obvious organic cause may be challenging for the clinician, particularly because specific physical findings are rare in these patients. Nevertheless, several common facial pain syndromes can be identified, usually by determining the characteristics, location, and distribution of the pain (1–3).

Relevant Anatomy and Physiology

Pain perception (nociception) in the head and neck is relayed by cranial nerve (CN) V, VII, IX, and X as well as by spinal nerves C2 and C3. Nociceptive pain fibers within these nerves include A-delta and C fibers. The A-delta fibers are small and finely myelinated, conveying sharp, pricking pain sensations. They are typically located in the skin and mucous membranes and have a conductance speed of 5 to 30 m/s. C fibers are small and unmyelinated, conveying high-intensity mechanical, chemical, and thermal stimuli as burning sensations. C fibers typically are located deep within tissue and skin and have a conductance speed of 0.5 to 2.0 m/s.

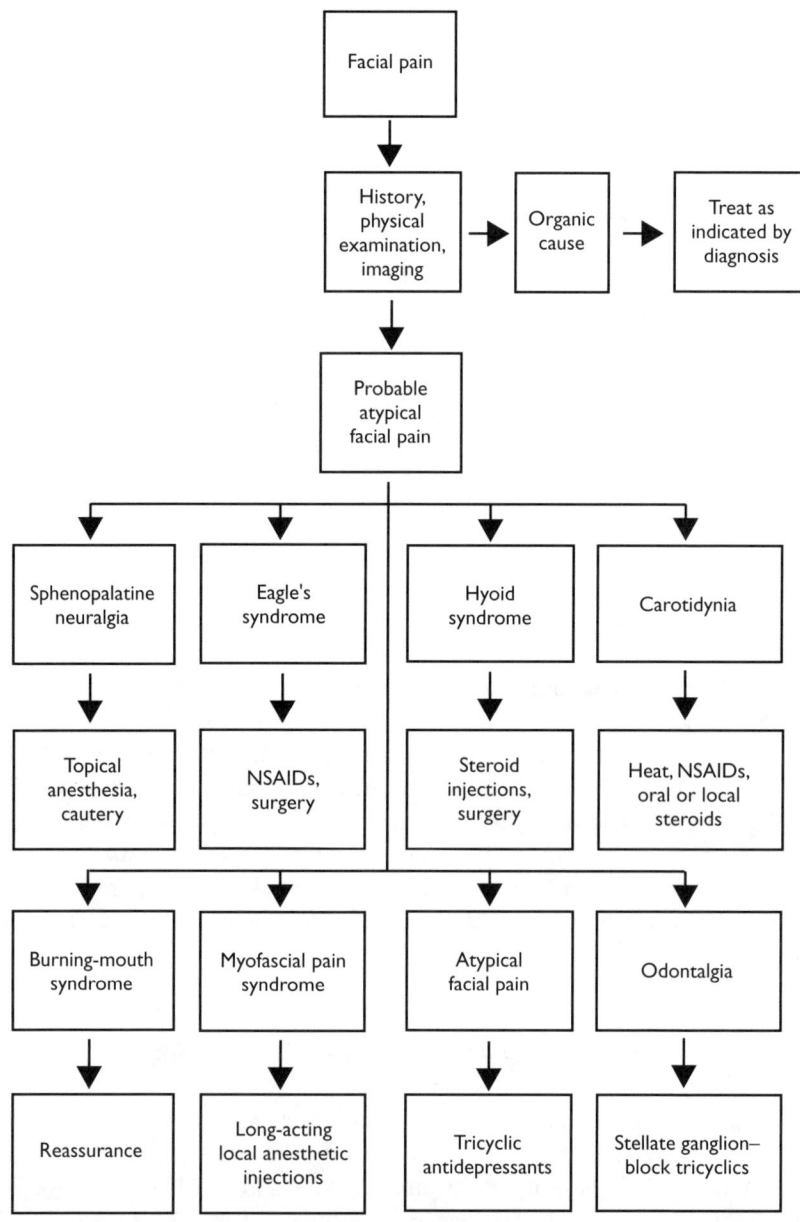

Algorithm Management of atypical facial pain. NSAIDs = nonsteroidal anti-inflammatory drugs.

Within the head and neck, there is little overlap of the primary sensory neurons; however, convergence does occur at the second- and third-order projections. The second-order projection is within the brainstem and spinal cord; the third-order projection is in the thalamus. The medial thalamus conveys emotional and perceptual responses to pain, and the lateral thalamus allows for discriminating the location of painful stimuli. From the lateral thalamus, projections are made to Brodmann's areas 3, 1, and 2 for location-specific pain sensation.

Nociception can be separated into four categories: local, referred, deafferentation, and psychogenic. The category of pain that a patient experiences depends on the neurological level at which the pain is sensed (4). The higher the neurological level is, the more complex the processing and, hence, the less well it is understood. In referred nociception (e.g., TMJ disease, in which painful stimuli from deep within the TMJ crosses over at the secondary or tertiary neurons), the brain perceives the pain as originating from an adjacent structure rather than its true location (e.g., the ear instead of the TMJ). A more complex level of painful sensation is deafferentation pain, which is discussed in some detail below. Psychogenic pain (or pain without organic basis) is perceived as originating within the head and neck despite its cerebrocortical origin.

Deafferentation pain is a complex and poorly understood process. After an injury, human beings undergo a hyperesthetic response in which the hyperesthestic region normally progresses to hypoesthesia and then to normal sensation over a variable length of time. In some instances, patients can develop a continued cycle of hyperesthesia caused by plasticity within the nervous system. A "loop" between the sympathetic nervous system and the spinal column develops, allowing aberrant communication of A-beta and C fibers. Because of the interaction between pain (C) fibers and touch-perception (A-beta) fibers, benign stimuli are perceived as painful. Patients with deafferentation pain (e.g., phantom limb pain, atypical odontalgia, reflex sympathetic dystrophy) have difficulty explaining it. Their pain, which usually has an affective quality, frequently is described as a "drawing" or "pulling," and patients may use such terms as "tearing the life out of me." These complaints typically exaggerate their observed level of discomfort. Deafferentation pain tends to respond best to tricyclic antidepressants (TCAs).

History

The first important focus of the history in a patient with facial pain is determining whether there is an organic cause for the pain. For example, there are some obvious infectious causes of facial pain: acute sinusitis, acute pharyngotonsillitis, and dental abscess; this type of pain is expected to resolve when the underlying cause is treated (5). There are also the more common types of headaches and facial pain complexes, including tension, migraine and cluster headaches; TMJ pain; and trigeminal, glossopharyngeal, postherpetic, and posttraumatic neuralgias. Causes of facial pain that are less common but extremely important to the diagnosis include brain tumors, subdural hematoma, subarachnoid hemorrhage, temporal arteritis, and hypertension. These organic causes of facial pain must be ruled out before the patient is diagnosed with "atypical facial pain."

Pain without a detectable underlying cause is more difficult to diagnose and treat. Determining the major characteristics of the pain is the starting point in discovering its cause. Important components include when the pain first started, whether it is constant or intermittent, and what makes it better or worse. The specific character of the pain can be described as "burning," "boring," "stinging," "pressing," "irritating," etc., and its exact distribution must be determined in detail.

Although *atypical facial pain*, by definition, means pain without an obvious source, the exact location and distribution of the pain can help determine its origin. Some of the more common pain syndromes in the head and neck include sphenopalatine neuralgia, Eagle's syndrome, hyoid syndrome, carotidynia, burning-mouth syndrome, and myofascial pain syndrome.

Sphenopalatine neuralgia was first described in 1915 by Dr. Sluder and is sometimes called "Sluder's neuralgia." This sharp pain is presumed to originate within the vidian nerve or sphenopalatine ganglion, which is located behind the posterior wall of the maxillary sinus (6). A patient with sphenopalatine neuralgia has pain behind the eye, upper jaw, palate, nose, and teeth that sometimes extends to the temple, occiput, and neck. In its most severe form, the pain can radiate down the arm.

Eagle's syndrome was first described by Dr. Eagle, who attributed throat pain to an elongation of the styloid process. This pain is usually a dull, nagging pharyngeal pain that worsens with deglutition, often radiating to the ear and the mastoid region. Treatment consists of surgically removing the styloid process (7).

Another vague head and neck pain syndrome is **hyoid syndrome** (Brown's or greater cornu syndrome) that is attributed to bursitis near the greater cornu of the hyoid with irritation of nearby neural structures (i.e., the sympathetic carotid plexus or, possibly, CN IX). A patient with hyoid syndrome describes a dull, stabbing, sore-throat pain that is triggered by talking, yawning, and swallowing. These patients also have point tenderness at the greater cornu of the hyoid bone. Surgical removal of the greater cornu of the hyoid bone and steroid injection have been used with moderate efficacy (8).

Carotidynia is a type of pain that shares its distribution with the styloid and hyoid pain syndromes. It consists of pain and tenderness in the region of the carotid bifurcation that is attributed to irritation of the carotid sympathetic plexus. Pain can be intermittent or constant, throbbing or lancinating, and can radiate to the ear, temple, or lateral neck. The pain persists for weeks or months, remitting spontaneously. Injecting steroids into the carotid sinus area may help.

Burning-mouth syndrome is characterized by oral pain without evidence of mucosal lesion; it occurs three times as often in women as in men. Patients describe a burning and tender sensation (usually bilateral) that encompasses the anterior tongue, anterior hard palate, and lower lip. They also may report dry mouth or a metallic taste. No defined treatment works well.

Myofascial pain syndrome is sometimes called myalgia, fibrositis, or fibromyalgia and is attributed to acute trauma or chronic muscle fatigue (e.g. typing) that leads to nerve sensitization and produces taut muscle bands. Patients describe a constant dull ache with a "trigger area" that refers pain to the general vicinity.

Atypical facial pain occurs in a female-to-male ratio of approximately 19 to 1, and its mean age of onset is 40 years. These patients report years of deep, poorly localized facial pain that crosses anatomical boundaries, does not respect normative distributions of the sensory nerves, and is bilateral in 20% to 35%. Patients with atypical facial pain describe it as a "pulling," "tearing," or "drawing" sensation. Treatment is not well defined, and patients should be referred to a chronic pain facility.

Atypical odontalgia is pain in apparently normal teeth and phantom pain after tooth extraction (reported in 3% to 6% of patients). Patients generally are women between 40 and 49 years of age. This is deafferentation pain because the physician perceives an emotional undercurrent and the patient has difficulty locating the origin of the pain.

Physical Examination

Complete head and neck and neurological examinations are the starting point with these patients. Specific physical findings that support a particular diagnosis of atypical facial pain are rare. In **sphenopalatine neuralgia**, there may be inflammation of the mucosa of the posterior nasal cavity overlying the sphenopalatine ganglion. In **Eagle's syndrome**, the tip of an elongated styloid process may be palpable in the tonsillar fossa. A patient with **hyoid syndrome** may have an enlarged greater cornu of the hyoid. In **carotidynia**, there is often tenderness on palpation of the carotid artery. **Burning-mouth syndrome** elicits no specific physical findings. **Myofascial pain syndrome** has four specific physical findings: 1) the jump sign (i.e., a patient who jumps when his or her trigger point is palpated), 2) the rope-muscle sign (i.e., the adjacent muscle fibers feel like rope), 3) dermatographism (i.e., stroking of the painful area produces blanching followed by hyperemia), and 4) pain elimination by local anesthetic injection or topical evaporative coolant.

As with the typical history in a patient with atypical facial pain, the key factor is the absence of findings that support other specific diagnoses.

Diagnosis and Management

Many of the syndromes in this category of atypical facial pain are predominantly diagnoses of exclusion (Table 23.1). In addition to the symptoms described in the preceding section, other clues that assist in the diagnosis of **sphenopalatine neuralgia** are 1) its similarity to lower-half cluster headache, and 2) the fact that it is more common in women. Treatment consists of cauterization of the ganglion or topical anesthetics placed intranasally in the region of the sphenopalatine ganglion (Case 23.1).

In **Eagle's syndrome**, lateral skull radiographs may show an elongated styloid process (usually 1.52–4.20 cm in length) (Fig. 23.1) or a calcified stylohyoid ligament. Not all patients with these radiographic findings are symptomatic. The pain due to an elongated process or calcified ligament is attributed to a fracture of this process, nerve compression of CN IX or X, mucosal irritation, or impingement of the carotid artery. The syndrome is more common in women between 20 and 39 years of age. Differential diagnosis includes CN IX neuralgia, TMJ disease, and carotidynia. Conservative treatment of Eagle's syndrome includes reassurance, nonsteroidal anti-inflammatory drugs, and local injection of a corticosteroid. The following surgical treatments have exhibited only variable success: fracturing of the styloid, transoral resection of the elongated styloid process (Case 23.2), and an external neck–incision approach to the styloid process.

Patients with **hyoid syndrome** may have a prominent greater cornu on radiography. Treatment includes local corticosteroid injection as well as surgical resection of the greater cornu through an incision in the neck.

The differential diagnosis of **carotidynia** includes a dissecting aneurysm of the cervical portion of the carotid artery. Treatment consists of reassurance, heat, nonsteroidal anti-inflammatory drugs, and corticosteroids administered orally or by local injection.

Table 23.1 Differential Diagnosis of Atypical Facial Pain

Sphenopalatine neuralgia	Burning-mouth syndrome
Eagle's syndrome	Myofascial pain syndrome
Hyoid syndrome	Odontalgia
Carotidynia	Atypical facial pain

> **Case 23.1** **Woman with Sphenopalatine Neuralgia**
>
> A woman 32 years of age presents with a 3-year history of retro-orbital pain that often extends to include her nose, palate, and occasionally her occiput. The pain is generally worse on the right side. She has had a thorough evaluation of her sinuses and has undergone limited endoscopic sinus surgery, with mild symptom improvement of brief duration. Several computed tomography and magnetic resonance imaging scans over the past 3 years failed to reveal any other pathology, and she has no focal neurological signs on physical examination.
>
> Because her physician notices moderate mucosal erythema over the right posterior lateral nasal wall, a trial of topical anesthesia is carried out. Pledgets soaked in pontocaine are placed in this area. After 10 minutes, the patient's pain eases. Later in the day, as the local anesthesia wears off, the pain returns. A presumptive diagnosis of sphenopalatine neuralgia is made
>
> The patient undergoes a chemical cauterization of the sphenopalatine ganglion. The symptom relief from this lasts 5 to 7 months, and the symptoms continue to respond to periodic cauterization.

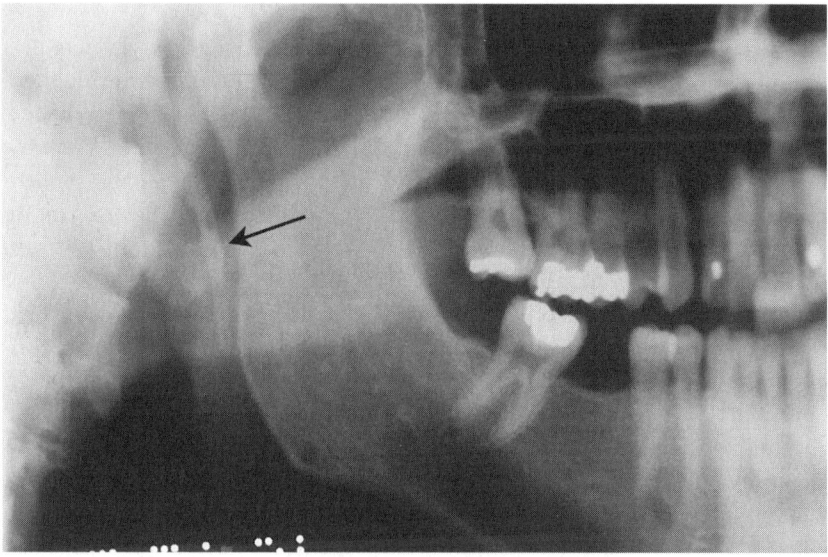

Figure 23.1 Panoramic mandibular radiograph of the elongated styloid process (*arrow*) associated with Eagle's syndrome.

The differential diagnosis of **burning-mouth syndrome** includes Plummer–Vinson syndrome (with its associated iron-deficiency anemia, diabetes mellitus, esophageal webs, and glossitis), which suggests the use of a complete

> **Case 23.2 Young Woman with Eagle's Syndrome**
>
> A woman 21 years of age presents with an 18-month history of a dull, left-sided throat pain that worsens when she swallows (especially hot beverages) and occasionally radiates to the ear. She underwent a tonsillectomy approximately 6 months ago for the presumptive diagnosis of chronic pharyngotonsillitis, but her pain has not improved.
>
> On physical examination, palpation of the left tonsillar fossa recreates her pain. There is a suggestion of a small hard mass that is palpable within the tonsillar fossa. Skull radiography reveals an elongated styloid process on the left side.
>
> The patient is started on ibuprofen, with moderate symptom improvement. Several months later, when she reports a great deal of stress at her workplace, the pain worsens, despite the ibuprofen. A local steroid injection yields only mild improvement. Finally, a transoral resection of the elongated styloid process is undertaken. After the postoperative pain resolves, the patient finds that her throat pain has improved significantly. She still requires ibuprofen at times of high stress but is otherwise free of symptoms.

blood count, glucose tolerance test, and contrast esophagography. Ninety percent of the women with this syndrome are postmenopausal, but hormone replacement does not relieve the pain. Gastroesophageal reflux disease may be a contributory cause, and a therapeutic trial of antireflux agents may be in order. A combination of Mycostatin, hydrocortisone, tetracycline, and diphenhydramine elixir may be helpful. Burning-mouth syndrome tends to subside as mysteriously as it arises.

The goal of **myofascial pain** treatment is to interrupt the pain cycle with a series of intramuscular injections of a long-acting local anesthetic with or without a corticosteroid. The patient experiences a decrease in referred pain lasting hours to days—much longer than the local anesthetic's putative duration of action.

Although analgesics are reported to be of no help in atypical facial pain syndrome, they are still used frequently by patients. The patient often denies a psychological contribution, even though the physician may suspect underlying depression, obsessive-compulsive disorder, or hysteria. Atypical facial pain often follows an episode of trauma. Patients describe discomfort reminiscent of deafferentation pain, which may imply plasticity in the third-order neurons (i.e., the thalamus), explaining the affective dimension of the patient's pain. Patients with atypical facial pain respond well to TCAs but poorly to surgery or psychotherapy. Cutaneous electric nerve stimulators and alternative health practices (e.g., cranial manipulation, acupuncture, self-hypnosis) may be beneficial.

Local anesthetic injection typically relieves odontalgia from dental caries but not the pain of **atypical odontalgia**. However, stellate ganglion–block TCAs benefit only 10% of patients with typical odontalgia but 70% of patients with atypical odontalgia. Treatment for atypical odontalgia includes amitriptyline 80 mg/d. The management of atypical facial pain is summarized in the Algorithm.

Danger Signs

The chief danger in treating atypical facial pain is mistaking a life-threatening organic cause (e.g., brain tumor, subarachnoid hemorrhage) for atypical facial pain and, thus, delaying treatment of the organic pain cause. Specific abnormalities in the neurological examination (e.g., CN deficits, anisocoria, gait abnormalities, visual changes) indicate that something other than atypical facial pain is occurring. Such signals warrant immediate in-depth neurological evaluation and appropriate radiographic imaging.

Summary

Atypical facial pain and related pain syndromes adversely affect quality of life and emotional stability. Patients typically have consulted numerous physicians, many of whom have concluded the pain to be psychogenic and have suggested psychiatric counseling. Unfortunately, psychiatric treatment gives little relief. Patients with deafferentation pain often benefit from TCA therapy and an interruption of the pain cycle. The physician who acknowledges the physical rather than psychological basis for this pain is already in a position to offer great support to the patient through a difficult course of diagnosis and treatment.

Although individuals with atypical facial pain and related syndromes are among the most challenging of patients, they offer the greatest satisfaction when the physician is equipped by knowledge and temperament to offer treatment, reassurance, and hope.

REFERENCES

1. **Clark JL.** An overview of face pain. *Postgrad Med.* 1984;72:90–172.
2. **McDonald JS, Pensak ML, Phero JC.** Part I: Differential diagnosis of chronic facial, head, and neck pain conditions. *Am J Otol.* 1990;11:299–303.
3. **Klausner JJ.** Epidemiology of chronic facial pain: diagnostic usefulness in patient care. *J Am Dent Assoc.* 1994;125:1604–11.
4. **Maciewicz R, Mason P, et al.** Organization of trigeminal nociceptive pathways. *Semin Neurol.* 1988;8:255–338.

5. **Schon DI.** Headache and facial pain: the role of the paranasal sinuses—a literature review. *J Craniomandib Prac.* 1993;11:36–49.
6. **Hardebo JE, Elner A.** Nerves and vessels in the pterygopalatine fossa and symptoms of cluster headache. *Headache.* 1987;27:528–32.
7. **Murthy PS, Hazarika P, et al.** Elongated styloid process: an overview. *Int J Maxillofac Surg.* 1990;19:230–1.
8. **Kunachak S.** Anterior cervical pain syndromes: hyoid, thyroid, and cricoid cartilage syndromes and their treatment with triaminalone acetamide. *J Laryngol Otol.* 1995;109: 49–52.

SUGGESTED READINGS

Acquadro MA, Montgomery WW. Treatment of chronic paranasal sinus pain with minimal sinus disease. *Ann Otol Rhinol Laryngol.* 1996;105:607–14.
  This article gives a detailed discussion of deafferentation pain and its role in facial pain presumed to be of sinus origin.
Baugh RF, Stocks RM. Eagle's syndrome: a reappraisal. *ENT J.* 1993;72:342–4.
  This article provides an excellent overview of styalgia.
Brass LS, Amedee RG. Atypical facial pain. *J LA State Med Soc.* 1990;142:15–8.
  This article gives a brief overview and differential diagnosis of facial pain.
Goebel J. The chronic headache. *ENT J.* 1987;66:383–98.
  This article is a good overview of headaches, including Wolff's pain maps (i.e., referred head pain of nasal origin).
Heir GM. Facial pain of dental origin: a review for physicians. *Headache.* 1987;27:540–7.
  This article contains a thorough discussion of tooth-associated and TMJ pain written by a dentist for physicians.
Mori H, Nishimura Y, et al. Reconsideration of the hyoid syndrome. *Otol Head Neck Surg.* 1994;110:324–9.
  This is an excellent review and discussion of this poorly understood malady.
Solomon S, Lipton RB. Facial pain. *Neurol Clin.* 1990;8:913–28.
  This article provides an overview, explaining the International Headache Society classifications.

24

Facial Asymmetry

Brian P. Driscoll, MD

The differential diagnosis of disorders that cause facial asymmetry include an exhaustive list of congenital anomalies, malformations, deformations, and disruptions (1). However, rather than focus on abnormal embryogenesis, this chapter concentrates on the general approach to the patient with facial asymmetry and discusses the treatment of common problems, including facial paralysis, hemifacial atrophy, fibrous dysplasia, tumors, and infection.

Facial Paralysis

This discussion focuses on patients who present with a unilateral or bilateral (uncommon) facial paralysis of peripheral origin (i.e., there is no central sparing of the forehead that would indicate a supranuclear lesion such as a stroke or brain tumor). A lesion is assumed to be present somewhere along the course of the facial nerve after it leaves the brain stem. Patients report movement that has decreased (paresis) or is absent (paralysis) on the involved side of the face. They also may describe pain and symptoms that, depending on the cause of the paralysis, indicate other cranial nerve involvement.

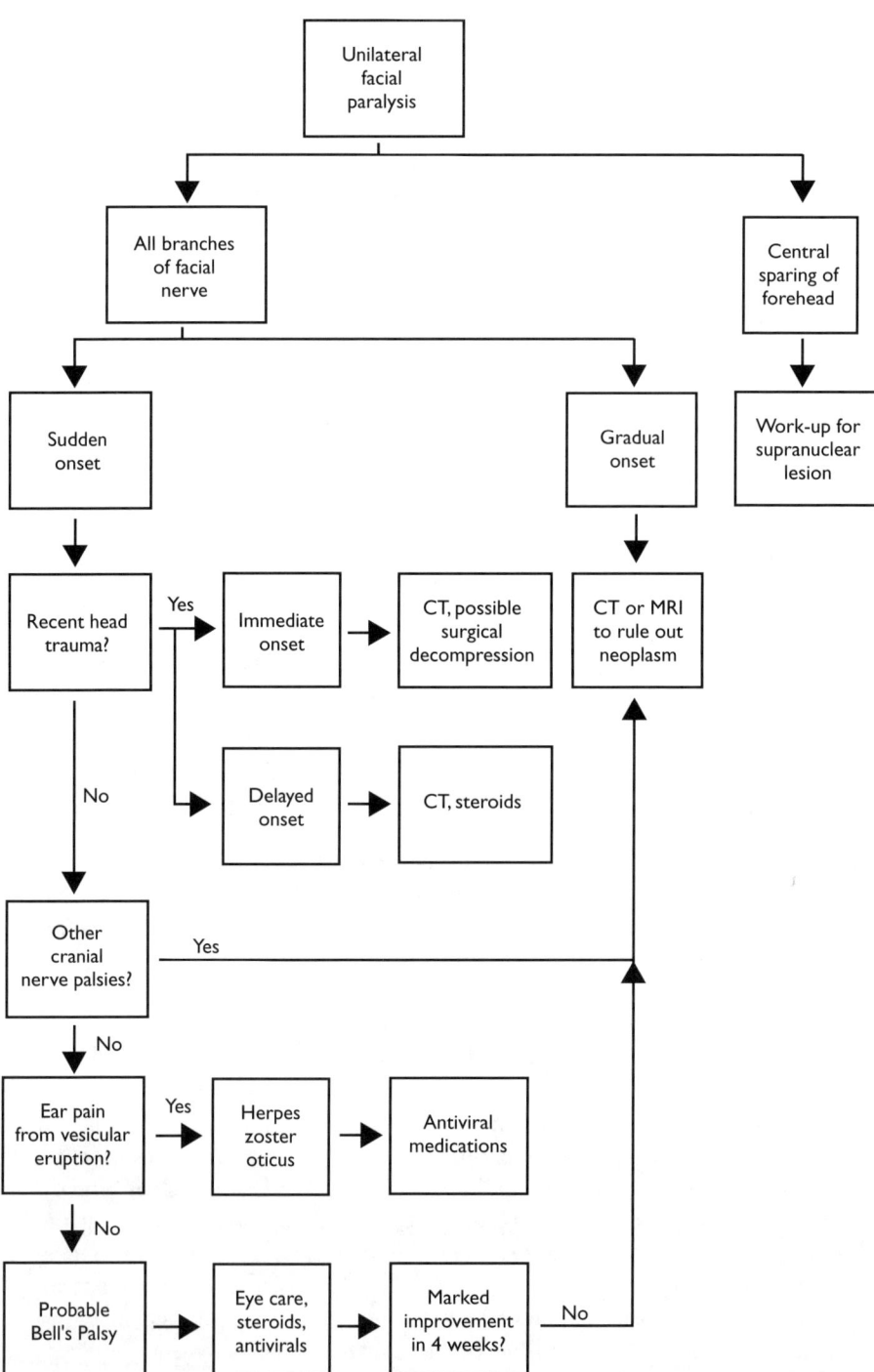

Algorithm Management of facial asymmetry. CT = computed tomography; MRI = magnetic resonance imaging.

Anatomy and Physiology

The facial nerve is a complex sensorimotor nerve that combines special afferent fibers, general efferent fibers, special efferent fibers, and possibly sensory afferent fibers that supply sensation to a small portion of the external auditory canal. After exiting the brainstem, the nerve crosses the cerebellopontile angle to enter the internal auditory canal. It then exits the canal via the meatal foramen and begins its serpiginous course through the temporal bone in its fallopian canal. The meatal foramen is the narrowest portion of this canal and, thus, is thought to be the site of injury to the nerve secondary to swelling in Bell's palsy and herpes zoster oticus (HZO). The first intratemporal portion is called the labyrinthine segment and is 2 to 4 mm long, ending at the geniculate ganglion. At the ganglion, the greater superficial petrosal nerve branches off, supplying general efferent parasympathetic fibers to the lacrimal and palatine glands. The nerve then makes a 40° to 80° turn posteriorly to enter the middle ear, beginning the tympanic segment (2). In 50% of the population, the bony canal is dehiscent in this area, increasing the chance of paralysis secondary to pressure during acute otitis media. As the nerve courses inferiorly to the lateral semicircular canal, it makes a 110° to 120° turn inferiorly to begin the mastoid segment. In the mastoid segment, the chorda tympani nerve branches off, supplying parasympathetic general efferents to the submandibular and sublingual glands and special afferents to the anterior two thirds of the tongue for taste and sensation. Additionally, a small motor nerve to the stapedius muscle branches off here. The nerve then exits the stylomastoid foramen as a motor nerve that supplies special efferents to the muscles of facial expression as well as to auricular, digastric (posterior belly), stylohyoid, and platysma muscles (2). The mastoid segment is most likely to be involved with chronic ear disease and cholesteatoma.

History

As noted above, most patients who present with acute unilateral facial paralysis have Bell's palsy. Although classically considered idiopathic in nature, there is growing support that most Bell's palsy cases are actually herpes simplex neuritis caused by herpes simplex virus type I (HSV I) (3,4). However, Bell's palsy remains a diagnosis of exclusion that is made only after an exhaustive search for other causes (Table 24.1). Most of the history and physical examination is directed toward elucidating these other causes. The typical patient with Bell's palsy presents with a sudden unilateral weakness of all facial muscles (Case 24.1) and may complain of otalgia, hyperacusis, alteration of taste, and numbness in the middle and lower face (2). Patients with HZO can present in a similar fashion, but the ear pain is usually more intense and a

Table 24.1 Differential Diagnosis of Facial Paralysis

Bell's palsy (60%–75%) (2)	Lyme disease*
Trauma (17%) (10)	Melkersson–Rosenthal syndrome*
Herpes zoster oticus (4.5%–8.9%) (5)	Sarcoidosis*
Acute suppurative otitis media	Guillain–Barré syndrome*
Chronic otitis media	Tuberculosis
Cholesteatoma	Facial nerve tumors (neuroma or hemangioma)
Parotid tumors	

* May cause bilateral facial paralysis. Guillain–Barré syndrome is the most common cause of bilateral facial paralysis.

Case 24.1   Woman with Bell's Palsy

A woman 33 years of age awakens with a total left peripheral facial paralysis and seeks urgent care from her physician. She has been otherwise healthy but had noted some minimal discomfort behind her left ear the day before onset of the paralysis. She denies hearing loss, tinnitus, paresthesias, dysphagia, and any other symptoms of cranial neuropathy. She complains of tearing from her left eye but has no diplopia or headache. She does not have diabetes, is not pregnant, and has not been in a region known to be infested with deer ticks.

Physical examination reveals a total left facial paralysis (House–Brackman grade 6) and left epiphora with good Bell's phenomena. She has no evidence of other cranial neuropathy or weakness, and her tympanic membrane is normal. There is no evidence of parotid swelling. An audiogram was normal; topognostic testing was not performed. She is diagnosed with Bell's palsy

The patient is begun on prednisone 30 mg/d for 3 weeks with a planned taper. Artificial tears and Lacrilube were prescribed, and she was instructed to tape her eye closed at night to prevent corneal exposure. An earlier taper is begun after the patient calls the office five days later to say that her nerve function is beginning to return.

Discussion

This patient presented with classic Bell's palsy, which responded rapidly to oral steroids. She had no particular risk factors, and there was no history or finding on her physical examination to suggest facial paralysis due to ear disease, parotid tumor, or Lyme disease. In retrospect, her paralysis most likely would have resolved without steroids, but the potential benefit of the treatment clearly outweighed the risks.

---

vesicular eruption may occur on the ear (2,5) (Case 24.2). Additionally, patients with HZO may experience hearing loss and vertigo, whereas patients with Bell's do not (2). If the paralysis is slowly progressive and associated with twitching, then neoplasm should be strongly suspected. Any patient with pre-

> **Case 24.2** **Man with Facial Paralysis Caused by Herpes Zoster Oticus**
>
> A man 47 years of age develops severe pain in his right ear, and his examination is initially normal. His physician prescribes topical eardrops. The following day, the patient notes blisters in his ear canal and awakens the morning after with total ipsilateral facial paralysis.
>
> Physical examination reveals multiple vesicles in his right ear canal and conchal bowl and total right facial paralysis. Herpes zoster oticus is diagnosed.
>
> The patient is begun on acyclovir 800 mg five times daily and prednisone 60 mg/d for 3 weeks with a planned slow taper. He has no improvement for 2 weeks and then notes some minimal motion of the corner of his mouth. The prednisone taper was extended over an additional 3 weeks, with gradual return of function over 3 months.
>
> **Discussion**
>
> Herpes zoster oticus results in a greater risk of permanent facial nerve damage than does the more common Bell's palsy. As a result, higher doses of steroids and antiviral medication are administered routinely. Dosages chosen are higher than those for more benign herpetic infections, and investigational dosages as high as 800 mg five times daily have been used. However, even with aggressive treatment, one third to one half of affected individuals may not achieve a complete recovery.

vious otologic surgery or chronic ear disease is assumed not to have Bell's palsy.

The duration of the paralysis is also important. Patients with partial facial paralysis that does not resolve within 3 to 6 weeks or total paralysis with no evidence of return of movement by 4 months should undergo a search for another cause (e.g., tumor). Family or personal history of previous facial paralysis is important. Patients with Bell's palsy and Melkersson–Rosenthal syndrome (i.e., the triad of recurrent facial paralysis, facial edema, and fissured tongue) can have both personal and family histories of facial paralysis (2).

Physical Examination

The physical examination centers on determining the extent of the facial paralysis and its possible causes, beginning with a complete head and neck examination. Complete versus partial paralysis is noted because this relates to prognosis. A patient with facial palsy that does not progress to complete paralysis has a much better chance for complete recovery (2,5,6). When the face is examined, the examiner carefully documents whether the paralysis is partial or complete and where motion is occurring. The most commonly used system for classifying the level of facial paralysis is the **House–Brackman Scale** (Table 24.2). Figure 24.1 is an example of a grade 6/6 paralysis.

Eye opening is mediated primarily via the levator (oculomotor nerve, cranial nerve III), whereas **eye closing** is a function of levator relaxation and orbicularis (facial nerve, cranial nerve VII) contraction. In a paralyzed face, the eyelid opens fully and easily, but the patient is usually unable to close it. The ability of the patient to protect the eye (e.g., eye closure, intact Bell's phenomenon, intact corneal sensation) is assessed carefully. If closure is incomplete, eye care (e.g., lubricating eye drops, taping or patching the eye closed at night) is needed to avoid exposure keratitis. Implanting a gold weight in the upper eyelid is a reversible surgical procedure that can obviate the need for drops and patching when several months or more are expected to elapse before function returns. Placing the gold weight can be performed under local anesthesia and can be removed easily after facial function returns.

The parotid gland is palpated carefully to search for tumor. Pneumatic and microscopic otoscopy, if available, are used to search for otologic infection as the cause of the paralysis. Otoscopy also may disclose a middle ear mass from a facial nerve neuroma. Any suspicion of otologic disease in the presence of a facial paralysis should prompt an evaluation by an otologist, because treatments for otologic facial palsy and for Bell's palsy are quite different.

Careful intraoral examination searches for inflammation of the fungiform papillae of the tongue (on the anterior two thirds of the tongue and involving chorda tympani innervation), which Adour and coworkers (3) found in 100% of patients with Bell's palsy, making this a "tongue blade" diagnosis. Complete neurological examination seeks other cranial neuropathies. Multiple cranial neuropathies may indicate tumor, infection, or other disorders.

Additional Diagnostic Evaluation

All patients who present with a facial paralysis should undergo **audiologic testing**, which documents normal or abnormal hearing (suggesting a possible

Table 24.2 House–Brackman Facial Nerve Grading System

Grade	Dysfunction	At Rest	With Motion
1	Normal	Normal	Normal
2	Mild	Normal	Slight weakness on close inspection
3	Moderate	Normal	Obvious weakness, no disfiguring asymmetry, mild synkinesis (eye closure)
4	Moderately severe	Normal	Obvious weakness, disfiguring synkinesis (incomplete eye closure)
5	Severe	Asymmetric	Only minimal movement
6	Total paralysis	Asymmetric	No movement

otologic source of the paralysis), tests the stapedius muscle (facial nerve), and evaluates cranial nerve VIII. Concurrent eighth-nerve involvement makes Bell's palsy unlikely. If the presentation is atypical, the paralysis complete, or the diagnosis uncertain, then **magnetic resonance imaging with gadolinium** can rule out tumors and infection and shows enhancement of the facial nerve at the meatal foramen in both Bell's palsy and HZO. Patients with HZO also may show enhancement of the eighth nerve and labyrinth (7). At times, laboratory tests for Lyme disease, diabetes mellitus, sarcoidosis, and autoimmune disorders may be helpful.

Patients with complete paralysis should undergo **electrical testing of the facial nerve**. Surgical decompression may be indicated in selected cases. There are many methods of electrical testing, but the most widely accepted is **electroneurography**, which provides a quantitative measure of neural degeneration. According to Fisch (8), if the electroneurography falls to 10% of the

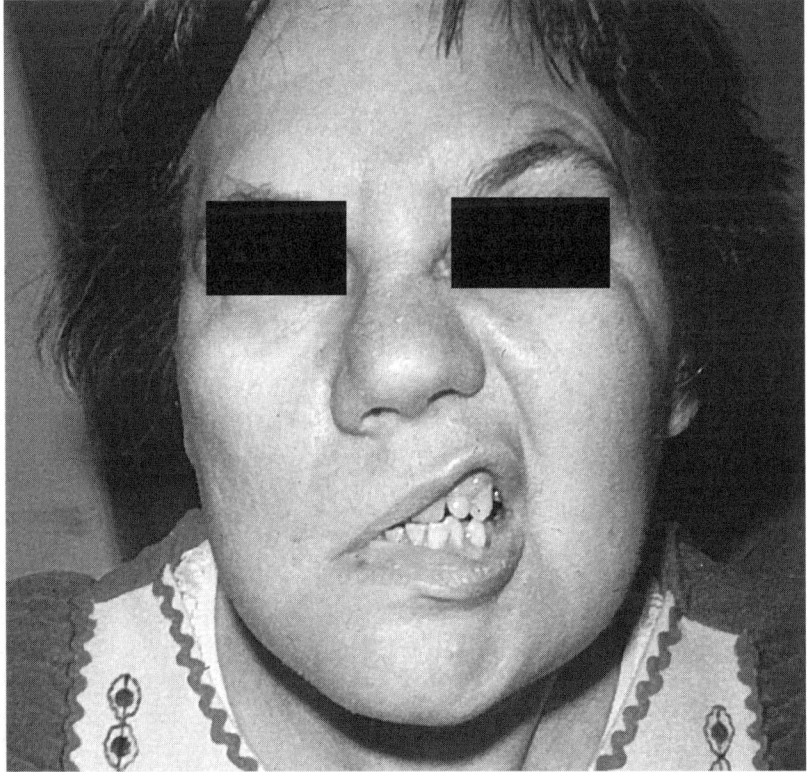

Figure 24.1 Total right facial paralysis with asymmetry at rest (not shown) and no motion on the right. This is classified as a grade 6/6 paralysis. (Courtesy of Dr. David E. Eibling.)

contralateral normal side within 3 weeks of the onset of weakness, then surgical decompression of the facial nerve is recommended within 24 hours of the abnormal electroneurographic result. Because this procedure requires opening the meatal foramen at the internal auditory meatus, the potential risks and benefits of such surgery must be considered individually.

Management and Follow-Up

The management of facial paralysis (*see* Algorithm) falls into two categories: managing the cause of the paralysis and preventing further complications.

The most common and preventable complication of facial paralysis is **exposure keratitis**. The primary cause of this condition is the inability to fully close the eye, which is often aggravated by decreased tear production, lack of Bell's phenomenon (i.e., upward gaze of the eye with attempted closure, which protects the cornea), and decreased corneal sensation (9). Any patient with a diminished ability to close an eye should be started on an eye-care program and educated about exposure keratitis. A minimal eye-care program consists of frequent application of artificial tears (at least four times daily) during the day and petrolatum-based ointment at night (9). If the eye examination is abnormal, showing redness or irritation, or if there are any vision changes, urgent ophthalmologic evaluation is recommended.

The specific management of facial paralysis varies with the cause. Most Bell's palsy is likely secondary to HSV I; however, the best treatment remains controversial. In 1982, Peitersen (6) published the natural history of the disease in 1011 patients, showing that 85% of patients had a return to normal or near normal function without treatment. Findings that indicate a poorer outcome included complete paralysis at presentation, recovery beginning later than 3 weeks after onset, postauricular pain, and increasing patient age.

Treatment options include observation only or systemic steroids with or without acyclovir or a similar antiviral. The definitive study that proves the efficacy of steroids or antivirals has yet to be done. Adour and coworkers (3) demonstrated that steroids are better than no treatment and that steroids plus acyclovir are better than steroids alone. They recommended prednisone (0.5 mg/kg/d bid for 5 days, tapered to 5 mg/d bid for 5 days) and oral acyclovir (400 mg five times daily for 10 days). They acknowledge that the usual dosage of 200 mg five times daily for HSV I also may be effective but did not use this dosage in the study.

As with any other disease, the decision to treat a given patient is based on risk-to-benefit considerations, keeping in mind the favorable natural history in most patients. Patients with relative contraindications to such treatment include those with diabetes mellitus, peptic ulcer disease, connective tissue disease, renal or hepatic dysfunction, malignant hypertension, or immunodeficiency states (3). Because the damage from Bell's palsy peaks at 2 to 3 weeks (8), treatment initiated after this time is of questionable benefit.

Trauma in the form of temporal bone fractures is the second most common cause of facial paralysis, accounting for 17% of cases (10) (Fig. 24.2). Although it is unlikely that such patients present primarily to an internist, the most important piece of information about such patients is whether the palsy or paralysis is immediate or delayed. If the facial nerve functions normally immediately after the trauma and develops paralysis gradually after that, then anatomical disruption of the nerve is unlikely. In such a circumstance, the most common cause of paralysis is edema, and reversibility with good return of function is likely (2). (Case 24.3 provides an example of deciding on a course of treatment when information about immediate or delayed paralysis is not available.) In cases in which the facial paralysis is noted to be immediate, the investigation of surgically treatable causes should be undertaken. Scan the temporal bone to rule out an impingement of bony fragments from a fracture, and seek out lacerations that may have severed the nerve. If one of these causes is found, then surgery with repair of the nerve may help. If no cause is found, the treatment is the same as for delayed paralysis.

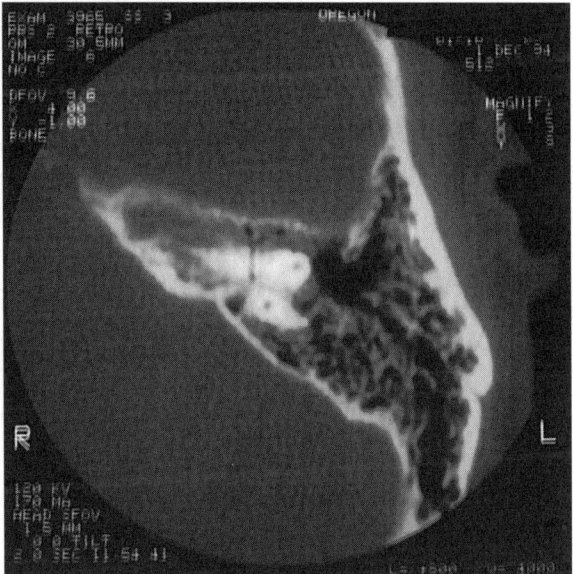

Figure 24.2 Computed tomography scan showing a transverse temporal bone fracture on the left. This type of fracture more commonly results in facial nerve paralysis. Early examination of facial function is important, because the prognosis is worse and the treatment is significantly more involved for immediate-onset facial paralysis than for delayed-onset facial paralysis. (Courtesy of Dr. Sean McMenomey.)

> **Case 24.3** **Boy with Left Peripheral Facial Nerve Paralysis After a Closed Head Injury**
>
> A boy 14 years of age is brought to the trauma unit after having suffered a closed head injury caused in an accident with an all-terrain vehicle. He is unconscious at the scene and has a Glasgow Coma Scale score of 8 in the trauma unit. A computed tomography scan demonstrates a longitudinal temporal bone fracture through the left temporal bone. Four days later he is noted to have total left peripheral facial nerve paralysis with inadequate Bell's phenomenon. Review of the records fails to indicate whether facial motion had been noted on arrival in the trauma unit. Electroneurography is normal.
>
> Nursing service is instructed in careful eye taping with liberal use of sterile eye lubricant. Steroids, instituted previously, are continued. Over the next 4 weeks, the patient regains some motion on the left side of his face. Six months later, when seen on follow-up for repair of his conductive hearing loss, his facial function was normal.
>
> **Discussion**
>
> This case points out the difficulty that could have developed by facial function not being noted in the trauma unit. Fortunately, facial function returned, as was suggested by the normal electroneurography and the computed tomography scan that demonstrated a longitudinal fracture. Nevertheless, there would have been much less concern if someone had documented normal facial function in the trauma unit.

The third most common cause of facial paralysis is **otologic disease**. Patients with facial paralysis secondary to acute otitis media, acute or chronic mastoiditis, or cholesteatoma may be misdiagnosed as having Bell's palsy. This misdiagnosis has the unfortunate effect of delaying the required antibiotic therapy or surgery, which can affect recovery and lead to other complications from the infectious process (e.g., brain abscess, meningitis). HZO that results from the reactivation of a previous herpes zoster infection accounts for approximately 4.5% to 8.9% of peripheral facial palsies (5). Unlike Bell's palsy, only approximately 50% of these patients recover satisfactory facial function. Murakami and coworkers (11) found that HZO patients who were treated with oral acyclovir (800 mg five times daily) plus steroids (in similar doses to that used for Bell's palsy) within 3 days of the onset of palsy had a 75% chance for full recovery, compared with only 30% if medications were begun after 7 days. Treatment delay is sometimes due to paralysis that precedes vesicular eruption, leading to the misdiagnosis of Bell's palsy. Magnetic resonance imaging is sometimes helpful in distinguishing these lesions. Many surgeons think that surgical decompression does not benefit patients with HZO (2).

All patients should be followed until the facial paralysis resolves or stabilizes.

Danger Signs

Danger signs in the evaluation of facial paralysis include the following:
- Incomplete paralysis
- Concurrent ear disease
- Otalgia
- Vertigo or hearing loss
- Vesicles in the external canal or the auricle
- Multiple cranial neuropathies
- Slowly progressive paralysis (>2–3 weeks)
- Recurrent paralysis

Fibrous Dysplasia

Fibrous dysplasia is a disease of unknown etiology in which normal medullary bone is replaced by fibrous and osseous tissue. The disease presents in three forms: monostotic (one bone), polyostotic (two or more bones), and the McCune–Albright syndrome (a subset of the polyostotic form that includes endocrine disturbances [precocious puberty and/or hyperthyroidism] and skin hyperpigmentation) (12).

The monostotic form accounts for over 75% of the presentations and occurs equally in men and women, usually in the second and third decades of life. The head and neck is involved in approximately 25% of cases, with the zygomatic process of the maxilla most commonly involved (followed by the angle of the mandible, frontal bone, ethmoid and sphenoid sinuses, and temporal bone). The polyostotic form accounts for 20% to 25% of fibrous dysplasia cases. McCune–Albright syndrome accounts for approximately 5% to 25% of cases of the polyostotic form. It is three times more common in women, typically manifesting in the first decade of life. The primary differential for fibrous dysplasia is bone neoplasms.

History

Fibrous dysplasia generally presents as asymptomatic swelling, but the patient may complain of pain, displaced teeth, malocclusion, headaches, proptosis, nasal obstruction, or symptoms secondary to nerve compression. The diagnosis is suggested by the presentation and radiologic appearance (12,13).

Physical Examination

Examination reveals a variably asymmetric face, depending on the bone involved. The mucosa overlying the bone is typically intact. A complete head and neck examination includes intranasal examination and an assessment of cranial nerve function. Palpation is important and confirms the bony nature of the lesion.

Additional Diagnostic Evaluation

Computed tomography scan with bone and soft tissue windows shows a radiographic appearance that varies with the form of fibrous dysplasia. Predominately osseous lesions are radiodense, whereas fibrous lesions are radiolucent. The usual combination of bony and fibrous tissue gives a typical "ground glass" appearance. The expanded cortex is usually thin and intact (12).

Management and Follow-Up

The goal of treatment is to achieve facial symmetry. Unless the lesion is very small, total removal is impractical; instead, the area should be surgically contoured. This procedure may need to be repeated many times because regrowth may occur (12,13).

Danger Signs

There is a 1 in 200 chance of the malignant transformation of fibrous dysplasia (usually to osteosarcoma), occurring mostly with the polyostotic form. A rapid increase in size or pain in a preexisting area of fibrous dysplasia should precipitate a work-up. Laboratory examinations may indicate increased serum alkaline phosphatase, and radiologic examination may show periosteal reactions (12,13).

Progressive Hemifacial Atrophy

Progressive hemifacial atrophy (Parry–Romberg syndrome) is a rare disease of unknown etiology that results in a progressive atrophy of the subcutaneous tissues of the face, with subsequent wasting of the associated muscle, skin, bone, and connective tissue (13,14). The disease usually affects the distribution of the trigeminal nerve and can involve one or all divisions; rarely does it involve the lower body. Progressive hemifacial atrophy is characterized by onset in the first or second decade of life and an active progressive phase of 2 to 10 years followed by a phase of stability (14).

History and Physical Examination

The disease may begin with irregular hyper- or hypopigmentation of the cheeks, forehead, or lower jaw. Rarely, the patient presents with premonitory muscle spasm or neuralgia followed by progressive atrophy that may extend in area or depth as the active phase ensues. A variety of other signs may be present, including enophthalmos, lower-lid atrophy, headaches, learning difficulties, and epilepsy (14).

Management and Follow-Up

There is no cure for progressive hemifacial atrophy. When the disease enters the stable phase, surgery to restore facial symmetry and bulk can be performed (14).

Tumors and Infection

Although neoplastic and infectious processes are beyond the scope of this chapter, they also may lead to facial asymmetry. When considering such processes, an anatomical approach that divides the face into thirds from top to bottom can be helpful. In all layers, tumors or infection may arise from skin, subcutaneous tissue, superficial muscles of facial expression, or deep muscles of mastication (temporalis or masseter).

The upper third of the face (from hairline to glabella) includes the frontal sinuses; thus, tumors and infectious processes of the frontal sinuses can cause localized swelling of the forehead that is associated with inferior displacement of the eye.

The middle third of the face (from glabella to subnasale) includes the orbits, eyes, ethmoid and maxillary sinuses, and the parotid glands laterally. Tumors and infection of the maxillary sinus can lead to a recontouring of the normally concave surface of the maxilla, making it convex and presenting as puffiness of the involved cheek. Processes that involve the ethmoid sinuses tend also to involve the eye, beginning with swelling in the medial canthus area and progressing to lateral deviation of the eye, with movement restriction and visual loss. Involvement of the parotid gland causes unilateral (or bilateral) swelling of the pre-auricular area or angle of the mandible.

The lower third of the face (from subnasale to menton) includes the upper and lower teeth, the mandible, and the submandibular glands. Any dental neoplasm or infection can lead to asymmetry, trismus, and pain. Any dental infection that causes visible asymmetry in the facial appearance may be spreading to the deep facial spaces and may require urgent surgical drainage.

Danger Signs

Patients with wasting of their facial form need to have systemic diseases ruled out. Any disease that causes muscle weakness or progressive weight loss should be considered. In facial asymmetry associated with normal or minimally abnormal facial nerve function, any underlying process that involves the facial skeleton needs to ruled out.

REFERENCES

1. **Cohen MM Jr.** Perspectives on craniofacial asymmetry. Part I: The biology of asymmetry. *Int J Oral Maxillofac Surg.* 1995;24:2–7.
2. **Coker NJ.** Acute paralysis of the facial nerve. In Bailey BJ (ed). *Head and Neck Surgery–Otolaryngology.* Philadelphia: JB Lippincott; 1993:1711–28.
3. **Adour KK, Ruboyianes JM, Von Doerstein PG, et al.** Bell's palsy treatment with acyclovir and prednisone compared with prednisone alone: a double-blind, randomized, controlled trial. *Ann Otol Rhinol Laryngol.* 1996;105:371–8.
4. **Murakami, S, Mutsuhiko M, Nakashiro Y, et al.** Bell's palsy and herpes simplex virus: identification of viral DNA in endoneurial fluid and muscle. *Ann Intern Med.* 1996;124:63–5.
5. **Devriese PP, Moesker WH.** The natural history of facial paralysis in herpes zoster. *Clin Otolaryngol.* 1988;13:289–98.
6. **Peitersen E.** The natural history of Bell's palsy. *Am J Otol.* 1982;4:107–11.
7. **Branndle P, Satoretti-Schefer S, Bohmer A, et al.** Correlation of MRI, clinical, and electroneurographic findings in acute facial nerve palsy. *Am J Otol.* 1996;17:154–61.
8. **Fisch U.** Surgery for Bell's palsy. *Arch Otolaryngol.* 1981;107:1–11.
9. **Handler LF, Galetta SL, Wulk AE, Popp JC.** Facial paralysis: diagnosis and management. In Bosniak S (ed). *Principles and Practice of Ophthalmic Plastic and Reconstructive Surgery.* Philadelphia: WB Saunders; 1996:465–83.
10. **Selesnick SH, Patwardnah A.** Acute facial paralysis: evaluation and early management. *Am J Otolaryngol.* 1994;15:387–408.
11. **Murakami S, Hato N, Horiuchi J, et al.** Treatment of Ramsay Hunt syndrome with acyclovir and prednisone: significance of early diagnosis and treatment. *Ann Neurol.* 1997;41:353–7.
12. **Wenig BM.** Neoplasms of the nasal cavity and paranasal sinuses. In Wenig BM (ed). *Atlas of Head and Neck Pathology.* Philadelphia: WB Saunders; 1993:44–5.
13. **Mazzeo N, Fisher JG, Mayer MH, Mathieu GP.** Progressive hemifacial atrophy (Parry–Romberg syndrome): case report. *Oral Surg Oral Med Oral Pathol Oral Radiol Endod.* 1995;79:30–5.
14. **Burton JL.** Disorders of connective tissue. In Champion RH, Burton JL, Ebling FJG (eds). *Textbook of Dermatology.* London: Blackwell Scientific; 1992:1781–2.

SUGGESTED READINGS

Matthias C, Terstegge K, Siemes H. Otorhinolaryngological complications of progressive facial hemiatrophy (Romberg's disease). *Ann Otol Rhinol Laryngol.* 1995;104:853-7.

This article contains a comprehensive description of the presentation of facial hemiatrophy, including hearing loss, localized bone destruction, parotid gland shrinkage, and masticatory spasm.

Murakami S, Hato N, Horiuchi J, et al. Treatment of Ramsay Hunt syndrome with acyclovir and prednisone: significance of early diagnosis and treatment. *Ann Neurol.* 1997;41:353-7.

This article contains an excellent summary of the arguments for the treatment of Ramsay Hunt syndrome with both steroids and antiviral medications.

Selesnick SH, Patwardnah A. Acute facial paralysis: evaluation and early management. *Am J Otolaryngol.* 1994;15:387-408.

This article details a systematic approach to early evaluation of new-onset facial paralysis and suggests management approaches.

Stanton RP, Montgomery BE. Fibrous dysplasia. *Orthopedics.* 1996;19:679-85

Although this excellent review article deals with the entire skeleton rather than just the face and neck, its explanation of the physiology of this disease and the overview of functional and aesthetic constraints of management make it well worth reading.

25

Lesions of the Face and Scalp

Luke K.S. Tan, MD

This chapter focuses on common skin lesions of the head and neck, including the scalp. Although many skin lesions are benign, some malignant lesions can be mistaken easily for benign lesions; therefore, the use of liberal criteria for biopsy is crucial. The emphasis is on skin malignancies, because these account for the greatest number of cancer cases in the United States today (1). Prompt biopsy and treatment aimed at complete eradication of tumor cells often result in a high cure rate and normal life expectancy.

Anatomy and Physiology

The mnemonic **S**kin, sub**C**utaneous, **A**poneurosis, **L**oose areolar tissue, and **P**eriosteum describes the soft tissue layers of the scalp. Although the skin over the face and neck is attached loosely to the underlying deep tissues, the skin of the cranial vault is firmly affixed to the underlying periosteum. Thus, the closure of scalp defects by mobilization and undermining is more difficult than is the closure of face and neck defects. The periosteum is a significant barrier to the deep extension of tumors.

The lymphatic drainage of head and neck skin is of great importance in determining the spread of malignancy. Because the scalp has no lymph nodes, its lymphatic fluid drains into the mastoid, occipital, pre-auricular, postauricular and upper neck nodes. The pre-auricular nodes can be superficial to or within the parotid gland, which explains the occasional appearance of metastatic lesions in the parotid gland. The skin of the face drains into the submental, sub-

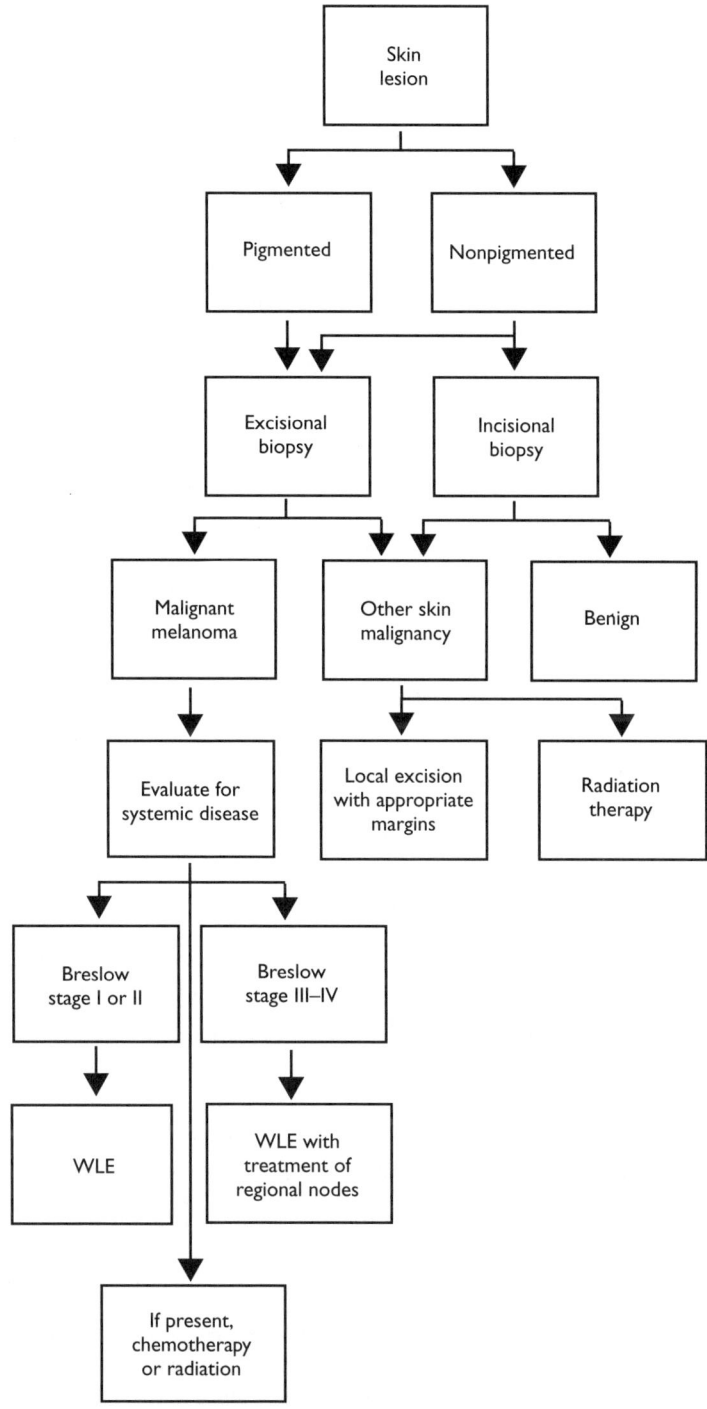

Algorithm Management of skin lesions. WLE = wide local excision.

mandibular, anterior cervical, pre-auricular, and buccal nodes. The buccal nodes lie on the buccinator muscle near the marginal mandibular branch of the facial nerve. All lymphatic fluid ultimately reaches the deep cervical nodes that surround the internal jugular vein.

The facial skin lines are important in the reconstruction of defects. Facial lines run at right angles to the facial musculature. Forehead lines are horizontal, cheek lines are oblique to the nasolabial folds, and neck creases are horizontal to the pull of the platysma. Although the main purpose of tumor resection is to obtain clear margins, consideration for achieving aesthetically pleasing results is also important. This is especially so in lesions that have a good prognosis, such as basal cell carcinoma (BCC).

History

Any lesion of recent onset or that which has exhibited a change in behavior may herald a malignancy. Squamous cell carcinoma (SCC) and malignant melanoma can have a rapid rate of growth. Most benign lesions grow slowly; however, keratoacanthoma and papilloma (viral warts) can grow rapidly. Abnormal growth patterns, such as asymmetrical growth (especially in pigmented lesions), often indicate malignancy. Lesions that grow so rapidly that they outgrow their blood supply often necrose, leading to ulceration and bleeding. Pigmented basal cells may be confused with melanomas. Because pain is uncommon in skin lesions, its presence may indicate involvement of the underlying neural structures.

Other relevant history features include 1) sun exposure, sunburn, and the use of sunscreens, 2) previous or concurrent skin lesions, 3) cigarette use, and 4) family history of similar skin lesions.

The differential diagnosis of common skin lesions is shown in Table 25.1.

Physical Examination

Examining the skin of the face and neck can be complex. A systematic approach that focuses on the scalp and other common sites of skin cancer makes for a more efficient and effective examination. Scalp lesions often are not read-

Table 25.1 Differential Diagnosis of Common Facial Skin Lesions

Actinic keratosis	Squamous papilloma
Seborrheic keratosis	Basal cell carcinoma
Keratoacanthoma	Squamous cell carcinoma
Nevus	Malignant melanoma

ily apparent. A scalp covered with plentiful hair requires more detailed scrutiny than a bald scalp to detect the same lesion. Facial areas that receive maximum sun exposure (e.g., forehead, temple, pre-auricular region, nose) are most prone to developing skin cancers.

Diagnosis and Management

Four general principles guide the treatment of facial skin lesions:
1. Whenever malignancy seems possible, lesions of the face and scalp are **biopsied** to exclude malignancy.
2. The aim of treatment for skin malignancy is the **complete eradication of tumor cells**. The specific treatment modality is less important; however, inadequate eradication leads to recurrence and metastasis.
3. Postexcision defects of the face and scalp present a **reconstructive challenge**. The goal of reconstruction is to restore any compromised function with the best possible aesthetic appearance.
4. **Prevention (i.e., protection against the sun)** is the key to avoiding most skin lesions of the face. Patient education about carcinogenic sun exposure is helpful.

The management of skin lesions is summarized in the Algorithm.

Biopsy

The two main types of skin-lesion biopsies are **excisional biopsy**, which removes the entire lesion without violating any margins, and **incisional biopsy**, which provides tissue for diagnosis but must be followed by total tumor eradication to avoid locoregional recurrence and distant metastasis (3,4). Both procedures are quick and easy to perform. Examples of incisional biopsy include punch biopsies, shave biopsies, and small excisions.

Punch biopsy is performed with a biopsy punch, an instrument that is available in different diameters (Fig. 25.1). The disposable biopsy punch has the advantage of not needing to be cleaned. The punch is circular in shape, with a sharp bottom edge of the circle. After appropriate numbing of the skin, the punch is held against the skin and twisted firmly in a back-and-forth motion until the entire dermis is penetrated. The punch is removed, and surgical forceps are used to pick up the core of skin and elevate it above the surrounding tissue. Scissors are used to sever this biopsy material in the subdermal plane.

Actinic Keratosis

Actinic keratosis (AK), also known as solar or senile keratosis, is a common lesion of the face and scalp that is more prevalent on sun-exposed areas of the

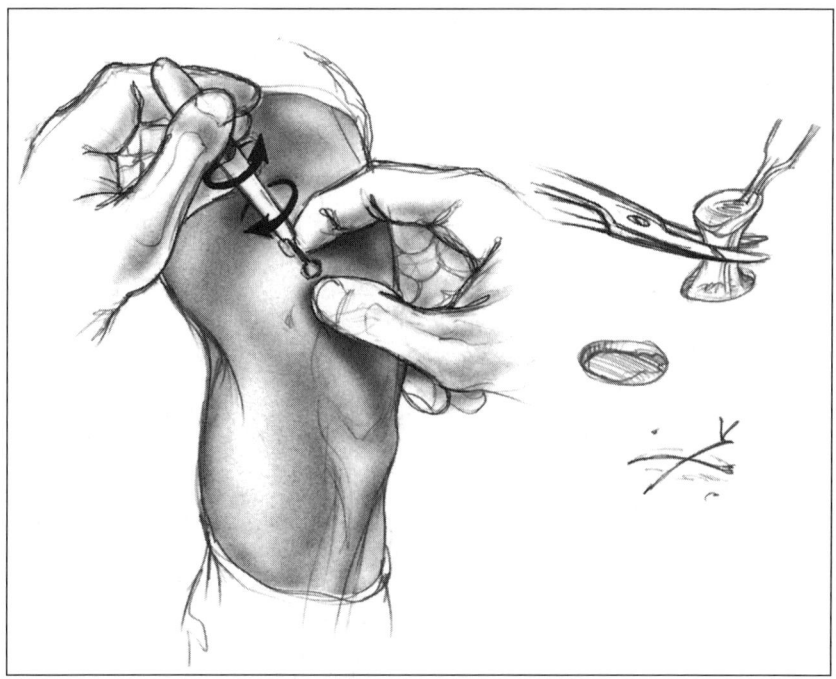

Figure 25.1 Punch biopsy technique. (Reprinted with permission from Bailey BJ [ed]. *Head and Neck Surgery–Otolaryngology*, ed 1. Philadelphia: JB Lippincott; 1993.)

face and scalp. It appears as a warty, rough, or scaly "sand paper"–like lesion and often is present in more than one site (Fig. 25.2). Ultraviolet-B waves—most intense between 10 AM and 3 PM in the summer in the northern hemisphere—are thought to cause this lesion. AK typically occurs in men in their fifth decade of life who have a history of significant sun exposure. The differential diagnosis includes seborrheic keratosis (SK), BCC, and SCC. Because AK cannot always be differentiated clinically from a malignant lesion, and because malignant change of AK to SCC can occur, many of these lesions are biopsied. The typical pathologic feature of AK is the presence of dysplastic keratinocytes of varying degrees. There should be no evidence of a basement-membrane breach, for this finding indicates a squamous cancer. The patient with AK should be followed regularly because of the malignant potential of these lesions. The treatment options for AK include cryosurgery, curettage, electrodesiccation, dermabrasion (5), topical chemotherapy (6), and surgical excision. Cryosurgery with liquid nitrogen or electrodesiccation can result in permanent skin hypopigmentation. Topical 5-fluorouracil (5-FU) at concentra-

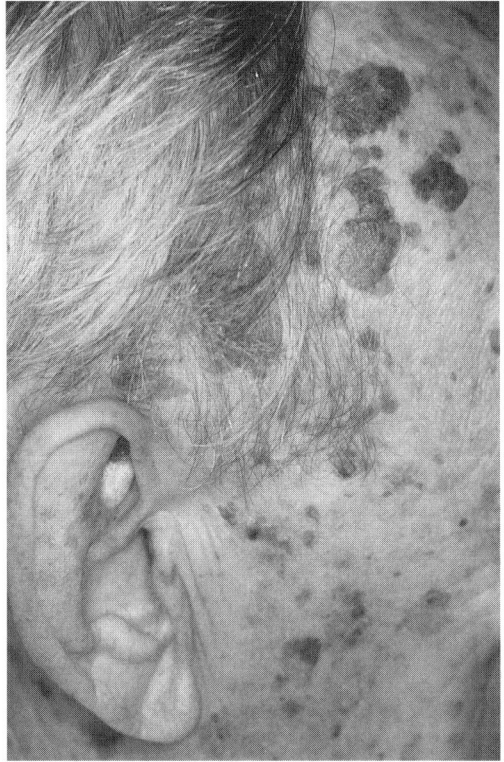

Figure 25.2 Facial actinic keratosis.

tions of 1% or 5% (both equally effective) has been used twice daily for 4 to 8 weeks. Combination therapy of topical 5-FU with other cutaneous topical agents (e.g., trichloroacetic acid) also may be used; tretinoin enhances the effects of 5-FU (7) (Table 25.2).

Seborrheic Keratosis

A raised lesion of variable size, SK is round to oval in shape, friable, and dry looking, with an overlying crust; it also may be inflamed. Histologically, several subtypes of SK show varying degrees of acanthosis, hyperkeratosis, and papillomatosis. As with AK, a biopsy may be required to rule out malignancy. The sudden onset of multiple SKs (Leser–Trélat sign) may indicate a possible internal malignancy, most commonly large-bowel adenocarcinoma (8,9). Treatment (excision) is reserved for aesthetic or functional reasons.

Keratoacanthoma

Keratoacanthoma (KA) is a benign lesion that grows rapidly (up to 10–25 mm over 4 to 8 weeks) and appears similar to BCC or SCC (10). Histologically, KA can be difficult to differentiate from SCC and may also have central necrosis and a keratinous core that mimics the "rodent bite" appearance of BCC. Unlike malignant lesions, the natural history of KA is a gradual resolution over several months, leaving an atrophic scar. During the growth phase, KA can be very destructive (Table 25.3) (11). Because its behavior can mimic that of a malignant lesion, and because the histology can be confused with SCC, excisional biopsy is the treatment of choice in most circumstances. The margins for excisions need to be clear of disease (2–4 mm). A high cure rate can be expected. The cause and trigger for KA are not understood clearly.

Histologic findings of KA include pseudoepitheliomatous hyperplasia with an exophytic keratinized growth pattern. There is no evidence of basement-membrane involvement. Distinguishing KA from SCC is the main purpose of the biopsy and can be difficult because perineural, perivascular, and muscle invasion have been reported (12). Mohs' micrographic surgery (13) and curettage (14) have high success rates (95%). The few indications for radiotherapy treatment include giant, aggressive KA and patients who are not willing to undergo surgical treatment. KA lesions are radiosensitive, and the cure rates are

Table 25.2 Treatment Options for Actinic Keratosis

Topical chemotherapy (5-FU and others)	Dermabrasion
Cryosurgery	Excision
Curettage and electrodesiccation	Combination (topical 5-FU and other cutaneous topical agents)

5-FU = 5-fluorouracil.

Table 25.3 Comparison of Keratoacanthoma, Squamous Cell Carcinoma, and Basal Cell Carcinoma

	KA	SCC	BCC
Classification	Variable	Malignant	Malignant
Growth Pattern	Expansile	Invasive	Locally invasive
Metastasis	None	Higher potential	Lower potential
Number	Can be multiple	Usually single	Can be multiple
Prognosis	Excellent	Variable	Good

BCC = basal cell carcinoma; KA = keratoacanthoma; SCC = squamous cell carcinoma.

high (15). Topical 5-FU (20%) causes resolution of KA; however, confusion can arise because 5-FU can cause initial improvement and, thus, masking of SCC (16). Systemic agents such as retinoids and methotrexate may be indicated for aggressive forms of KA (giant or multinodular types) (17).

Nevus

Most nevus types are acquired, usually presenting during childhood, the teen years, or early adulthood. The three primary varieties are junctional, dermal, and compound. A junctional nevus is usually flat and pigmented, whereas a dermal nevus is nonpigmented and rises well above the surface of the surrounding skin. A compound nevus has characteristics of both junctional and dermal types. An elevated nevus often can be removed with shave techniques, although this leaves a small chance of recurrence (Fig. 25.3). Complete excision (excisional biopsy) is a better choice for a junctional nevus.

Many other variants of nevus exist, many of which are pigmented. The primary risk in treating such lesions arises when an early melanoma is thought to be a benign lesion and a biopsy is not performed. The safest approach is to use liberal criteria for excisional biopsy, especially of pigmented skin lesions that recently have changed in character or appearance.

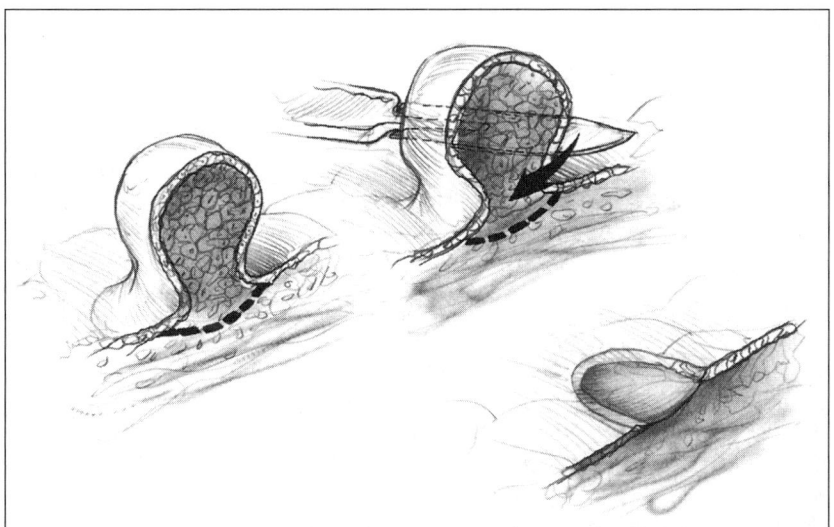

Figure 25.3 Shave biopsy technique. (Reprinted with permission from Bailey BJ [ed]. *Head and Neck Surgery–Otolaryngology*, ed 1. Philadelphia: JB Lippincott; 1993.)

Squamous Papilloma

Squamous papilloma is a usually soft, benign, sessile lesion caused by a local infection with the human papilloma virus. It typically occurs over the neck or scalp, appearing as single or multiple lesions (Fig. 25.4). Single lesions are usually present for many years and typically grow slowly. Surgical excision, either by shave technique or complete excision, usually is advised. Squamous papilloma has a low incidence of malignant transformation.

Basal Cell Carcinoma

The most common malignant skin lesion (Fig. 25.5), BCC has a incidence in excess of 600,000 new cases annually in the United States. A major contributing cause is photodamage from ultraviolet-B light exposure secondary to work or leisure activities; hence, prevention with the use of sunscreen is encouraged. The Fitzpatrick scale (Table 25.4) is a method used to classify skin types and their respective sensitivity to sun exposure. Skin identified as Fitzpatrick I or II is prone to develop multiple skin cancers if subjected to unprotected exposure to sunlight. Individuals who have these skin types should be counseled to use sunscreens and practice avoidance. Although BCC is locally aggressive, it rarely metastasizes. Occasionally, large neglected lesions can become invasive and can metastasize (Fig. 25.6). Although most BCCs are

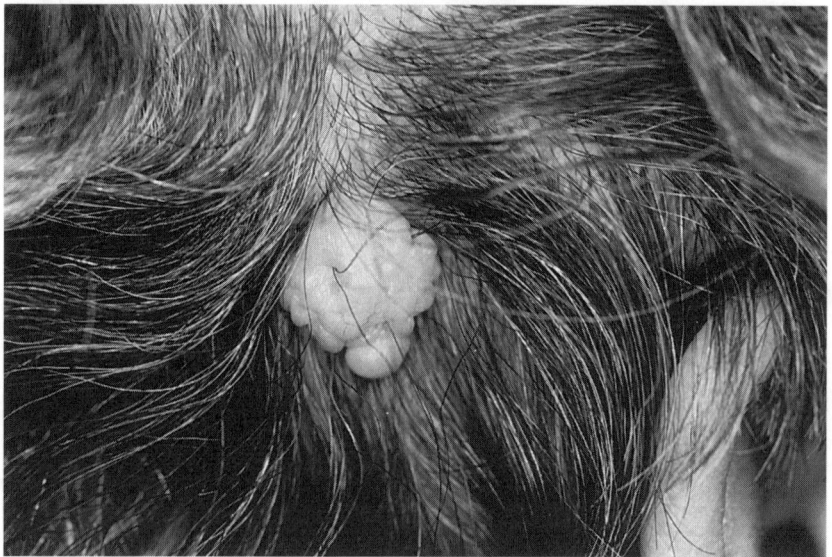

Figure 25.4 Squamous papilloma of the scalp.

nodular, a diffuse form exists that has a high rate of recurrence due to islets of tumor in the dermis. When encased in dense fibrous tissue, this BCC subtype is called "sclerosing" or "morpheic." The presence of these variants on a pathology report should alert the physician to expect more biologically aggressive behavior.

The treatment of BCC is usually surgical excision. Clear margins are important, because incomplete excision leads to recurrence; hence, excision margins should not be altered because of reconstructive concerns. The 5-year cure rates for standard surgical resection of BCC range from 90% to 95%.

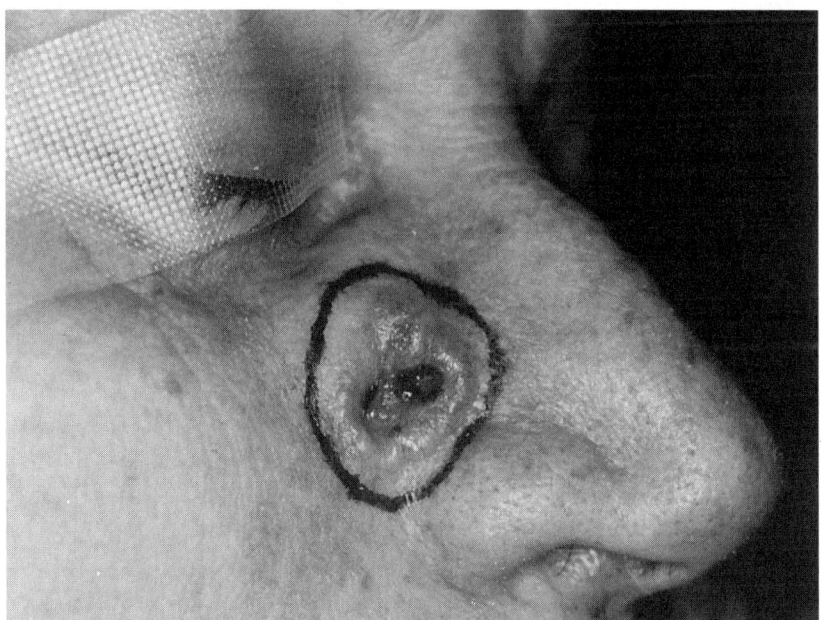

Figure 25.5 Basal cell carcinoma of the melolabial fold.

Table 25.4 Fitzpatrick Sun-Reactive Skin Types

Skin Type	Skin Color	Tanning Response
I	White	Always burns, never tans
II	White	Usually burns, tans with difficulty
III	White	Sometimes burns mildly, tans normally
IV	Brown	Rarely burns, tans with ease
V	Dark brown	Very rarely burns, tans very easily
VI	Black	Never burns, tans very easily

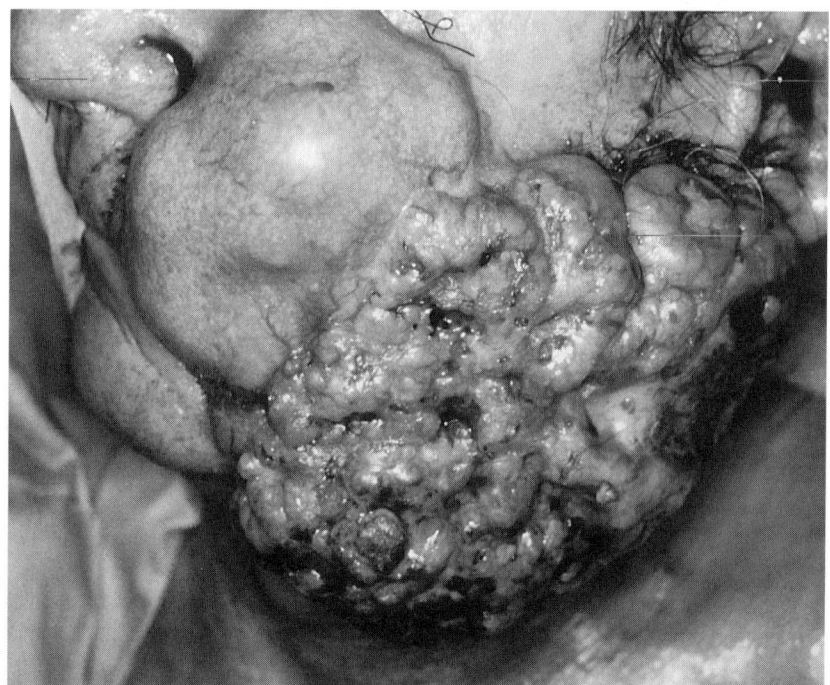

Figure 25.6 Large basal cell carcinoma over the cheek developed over 8 years.

Dr. Frederic Mohs developed a more time-consuming but effective method of micrographic surgery. Cure rates up to 99% are reported. Mohs' micrographic surgery (MMS) involves a careful marking of the excised specimen and a histologic examination of the entire patient–tumor interface. The specimen is divided (usually into quadrants); if additional tumor is detected, further excision is performed in the quadrant(s) involved. Each stage of excision is similarly marked and examined. In this way, spreading "fingers" of the tumor are followed and excised completely.

An excellent treatment for all types of BCC, MMS is particularly recommended for those with a high potential for recurrence, including all sclerosing or morpheic variants. In addition, MMS should be considered for BCC located in the "H" zone (i.e., the skin around the eyes, nose, upper lip, and ear and a strip of pre-auricular skin between the angle of the mandible and the temple). BCC in the "H" zone—much of which is composed of embryonic fusion planes—is often more aggressive.

Radiotherapy is an alternate therapeutic option in patients who are deemed unsuitable for surgery or as a form of adjuvant therapy. Because BCC is highly curable and frequently occurs in relatively young patients, a

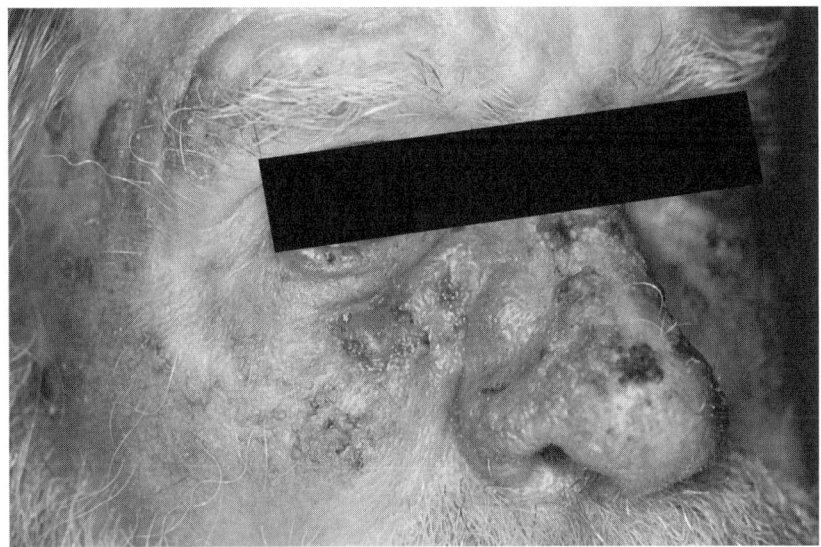

Figure 25.7 Squamous cell carcinoma of the cheek and dorsum of nose.

long-term, aesthetically pleasing outcome is the aim. (*See* section on Reconstructive Outcomes below for a discussion of facial plastic reconstructive procedures.) Regional neck dissection is reserved for large aggressive lesions or for clinical evidence of metastasis; however, eradication of regional lymph nodes is rarely necessary for BCC.

Squamous Cell Carcinoma

The second most common form of nonmelanoma skin cancer, SCC is epidermal in origin and is associated with exposure to ultraviolet light. There are several histologic variants of SCC, each with a different level of aggressiveness. Verrucous carcinoma is less aggressive, whereas clear cell and signet-ring cell SCC are very aggressive (18,19). SCC can be difficult to differentiate from pseudoepitheliomatous hyperplasia and keratoacanthoma. SCCs of the face and scalp are typically ulcerative lesions that spread in the path of least resistance. SCCs of the face tend to spread superficially as well as deeply, often with bony involvement (Fig. 25.7). In contrast, scalp lesions usually do not involve the underlying bone because of the thick layer of periosteum over the scalp (Fig. 25.8). SCC has a high propensity for regional metastasis, even small lesions. Typical examples include small medial canthal or lower eyelid lesions that sometimes present later as nodal metastasis in the parotid or upper jugular chain. A computed tomography scan of larger facial lesions is indicated if the depth of the lesion is difficult to assess.

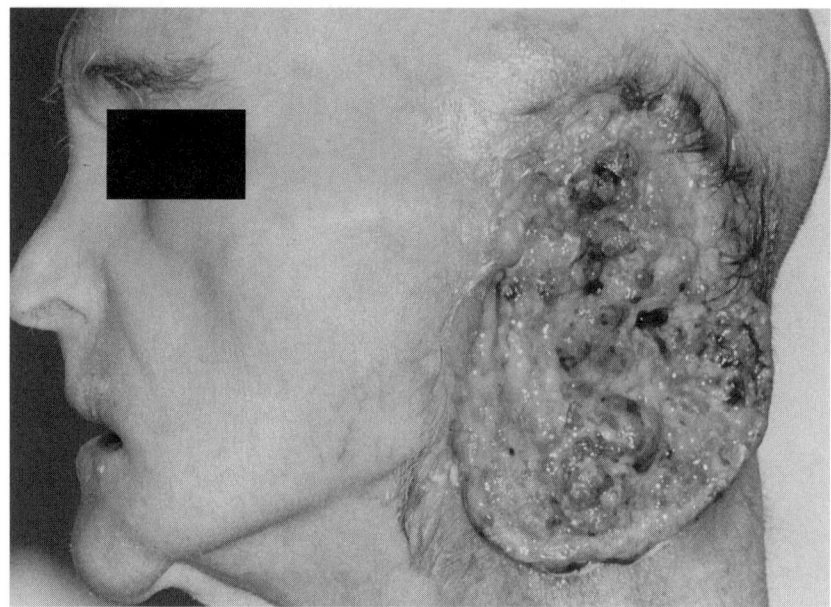

Figure 25.8 Large squamous cell carcinoma of the ear, presenting with facial paralysis from facial nerve invasion. (Courtesy of Dr. Gary Clayman.)

Adnexal Lesions

Neoplasms of adnexal origin are rare, comprising less than 1% of all head and neck cancers. The varied origin and behavior of these lesions can be a dilemma in both diagnosis and treatment. Adnexal lesions can be classified broadly by their cells of origin: hair follicles, sweat glands (apocrine and eccrine), sebaceous glands, vascular tissue, and subcutaneous tissue.

Malignant Melanoma

Most malignant melanomas of the head and neck arise de novo. A preexisting mole has been known to be present in up to 70% of cases. Malignant melanoma that is associated with melanocytic nevus occurs more often in the trunk and limbs. In a study of 1002 cases, malignant melanoma of the head and neck accounted for 14% of all malignant melanomas (20). These lesions occur mainly in adults with peak incidence in the fifth to seventh decades and are especially prevalent in outdoor workers or in patients with a history of multiple sunburns (especially during childhood). Malignant melanoma of the head and neck is similar to that of the trunk and limbs, usually presenting as a slow-growing, macular, pigmented lesion. A recent change in color, shape, and size and the ulceration or bleeding of a preexisting mole are presenting complaints in most cases. A complete head and neck examination, including all mucosal surfaces of the upper aerodigestive tract and the cervical lymph node, should be performed. All patients with malignant melanoma should be evaluated for systemic disease.

An excisional biopsy should be performed for all suspected cases of malignant melanoma. Curettage and shave biopsies are not useful because the prognosis of malignant melanoma depends largely on the depth of invasion. Malignant melanoma can be staged by thickness (Breslow) or depth of invasion (Clark), and treatment is based on this staging (Tables 25.5 and 25.6). A thickness of less than 0.76 mm (Breslow stage I) indicates early disease, and local wide excision with a margin of 1 cm results in a low rate of local recurrence or metastasis (21,22). Thicker lesions should be resected with wider margins, typically 2 cm for a lesion 1 to 2 mm thick and 3 cm for a tumor thicker than 2 mm. Obtaining such margins occasionally is limited by vital structures in the head and neck. Alternate treatments include radiotherapy and locoregional chemotherapeutic perfusion; immunotherapy has proved useful in some studies.

Management of the lymph nodes is controversial in malignant melanoma of the head and neck. Generally, neck dissection is unnecessary in Breslow stage I lesions. In lesions greater than 4 mm, neck dissection is used therapeutically for the removal of involved nodes. In lesions between 0.75 and 4.0 mm, the rule of neck dissection is unknown. Sentinel-node mapping is being tested with good success in patients with no palpable nodes and medium-depth lesions.

Table 25.5 Breslow's Staging for Malignant Melanoma

Stage	Thickness (mm)
I	<0.75
II	0.75–1.50
III	1.5–4.0
IV	>4.0

Table 25.6 Clark Staging for Malignant Melanoma

Level	Depth of Invasion
1	Basement membrane
2	Through basement membrane
3	Into papillary dermis
4	Into reticular dermis
5	Into subcutaneous tissue

Reconstructive Options

The first principle of skin cancer treatment is complete tumor resection. After the tumor has been removed completely, aesthetic considerations are crucial,

Table 25.7 Reconstructive Options

Second Intent Healing
    Useful only in small defects
    Primarily used in medial canthus and the temple areas

Grafting
  Split-Thickness Skin Graft
    Rarely used, except for temporary coverage during tissue expansion
  Full-Thickness Skin Graft
    Used for small defects
    Has poor texture, color, and surface-level match
  Composite Graft
    Auricular skin, subcutaneous tissue, perichondrium, and cartilage
  Combination
    Cartilage graft for nasal reconstruction can be used in combination with regional flaps (e.g., melolabial or forehead flaps)

Local Flaps
  Advancement
    A-to-T useful in forehead and temple defects
    Cheek-advancement flaps
  Rotation
    Bilobed
    V-to-Y
    Transnasal (bridge)

Regional flaps
  Locoregional
    Nasolabial
    Forehead
      Median or paramedian
      Particularly useful for reconstruction of large significant nasal defects
  Distant
    Latissimus dorsi musculocutaneous flap
    Pectoralis major myocutaneous flap
    Trapezius
    Reserved for large defects of the head and neck, especially the pre-auricular region; the latissimus dorsi has a longer pedicle and larger skin paddle and, thus, is more versatile

Free-Tissue Transfer
    Used for large defects that involve the scalp and the upper and mid-face
    Common donor sites include rectus, radial forearm, and scapula

Lesions of the Face and Scalp 519

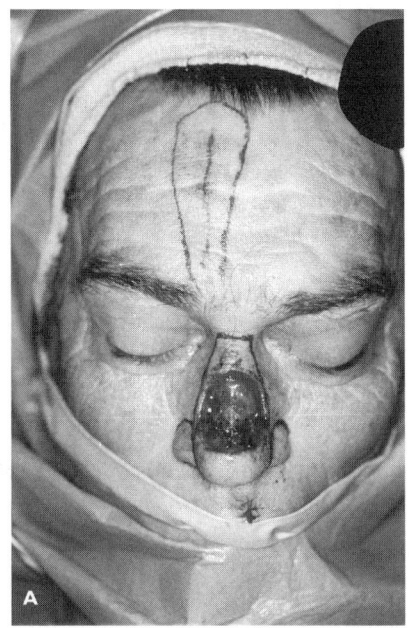

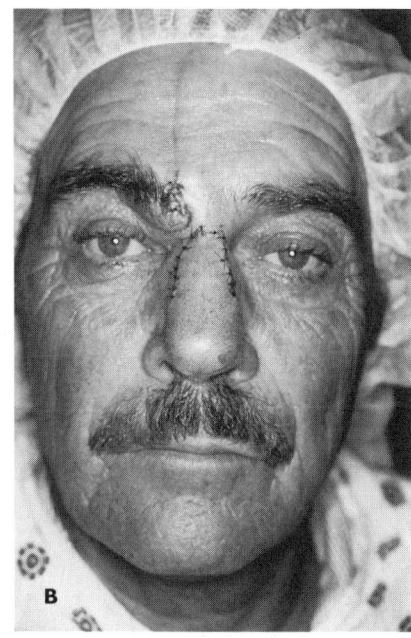

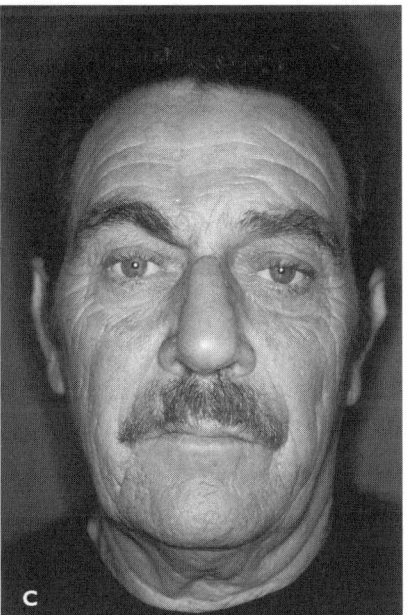

Figure 25.9 Stages of reconstruction in a patient with basal cell carcinoma over the nasal dorsum. **A,** Mohs' defect over the dorsum of nose that is to be reconstructed with a forehead flap. **B,** Early results after division of pedicle of forehead flap. **C,** Results at 2 months. The patient was satisfied and declined further aesthetic refinement.

especially in dealing with face and scalp lesions. Alterations to normal anatomy in these areas should be apparent. Many of these patients have curable disease and a normal life expectancy.

Reconstructive options depend on the size and site of the tumor and on the importance of appearance to the patient. A wide variety of the reconstructive options exist (Table 25.7). For larger tumors that require more complex reconstruction, having separate teams for resection and reconstruction makes good sense. In many centers, a dermatologist performs MMS for excision, and a surgeon performs the reconstruction (Fig. 25.9). MMS is labor intensive and is not readily available everywhere.

Small defects in favorable locations (e.g., forehead, mid-cheek) often can be closed primarily. Small defects in selected locations (e.g., medial canthus, temple) can be allowed to heal by secondary intent. Reconstruction of medium-sized facial defects with local flaps often yields good results. For larger face or neck defects or many scalp defects (because scalp skin has poorer elasticity), regional flaps or tissue expanders are frequently required. For lesions that extend into the orbit, orbital exenteration is sometimes indicated. Although skin grafting remains an option for many defects created by skin-tumor removal, the poor matching of texture, color, and surface level makes these unacceptable to most patients. In some large, complex defects, free-tissue transfers (e.g., radial forearm flaps) are necessary. Radiation therapy remains a viable alternative for the patient who is an unacceptable medical risk for surgery or who does not want surgery. Photodynamic therapy is being investigated for use in SCC, although the side effects of prolonged photosensitivity may limit its practical application.

Danger Signs

Danger signs for skin lesions include the following:
- Recent appearance with rapid growth
- Recent change in the size, shape, or color of a preexisting lesion
- Ulceration or bleeding of a facial lesion

Summary

When in doubt about a skin lesion, biopsy it. Incisional biopsies are acceptable for many lesions; however, lesions suspected of being malignant melanoma should be biopsied excisionally, because the thickness of the lesion determines the prognosis. After all tumor cells have been eradicated, the next goal of treatment is successful reconstructive surgery, for which there are many options.

REFERENCES

1. **American Cancer Society.** Cancer statistics; 1996.
2. **Redden EM, Baker DC.** Medicolegal problems in the management of patients with skin cancer. *Cancer of the Skin.* Philadelphia: WB Saunders; 1991:603.
3. **Austin JR, Byers RM, Brown WD, Wolf P.** Influence of biopsy on the prognosis of cutaneous melanoma of the head and neck. *Head Neck.* 1996;18:107–17.
4. **Dellon AL, DeSilva S, Connolly M, Ross A.** Prediction of recurrence in incompletely excised basal cell carcinoma. *Plastic Reconstr Surg.* 1985;75:860–71.
5. **Winton GB, Salasche SJ.** Dermabrasion of the scalp as a treatment for actinic damage. *J Am Acad Dermatol.* 1986;14:661–8.
6. **Jansen TG.** Use of topical fluorouracil. *Arch Derm.* 1983;119:784–5.
7. **Resnik SS, Resnik BI.** Management of actinic keratosis. In Wheeland RG (ed). *Cutaneous Surgery.* Philadelphia: WB Saunders; 1994.
8. **Holdines MR.** The sign of Leser–Trélat. *Int J Derm.* 1986;25:564–72.
9. **Liddell K, White JE, Caldwell JW.** Seborrheic keratosis and carcinoma of the large bowel. *Br J Derm.* 1975;92:449–52.
10. **Jackson IT.** Diagnostic problem of keratoacanthoma. *Lancet* 1969;1:490–2.
11. **Iverson RE, Vistnes Lm.** Keratoacanthoma is frequently a dangerous diagnosis. *Am J Surg.* 1973;126:359–65.
12. **Janecka IP, Wolff M, Crikelair GF, et al.** Aggressive histological features of keratoacanthoma. *J Cutan Pathol.* 1978:4;342.
13. **Larson PO.** Keratoacanthoma treated with Mohs' micrographic surgery (chemosurgery): a review of forty-three cases. *J Am Acad Dermatol.* 1987;16:1040–4.
14. **Reymann F.** Treatment of keratoacanthoma with curettage. *Dermatologica.* 1977;155:90–96.
15. **Caccialanza M, Sopelana N.** Radiation therapy of keratoacanthoma: results in 55 patients. *Int J Radiat Oncol Biol Phys.* 1989;16:475–7.
16. **Cobb MW, Pellegrini AE.** Squamous cell carcinoma following fluorouracil-responsive "keratoacanthoma." *Arch Dermatol.* 1987;123:987–988.
17. **Kestel JL Jr, Blair DS.** Keratoacanthoma treated with methotrexate. *Arch Dermatol.* 1973;108:723–4.
18. **Kuo T.** Clear cell carcinoma of the skin: a variant of the squamous cell carcinoma that stimulates sebaceous carcinoma. *Am J Surg Pathol.* 1980;91:488–91.
19. **Cramer SF, Heggeness LM.** Signet-ring squamous cell carcinoma. *Am J Surg Pathol.* 1980;4:573–83.
20. **Friedman RJ, Heilman ER, Waldo ED, et al.** Malignant melanoma: clinicopathologic correlations. In Friedman RJ, Rigel DS, Kopf AW, et al. (eds). *Cancer of the Skin.* Philadelphia: WB Saunders; 1991.
21. **Breslow A, Macht SD.** Optimal size of resection margin for thin cutaneous melanoma. *Surg Gynecol Obstet.* 1977;145:681.

22. **Day CL, Harris TJ, Gorstein F, et al.** Malignant melanoma : prognostic significance of "micro satellites" in the reticular dermis and subcutaneous fat. *Ann Surg.* 1981; 194:108.

SUGGESTED READINGS

Larrabee WF Jr, Sherris DA. *Principles of Facial Reconstruction.* Philadelphia: Lippincott-Raven; 1995.

This well-organized and readable book gives simple and clear diagrams as well as good illustrative clinical photographs and excellent reconstructive algorithms for approaching defects of the face and scalp.

Weber RS, Miller MJ, Geopfert H. *Basal and Squamous Cell Skin Cancers of the Head and Neck* Baltimore: Williams & Wilkins; 1996.

This comprehensive well-organized book covers in depth the various issues surrounding this topic. Chapters are divided into the relevant clinical foci (e.g., peri-auricular disease, periorbital disease, role of Mohs' surgery, neck dissections).

26

Facial Trauma

Karen T. Pitman, MD

Patients who have suffered facial trauma usually have been involved in motor vehicle accidents or have sustained industrial injuries, sports injuries, or physical assaults. Multisystem traumatic injuries are common in major accidents and can require evaluation by a general surgeon or trauma team. An otolaryngologist, plastic surgeon, or oral-maxillofacial surgeon usually treats maxillofacial trauma, with referral patterns determined by local customs within the medical community.

History

In the initial care of maxillofacial trauma, the first question to be answered is "What is the mechanism of injury (i.e., blunt or penetrating trauma of high or low velocity)?" followed by "Was only the head involved, or were the torso and/or extremities affected as well?" The patient or bystanders should be asked about loss of consciousness, and an attempt should be made to ascertain a basic medical history (e.g., major medical problems, current medications, drug allergies, pregnancy), which affects treatment of the trauma. This history is usually obtained while initial treatment is taking place.

Patients with an unstable or marginal airway require endotracheal tube insertion or tracheostomy, depending on the potential for a continuing increase in edema of the face, oral cavity, or oropharynx. **Orotracheal intubation should be attempted only after it has been determined that there is no in-**

jury to the cervical spine or when there is minimal distortion of the upper airway structures from edema, bleeding, or laryngeal trauma. **Nasotracheal intubation should *not* be performed in patients with trauma to the midface or with suspected basilar skull fracture because of the risk of inadvertently introducing the endotracheal tube into the cranium**; under these circumstances, tracheostomy or emergent cricothyrotomy should be performed. The amount of time until the facial injuries are repaired is also a consideration; if several days are required to stabilize the patient, a tracheostomy should be preferred to minimize the sequelae of prolonged intubation. A conscious patient with a tenuous airway may be served most optimally by a tracheostomy, because the sedation required to keep an intubated patient comfortable is not necessary with this procedure, allowing the patient to communicate and remain fully conscious. Definitive management of facial injuries often produces additional edema, making early extubation dangerous; hence, tracheostomy is often performed perioperatively.

Physical Examination

As with all trauma patients, the first part of the physical examination is to determine airway adequacy. Facial fractures may weaken bony support of the oral cavity or oropharynx and may compromise the upper portion of the airway. Edema and hemorrhage that results from facial fractures can compromise the upper airway if the patient cannot clear blood and secretions adequately. Dislodged teeth or broken dentures may become foreign bodies in the airway.

Once the airway has been secured, the condition of the circulatory and neurological systems must be determined. Shock and loss of consciousness require immediate attention. The neurological status of the patient should be monitored because intracranial injuries are common in maxillofacial trauma. Facial trauma should be evaluated and treated after the airway, cervical spine, and the hemodynamic and neurological status of the patient have been stabilized.

Patients with a history of facial trauma and suspected facial injuries require a complete head and neck examination, including an assessment of the orbits, ocular function, periorbital tissues, nose, bony skeleton, soft tissues, intraoral structures, and cranial nerves. Flexible fiberoptic evaluation of the laryngopharynx is often necessary. The following is an overview of the focused head and neck examination for the facial trauma patient. Physical findings associated with a particular type of injury are detailed in the section on Diagnosis and Management.

Extraocular muscle mobility, pupillary light response, and visual acuity are assessed for the orbit and globe. The position of the globe within the orbital cavity is evaluated, and enophthalmos or exophthalmos is noted. The orbit and periorbital tissues are inspected, and subconjunctival hemorrhage, periorbital edema, and ecchymosis are noted. Treatment of ocular emergencies (e.g., retrobulbar or optic nerve hematoma, ruptured globe, detached retina) requires immediate evaluation by an ophthalmologist. These injuries take precedence over the definitive management of facial fractures.

The nasal examination evaluates the shape and symmetry of the nose and the patency of the nasal airway. Preinjury photographs (e.g., driver's license) assist in determining if a new nasal deformity is present. The presence of intranasal blood, cerebrospinal fluid (CSF), or both is noted. Palpation may reveal mobile or misplaced nasal bones.

The middle third of the face—the area between the zygomaticofrontal suture and the occlusal plane of the teeth—is evaluated along with the mandible for integrity of bony structure, symmetry, contour, dental occlusion, and edema.

A complete evaluation of the cranial nerves should be performed. Flexible fiberoptic examination provides additional information about the status of the nasopharynx, hypopharynx, and larynx. Intraoral examination describes any interdental occlusion, the condition of the dentition and soft tissues, and the integrity of the hard palate.

Differential Diagnosis

The differential diagnosis in maxillofacial trauma is vast and includes purely soft tissue injuries, cartilaginous and bony injuries, major vessel and nerve damage, and trauma to the intracranial contents. Consequences of these injuries can range from mild deformity (e.g., unrepaired, mildly displaced nasal fracture) to major life-threatening problems (e.g., CSF rhinorrhea with meningitis, globe injury causing blindness, cervical spine injury causing quadriplegia, vascular injury causing a carotid–cavernous sinus fistula). A physician or oral surgeon who is well-versed and experienced in maxillofacial trauma should perform the evaluation of these patients—even ones with apparently minor injuries. A multidisciplinary team (i.e., general surgeon, otolaryngologist, ophthalmologist, vascular surgeon, neurosurgeon, and oral surgeon) provides optimal care.

Radiographic Studies

A physician who is consulted about a patient with facial injuries should check with the physician who is coordinating the patient's care before ordering any radiographic studies. This minimizes overall cost and patient inconvenience by avoiding repeated visits to the radiology suite. Specific computed tomography (CT) examinations and algorithms are used for evaluating facial fractures and for surgical planning. For example, plain radiographs of the nose for a suspected nasal fracture may not be required for diagnosis or treatment planning. A panoramic radiograph (Panorex) of the mandible may be the sole preoperative study for patients with straightforward mandible fractures. Patients with multiple facial fractures require axial and coronal fine-cut CT for preoperative planning.

Diagnosis and Management

Facial Fractures

Mandible Fractures

Mandible fractures should be suspected in patients with a history of trauma to the lower face who complain of pain, malocclusion, or a sensation of the teeth not fitting together correctly. Over 50% of patients with mandible fractures have breaks in more than one place owing to the shape and attachments of the mandible. When a mandible fracture is discovered, a second fracture site should be sought. Mandible fractures are the second most common facial fracture after nasal fractures (which are discussed below). The distribution of mandibular fracture sites are shown in Figure 26.1.

Physical findings that indicate a mandible fracture include trismus (difficulty opening the mouth) secondary to muscle splinting of the fracture. The normal interincisional opening between the upper and lower first teeth is greater than 40 mm, but a patient with mandible fractures typically cannot open his or her jaw more than 35 mm. On jaw opening, there may be deviation of the chin toward the side of the fracture. The intraoral examination may demonstrate a hematoma on the floor of the mouth or laceration of the gingiva. There may be lower lip or chin anesthesia secondary to injury to the inferior alveolar nerve. Often there is palpable mobility of the fracture fragments (Fig. 26.1).

The initial management of an uncomplicated mandible fracture includes pain control and a soft or liquid diet. Emergency conditions that are related to mandible fractures include airway impairment, displacement of the mandibular condyle into the middle cranial fossa, injury to the internal carotid artery, and severe hemorrhage.

Plain radiographs are usually adequate for assessing an isolated mandible fracture; views that should be requested include panoramic, lateral Towne's, and posteroanterior views. CT or additional studies are helpful in some com-

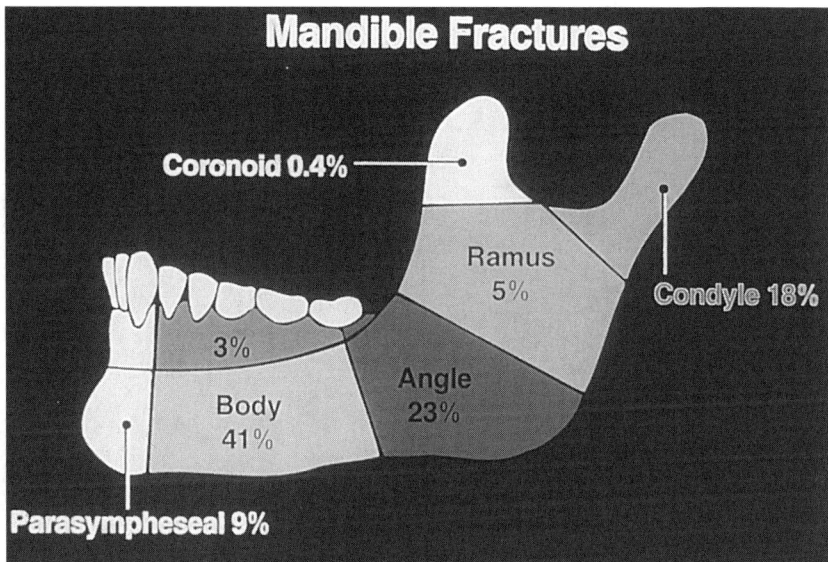

Figure 26.1 Distribution of mandibular fracture locations. (Republished with permission from Calhoun K. *Maxillofacial Trauma Slide Lecture Series*. Alexandria, VA: American Academy of Otolaryngology–Head and Neck Surgery Foundation; 1994.)

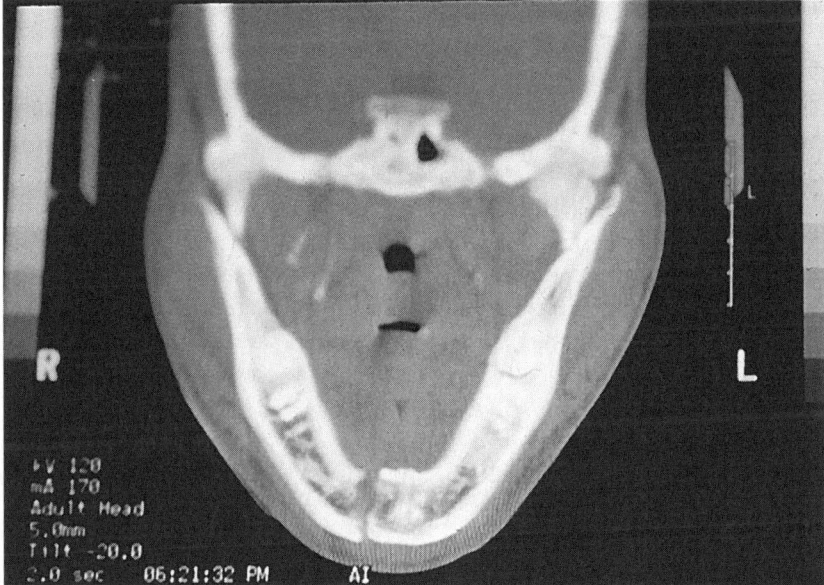

Figure 26.2 Computed tomography scan showing a parasymphaseal fracture of the mandible. (Republished with permission from Calhoun K. *Maxillofacial Trauma Slide Lecture Series*. Alexandria, VA: American Academy of Otolaryngology–Head and Neck Surgery Foundation; 1994.)

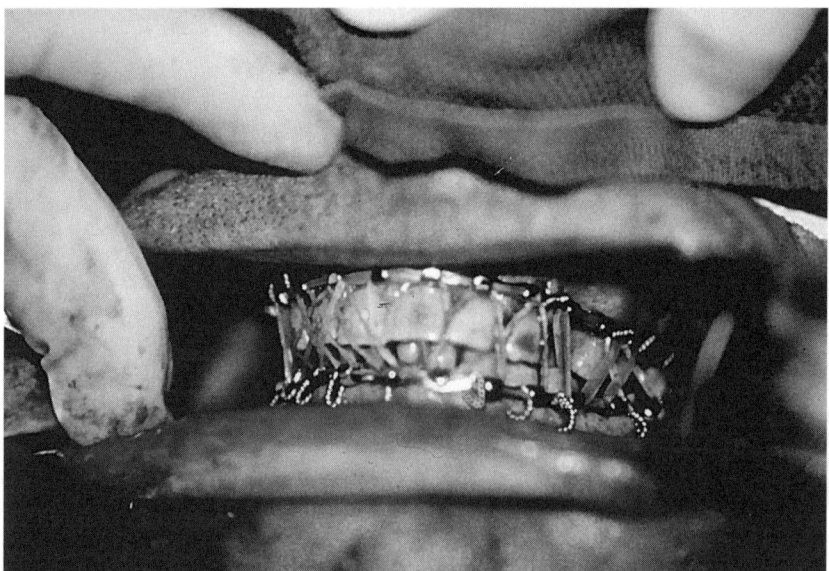

Figure 26.3 For some mandibular fractures with stable teeth on both sides of the fracture line, intermaxillary wiring (sometimes called maxillomandibular or interdental wiring) is sufficient treatment. (Republished with permission from Calhoun K. *Maxillofacial Trauma Slide Lecture Series.* Alexandria, VA: American Academy of Otolaryngology–Head and Neck Surgery Foundation; 1994.)

plex cases (Fig. 26.2). Preoperative dental impressions may assist in estimating preinjury dental occlusion.

Definitive treatment of isolated mandible fractures is recommended within 7 to 10 days of the injury. Injuries that are more life threatening should be addressed first; however, if the patient is taken to the operating room for repair of these other injuries, the mandible and other facial fractures can be treated concurrently. **Intermaxillary fixation** (wiring the teeth together), **open reduction with internal fixation, circumandibular wiring**, and **splinting** are all methods that can be used (Figs. 26.3 and 26.4). Both the timing of the operation and the specific technique used for repairing the fracture depend on fracture location in the mandible, patient age, and dentition status. **Waiting more than 7 to 10 days for definitive repair can lead to fixation of the malpositioned bone fragments.**

Zygomatic Trauma

Trauma to the **malar eminence** or cheekbone can result in fractures of the zygomatic complex. The zygoma forms the most lateral and inferior aspect of the orbital rim and consists of the malar bone and zygomatic arch. Skeletal su-

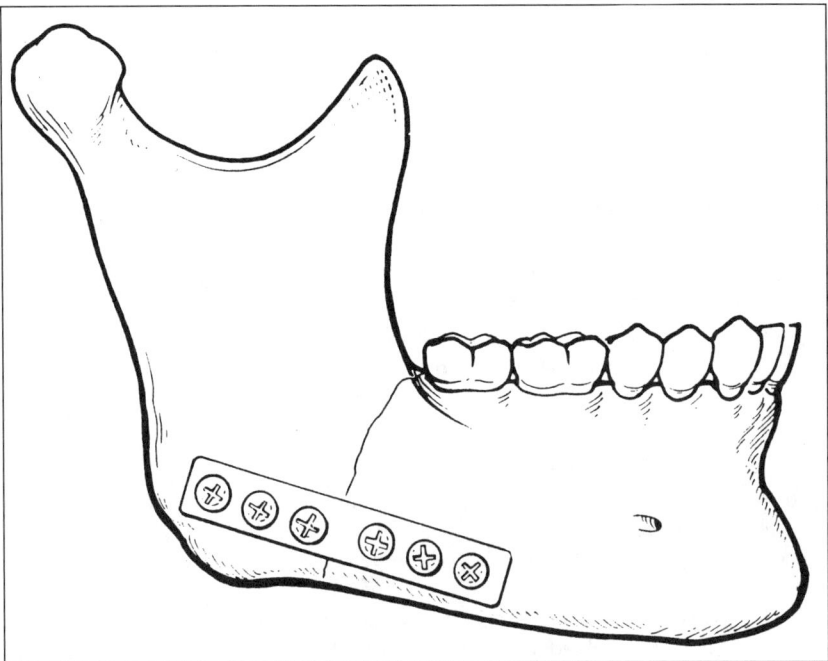

Figure 26.4 A mandibular fixation plate can be screwed to both sides of the fracture, immobilizing the bone fragments while healing takes place. Usually these plates do not need to be removed. Absorbable plates are now available for mid-face fractures and may soon be available for mandibular fractures. (Republished with permission from Komisar A, Blitzer A, Valdes M. *Maxillary and Trimalar Fractures SIPac: Applied Physiology.* Alexandria, VA: American Academy of Otolaryngology–Head and Neck Surgery; 1994.)

tures form the attachments of the zygoma to the frontal, maxillary, and temporal bones. Each of these attachments should be evaluated if a zygomatic injury is suspected.

Depending on the type of trauma to the zygomatic complex, several fracture patterns are possible. An isolated zygomatic arch fracture results from localized trauma to the arch. When all three attachments—maxillary, frontal, and temporal—are disrupted, it is called a **tripod or trimalar fracture** (as distinct from the trimalleolar ankle fracture) (Case 26.1). A disruption of the orbital floor or medial orbital wall may occur as an isolated injury or with a **"blow out" fracture**, which results from a rapid increase in intraorbital pressure (e.g., by a racquetball striking an unprotected eye [Fig. 26.5]).

A depressed or flattened malar eminence is a characteristic physical finding of a **zygomatic complex fracture**. Other physical findings include ecchymosis and edema of the periorbital region, decreased range of motion of the

Case 26.1   Young Woman with Fracture of the Anterior Wall of the Frontal Sinus

While playing basketball, a woman 18 years of age leaps to make a basket, hanging for a moment on the rim. The rim and basket come loose from the backboard and hit her in the upper face. She has a momentary loss of consciousness, then complains of severe facial pain and begins to bleed from her nose.

A thorough evaluation in the hospital emergency department shows only a displaced fracture of the anterior table of her frontal sinus, although by this time the swelling is sufficient that no forehead indentation can be seen. In 4 days, when much of the swelling has resolved, a moderate indentation is noted in the center of her forehead, just above the eyebrows. A computed tomography scan confirms an anterior wall fracture with an intact posterior table of the sinus.

In the operating room, a small drill hole is made in the bone just below the medial end of her left eyebrow, entering into the frontal sinus through its floor. First, a rigid 70° endoscope was passed into the sinus. It is possible to see the nasofrontal duct, which appears open. A urethral sound is then inserted into the sinus via this trephine hole. Using judicious pressure, the posteriorly displaced fragment of the anterior frontal sinus table is elevated back into its normal position with an audible "snap." The soft tissue over the trephine hole is closed, the forehead is protected from any pressure or blows for 3 weeks, and uneventful healing with a normal forehead contour occurs.

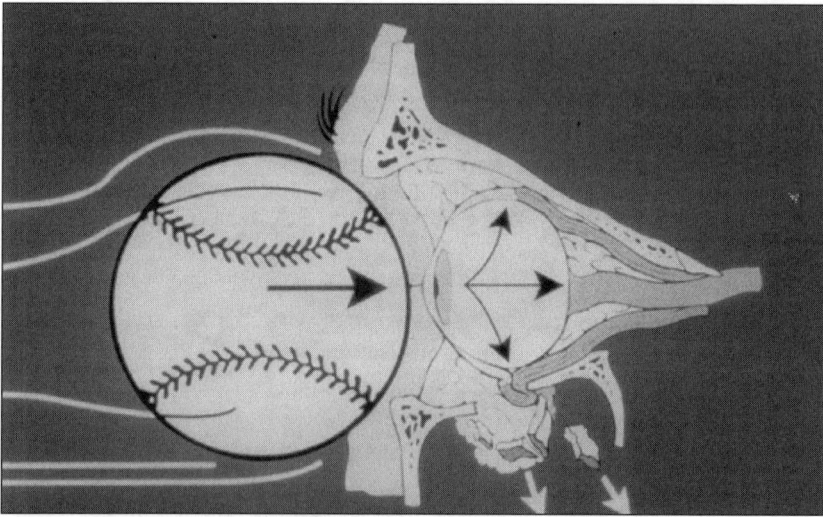

Figure 26.5 A direct blow to the globe can cause a "blow out" fracture, i.e., a fracture of one of the orbital walls (usually inferior) in which the orbital rim remains intact. (Republished with permission from Calhoun K. *Maxillofacial Trauma Slide Lecture Series.* Alexandria, VA: American Academy of Otolaryngology–Head and Neck Surgery Foundation; 1994.)

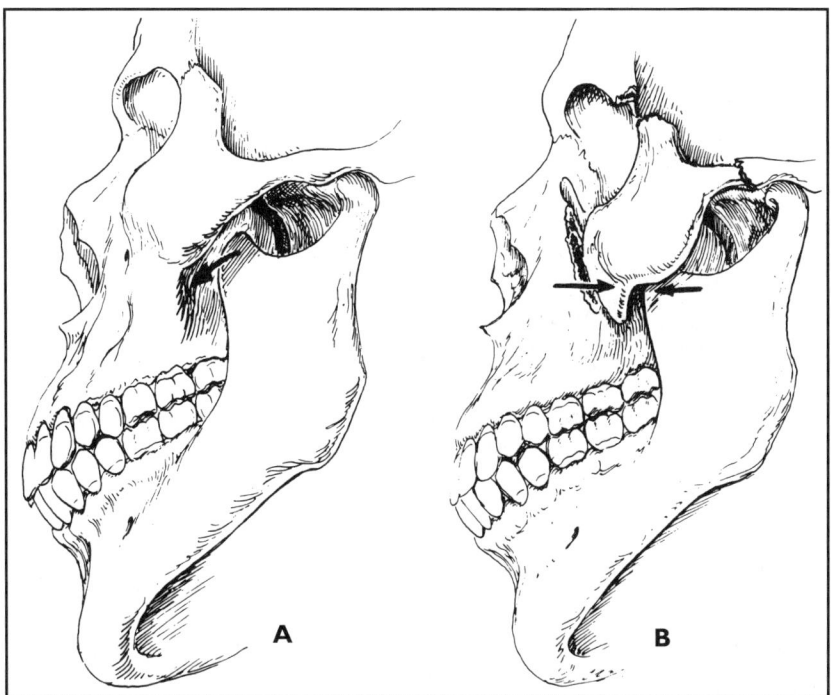

Figure 26.6 When a trimalar fracture is displaced, it impinges on the coronoid process of the mandible and prevents full opening of the mouth. **A**, Normal anterior movement of the coronoid process on opening the jaw. **B**, Impaction of the coronoid process into the fractured zygoma with resultant trismus. (Republished with permission from Komisar A, Blitzer A, Valdes M. *Maxillary and Trimalar Fractures SIPac: Applied Physiology*. Alexandria, VA: American Academy of Otolaryngology–Head and Neck Surgery; 1994.)

mandible and trismus caused by impingement of the coronoid process on the displaced zygoma (Fig. 26.6), infraorbital nerve hypoesthesia, and palpable defects of the infraorbital rim and zygomaticofrontal suture. Diplopia may be present, resulting from edema of nerves or muscles or from the entrapment of extraocular muscles in the fracture. Enophthalmos results from displacement of the orbital contents into the maxillary or ethmoid sinus cavities. Extension of the fracture to the orbital apex can cause immediate blindness or progressively decreasing visual acuity and requires immediate ophthalmologic consultation.

Fine-cut CT of the orbits shows the displaced bony segments, the floor and medial wall, and the apex of the orbit.

Asymptomatic, nondisplaced fractures of the zygomatic arch and orbital rim do not require treatment. Patients with enophthalmos and persistent impairment of extraocular muscle function require definitive reduction of the bones into their proper position, usually with surgical fixation with wires and plates.

Mid-face Fractures

The middle third of the face is the area between the zygomaticofrontal sutures and the occlusal plane of the teeth. It includes the zygoma, maxilla, and the nose. The maxilla acts as the shock absorber for the skull and intracranial contents and is often injured in motor vehicle accidents (Fig. 26.7). Mid-face fracture topology depends on the direction and strength of the force that caused the injury. Fractures of the maxilla are usually bilateral and often involve its attached nasal and zygomatic bones (Fig. 26.8).

Patients with mid-face injuries display facial asymmetry and edema, a flattened or "dishpan" face, and bilateral periorbital edema and ecchymosis. An

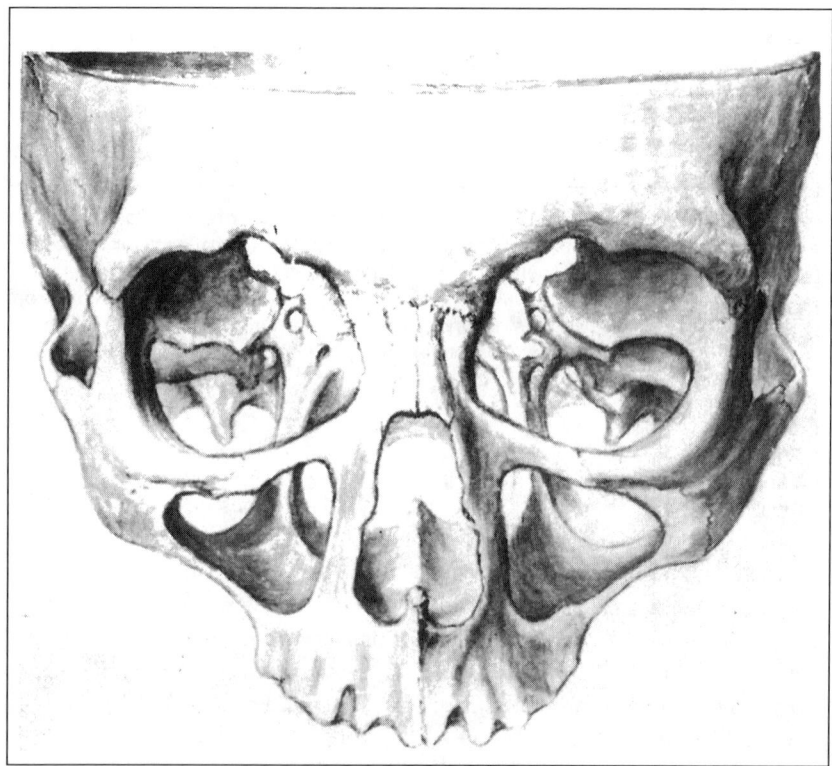

Figure 26.7 The mid-face bones form a buttress that can absorb some of the energy of blunt trauma, protecting the cranial contents. (Republished with permission from Komisar A, Blitzer A, Valdes M. *Maxillary and Trimalar Fractures SIPac: Applied Physiology.* Alexandria, VA: American Academy of Otolaryngology–Head and Neck Surgery; 1994.)

open-bite malocclusion is apparent when the front teeth cannot be brought together as the patient attempts to bite down and the molars meet sooner than usual (Fig. 26.9). Palpating the orbital rim may reveal a "step off" displacement of the fracture. Clear fluid running from the nose suggests CSF rhinorrhea. Emergencies associated with mid-face fractures include airway obstruction, decreased or absent visual acuity and function, and severe hemorrhage. Hemorrhage may require prompt operative intervention.

Fine-cut axial and coronal CTs show the extent of injury and can give information about the status of the optic nerves and intracranial contents; these are the studies of choice for operative planning. Repairing mid-face fractures requires adequate surgical exposure and accurate three-dimensional reduction and stabilization of fractures. Repairs that are performed within 7 days of the injury have greater overall success.

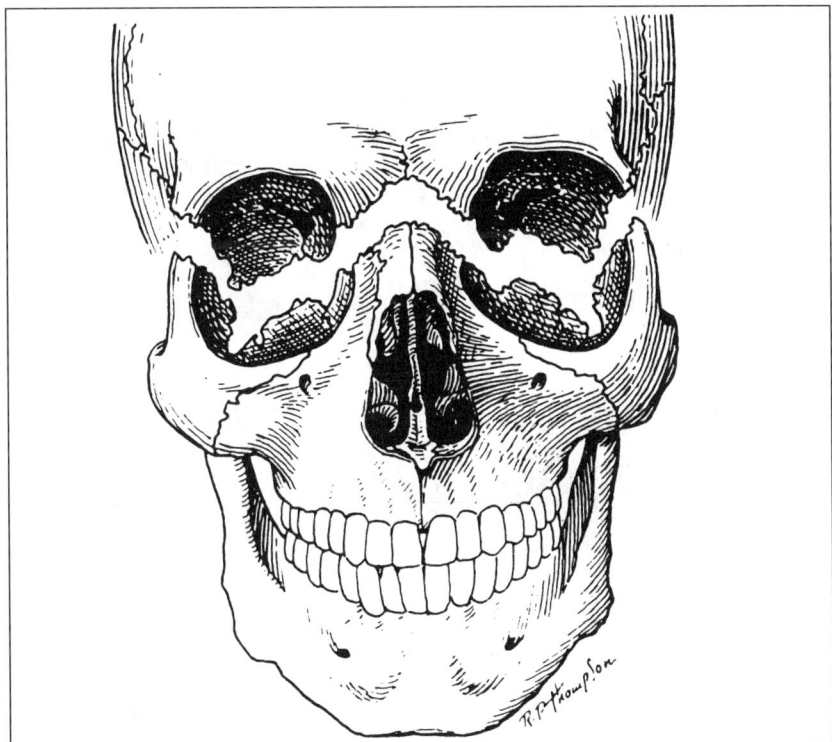

Figure 26.8 The most severe mid-face fracture is craniofacial disjunction in which the facial bones are disconnected completely from the cranial vault. (Republished with permission from Komisar A, Blitzer A, Valdes M. *Maxillary and Trimalar Fractures SIPac: Applied Physiology.* Alexandria, VA: American Academy of Otolaryngology–Head and Neck Surgery; 1994.)

Nasal Fractures

Fractures of the nasal bones and cartilaginous septum are diagnosed by history and appearance of the nose and nasal septum. Ecchymosis and edema over the nasal dorsum and epistaxis are the hallmarks of a nasal fracture. Intranasal examination should be performed to rule out a septal hematoma and intranasal lacerations. If present, a septal hematoma must be drained to prevent septal abscess and eventual saddle-nose deformity. Radiographs are not helpful in either diagnosis or treatment planning. Nasal fractures usually are treated with closed reduction within 7 days of injury to allow the edema to subside; septal fractures often require open surgical reduction. Untreated nasal fractures account for a number of subsequent corrective procedures for nasal deformity and nasal obstruction.

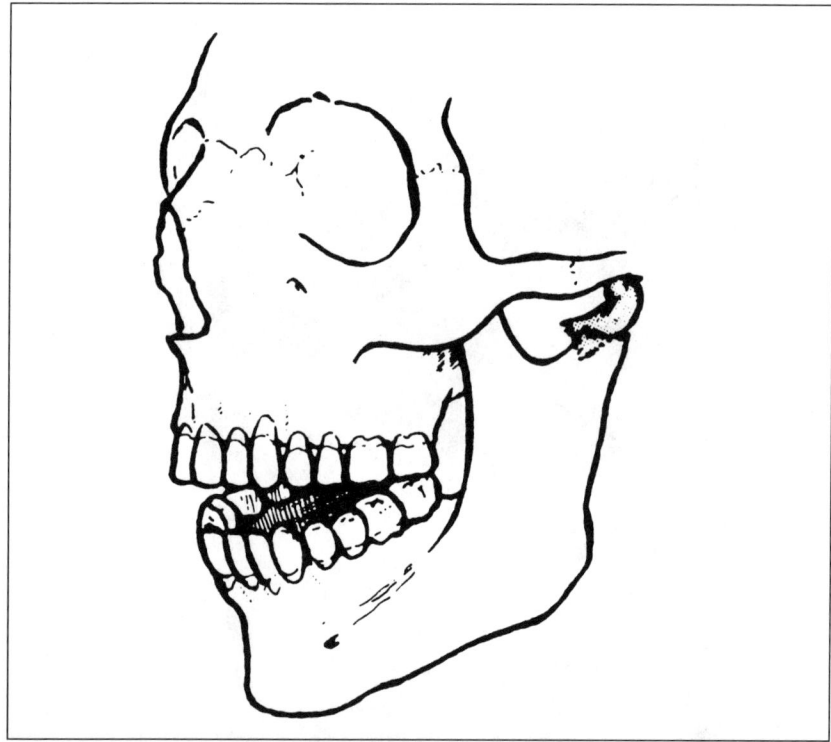

Figure 26.9 When the condyle is fractured, the muscle forces that act on the mandible pull it up and back, resulting in an "open bite" deformity, wherein the molars meet before the anterior teeth are able to come together in their normal position. (Republished with permission from Komisar A, Blitzer A, Valdes M. *Maxillary and Trimalar Fractures SIPac: Applied Physiology.* Alexandria, VA: American Academy of Otolaryngology–Head and Neck Surgery; 1994.)

Trauma to the nose and interorbital area can result in fractures of the nasal bones, medial orbital wall, and ethmoid bone; hence, the term **naso-orbital-ethmoid complex fracture**. Included in this region are the **medial canthal ligaments** and **nasolacrimal apparatus**. A patient with this fracture demonstrates bilateral periorbital ecchymosis, flattening of the nasal dorsum, and possibly widening of the intercanthal distance (traumatic telecanthus). CSF rhinorrhea and anosmia may be present if the cribriform plate is fractured. A **frontal sinus fracture** is also sometimes seen in this type of injury.

Computed tomography is used to rule out associated fractures and to visualize the intracranial contents. Repair of naso-orbital-ethmoid fractures consists of reconstituting the bony anatomy of the region and the integrity of the medial canthal ligament and the lacrimal apparatus; it is often performed with an ophthalmologist as a combined procedure.

Disruption of the anterior and/or posterior wall of the frontal sinus implies that the trauma was inflicted with considerable force, and associated injuries are common (Case 26.2). Complications include **meningitis, pneumocephalus, mucopyocele**, and major cosmetic deformity. Suspicion of a frontal sinus fracture requires CT to determine whether the anterior table, posterior table, or nasofrontal ducts are fractured.

Management includes observation, open reduction, and sometimes obliteration of the sinus, depending on extent and location of the fracture, injury to

---

Case 26.2 **Man with a Zygomaticomaxillary Fracture Accompanied by Facial Parlaysis**

A man 32 years of age is an unrestrained driver in a motor vehicle accident. After an emergency splenectomy is performed and he awakens from anesthesia, it is noted that he has a swollen ecchymotic area over his right cheekbone and that the right side of his face does not move.

Ophthalmologic evaluation reveals no signs of ocular injury. Computed tomography reveals a moderately displaced zygomaticomaxillary complex fracture. There is concern that the facial paralysis might be caused by a traumatic disruption of the facial nerve, which would require surgery to expose and repair the nerve. Fortunately, rechecking of the notes of the alert emergency medical technician who had brought the patient to the hospital reveals documentation that both sides of the patient's face had been moving normally at the scene of the accident. This means that the patient is suffering instead from delayed-onset facial paralysis, probably related to posttraumatic edema.

Four days later, the patient undergoes open reduction and internal fixation of his zygomaticomaxillary fracture. Six weeks later, both his facial appearance and movement are back to normal. Now, he never drives without wearing a seatbelt.

the nasofrontal ducts, and the presence of a CSF leak. For example, a nondisplaced minimal fracture of the anterior table without damage to the frontal nasal duct may require no treatment, whereas a severe injury that involves the posterior wall may require **cranialization** of the frontal sinus (i.e., removal of the posterior table of the sinus, which allows the frontal lobe to settle forward and occupy the space that was once the frontal sinus). (*See* Chapter 12 for a more detailed discussion of nasal fractures.)

Soft Tissue Injuries

Penetrating trauma to the lateral face and fractures of the face and temporal bone can result in **damage to the facial nerve** (Fig. 26.10). Impaired facial nerve function requires prompt evaluation, because the best possible outcome occurs with timely repair of neuronal integrity–from temporal bone to motor endplates. However, not all facial nerve injuries require surgical repair. Severed zygomatic and buccal branches to the upper and lower cheek that are anterior to a line dropped vertically from the lateral canthus of the eye do not require repair due to the abundant anastomotic branching in this region and the high likelihood of cross-innervation from other peripheral branches (Fig.

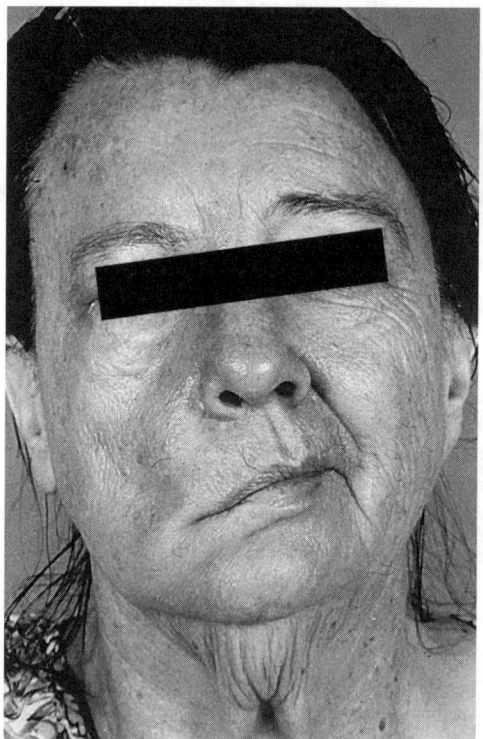

Figure 26.10 Complete facial paralysis is a devastating injury. (Republished with permission from Calhoun K. *Maxillofacial Trauma Slide Lecture Series*. Alexandria, VA: American Academy of Otolaryngology–Head and Neck Surgery Foundation; 1994.)

26.11). Injuries proximal to the lateral canthus do require reanastomosis. The distal frontal and marginal mandibular branches also should be repaired because these control eye closure and mouth movement. For optimal results, repair should be performed within 2 to 3 days of injury.

Lacerations to the face in the region of the masseter muscle are likely to injure **Stensen's (parotid) duct** and branches of the facial nerve. If the duct is severed, saliva can be seen in the wound. Duct repair is performed in the operating room at the same time as soft tissue repair.

Soft tissue injuries to the **eyelid** and **lacrimal system** disrupt the protective function that these structures provide for the globe. Injury to the **canalicular apparatus** should be evaluated in any medial eyelid injury. Damage to the medial canthal ligament must be repaired surgically to prevent permanent telecanthus. Prompt ophthalmologic consultation is needed for all suspected orbital injuries.

Twenty-five percent of patients with head injury have associated orbital or ocular injury. Prompt ophthalmologic consultation is appropriate for all suspected orbital injuries. The physical evaluation rules out lid or orbital hematoma, foreign body, hyphema, and traumatic optic neuropathy after a closed head injury.

Leaks of CSF are seen with fractures of the temporal bone, orbit, frontal sinus, cribriform plate, and floor of the anterior cranial fossa. CSF rhinorrhea

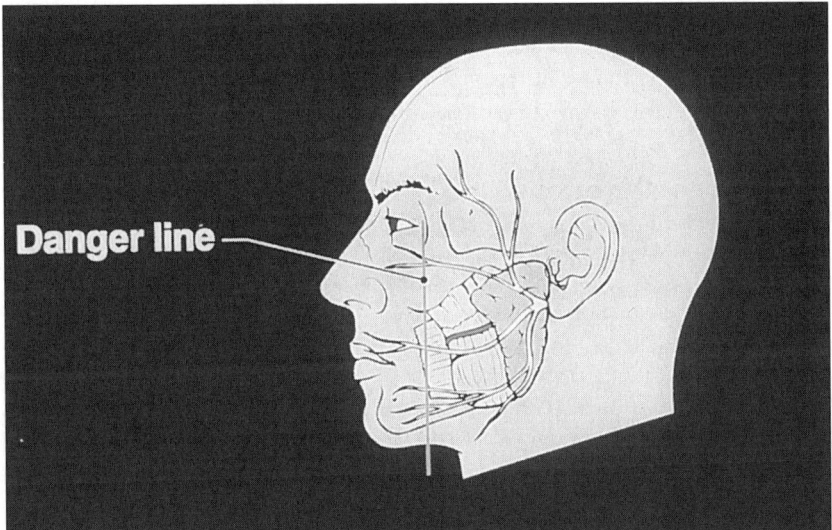

Figure 26.11 An injury to the facial nerve anterior to a line dropped vertically from the lateral canthus usually does not require repair. (Republished with permission from Calhoun K. *Maxillofacial Trauma Slide Lecture Series*. Alexandria, VA: American Academy of Otolaryngology–Head and Neck Surgery Foundation; 1994.)

or otorrhea can lead to meningitis and death. Traumatic CSF leaks may heal spontaneously with conservative management; however, persistent leaks require surgical closure. Trauma patients who report clear fluid draining from the nose (unilateral or bilateral) or ear or salty fluid draining down the back of the throat require evaluation by an otolaryngologist, neurosurgeon, or both.

Human and animal bites to the face can cause severe infection and cosmetic deformity. Treatment includes thorough cleansing, minimal debridement, evaluation for possible primary closure, and antimicrobial drugs known to be effective against gram-positive and -negative organisms. In general, **human bites** are treated with delayed secondary closure (i.e., closure after several days of intravenous antibiotics and local wound care); many animal bites, if evaluated within 5 to 10 hours, can be safely closed primarily.

Anosmia (the loss of the sense of smell) after head injury occurs in an estimated 7% of patients. The mechanisms of this injury include trauma severe enough tear the olfactory filaments at the cribriform plate, causing hematoma or edema of the olfactory bulb or contusion of the central olfactory pathways. Spontaneous recovery occurs in approximately 10% of cases.

Summary

Maxillofacial trauma produces complex injuries and can require a multidisciplinary team for best functional and cosmetic results. Injuries may range from mild deformity to life-threatening trauma, and even patients with seemingly minor injuries should be evaluated by a physician who is experienced in maxillofacial trauma. The timing of repair is crucial, and attention to the report of the emergency medical technician is often important in guiding treatment decisions.

SUGGESTED READINGS

Greenberg AM. Management of facial fractures. *NY State Dent J.* 1998;64:42–7.
This nicely written article discusses new horizons in treatment of facial fractures, including updated surgical approaches and newly available biomaterials.

Josell SD. Evaluation, diagnosis, and treatment of the traumatized patient. *Dent Clin North Am.* 1995;39:15–24.
This article reviews the initial evaluation of patients with maxillofacial fractures, including general evaluation of the entire patient and assessment of the urgency of treatment of their various injuries.

King HK. Airway management of patients with maxillofacial trauma. *Acta Anaesthesiol Sin.* 1996;34:213–20.
One of the difficult aspects of treating patients with maxillofacial trauma is that the bony trauma and its associated injuries can compromise the airway. Normal anatomy is distorted, making laryngoscopy for endotracheal tube placement difficult or impossible. The article reviews airway-management options, with recommendations for the situations in which each technique should be used.

27

Facial Rejuvenation

J. Gregory Staffel, MD

Scientific advancements, widespread media coverage, social acceptance, and an aging "baby boom" generation have made basic knowledge of wrinkle treatment and facial rejuvenation necessary for the internist. Skin-resurfacing procedures now include laser resurfacing, with laser technology progressing rapidly. Other advances are being made in facial rejuvenation surgery as well, including minimally invasive endoscopic procedures. This chapter discusses the indications, techniques, and complications of these treatments.

Pathophysiology of Skin Damage

Although there are a few medical causes of wrinkling (notably, pseudoxanthoma elasticum), most wrinkles are a form of photodamage; smoking is another major cause of premature wrinkling. However, the exact ultrastructural cause of wrinkles remains unclear. When skin is exposed to light, photodamage occurs. Certain wavelengths of light, such as ultraviolet B (UVB) light (i.e., wavelengths of 280–320 nm; "burning rays") are known to be particularly damaging. Longer-wavelength ultraviolet A (UVA) light (i.e., wavelengths of 320–360 nm; "tanning rays") passes through windows, penetrates more deeply into skin, and also has been implicated recently in photodamage.

Histologically, photodamage consists of a thickening of the stratum corneum, thinning of the stratum spinosum, disorganization in the epidermal maturation process, irregular melanin dispersion, a decrease in collagen, and a decrease in the organization of elastin in the dermis. Clinically, these changes result in rough, scaly skin with mottled hyperpigmentation, decreased elasticity, and wrinkling. The Glogau classification system is often used among clinicians to communicate the degree of photodamage (Table 27.1). A person 20 years of age who has not been exposed to any excess sun while growing up typically has Glogau type I skin, whereas an older, wrinkled, weathered gardener might have Glogau type IV skin (Fig. 27.1).

Table 27.1 Treatment Approaches for Different Types of Rhytidectomy Patients

Type	Findings
I	Laxity of skin envelope only; minimum sagging of jowls and platysma
II	More advanced laxity of facial skin; more prominent jowls and nasolabial folds
III	Similar to types I and II, but presents with visible platysmal bands in the anterior neck
IV	Findings as above plus a variable amount of cervical and submental fat

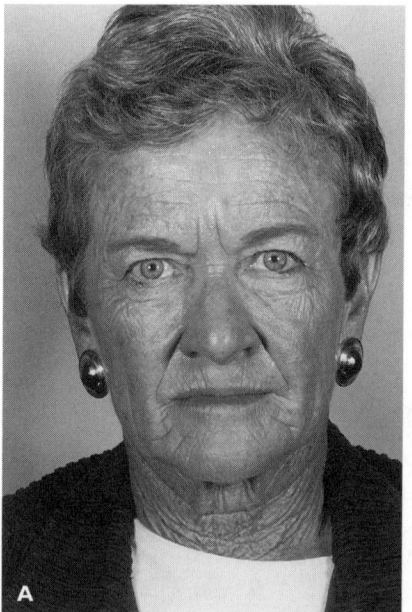 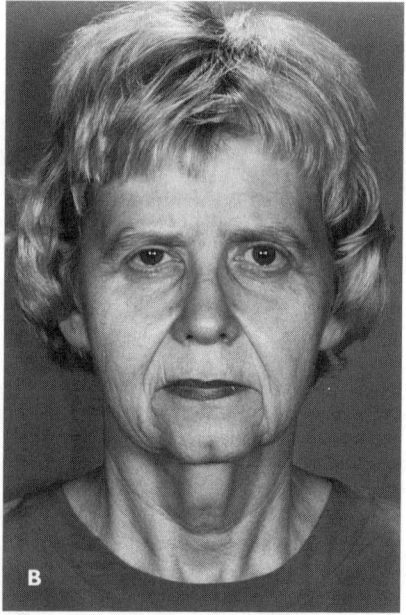

Figure 27.1 Comparison of patients who are similar in age with different skin problems. **A,** Skin that has undergone severe photodamage from years of sun exposure benefits most from a resurfacing procedure. **B,** Skin that is relatively undamaged but shows the stigmata of gravitational changes (e.g., ptotic brow, ptotic malar fat pad, prominent melolabial folds, jowling) benefits most from a resuspending procedure.

The first line of defense in the treatment of wrinkles is sun protection. Sunscreens come in two classes. The first class physically blocks light from hitting the skin. Zinc oxide and titanium dioxide are examples that can be fun on the beach, but many patients find the opaque appearance unacceptable for daily wear. The second class of sunscreens contains chemicals that bind to the stratum corneum and absorb the damaging rays. The prototype of this was para-aminobenzoic acid (PABA); however, better compounds (e.g., dioxybenzones, oxybenzones) that react less with the skin and absorb a broader spectrum of light (including UVA and UVB) are now widely available. Daily use forms the basis for any skin rejuvenation and repair regime.

Skin Resurfacing

Topical Therapy

Since 1969, tretinoin (Retin-A, Renova) has been used topically to treat acne, but many patients also noted improvement in their fine wrinkles with prolonged treatment, causing intense media coverage of the new "antiwrinkle cream." Studies have shown that tretinoin thins the stratum corneum, thickens the stratum spinosum, disperses melanin, restores order to the keratinocyte maturation process, and can cause deposition of new collagen, elastin, and blood vessels in the skin. This decreases the appearance of fine wrinkles and the roughened texture of the skin. One drawback to tretinoin is that it can be irritating to some patients, especially at the beginning of treatment. Irritation often decreases with continued use.

A class of weak acids found in foods (alpha-hydroxy acids) has been noted to have similar beneficial effects on photodamaged skin as tretinoin, without as much irritation. These acids, applied daily in low concentrations, form the basis for many over-the-counter products and cosmetics that claim antiwrinkle activity. The concentration of alpha-hydroxy acids in these products is relatively low, and the efficacy may vary significantly from person to person. Higher-strength products are available by prescription only. The pH of the product is important, with the most effective products having a pH of 2.5 to 3.5.

Chemical Peeling

After the benefits of topical therapy have been achieved, chemical peeling may be considered the next step in the treatment of photodamaged skin. Throughout the years in various countries, many different chemicals have been applied in attempts to rejuvenate the skin. The basis for any of these is the destruction of the skin's superficial layer, regenerating a more youthful appearance. The histologic changes seen with chemical peeling are similar to those caused by tretinoin and alpha-hydroxy acids but are more pronounced. They include an increase in the thickness of the epidermis and in the amount of collagen, elastic fibers, and glycosaminoglycans in the papillary and reticular dermis. Because these changes are directly proportional to the depth of the peel, the deepest layer affected classifies peels. Most patients are treated for at least 2 weeks before the peel with tretinoin or an alpha-hydroxy acid to thin the stratum corneum (which allows more uniform penetration of the peeling agent) and to speed reepithelialization.

The most superficial peels involve only the upper layer of the epithelium and may be performed with 30% to 50% glycolic acid, one to three coats of Jessner's solution (a combination of salicylic acid, resorcinol, lactic acid, and ethanol), or 10% to 15% trichloroacetic acid (TCA) left on the skin for 1 to 2 minutes.

The next most superficial peels involve the deeper layers of the epidermis. These **"micropeels"** are performed with 50% to 70% glycolic acid, four to 10 coats of Jessner's solution, or 15% to 20% TCA for 2 to 20 minutes. Typically, the skin shows some erythema; however, the patient can go back to work the same day, and no anesthesia is required. The remodeling of the epidermis gives a smoother texture to the skin. These peels, often performed by trained personnel in a physician's office, may be repeated quite regularly.

If a peel goes through the epidermis into the papillary dermis, it is called a **medium-depth peel** and often are performed with 70% glycolic acid or 30% to 50% TCA for 3 to 30 minutes. These are perhaps better peels when dyschromia is present, because melanocytes typically lie at the bottom of the basement membrane of the epidermis. Because these treatments cause marked peeling, the patient should allow 7 to 9 days between the peel and any major business or social commitments.

Medium-depth peels can cause scarring or hypopigmentation, which is usually related to the concentration of the peeling acid. In an attempt to obtain deeper peels with fewer complications, certain combinations of agents have been used. The most popular of these combinations is probably a peel consisting of Jessner's solution and 25% to 35% TCA. Another popular combination involves using solid carbon dioxide to treat the deepest wrinkles followed by a peel of 25% to 35% TCA.

One of the problems with medium-depth TCA peels is variable penetration of the agent, causing "hot spots." To obtain even penetration, Dr. Obagi has added a saponin to the TCA, and Dr. James Fulton has added methyl salicylate. Only experienced personnel who have extensive experience with milder peels should use these modified TCA peels.

The deepest peels involve penetration to the reticular dermis and are performed with phenol, either as an 88% solution or a 55% solution (e.g., Baker's formula). Phenol stops its own penetration by coagulating protein as it penetrates the skin. The higher the concentration of phenol, the quicker the protein turns into an impenetrable coagulum. Paradoxically, phenol in lower concentrations doesn't coagulate protein as quickly and, therefore, does not stop its own penetration as well. Hence, the lower the concentration of phenol is, the deeper the peel (to a point)—e.g., a peel consisting of a 55%-phenol Baker's solution is actually a deeper peel than an 88% phenol peel.

A phenol peel to the reticular dermis causes collagen remodeling and thickening, and the benefits can last a lifetime. These peels are for severely photodamaged skin, and the results are often dramatic, with the skin becoming quite smooth. Because phenol is toxic to melanocytes, hypopigmentation can cause a visible demarcation between the color of the facial skin and the color of the neck skin. Compared with facial skin, neck skin has a paucity of appendages and, thus, a propensity to scar; hence, it cannot be peeled deeply. The face has 30 to 40 times the density of pilosebaceous units as does the neck, and these units serve as reservoirs of skin cells that rapidly regenerate new epidermis.

Phenol, when applied to the skin, is absorbed fairly well. Eighty percent of absorbed phenol is excreted unchanged by the kidneys, and the liver detoxifies the remaining 20%. For this reason, preoperative renal- and liver-function studies are required. Furthermore, because phenol in the bloodstream can cause cardiac arrhythmias, all patients should receive a preoperative electrocardiogram and intraoperative monitoring. Hydration decreases the concentration of phenol in the blood and speeds its excretion by the kidneys, so patients are given intravenous fluids and are encouraged to drink plenty of water before, during, and after the peel. Phenol is excreted fairly quickly via the kidneys, and most cardiac arrhythmias that occur during phenol peels are related to the speed of the phenol application. In current practice, phenol is applied only to one section of the face at a time, and 15 to 30 minutes must pass before more phenol is applied to a different section. This systematic approach prevents the blood concentration of phenol from rapidly increasing, causing arrhythmias.

Complications of Chemical Peels
Uneven Peels
Because oil on the skin can prevent many peeling agents from penetrating, the skin is often washed with soap several times and then degreased with alcohol or acetone. If any areas of apparently uneven frosting are noted during the peel, immediate retreatment of these areas may help equalize the final peel depth.

Inadequate Depth of Peel
Both superficial and medium-depth peels are used for improving skin texture and for treating many pigmentation problems and very fine wrinkles. Despite

counseling, some patients may be disappointed that not all the wrinkles have disappeared after a peel. Repeat peels can treat fine wrinkles in some cases, but many wrinkles simply require treatment of a deeper level than the papillary dermis.

Hyperpigmentation

Most physicians use the Fitzpatrick skin type classification to communicate the level of pigment in a person's skin. The scale ranges from type I (white skin that always burns and never tans) to type VI (black skin that never burns and is deeply pigmented) (*see* Table 25.4). Many people's skin responds to injury (or inflammation) by producing more melanin. The darker a person's native skin tone is, the more likely this postinflammatory hyperpigmentation. Typically, this is expected in Fitzpatrick types III to VI. Because melanin is produced from tyrosine by melanocytes and then is released in melanosomes, some authors believe that inhibiting melanin production can reduce postinflammatory hyperpigmentation. Several compounds (e.g., hydroquinone, kojic acid, azelaic acid) inhibit tyrosinase, a critical enzyme in the production of melanin. These compounds are often applied to the skin for 2 to 6 weeks before a peel and for up to 3 months after the peel (but only after the epithelium has regenerated enough to allow nonirritative application of the compounds, usually after 3–4 weeks). This application is often in combination with a steroid (to decrease the inflammation and, therefore, the stimulus to increased melanin production) and tretinoin or an alpha-hydroxy acid (for more even dispersion of the melanin). Sunscreens are also of paramount importance in preventing melanocyte stimulation.

Hypopigmentation

The number of melanocytes may be reduced significantly by a peel, causing areas of decreased pigment that often become worse with time. **Phenol is toxic to melanocytes**, and hypopigmentation is expected, leaving noticeable changes in pigmentation at the border of the peel. Some patients can cover this with makeup. Peeling the whole face can efface subunit demarcation, but occasionally the neck pigmentation is different from that of the face. Blending a peel with TCA may be necessary to minimize these color changes.

Infection

Whenever a medium to deep peel is performed, infection is a possibility, usually in a wound that has received inadequate care. *Staphylococcus* and *Streptococcus* are common pathogens, and many physicians treat patients prophylactically with antibiotics such as Cephalexin. *Pseudomonas* can thrive in a wet environment but not in an acidic one, so diluted-vinegar washes are sometimes recommended. *Candida* is another organism that can live in these types of wounds. Type I herpetic recrudescence can be expected in patients with a history of fever blisters who are not treated with prophylactic medication before and after the peel. In fact, most surgeons treat all patients prophylactically with acyclovir, because many people do not remember having an attack but do indeed carry the herpes virus. Patients who develop small blisters on the peeled surface a few days after the peel have a herpetic infection and should be treated immediately with high-dose acyclovir or a similar medication.

Any wound that is not healing properly should be cultured immediately for bacteria and yeast. Aggressive local wound care should be instituted so that scarring from infection can be avoided.

Scarring

As mentioned above, a severe infection may cause scarring; however, a more common cause is an overly deep peel. Aggressive treatment is deemed appropriate at the first hint of delayed wound healing and usually can prevent a cosmetic disaster. A persistent area of redness in the middle of peeled skin that is otherwise healing well is considered an incipient hypertrophic scar. **Topical steroids** and **topical silicone gels** are good initial therapies, followed by **injections of steroids** if a scar begins to mature. The passing of time does much for these wounds if they are treated appropriately early on; however, the patient requires much counseling and reassurance.

Laser Resurfacing

Laser resurfacing is quickly becoming the mainstay of wrinkle treatment. The treatment principle (i.e., the destruction of epithelium resulting in skin regeneration) is the same as that of peeling (and of dermabrasion, which is discussed below). The histologic changes in the new skin (i.e., a thicker, more orderly epidermis, with new collagen and elastin in the dermis) are also similar to that seen with peeling. The new collagen undergoes remodeling over time, and the effects seem to be long lasting. All of these changes occur with whatever modality (chemical, dermabrasion, or laser) is used to destroy the upper layer of skin. Some physicians believe that, because of its thermal effects, a laser causes collagen shrinkage that may be longer lasting.

Laser technology progresses almost as quickly as does computer technology. The carbon-dioxide laser has a wavelength of 10,600 nm and is absorbed by water. When the laser hits the skin, intra- and intercellular water is heated to steam, exploding the cells. This hot water also heats up the surrounding tissue, causing protein denaturation (by thermal damage), which may be significant and can penetrate much deeper than the vaporization depth of the laser beam itself. However, because thermal damage is temperature and time dependent, it can be prevented. Have you ever passed your finger through a candle flame and not felt any pain? You can do this because your finger must be exposed to heat for a certain amount of time before its own temperature rises. In the same manner, a laser beam that hits water and boils it quickly, vaporizes the water but barely warms the surrounding tissue. Hence, the perfect facial resurfacing laser is one that is absorbed by water, is able to be turned on and off quickly, and is powerful enough to heat a certain area of skin rapidly to over 100°C.

The first laser that meets these criteria is the **UltraPulse 5000** (Coherent), which has exposure times on the order of a millisecond and is powerful enough to cause tissue vaporization over an adequate spot size. Other lasers attempt to minimize thermal damage by coupling two less-powerful pulses very quickly or by rapidly scanning a continuous-wave beam over the skin with the use of a microprocessor-controlled scanner. All of these techniques may be effective.

Resurfacing with a carbon-dioxide laser requires a similar skin-pretreatment regimen as does chemical peeling. Reepithelialization can require 7 to 14 days after treatment, and wound care during this time can be intense. Redness often persists for several months after laser treatment. The complications associated with laser resurfacing include the same ones associated with chemical peeling (*see* above); treatment is also similar. Prophylactic antibiotics and antivirals are indicated.

Temporary hyperpigmentation occurs in many patients and is treated with **prophylactic bleaching compounds** (e.g., hydroquinone, kojic acid), retinoic acid, and steroids. Incidences of long-term, mild hypopigmentation are just starting to be reported; however, at this point, the problem does not seem to be as severe after laser resurfacing as it is after phenol peeling.

The latest laser technology to be used for resurfacing is the **erbium: yttrium-aluminum-garnet (Er:YAG)** laser. The 2940-nm wavelength of this laser is absorbed much more specifically by water, allowing the water in the skin to vaporize with even less collateral thermal damage. This lack of thermal damage also allows quicker healing with less redness. However, because the Er:YAG generates so little heat in the surrounding tissue, some tiny blood vessels in the skin do not coagulate. Thus, patients may have pinpoint bleeding after this treatment. Additionally, the Er:YAG laser has difficulty treating deeper wrinkles. Because each pass with the Er:YAG affects a much shallower region of tissue, multiple passes are needed to attain the depth of penetration of one pass of the carbon-dioxide laser. The more passes that are necessary, the more difficult it is to create a uniform depth of wound. The lack of heat also may reduce collagen shrinkage. Techniques are currently evolving, and we should know fairly soon how the Er:YAG laser fits in to the resurfacing armamentarium.

Dermabrasion

Although lasers represent the latest in resurfacing technology, interest recently has been renewed in an older form of resurfacing–dermabrasion. Remember that resurfacing simply involves destroying the epidermis and part of the dermis to induce reepithelialization and dermal changes. The epithelium can be destroyed by chemicals, light, and heat or by mechanically abrading the skin's surface, i.e., dermabrasion. In the past, high-speed, rotating fraises and wire brushes have been used; however, more recently, interest has been renewed in using sandpaper, diamond fraises, or wire brushes by hand. Some physicians freeze the skin with a refrigerant spray to provide a firmer surface and to control of the depth of dermabrasion better, but this can be tricky and can cause scarring. Dermabrasion is most useful in treating deep acne, posttraumatic, and postoperative scars but also can be used to treat rhagades (Fig. 27.2). The level of dermis affected is usually the same as with a deep peel. Hypopigmentation is a known side effect, occurring less often than with a deep phenol peel but probably more often than with laser resurfacing.

Facial Rejuvenation Surgery

Aside from photodamage, facial changes with aging are due largely to gravitational and muscular effects (*see* Fig. 27.1). Facial rejuvenation surgery may be performed to minimize the appearance of aging caused by such muscular effects.

Forehead and Eyebrows

Horizontal lines caused by the chronic contraction of the frontalis muscles often mark the aging forehead. The muscular contraction often is worsened as the eyebrows fall below the orbital rim and begin to obstruct the vision, but this just makes the horizontal forehead creases deeper. The procerus and corrugator muscles also can cause vertical and horizontal rhytids at the top of the nose due to chronic contraction.

The fallen (ptotic) brows may be treated by one of several methods of brow lifting. In a **coronal lift**, an incision is made from ear to ear across the top of the head, the brow is pulled up while excess scalp is excised, and the frontalis muscles are incised to soften the horizontal rhytids. This approach allows excision of the corrugator and procerus muscles under direct vision. The incision for this operation also may be made in the anterior hairline (a pretrichial incision). More recently, some surgeons have been using the **endoscopic approach**, in which three to four small incisions are made just behind the hairline and the scalp and forehead are undermined. Through these incisions, under visualization with endoscopes, the muscles are incised and sutures are placed to pull the brows up. These sutures are then anchored to small screws placed into the bone at the site of the incisions. Initial results with this endoscopic approach are encouraging, especially in younger patients, but long-term effects must be evaluated.

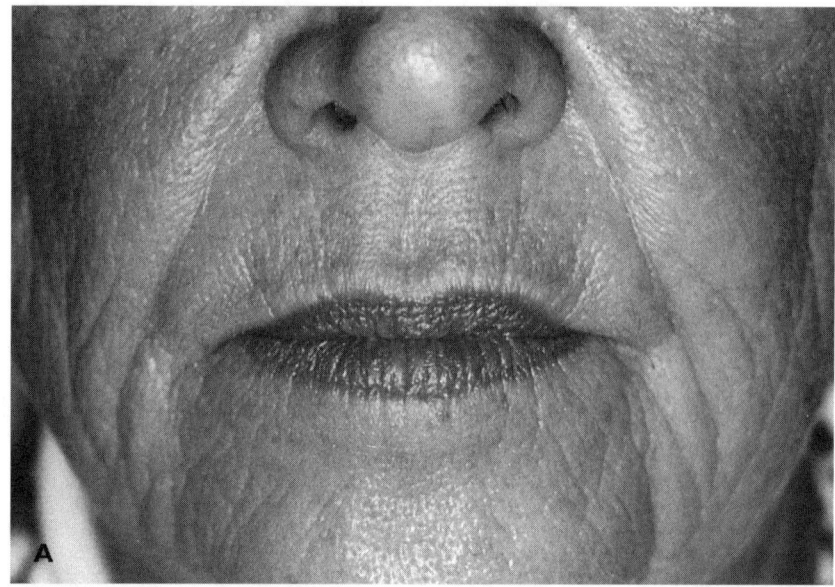
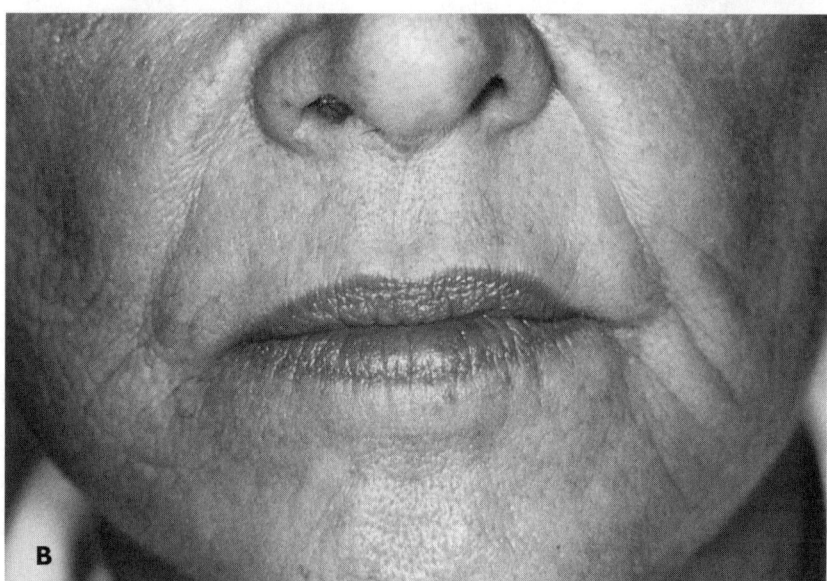

Figure 27.2 A woman before (*part A*) and after (*part B*) her upper lip wrinkles were treated with hand dermabrasion using a wire brush.

Some surgeons prefer to treat forehead rhytids with **injections of botulinum toxin** into the muscles causing the wrinkling (e.g., frontalis, procerus, corrugator). This toxin also is being used to treat spasmodic dysphonia and blepharospasm, with the end point of weakening or paralyzing these muscles the same in all uses. The effect lasts approximately 4 to 6 months, after which a full return to the original state occurs and subsequent injections are needed.

Eyes

Excess upper eyelid skin and fat herniation can make one look older and more "tired." A youthful, "fresher" appearance can be achieved with an **upper eyelid blepharoplasty**, during which excess upper eyelid skin, muscle, and sometimes fat is removed. The upper lid crease is better defined after this operation, but care must be taken not to remove too much skin because lagophthalmos and subsequent corneal ulceration may result. Patients often have to use lubricating drops or ointment for a while after the surgery, and dry eyes (as determined by the Schirmer's test) are a relative contraindication. Of the many techniques for performing upper lid surgery, almost all of them work well and have minimal morbidity.

Wrinkles that an upper blepharoplasty cannot improve are the so-called "crow's feet" lines that appear just lateral to the orbit. These are caused by contraction of the orbicularis oculi when smiling or squinting. These lines may be treated with laser resurfacing, direct excision of redundant muscle, or even injection of botulinum toxin.

Skin laxity and herniation of fat in the lower eyelids give a "baggy" and "tired" appearance that can be corrected by **lower-eyelid blepharoplasty**. Initially designed to remove excess lower-eyelid skin and pseudoherniated orbital fat, this procedure has evolved into a sophisticated recontouring operation. An incision is made either in the conjunctiva or just below the lashes, and usually a flap of skin and muscle (or just skin) is elevated. The orbital septum is penetrated; excess fat is expressed, clamped, and excised; and the base is cauterized to prevent an orbital hematoma from developing from the vessels that retract with the remaining fat. Removing too much fat can result in a hollow-eyed cadaveric appearance, whereas removing too little may cause bulges to appear in the lower lid. Removing excess skin may cause scleral show or, worse, ectropion. These complications are more likely in patients with extremely lax lower lids as determined by the preoperative pinch and snap tests. Performing the blepharoplasty through a transconjuctival approach minimizes the risks of these complications.

Traditional lower-eyelid blepharoplasty removes the bulging in the lower lid but can replace it with a hollow if too much fat is removed. Recently, attention has been placed on recontouring the lower lid so that it has a smooth appearance, resembling the natural appearance in youth. This may involve suturing pedicles of fat into hollow areas (e.g., the nasojugal groove) and extending the dissection lower into the cheek where the suborbicularis oris fat and even the malar fat pad may be suspended from the periosteum of the infraorbital rim. Furthermore, with age and migration of the malar fat pad, the orbicularis oculi seems to move down and laterally. Sometimes, this muscle may be trimmed and resuspended to the malar bone periosteum to restore subtly a more youthful appearance. These advances have brought a new level of sophistication to this operation (Fig. 27.3).

In younger patients, skin may not need to be removed after the fat has been addressed; in other patients, only very fine wrinkling may be present. Some of these patients may benefit from a light chemical or laser peel performed in conjunction with or soon after lower blepharoplasty.

Cheeks and Jowls

Continuing down the face, the next common problem that people notice with aging is a deepening of the melolabial (or nasolabial) fold. Traditionally, this has been the hardest area of the aging face to treat. Corrective techniques used on these deep folds have included injecting fat or various alloplastic substances (e.g., silicone, collagen) and placing alloplastic implants deep to the folds. These techniques may improve the appearance initially but do not yield good long-term results because they do not address the sagging malar fat pad that is causing the fold in the first place.

Another area that is almost always affected at the same time as the cheeks are the jowls. The mandibulocutaneous ligament prevents the soft tissue from sliding forward off the chin; however, the skin and soft tissues just behind this ligament can sag, creating a jowling effect. The ptotic malar fat pad and the jowls may be treated with a **facelift**, during which the soft tissues are undermined and repositioned. The malar fat pad itself may be undermined and resuspended, carrying the dissection (above the zygomaticus muscles) beyond the melolabial fold and into the upper lip. The best way to support the jowls involves plicating or imbricating the **superficial musculoaponeurotic system**. The standard facelift generally gives a more youthful, rejuvenated look, but the melolabial folds remain difficult to treat even in the best of hands.

Neck

The next area of concern involves the aging neck. The platysma muscles may separate to create bands in the neck ("turkey gobbler" deformity), and excess skin also can accumulate here. The myriad treatment options for aging platysma muscles is a testimony to the variability of results. Some surgeons prefer undermining and resuspending the muscles posteriorly, whereas others prefer to excise excess muscle anteriorly and then suture the edges together like a corset; still others create geometric cuts in the muscle that are designed

Facial Rejuvenation 551

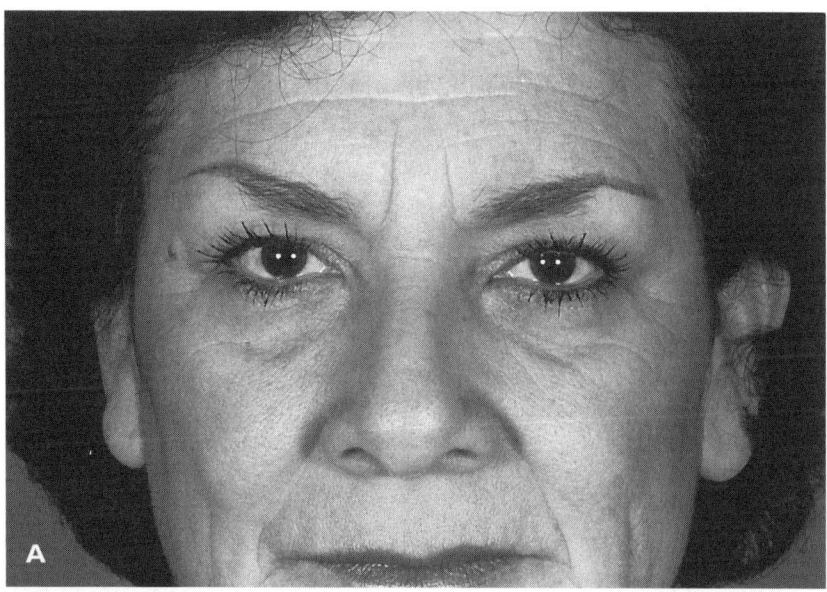

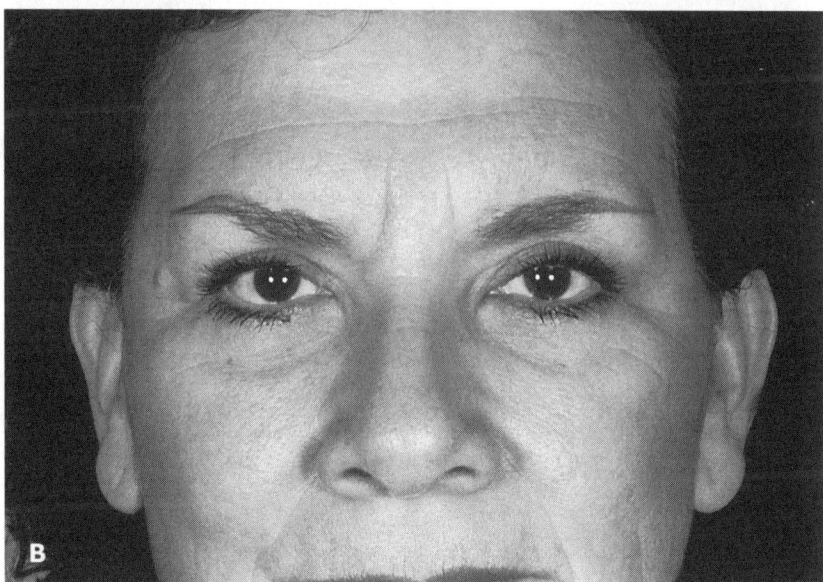

Figure 27.3 A woman before (*part A*) and 7 months after (*part B*) the sulcus between the orbicularis oculi and the malar fat pad were effaced significantly by trimming and re-suspending the muscle and by elevating the malar fat pad. Notice the difference in the contours of the lower eyelid.

to prevent recrudescence of the banding. The common denominator in all these techniques involves tightening the muscles and then redraping and excising the excess skin. The incisions for face and neck lifts are on the front of and behind the ears, extending into the scalp where they are inconspicuous. Care must be taken to create a natural hairline with no "tell tale" step-offs (Fig. 27.4).

Recently, interest has emerged in performing minimally invasive endoscopic procedures to treat the aging face. In some cases, periosteum is undermined from a remote entrance site and attempts are made to reposition the soft tissues to let the periosteum re-adhere in a new position. Results of these operations seem to be somewhat variable, depending on the patient's anatomy and the surgeon's technique. These procedures usually are performed on younger people who want to look "refreshed" without undergoing traditional surgery that involves large incisions.

Complications

Complications of facial rejuvenation surgery include an ever-present concern for both the patient and the surgeon. Whenever a flap of skin is elevated, the potential for the accumulation of a **hematoma** under the flap exists. When

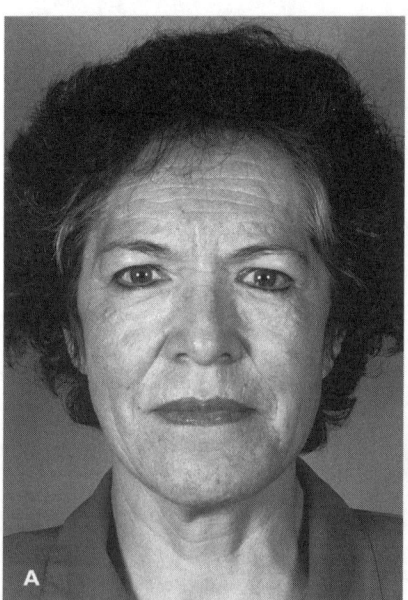 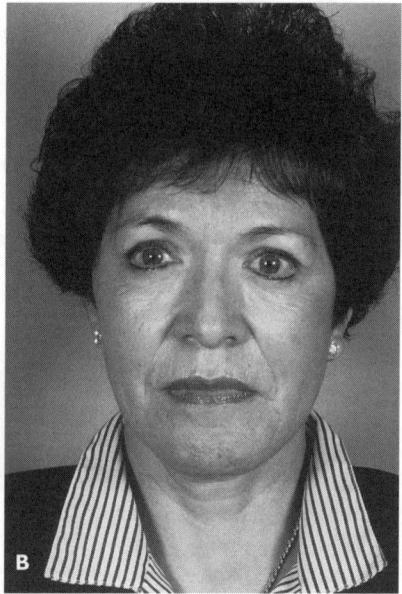

Figure 27.4 A woman before (*part A*) and 5 months after (*part B*) undergoing a full facelift with blepharoplasty.

this happens, the circulation to the skin over the hematoma is compromised, and sometimes skin **necrosis** can result. Treatment of an early hematoma consists of drainage and pressure dressing, and reexploration is indicated if the hematoma is expanding. Small delayed hematomas usually do not compromise distal cutaneous circulation but, if liquefied, should be aspirated approximately 9 to 10 days after surgery.

Microvascular disease, usually caused by cigarette smoking, makes distal circulation in skin flaps tenuous. When the acute vasoconstrictive effects of nicotine are added to chronic microvascular disease postoperatively, skin necrosis becomes an eminent threat. For this reason, patients are not allowed to smoke for 2 to 4 weeks before and 2 weeks after surgery. Nicotine replacement defeats the purpose and also is not allowed. Many surgeons create shorter skin flaps in smokers hoping to ensure better microcirculation.

Scarring after rejuvenation surgery may run the gamut from hypertrophic to widened and atrophic. Damage to the greater auricular nerve causes numbness of the earlobes. Damage to the branches of the facial nerve can cause paralysis. Lagophthalmos and ectropion already have been mentioned. Although orbital hematomas can occur, blindness from blepharoplasty is extremely rare.

Other Modalities

Two other direct ways of treating facial wrinkles involve **injecting collagen** and **implanting material** (e.g., expanded polytetrafluoroethylene) just below wrinkles. Although these techniques work in many cases, they each have their drawbacks.

Traditionally, injectable collagen has been made from a bovine source; although it can be cross-linked, allergic reactions can still occur. Obviously, those allergic to beef are not candidates, and test doses of the collagen should be placed on every patient. Some patients have a reaction even after a negative test dose; however, the collagen injections work well for most. Unfortunately, the human body tends to break down this material, and reinjection may be necessary every 4 to 6 months. Recently, genetic engineering has allowed the synthesis of collagen that is more biocompatible. (Collagenesis–the company that has pioneered this technique–can synthesize collagen similar to the patient's own skin tissue based on a biopsy of the patient's skin, thus overcoming some of the problems and limitations with bovine collagen.) In an effort to avoid the biological breakdown of bovine collagen, human collagen–in the form of processed acellular cadaveric skin (AlloDerm)–has been used. This material is not injectable and must be implanted surgically, seemingly providing a scaffold for the ingrowth of the patient's own tissue. Although early results are encouraging, long-term observation for eventual absorption is necessary.

Another method of treating wrinkles is to implant expanded polytetrafluoroethylene. As with any foreign-body implantation, some issues arise—infection is a concern, but extrusion is the most common complication. Research to design an implant that is more resistant to extrusion is ongoing.

Some surgeons prefer to implant the patient's own fat below the wrinkles, but graft retention seems to depend on many variables. Harvesting, washing, and injecting are technique sensitive. The fat must be injected through a needle large enough not to damage the fat cells but in small enough amounts to allow adequate neovascularization. Some investigators believe that perioperative hyperbaric oxygen therapy aids in graft retention.

Summary

Reconditioning, resurfacing, resuspending, peeling, abrading, filling, paralyzing, and muscle denervating comprise the antiwrinkle armamentarium. No doubt the list will become even longer in the years to come as our population comes face to face with the ravages of sun, fun, time, and life.

SUGGESTED READINGS

Beeson WH, McCollough EG. *Aesthetic Surgery of the Aging Face.* St. Louis: CV Mosby; 1986.
  This text provides a good overview of the various types of surgery that are useful in rejuvenating the signs of aging on the face.

Ellis DAF, Triman SJ, Ellis CS. The use of glycolic acid as a micropeel. *Facial Plast Surg Clin North Am.* 1994;2:15–20.
  This article details the use of glycolic acid peels as repeatable minimal-morbidity "fresheners" of the complexion.

Monheit GD. The Jessner's TCA peel: an enhanced medium-depth chemical peel. *Facial Plast Surg Clin North Am.* 1994;2:21–8.
  This article describes the use of Jessner's solution as a keratolytic before performing a TCA peel, resulting in medium-depth penetration of the dermis.

SECTION VII

Lower Aerodigestive Tract

28

Hiccups

David E. Eibling, MD

Hiccups affect almost everyone at one time or another. They even occur in utero and are relatively common in childhood, decreasing in occurrence with advancing age. Usually, hiccups last just a few minutes, resolving rapidly after some simple maneuver involving the pharynx or esophagus, such as eructation (a "burp"). Hiccups that last more than several minutes are unusual (Table 28.1). This chapter discusses the physiology and etiology of hiccups and details the evaluation and therapy for this disorder.

The term *hiccup* probably originated as a description of the sound made by a hiccup. *Singultus* is the formal appellation applied to the entity and is derived from the Greek word *singult*, which can be translated as "cough" or "choke."

Physiology

A hiccup is an unintentional diaphragmatic contraction. The resultant inspiration is interrupted by an almost instantaneous glottic (vocal cord) closure that occurs within 30 ms of the beginning of the diaphragmatic descent. This timing assures that there is no overall effect on respiration due to the limitation of inspiration by the closure of the glottis. The importance of glottic closure is illustrated by the alkalosis that develops from hiccups in a tracheostomy patient. Because glottic closure does not cut off airflow through the tracheostoma in the afflicted patient, unimpeded inspiration with each hiccup results in respiratory alkalosis.

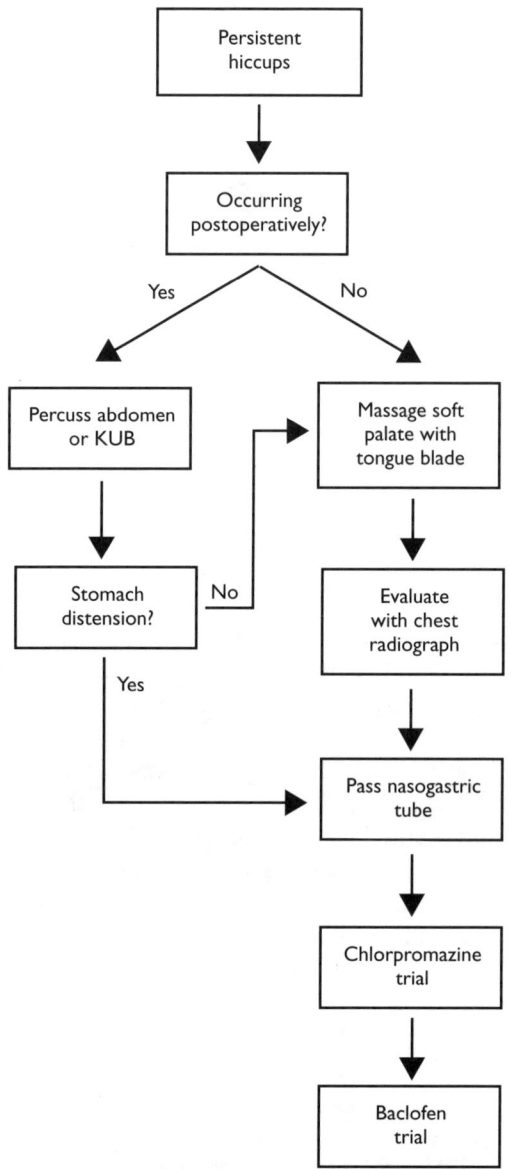

Algorithm Management of persistent hiccups. KUB = kidney and urinary bladder.

The short latency of the glottic closure reflex suggests that the central limb of the hiccup reflex does not lie within the respiratory center. The neural activity responsible for hiccups is probably at the level of the spinal cord or

Table 28.1 Classification of Hiccup by Duration

Type	Duration
Nonpathologic hiccups	Up to 48 hours
Persistent hiccups	48 hours–1 month
Intractable hiccups	>1 month

lower brainstem. The efferent component of hiccups involves both the phrenic and vagus nerves. Unilateral diaphragmatic contractions (usually left-sided) are more common than bilateral involvement.

A hiccup is an involuntary physiologic function that usually occurs in clusters, varying from four to 60 per minute. Persistent hiccupping may cease during sleep and resume on awakening, which suggests a relationship to generalized neuronal activity. The level of arterial carbon dioxide and alterations in serum sodium also suggest a relationship to the excitability of the central nervous system.

For reasons that are not known, intractable hiccups are more likely to be encountered in men. (However, in 1932, Dr. Mayo suggested that the male preponderance was due to chronic prostate infection!)

Etiology

A variety of factors can trigger hiccups. Vagal or phrenic irritation and stimulation of thoracic sympathetic fibers are common initiating stimuli. Metabolic changes, such a hyponatremia, can lower the excitability threshold. Hiccups can originate from both peripheral (more common) and central causes (Tables 28.2 and 28.3).

Among the peripheral causes of hiccups, gastrointestinal problems (e.g., gastric or bowel distention) are the most common. Gastric distention hiccups can be caused by aerophagia, excessive food consumption, ingestion of carbonated beverages, or gastric insufflation during mask ventilation under anesthesia or during upper gastrointestinal endoscopy. Gastric outlet obstruction also can result in distention and can present with hiccups as an early manifestation. Gastric distention should be suspected when hiccups develop postoperatively (Case 28.1). Spontaneous eructation may result in rapid resolution; however, if this does not occur, and if percussion of the abdomen suggests gastric distention, then the use of a nasogastric tube may be required to resolve the condition.

Any inflammatory process of the diaphragm, either thoracic or abdominal, can cause hiccups. Pneumonia, pericarditis, pleuritis, pleural effusion, and

Table 28.2 Peripheral Causes of Hiccup

Vagus Nerve Irritation	Abdominal Branches
Pharyngeal Branches	Distention of viscus
Pharyngitis	Gastritis
	Ulcer disease
	Abdominal abscess
Auricular Branches	Gallbladder disease
Hair or foreign body in ear canal	Tumors
	Traction on viscera during surgery
Thoracic Branches	
Pneumonia	**Diaphragmatic Irritation**
Pleuritis	Gastric distention (overeating, carbonated
Pleural effusions	beverages, air insufflation during endoscopy,
Empyema	gastric outlet obstruction)
Aortic aneurysm	Hiatal hernia (reflux)
Pericarditis	Splenomegaly
Chest tumors	Hepatomegaly
Myocardial infarction	Hepatitis
	Subphrenic abscess

Table 28.3 Central Causes of Hiccup

Toxic and Metabolic Disorders	Central Nervous System Disorders
General anesthesia	Neoplasms
Alcohol	Multiple sclerosis
Drugs	Brainstem tumors
Uremia	Arnold–Chiari malformation
Diabetes mellitus	Trauma
Electrolyte disorders (sodium, potassium, carbon dioxide)	Infection (meningitis, encephalitis)
	Vascular disease
	Brainstem or nerve compression
Psychogenic Disorders	
Stress	
Excitement	
Conversion reaction	
Hysterical neurosis	
Malingering	

empyema are the more common thoracic conditions that may present with hiccups caused by diaphragmatic inflammation. Subphrenic abscess and hepatic and renal diseases are the more common intra-abdominal inflammatory causes. Radiologic evaluation with chest radiographs, abdominal flat and up-

> **Case 28.1** **Woman with Gastric Distention Postoperatively Who Develops Hiccups**
>
> A woman 38 years of age develops hiccups one day after cholecystectomy. A laparoscopic procedure was attempted; however, because of intraoperative difficulties arising from scarring caused by previous cholecystitis, a laparotomy was performed instead. A nasogastric tube that was placed intraoperatively to decompress the stomach had been removed in the recovery room.
>
> Physical examination reveals a woman who is uncomfortable and has obvious hiccups. Palpation of the stomach is difficult due to tenderness, but percussion reveals an enlarged, gas-filled stomach. She is afebrile, and breath sounds are clear in both bases.
>
> A nasogastric tube is placed, and her stomach is decompressed of a large amount of air and 500 cm^3 of bilious drainage. The tube is left connected to intermittent low suction, and parenteral fluids are adjusted to replace the lost gastric drainage. Two days later, after it is demonstrated that she tolerates clamping of the tube, it is removed.
>
> **Discussion**
>
> Postoperative gastric outlet obstruction is probably the most common cause of hiccups in hospitalized patients. Gastric decompression with a nasogastric tube is both diagnostic and therapeutic.

right films, or computed tomography is warranted if the clinical scenario suggests a diaphragmatic process in a patient with hiccups.

Inflammation or compression of the vagus, phrenic, or thoracic sympathetic nerves can result in hiccups; hence, evaluating persistent hiccups should include an evaluation of the phrenic and vagus nerves. Hiccups caused by direct nerve involvement are extremely rare and are almost never encountered in a busy head and neck cancer practice.

Hiccups can be a response to emotional distress, such as those precipitated by crying in children. Because emotional stress lowers the hiccup threshold, hiccups that occur with emotional episodes may still have an organic basis and are unlikely to represent a conversion reaction.

Diagnostic Evaluation

Physicians must inquire about symptoms of the head and neck, chest, and abdomen in addition to discussing the hiccups. The presence of associated hoarseness and dysphagia suggests vocal cord paralysis due to recurrent laryngeal nerve injury (most likely from an intrathoracic cause). Ear symptoms

> ### Case 28.2 Boy with Intractable Hiccups Caused by Head Trauma
>
> A boy 15 years of age suffered a severe closed head injury when thrown from an all-terrain vehicle on which he was riding as a passenger. He was unconscious at the scene and presented as a 3 on the Glasgow Coma Scale. He was admitted to the neurosurgical intensive care unit for intracranial pressure monitoring and supportive care. He later recovered some cerebral function and was transferred to an inpatient rehabilitative facility for intensive rehabilitation. During his hospitalization he has developed intractable hiccups, which interfered significantly with his rehabilitation.
>
> The patient is treated initially with chlorpromazine at a dosage of 50 mg/d, but his hiccups do not improve. He is then started on baclofen 5 mg tid, which is slowly increased to 10 mg tid, lessening his hiccups to the point that they no longer interfered with his therapy.
>
> **Discussion**
>
> Intractable hiccups represent a therapeutic challenge. This patient was fortunate because baclofen controlled his hiccups at a dosage of only 30 mg/d. Head injury is commonly associated with intractable hiccups, which can present a significant problem during rehabilitation. Perhaps the most significant point of this case is that it shows the need to remind our patients of the dangers of using all-terrain vehicles, snowmobiles, etc., in an unsafe manner.

(even just a "tickle") suggest an oropharyngeal or hypopharyngeal process (usually a malignancy). Previous head trauma or known neurological disease may suggest an intracranial cause (Case 28.2). Abdominal (e.g., bloating, nausea, vomiting, pain, eructation) and thoracic (e.g., pleuritic chest pain, previous pneumonia, hemoptysis) symptoms suggest that diaphragmatic irritation is the cause (Case 28.3).

Physical examination includes laryngeal examination to rule out vocal cord paralysis or hypopharyngeal malignancy. Palpation of the neck identifies cervical masses in the regions of the phrenic and vagus nerves. Other evaluations include auscultation of the chest; percussion of the upper abdomen, diaphragm, and liver; and an abdominal examination.

Radiographic evaluation of intractable hiccups is guided by history and physical examination. Chest radiographs, abdominal flat plates, and barium studies of the upper gastrointestinal tract may diagnose thoracic causes, gastric distention, or reflux esophagitis. Magnetic resonance imaging of the upper spinal cord and the posterior fossa to evaluate the brainstem (to look for vessels compressing the brainstem) may be required. Computed tomography or magnetic resonance imaging of the neck, chest, and abdomen also may be re-

> **Case 28.3** **Man with Hiccups Caused by Diaphragmatic Irritation Due to Lung Cancer**
>
> A man 71 years of age presents with a 3-week history of intermittent hiccups. He thought that he had eaten something that had caused them, so he changed his diet and tried to "burp" frequently. His friends had advised him to eat granulated sugar, and one had even popped a paper bag behind him to startle the hiccups away. His past medical history is unremarkable with the exception of an 80-pack-year smoking history and some recent left-sided chest pain and coughing.
>
> Physical examination is unremarkable, but a chest radiograph reveals a 6-cm left-sided, pleural-based lung mass with a small pleural effusion. Pleural biopsy reveals non–small cell carcinoma of the lung.
>
> The patient is treated with palliative chemotherapy and radiotherapy.
>
> **Discussion**
>
> The list of differential diagnoses of persistent hiccups is extensive, but the most common etiologic process is diaphragmatic irritation—lung cancer in this case.

quired. **Endoscopy** can evaluate the esophagus and stomach and can identify potential sources of gastric outlet obstruction. Laboratory studies, such as blood-gas and electrolyte determinations, may be indicated because hyponatremia can cause and exacerbate hiccups.

Treatment

In most instances, patients have tried to induce eructation or have used one or more folk remedies before presentation. These remedies may include inducing a startle reflex with a sudden loud noise (traditionally by bursting an inflated paper bag); it has been postulated that the startle overrides the hiccup reflex and "resets" the neural driver. Other folk remedies include eating granulated sugar (probably a form of pharyngeal simulation) and breathing into a bag (to elevate the arterial level of carbon dioxide). Most of these probably have some degree of physiologic basis for their use.

During the initial examination, firmly massaging the soft palate with the tip of a tongue blade or cotton-tipped applicator may stop the hiccups immediately. It is thought that the strong stimulation or gag reflex produced by this maneuver may override the hiccup-generating neural center. Passing a nasogastric tube also can cure hiccups, both by stimulating the nasopharyngeal and esophageal mucosal receptors and by decompressing the stomach. Nasogastric tube decompression resolves most postoperative hiccups and should be used early.

Interesting reports on the effectiveness of these and other maneuvers abound, often with enthusiastic endorsement by the author of the case report. Forceful traction on the tongue, lifting the uvula with a spoon, sipping ice water, gargling with ice water, inhaling ammonia, irritating the tympanic membrane with a flexible object, and even digitally massaging the rectum have been reported to stop hiccups. Other unusual maneuvers include cooling the skin over the phrenic nerve with vapocoolant sprays and rhythmically tapping the fifth cervical vertebra.

Vagal stimulation (e.g., carotid massage, supraorbital massage) may be effective, with care taken to avoid bradycardia and asystole. Carotid massage also can result in embolic episodes in patients with vascular disease and, thus, should be avoided in these cases. Rhythmically tapping over the spinous process of the fifth cervical vertebra and applying ice to the anterior neck both have been reported to be effective and probably exert their effect through competing sensory input.

Pharmacologic Therapy

If hiccups persist despite common therapeutic maneuvers, then the use of a variety of pharmacologic agents can be considered (Table 28.4). Slow intravenous injection of **chlorpromazine** (Thorazine) has been the drug of choice

Table 28.4 Pharmacologic Management of Persistent or Intractable Hiccup

Drug	Dosage	Comments
Chlorpromazine	25–50 mg IV in 1 L saline infused slowly over several hours; maintenance 25–50 mg for 7–10 days	Usual drug of first choice
Baclofen	5 mg every 8–12 hours orally, increased as needed every 3 days to a maximum dose of 75 mg	Watch for hypotension and sedation
Diphenylhydantoin	200 mg IV infused slowly; maintenance 300 mg/d	Some physicians believe this to be the drug of first choice
Valproic acid	15 mg/kg/d	Watch for hepatotoxicity
Amitriptyline	10–100 mg/d	Watch for prolonged QT interval
Metoclopramide	10 mg orally every 6 hours	May cause gastrointestinal side effects

IV = intravenously.

for the treatment of persistent or intractable hiccups. Twenty five to 50 mg in a liter of saline is infused slowly over several hours, with close monitoring for hypotension or sedation. Daily doses of 25 to 50 mg usually are required for maintenance for 7 to 10 days. **Baclofen**, a derivative of gamma-aminobutyric acid (GABA), may be even more effective and is the drug of choice for some physicians. Therapy is initiated with low doses of 5 mg every 8 to 12 hours and increased as needed every 3 days to a maximum dose of 75 mg. Once the hiccups have resolved, the medication can be discontinued.

Anticonvulsants have been used in cases unresponsive to chlorpromazine. Intravenous phenytoin has been used with an initial dose of 200 mg and a maintenance dosage of 300 mg/d orally. Benzodiazepines are not successful in managing intractable hiccups and may even worsen them. The antidepressant **amitriptyline** and the motility stimulant **metoclopramide** have been reported to be effective in managing hiccups, probably through central and peripheral activity, respectively. **Valproic acid**, an anticonvulsant with central GABA-like neurotransmitter-inhibitory activity, also has been reported to be effective. It is postulated that the activity in hiccups is due to enhancement of the GABA inhibition of normal excitability within the hiccup-generating center. Starting dosages of 15 mg/kg/d are recommended, with incremental increases as necessary to control hiccups. One author noted that, in his experience, this drug was unsuccessful in controlling hiccups.

Phrenic nerve section has been reported to be effective but carries with it the risks of hypoventilation and dyspnea. On one occasion, intractable hiccups have been controlled by **microvascular decompression of an ectatic vertebral artery that was compressing the brainstem**. Newer, more-precise imaging techniques may reveal more anomalies as causes of hiccups that can be corrected.

Other Treatments

For "functional" hiccups (i.e., hiccups that seem to be a response to emotional distress), psychiatric referral may be considered but only after all possible organic causes have been excluded. Hypnosis, psychotherapy, and even acupuncture have been reported to effective. Occasionally, "nonorganic" therapeutic modalities such as these can cure hiccups that have known organic causes.

Summary

Hiccupping is a common physiologic condition usually caused by diaphragmatic stimulation by gastric distention. Typically self-limited, such hiccups often can be stopped by eructation or pharyngeal stimulation. However, persistent or intractable hiccups require investigation (e.g., radiologic imaging). Therapy for these types of hiccups is more challenging and often requires pharmacologic management with Thorazine or baclofen. Nonorganic stress-management therapy is occasionally beneficial.

SUGGESTED READINGS

Launois A, Bizec JL, Whitelaw WA, et al. Hiccup in adults: an overview. *Eur Respir J.* 1993;6:563–75.

This review article, with an extensive list of references, is a comprehensive discussion of the etiology and management of intractable hiccups. Perhaps Table 2 (a listing of common remedies) is the most interesting item. Examples include, "bilateral compression of radial arteries while gazing into the subject's eyes" (referenced!).

Loft LM, Ward RF. Hiccups: a case presentation and etiologic review. *Arch Otolaryngol Head Neck Surg.* 1992;118:1115–9.

The authors report a single case of hiccups occurring in a young man who developed hiccups secondary to an Arnold-Chiari malformation. The authors review the etiology, evaluation, and the therapeutic options available in a short, concise review article.

Hansen BJ, Rosenberg J. Persistent postoperative hiccups: a review. *Acta Anesthesiol Scand.* 1993;37:643–6.

The authors address the management of postoperative hiccups, beginning with the passage of a nasogastric tube for stimulation of the vagal receptors in the mucosa of the esophagus as well as for gastric decompression. Their algorithm suggests that this should be the first step before using a pharmacologic means of therapy.

Howard R. Persistent hiccups. *BMJ.* 1992;305:1237–8.

This brief report reviews the etiology and identifies chlorpromazine as the drug of choice in the management of intractable hiccups.

Ramirez FC, Graham DY. Treatment of intractable hiccup with Baclofen: results of a double-blind, randomized, controlled, crossover study. *Am J Gastroenterol.* 1992;87:1789–791.

The authors review the use of Baclofen in the management of hiccups in four patients studied in a double-blind, randomized, crossover trial. This recent report suggests that Baclofen should be considered in the management of intractable hiccups.

Rousseau P. Hiccups. *South Med J.* 1995;88:175–81.

The author reviews the history, physiology, evaluation, and therapy of hiccups. The section on therapy is particularly useful and serves as the basis for this chapter's therapy section.

29

Foreign Bodies

Gregory N. Postma, MD

Nearly 1500 people die annually from complications of foreign bodies in the upper aerodigestive tract, most of which occur in children. However, approximately 30% occur in adults, peaking in patients over 60 years of age, with a much higher incidence present in institutionalized patients (1). The history of foreign body ingestion or aspiration may be obvious, but more often the symptoms (either acute or chronic) are accompanied by minimal or subtle physical findings. This chapter discusses foreign bodies of the airway, esophagus, pharynx, ear canal, and nasal cavity.

Airway Foreign Bodies

Adults who aspirate foreign bodies into their airways are usually older and often have an underlying impairment of normal airway-protective mechanisms (1). This impairment may be due to sedative or alcohol use, primary neurological disorders (e.g., seizures, tumors of the central nervous system, mental retardation, dementia, cerebral vascular accidents), or head trauma. The use of dentures decreases functional palatal sensation when eating, impairing the management of the food bolus and predisposing the patient to swallowing a larger-than-intended food bolus that can lodge in the esophagus or can be aspirated.

Delay in the diagnosis of an airway foreign body is not unusual. Symptoms occur in three stages (2). The initial or acute stage, at the time of aspiration,

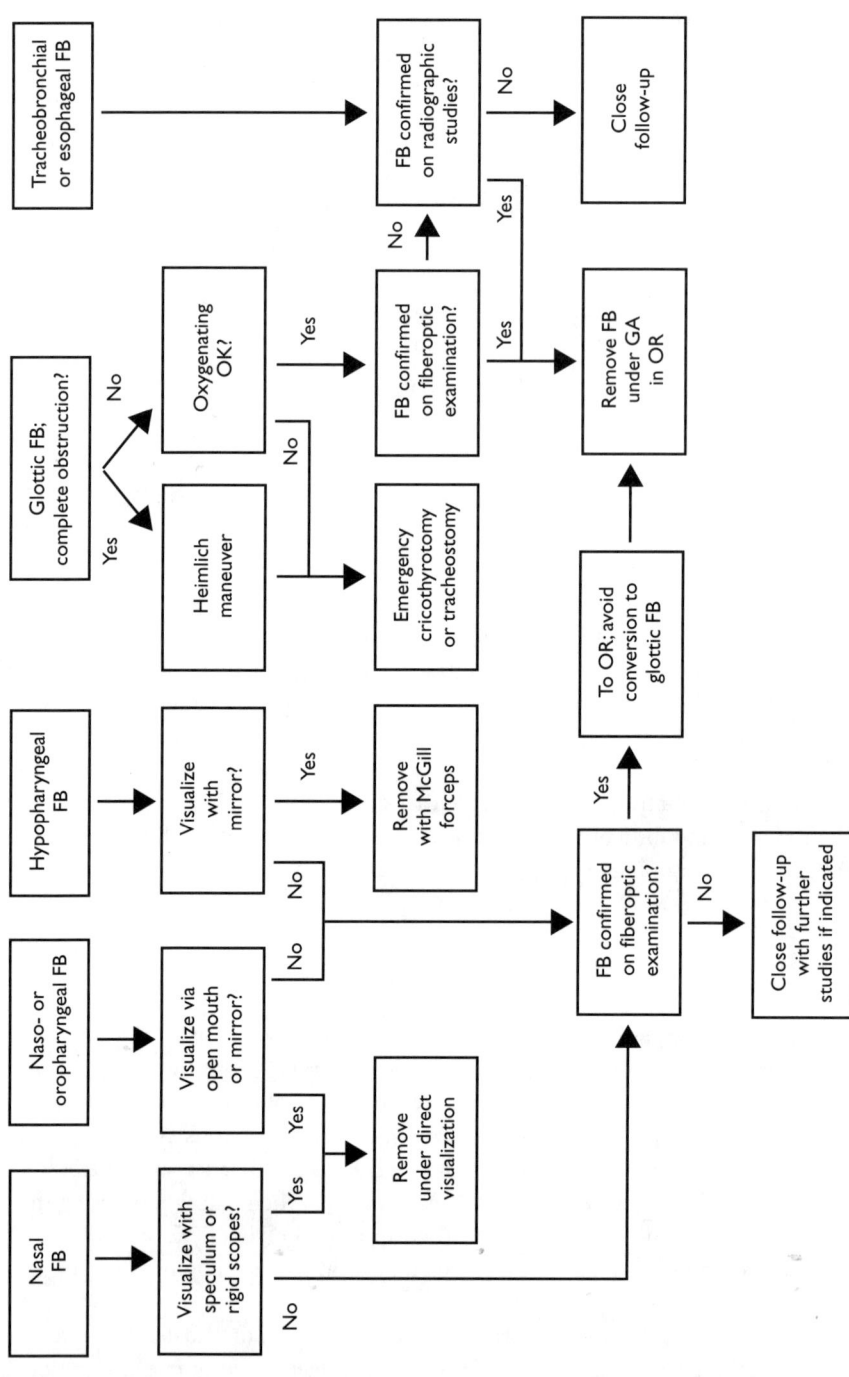

Algorithm Management of foreign bodies in the aerodigestive tract. FB = foreign body; GA = general anesthesia; OR = operating room.

consists of paroxysmal coughing, choking, gagging, wheezing, or rarely hemoptysis. Only approximately half of adult patients with an airway foreign body provide a history of coughing or choking (3). If undiagnosed at this time, there follows **a relatively asymptomatic interval during which diagnosis is difficult.** Laryngeal foreign bodies can cause hoarseness, a croup-like cough, aphonia, odynophagia, odynophonia, hemoptysis, wheezing, and shortness of breath. Displacement of the laryngeal foreign body to a more distal position in the airway is not uncommon if coughing does not expel it. Tracheal or bronchial foreign bodies are more common and are usually asymptomatic.

An undiagnosed foreign body eventually lodges in the airway, and any mild initial symptoms of irritation subside as the pulmonary reflexes fatigue. During this second or **asymptomatic phase,** the patient and family may be reassured falsely by the absence of symptoms for days or even months. The only symptom may be unexplained respiratory illness (recurrent or persistent) due to chronic airway foreign body. The possibility of an airway foreign body should be considered in patients with recurrent pneumonia, atypical asthma, chronic cough, or delayed resolution of pneumonia (1,2) (Table 29.1).

A third stage may occur weeks to months later from complications (e.g., mucosal erosion, secondary infection) caused by the continuous presence of the foreign body. A productive cough often is accompanied by fever or chest pain.

Physical Examination

The physical findings of an airway foreign body are often subtle; some patients have decreased breath sounds or localized wheezing. The classic findings of tracheal foreign bodies are an audible slap, palpable thud, and an asthma-like wheeze; however, most adults with an airway foreign body have a

Table 29.1 Symptoms of Airway Foreign Bodies

Laryngeal Foreign Bodies	Airway Foreign Bodies
Hoarseness	Unexplained respiratory symptoms
Croup-like cough	Persistent respiratory illness
Aphonia	Recurrent pneumonia
Odynophagia	Delayed resolution of pneumonia
Odynophonia	Progressive hoarseness
Hemoptysis	Atypical asthma or COPD
Wheezing	Chronic cough
Shortness of breath	
Presence or suspicion of airway foreign body	
Stridor	

COPD = chronic obstructive pulmonary disease.

Table 29.2 Differential Diagnosis of Airway Foreign Bodies

Airway foreign body	Reflux laryngitis
Malignant or benign tumor	Recurrent pneumonia in same area
Atypical asthma	Delayed resolution of pneumonia
Atypical COPD	Tuberculosis
Recurrent bronchitis	Cough secondary to ACE inhibitors

ACE = angiotensin-converting enzyme; COPD = chronic obstructive pulmonary disease.

normal physical examination. Conditions with symptoms similar to those seen with airway foreign bodies are listed in Table 29.2.

Diagnostic Evaluation

Radiologic evaluation is essential but not necessarily diagnostic. Inspiratory and expiratory chest radiographs can be helpful in evaluating a patient with a suspected airway foreign body. The cross-sectional area of the airway increases during inspiration, allowing foreign bodies to move distally. If the object allows air to flow during inspiration but blocks it during expiration (a one-way or ball-valve obstruction), then hyperinflation of the lung distal to the object occurs with depression of the ipsilateral hemidiaphragm and a mediastinal shift to the opposite side. (Fig. 29.1) If the object completely obstructs the airway, distal atelectasis occurs. Because a tracheobronchial foreign body can change location with coughing, repeat radiographs are obtained before endoscopy, if not immediately after the initial radiograph is obtained.

Meat and bones (e.g., meat, chicken, fish) are the most common foreign bodies, followed by dental appliances, teeth, and trauma-associated obstructions (1,3) (Figs. 29.2 and 29.3).

Management

Acute, completely obstructing airway foreign bodies are treated emergently with the **Heimlich maneuver** (*see* Algorithm), which increases intrathoracic pressure and forces the object from the airway. If the acute obstruction is incomplete (i.e., the patient is able to pass some air in and out) there is a danger of converting a partial airway obstruction to a complete obstruction by ill-advised, aggressive postural management or backslapping.

If a completely obstructing foreign body cannot be dislodged by the Heimlich maneuver, a method to "buy time" while setting up for an emergency cricothyrotomy or tracheostomy is to pass a **large-gauge Angiocath** through the cricothyroid membrane directed toward the feet. As soon as air is aspirated, the needle is withdrawn as the catheter is advanced into the airway.

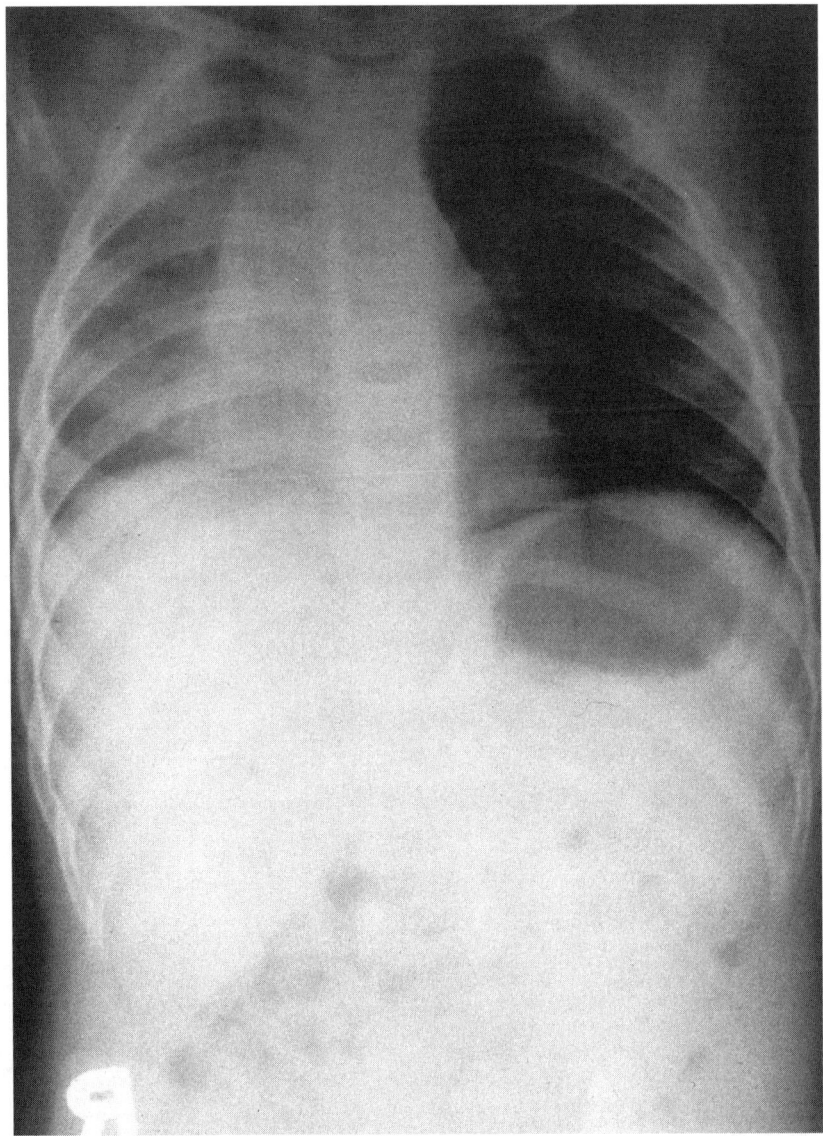

Figure 29.1 Hyperinflation of the left lung due to a "ball valve" foreign body in the left main bronchus. Note the mediastinal shift.

The tubing on most oxygen-supply bottles can be connected directly to the Angiocath, allowing instillation of some oxygen into the airway. Because the complete obstruction does not permit egress of instilled air, the tubing should

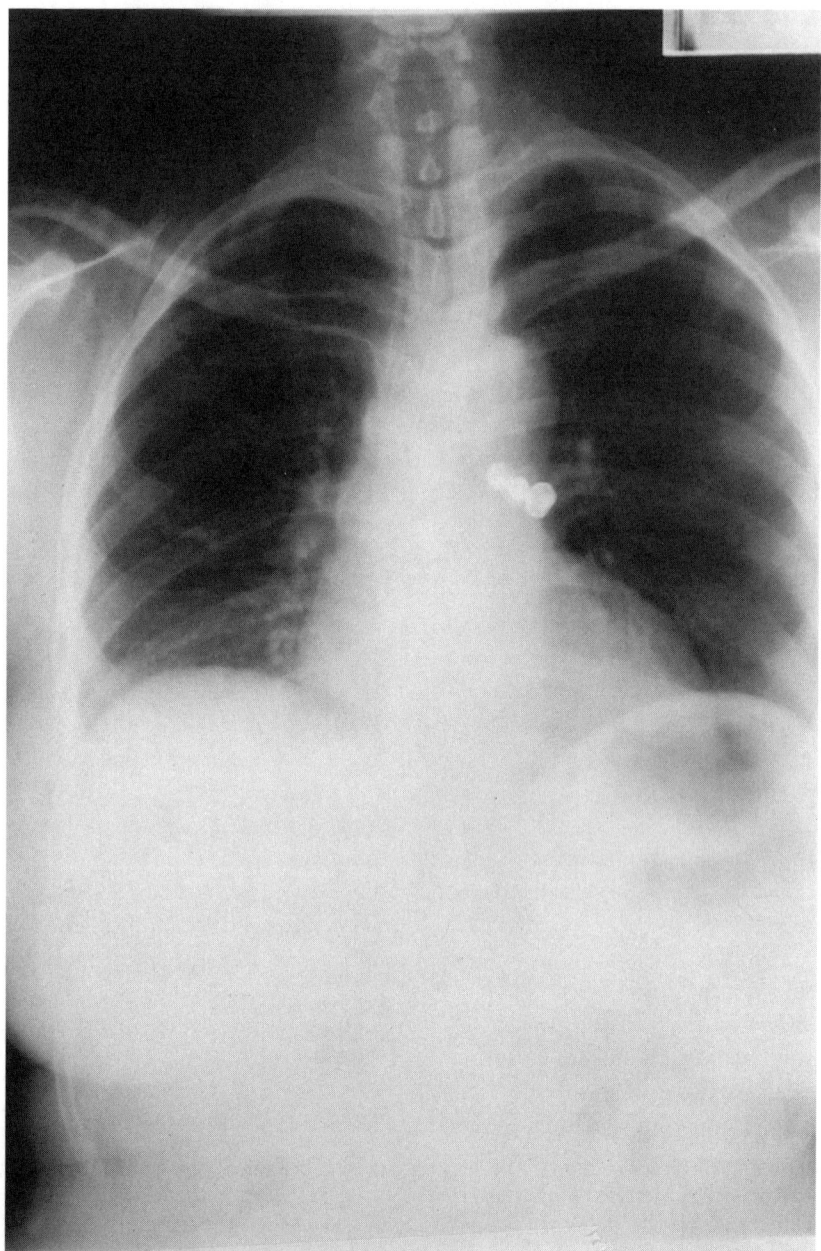

Figure 29.2 Dental appliance in the left main bronchus of a patient who presented with a chronic nonproductive cough 3 months after an assault.

be disconnected from the catheter frequently to permit egress through the catheter. However, this is merely a temporary measure useful only for 5 to 10 minutes while preparations are being made for placing a surgical airway. A tracheostomy is performed most optimally in the operating room by experienced personnel. If this is not possible, an emergency cricothyrotomy may be performed.

A patient with a laryngectomy presents another difficulty. Unlike the patient who merely has a temporary tracheostomy, **the laryngectomy patient has no opening between the mouth and the airway**; hence, mouth-to-mouth resuscitation, oral or nasal ventilation with a bag-valve mask, and attempts at oral or nasal intubation are unsuccessful. Many laryngectomy patients do not wear a tube in the stoma, whereas most tracheostomy patients do; however, this is not a completely reliable method of differentiating the two, because the reverse is possible. Some laryngectomy patients wear a laryngectomy tube in their stoma, and a few tracheostomy patients have a permanent tracheostoma that was fashioned by suturing the neck skin directly to the tracheal mucosa, obviating the need for a tube (Fig. 29.4). Because a thick mucus plug at the end of a tracheal tube can act as a foreign body, removing a possibly obstructed tube may be necessary. When this is done in a tracheostomy patient, the use of a lumen finder should be considered (particularly when replacing a recently placed tube) to ensure accurate tube replacement. A lumen finder is not necessary in a laryngectomy patient.

Prompt endoscopic removal of the foreign body is the treatment of choice (Case 29.1). Depending on the facilities available, the skills of the endoscopist, and the nature of the foreign body, either flexible or rigid endoscopy may be preferable in particular situations. The optical foreign body forceps that can be passed through a rigid bronchoscope are a major technical advance (Fig. 29.5).

Whichever technique is used, careful planning is important to ensure proper anesthetic control and appropriate instrumentation for a safe foreign body extraction. Having a family member obtain a duplicate of the foreign body (e.g., toy soldier, earring) allows the surgeon to use different types of instruments in a "dry run" to determine the best instrument for grasping and removing the object.

One of the perils of removing a tracheobronchial foreign body is capturing the foreign body and, during the removal process, losing control of it as the airway narrows at the subglottis and glottis, causing **complete glottic obstruction**. For smaller foreign bodies that lack the size to cause total airway obstruction (e.g., pin, fishbone), this is less of a concern. A rigid bronchoscope offers an advantage when extracting larger foreign bodies that can potentially obstruct the entire airway. Once the foreign body is brought into view and grasped with the forceps, it can be withdrawn completely into the bronchoscope; then the entire bronchoscope can be removed with the foreign body sheathed inside. Using this technique, one is less likely to lose control of the object at the glottis, thus decreasing the chances of total airway obstruction. In addition, rigid bronchoscopy usually is performed under general anesthesia;

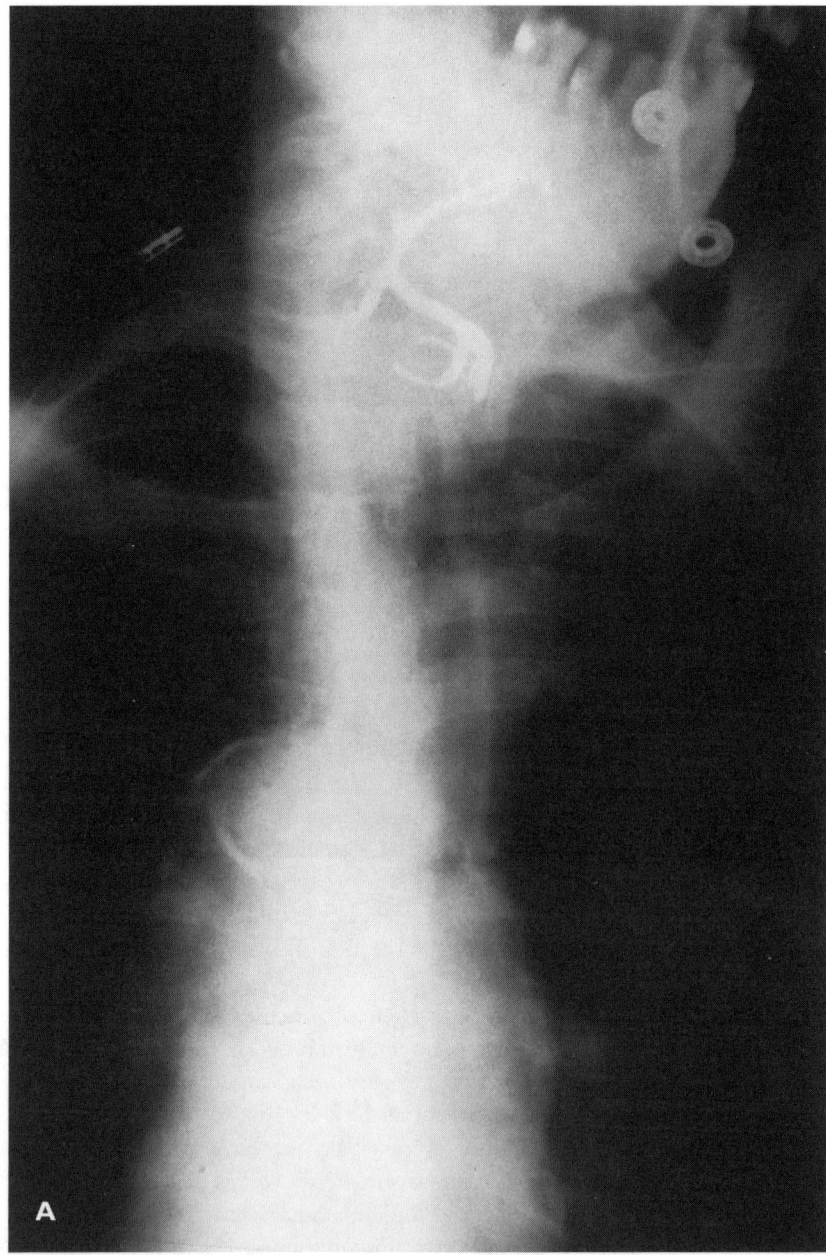

Figure 29.3 A, Lateral radiograph of an institutionalized patient who developed a cough after he "lost" his denture. **B,** Tip of the plastic edge of the denture (*dashed area*) can be seen, caught on the epiglottis. A tracheostomy was performed for airway control before removing the foreign body (see Case 29.3). (Courtesy of Dr. David Eibling.)

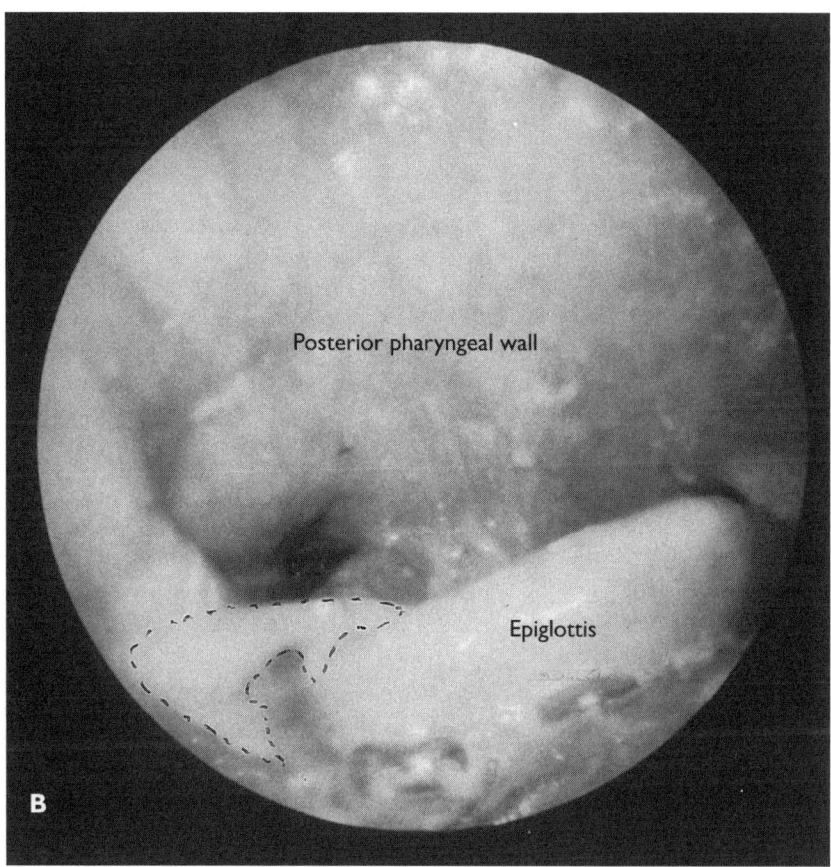

hence, controlled ventilation is possible through the rigid bronchoscope. However, because foreign bodies in the distal bronchi have to be smaller to have become lodged in the distal airway, they are often removed most optimally with flexible bronchoscopy (especially in the upper lobes of the lung, which can be difficult to visualize with a rigid endoscope) (1,3).

After removing the object, a complete reexamination of the tracheobronchial tree is essential when looking for a second foreign body or when visualizing the area of impaction or trauma (2,4). There may be more than one foreign body. In a review of 88 cases of foreign body aspiration in adults, McGuirt and coworkers (4) found multiple foreign bodies in 5% of patients.

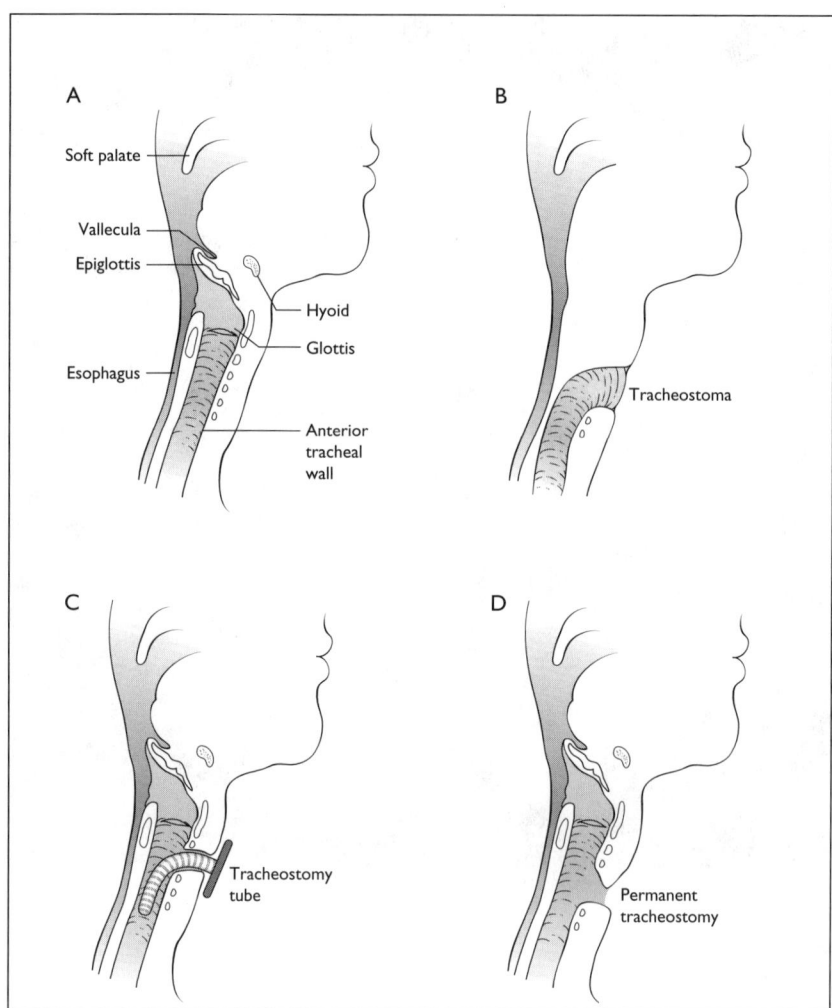

Figure 29.4 Lateral diagrams of the airway in the neck. **A,** Normal anatomy, with the airway entered via the glottis and the esophagus located just posteriorly. **B,** After a laryngectomy, there is no connection between the oral cavity and the airway. The larynx and hyoid bone have been removed, and the upper trachea opens directly into the neck. These patients sometimes wear "laryngectomy" tubes in the stoma, causing confusion with a tracheostomy. **C,** A tracheostomy, with the tube passing through the anterior neck skin to rest in the upper trachea. The connection of the airway with the oral cavity remains intact. **D,** Occasionally (as in sleep apnea patients), a permanent, skin-lined tracheostomy is created so that no tracheostomy tube is present; however, the connection of the oral cavity to the airway remains.

Postoperative care usually includes a brief period of antibiotics, chest physiotherapy, and humidification. If the foreign body has been present for weeks or months, chest physical therapy and antibiotics are particularly important.

> **Case 29.1** **Inhalation of a Foreign Body Resulting from the Impairment of Airway-Protective Mechanisms Caused by Intoxication**
>
> A college student 18 years of age was holding thumbtacks in his mouth while decorating for a Halloween party. He and his friends had already begun to drink alcohol, and he was mildly intoxicated. While laughing, he inhaled a tack, and began coughing. After several minutes the coughing stopped, but the tack could not be found. His friends were alarmed and thought that he might have swallowed it, so they brought him to the emergency department at the nearby university hospital.
>
> Physical examination at the hospital is essentially normal, with no unusual respiratory noise or evidence of pharyngeal laceration. Chest and abdominal radiographs are ordered, and the tack is found in the right lower lung. It is removed uneventfully via rigid bronchoscopy under general anesthesia. A postoperative chest radiograph is normal, and he is discharged the next morning to return to class, having missed only the Halloween party.
>
> **Discussion**
>
> This case is typical because the patient had an underlying reason for aspiration (in this case, he was talking and laughing while mildly intoxicated with a foreign body in his mouth). Moreover, the coughing stopped after several minutes, which could have led to a delayed diagnosis. The favorable outcome in this case is directly related to the suspicion of his fraternity brothers that all was not well and to the hunch that compelled the emergency department physician to obtain the diagnostic radiograph.

Complications

Complications of airway foreign bodies and their removal are fortunately rare (Table 29.3). Aside from the catastrophic potential for causing complete airway obstruction, laryngeal edema caused by instrumentation during foreign body removal is the most significant concern. This edema usually resolves when treated with humidified air, inhaled racemic epinephrine, and intravenous corticosteroids.

Esophageal Foreign Bodies

Acutely, esophageal foreign bodies are not as dangerous as airway foreign bodies. Meat impactions are the most common problems in adults, followed by bones that become lodged in the esophagus (5). The greatest concern with esophageal foreign bodies is **preventing conversion to airway foreign bodies**, particularly at the cricopharyngeus or cervical esophagus.

Most adults (65%–97%) who have impacted esophageal foreign bodies also have some esophageal pathology that varies from benign strictures or esophagitis to carcinoma (5) (Table 29.4). Because of the high prevalence of esophageal disease, diagnostic esophagoscopy is performed within several weeks, even if a food bolus passes after a brief obstruction.

Foreign body ingestions often occur in adults with underlying neurological abnormalities and in prisoners, psychiatric patients, and other institutionalized individuals. As with airway foreign bodies, wearing dentures is one of the more common predisposing factors associated with the ingestion of esophageal foreign bodies. An upper denture plate eliminates the palatal sensitivity that is critical to identifying pieces of bone and the size of a food bolus

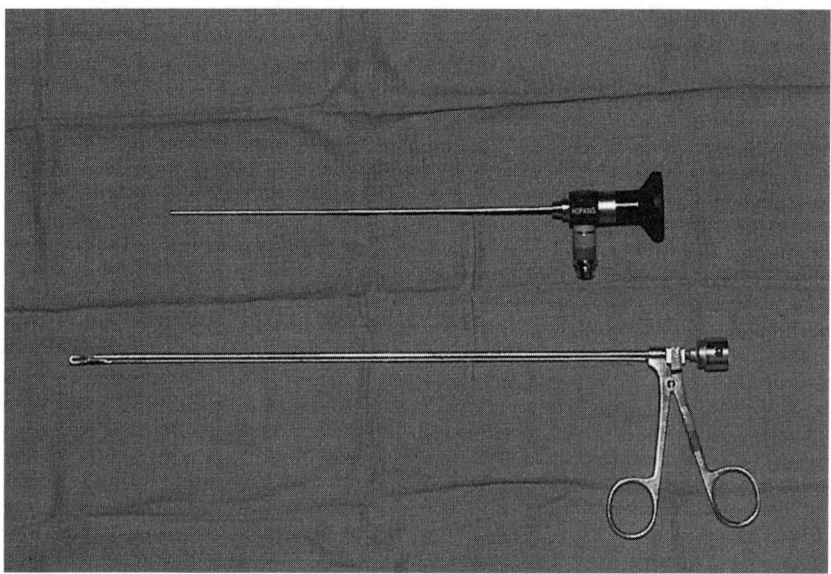

Figure 29.5 Optical forceps through which foreign bodies can be visualized clearly, facilitating their removal. (Courtesy of Dr. Kyle Kennedy.)

Table 29.3 Complications of Airway Foreign Bodies

Early	Late
Laryngeal edema	Hemoptysis
Hemoptysis	Inflammatory polyps
Laryngospasm	Granuloma formation
Perforation	Bronchial stricture
Pneumomediastinum	Bronchiectasis
Pneumothorax	
Asphyxia (death)	

(Fig. 29.6). Of all ingestions of esophageal foreign bodies, 80% to 90% pass through the gastrointestinal tract without difficulty. Only 10% to 15% lodge somewhere in the esophagus, and less than 1% cause viscus perforation (6).

Impaction usually occurs at areas of physiologic or pathologic narrowing (7). The esophagus has four areas of physiologic narrowing. The first and

Table 29.4 Causes of Obstruction of Esophageal Foreign Bodies

Stricture or esophagitis due to GERD	Diverticuli
Schatzki's ring	Esophageal motility disorders
Malignant or benign tumors	Sequelae of caustic ingestion, esophageal surgery, or tracheo-esophageal fistula repair
Intentional (e.g., in psychiatric prisoners)	

GERD = gastroesophageal reflux disease.

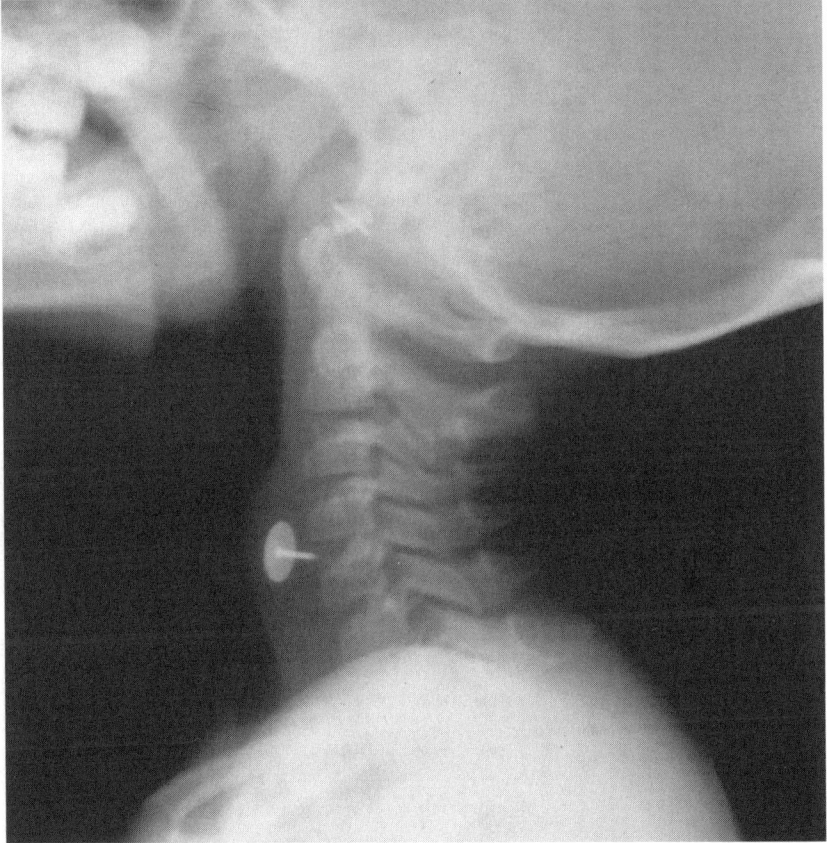

Figure 29.6 A tack lodged in the cervical esophagus.

narrowest is the cricopharyngeus muscle (upper esophageal sphincter) between the hypopharynx and the esophagus. Other areas of narrowing occur where the esophagus is compressed by the aortic arch and by the left main bronchus. The last area of narrowing is the gastroesophageal junction (lower esophageal sphincter). The most common types of pathologic narrowing are peptic strictures and Schatzki's ring.

History

Symptoms vary from partial obstruction in the distal esophagus with almost no symptoms to completely obstructed with drooling and aspiration (Case 29.2). The latter set of symptoms is a true emergency that requires immediate endoscopic removal of the foreign body.

The most common symptoms are dysphagia, odynophagia, foreign body sensation, excessive salivation, vomiting, and rarely chest pain (7,8) (Table 29.5). Odynophagia is often caused by mucosal trauma during passage of the foreign body. If it is large enough, a foreign body can displace the posterior wall of the trachea anteriorly, causing shortness of breath, wheezing, and stridor. Most adults with food impactions have significant symptoms, whereas only approximately half of those with non-food foreign bodies have acute symptoms.

Often, a patient with an upper esophageal foreign body impaction can point directly to the level of impaction. A foreign body in the lower esophagus, however, cannot be localized as accurately; referred pain to the sternum is common.

A history of caustic ingestion or long-standing gastroesophageal reflux disease suggests the possibility of stricture formation, predisposing the patient to foreign body impaction.

Physical Examination

The examination of patients with impacted esophageal foreign bodies is usually unremarkable, leading to a delay in diagnosis and treatment. The inability to communicate subtle symptoms puts some patients who have central nervous system abnormalities or psychiatric disorders at higher risk for delayed diagnosis.

Rarely, erythema and abrasions are seen in the pharynx. Stridor and wheezing occur occasionally, as does subcutaneous emphysema in the chest and neck, which should be considered evidence of perforation. Fever also may be evidence of a perforation, abscess formation, or mediastinitis.

Diagnostic Evaluation

All patients with possible esophageal foreign bodies undergo radiographic evaluation. The use of **posteroanterior and lateral chest and neck radiog-**

Case 29.2 Man with Complete Obstruction of the Esophagus and a History of Gastroesophageal Reflux Disease

A man 58 years of age with known gastroesophageal reflux disease is brought to the emergency department by his family after being unable to swallow after eating meat at a local steak house. The patient is edentulous and has no history of meat impaction. He is sitting up, spitting all of his saliva into a cup, and complains of significant substernal discomfort. Flexible fiberoptic examination of his pharynx is attempted but is not satisfactory due to the secretions in his pharynx. A small sip of barium is administered and identifies a complete block in the distal esophagus.

The patient is taken to the operating room urgently where he is anesthetized via a rapid-sequence technique (to prevent aspiration during induction) and undergoes removal of the impacted foreign body with rigid esophagoscopy. Repeat examination after removal demonstrates erythema and a suspicion of a stricture. He is observed overnight to rule out esophageal perforation and is discharged 12 hours after the procedure. Two weeks later, an esophagogram confirms the presence of a stricture, and the patient later undergoes esophagogastroduodenoscopy with balloon dilatation.

Discussion

This case is typical because the meat impaction occurred in an edentulous individual who was eating and talking in a restaurant. Furthermore, he had a preexisting esophageal abnormality that predisposed to obstruction, which illustrates the necessity of repeating the endoscopy after removing the impacted bolus. The complete obstruction with which he presented is typical, and many surgeons in such a situation would have bypassed the barium swallow and taken the patient directly to the operating room for removal. The impacted meat could have been removed via either rigid or flexible endoscope; however, sharp, pointed objects (e.g., bones) require rigid endoscopy. Balloon removal usually is not feasible in meat impactions because the catheter cannot be passed distal to the obstruction. There are other objections to balloon removal as well, particularly the risk that when the bolus is brought into the pharynx it could be lost and aspirated, resulting in total airway obstruction. Meat tenderizer should not be used in these cases, because the enzymes dissolve the esophagus as well, leading to perforation, particularly if instrumentation is required for removal.

Table 29.5 Symptoms of Esophageal Foreign Bodies

Presence or suspicion (e.g., sensation) of foreign body	Excessive salivation
Progressive dysphagia	Vomiting
Dysphagia with any voice or respiratory symptoms	Chest pain (rare)
Acute dysphagia	Shortness of breath
Odynophagia	Wheezing
Button battery ingestion	Stridor
Subcutaneous air	

raphy is recommended, because a single view cannot always identify the position or the number of foreign bodies. The position of a flat, metallic object (e.g., a coin) can provide a clue to the location of the foreign body; coins in the trachea usually are oriented in the sagittal plane, whereas those in the esophagus are oriented frontally (Fig. 29.7). Radiography also may detect a second radiopaque object. Because so many ingestible objects are not radiopaque, failure to detect an esophageal foreign body radiographically does not rule out a foreign body definitively. In many cases, the safest decision is for any patient with continued symptoms to undergo esophagoscopy.

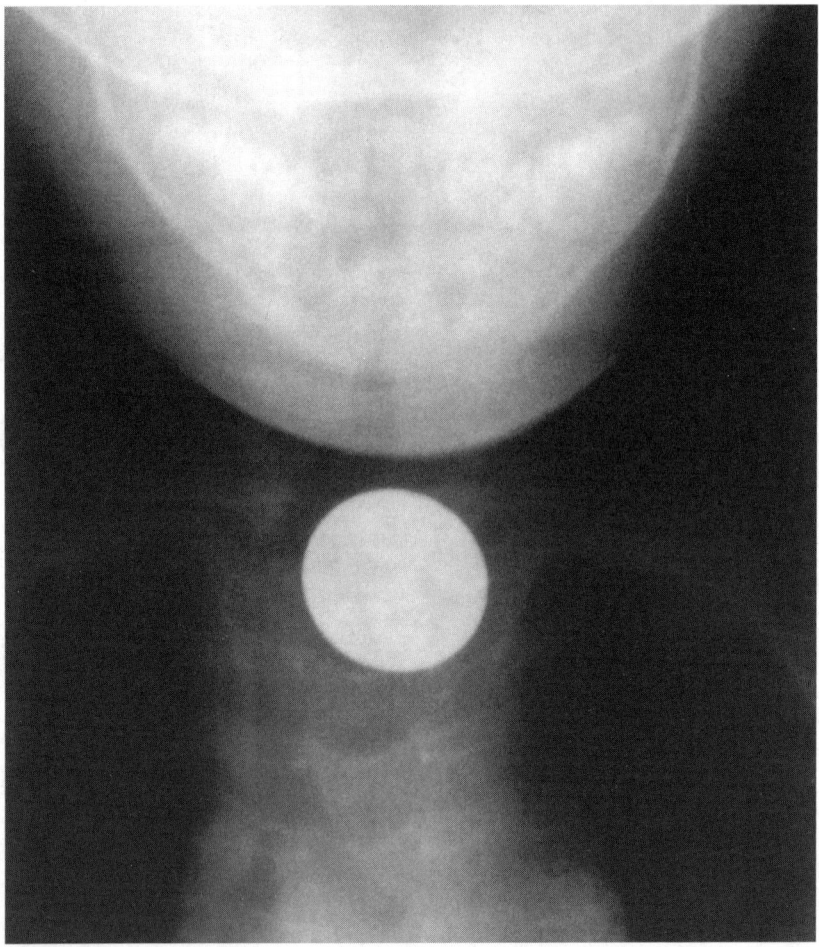

Figure 29.7 A coin in the esophagus. Note how it is located in the frontal plane, which is a clue to its position in the esophagus rather than in the airway.

A symptomatic adult who presents with a history of meat impaction does not necessarily require contrast studies. Barium is the optimal contrast medium, although its use requires removal by irrigation and suction. If perforation is suspected, a water-soluble contrast media (e.g., Gastrograffin) should be used because it induces less tissue inflammation. However, care is required in the use of these substances (especially Gastrograffin) because of their toxicity to lung tissue and because many patients with obstructing foreign bodies aspirate.

Radiolucent foreign bodies in the hypopharynx and esophagus may be difficult to diagnose if complete obstruction is not present. Some clinicians recommended a thin-barium suspension or barium-impregnated cotton to attempt to outline the object. Others think that if a high index of suspicion is present, then the patient should proceed directly to endoscopy. If radiographic studies are used, then endoscopy is performed when the radiograph is positive *or* when it is negative but the patient remains symptomatic.

Management

Management of the patient with an esophageal foreign body depends on the type and location of the foreign body and the degree of obstruction. **Airway protection is critical**. The patient with a complete esophageal obstruction is unable to swallow his own oral secretions, increasing the risk of aspiration. Asymptomatic coins in the distal esophagus should be allowed 12 hours to pass into the stomach, whereas coins in the mid- or upper esophagus are removed within hours to avoid swelling and regurgitation that might compromise the airway.

Endoscopic Treatment

The rate of successfully removing an esophageal foreign body is equal with either flexible or rigid esophagoscopy. Choosing which instrument to use should be based on the patient and the endoscopist involved. Rigid esophagoscopy under general anesthesia permits absolute airway control, which minimizes the risk of aspiration, whereas flexible esophagoscopy eliminates the need for general anesthesia, which is especially important if there is a comorbidity that might increase the rate of pulmonary or other sequelae to the general anesthesia. Additionally, the skill, training, and experience of the individual endoscopist also may make one technique a better choice in a given situation (5,6).

When a coin or similar foreign body is lodged in the upper esophagus, particularly in the area of the cricopharyngeus muscle, there is a much greater risk of it being converted inadvertently to an airway foreign body (8). As with bronchoscopy in the removal of airway foreign bodies, the ability to sheath the foreign body within the endoscope for removal minimizes the chance of losing a grip on it at the glottic inlet. Flexible esophagoscopy also can be performed under general anesthesia, decreasing the risk of patient movement at just the wrong moment.

Introducing the flexible scope into the hypopharynx without direct visualization risks perforation of the pharynx and esophagus and even displacement of the foreign body if it is impacted proximally in the esophagus. Safety can be enhanced by the use of a protective device to facilitate multiple passes of the instrument and to minimize the trauma to the tongue, hypopharynx, and upper esophagus.

Sharp or pointed foreign bodies may tear or perforate the esophageal wall during removal, and **complications are significantly higher**. These objects are often seen in prisoners and psychiatric patients (7). A rigid esophagoscope is usually the instrument of choice in patients with these types of foreign bodies, and using general endotracheal anesthesia is the safest method.

After removing an esophageal foreign body, most endoscopists obtain a routine chest radiograph and **observe the patient for at least 12 hours, watching for fever, tachycardia, and other signs of mediastinitis**. After the removal of a large or complex esophageal foreign body, which involves a significant amount of esophageal trauma, the patient usually is observed for 24 hours or more. A radiographic study with contrast material may be indicated to assess the integrity of the esophagus.

Button batteries are particularly dangerous—not only do they contain a heavy metal (i.e., mercury) and a concentrated alkaline electrolyte but they can also lodge in the esophagus at the level of the cricopharyngeus muscle. Direct corrosive action, low-voltage electrical burns, direct pressure necrosis, or rarely mercury toxicity can combine to damage the mucosa. Any button battery that is lodged in the esophagus is an emergency because it can cause severe damage in just 4 hours. Catastrophic complications that have been reported after battery ingestion include esophageal perforation, and tracheoesophageal and esophago-aortic fistulas.

Radiographs help distinguish button batteries from coins because, in the anterior projection, these batteries have a double-density shadow (or halo) due to their bilaminar structure. General endotracheal anesthesia is recommended for button-battery removal to ensure airway protection and to inhibit patient movement during extraction. After removing the battery from the esophagus, endoscopy is repeated to assess the damage. Barium swallow is recommended 24 hours after endoscopy to rule out a fistula, with a follow-up study 2 weeks later to check for early stricture formation.

Nonendoscopic Treatment

In some centers, a **balloon catheter** is passed just beyond the foreign body. Under fluoroscopic control, the balloon is inflated and the catheter is withdrawn in the hopes of bringing the foreign body out in front of it. Good success has been reported with this technique; however, it does not provide firm grasp and control of the object and therefore carries an increased risk of dropping the foreign body in the hypopharynx where it can be aspirated into the airway. In addition, balloon-catheter extraction is highly dependent on the skill of the operator and does not allow visual assessment of the condition of the esophageal mucosa or any pathology (which is nearly always present).

Further arguments against balloon-catheter extraction include a lack of airway protection, the possibility of missing other foreign bodies, and an increased risk of mucosal trauma or perforation when direct visualization is not used (10).

Although some authors report a lower complication rate with balloon-catheter extraction than with endoscopic techniques, patient selection introduces bias in this area (11). In centers that practice this technique, patients with larger, sharper foreign bodies present for a longer time, and patients who have failed attempts at balloon catheter extraction are the ones referred for endoscopic removal. Complications of extracting esophageal foreign bodies with a balloon catheter include laryngospasm, epistaxis, aspiration, dislodgment into the nasopharynx, and excessive patient discomfort (6).

Provided that the object has been lodged for less than 24 hours and that the obstruction is incomplete, balloon-catheter extraction of an esophageal foreign body is a useful option when operating facilities and endoscopic equipment are not available. Although there are cost savings with use of balloon-catheter extraction compared with endoscopy, firm contraindications to the use of the balloon-catheter technique are 1) a distressed or acutely unstable patient, 2) the existence of a complete obstruction (beyond which the balloon catheter probably will not pass), 3) known esophageal disease, 4) bleeding diathesis, and 5) impaction of an object that is not inert or smooth (10). In all situations, patient safety and comfort are the primary criteria when deciding which technique to use.

Several **nonmechanical removal methods** have been described for esophageal foreign bodies. Enzymatic digestion of meat with papain (meat tenderizer) is strongly discouraged because both fatal esophageal perforation and hemorrhagic pulmonary edema have occurred with its use (8). If enzymatic digestion fails, subsequent instrumentation of the now irritated and inflamed esophageal mucosa carries a higher risk of complications. Glucagon has been used to relax the lower esophageal sphincter, assisting the passage of an esophageal foreign body; however, this is effective only in patients with no additional esophageal pathology, because Glucagon has no effect on esophageal strictures, rings, or tumors (12). Even if successful, eventual endoscopy must be performed to rule out esophageal pathology. Glucagon used in combination with a gas-forming agent to increase intraluminal pressure may force the object into the stomach; however, because perforation and aspiration has been reported using this method, it is not recommended.

Complications

Esophageal perforation is a risk after the removal of any foreign body, particularly if the extraction was difficult or if the object was present for more than 24 hours (12,13). Signs and symptoms of perforation include fever, tachycardia, shortness of breath, chest or abdominal pain, and subcutaneous emphysema. After most foreign body removals, chest radiographs are obtained to look for free air, indicating a perforated viscus. In most cases, early diagnosis with surgical repair and drainage is the only option likely to prevent sepsis and possible death. Other complications of esophageal foreign bodies and their removal are listed in Table 29.6.

Pharyngeal Foreign Bodies

Fish and chicken bones are the usual culprits in foreign body injuries of the pharynx (Fig. 29.8), usually lodging in the lymphatic tissue of the pharyngeal or lingual tonsils.

History

Patients usually complain of a globus sensation or a sharp stabbing pain when attempting to swallow (8,11). A key question to ask the patient is whether he or she feels the pain with each swallow. Patients often present within a few hours because of the severity of the discomfort, and they usually are able to localize the level of the foreign body accurately. Mucosal trauma from the passage of a foreign body produces symptoms that may last for several days. As a result, only 25% of patients presenting with a foreign body sensation or pain after ingestion of chicken or fish have an endoscopically proven bone present

Table 29.6 Complications of Esophageal Foreign Bodies

Mucosal laceration	Dislodgement of foreign body into the nasopharynx
Esophageal stricture	
Esophageal perforation with possible neck abscess, mediastinitis, pneumothorax, pneumomediastinum, tracheoesophageal fistula, or catastrophic vascular injuries	Laryngospasm
	Epistaxis
	Aspiration
	Excessive patient discomfort
Esophageal necrosis (e.g., with button battery ingestion)	Balloon catheter

(12,14). Various contrast studies, plain radiography, and computed tomography have been advocated to identify such bones. In many cases, such studies delay appropriate intervention and incur extra expense. Moreover, normal calcifications of the laryngeal cartilages can result in confusion.

Physical Examination

Examination with a bright headlamp or head mirror facilitates complete evaluation of the oropharynx. Gentle finger palpation is also helpful in localization. Fiberoptic pharyngoscopy via the nose should be performed on patients in whom the initial evaluation is negative (Case 29.3). This procedure is usually well tolerated and provides optimal visualization of the oropharynx and hypopharynx. If there are abrasions or mucosal tears, then antibiotics and analgesics should be prescribed. If a complete examination (including flexible fiberoptic pharyngoscopy) fails to reveal a foreign body, the examination should be repeated in 24 hours. If symptoms persist, consideration for radiographic studies or endoscopy is appropriate.

Management

In cooperative adults, foreign bodies (if readily visualized) often can be removed directly in the emergency department or clinic with the use of topical

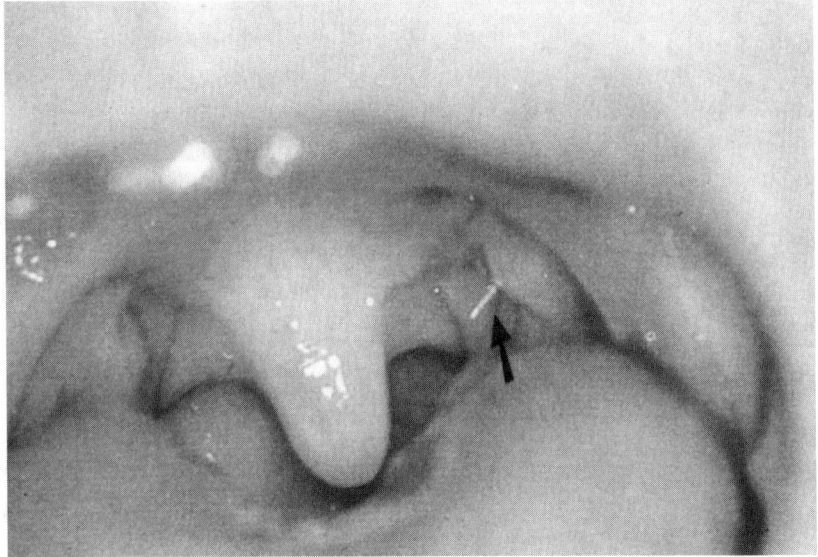

Figure 29.8 A fish bone (*arrow*) embedded in the left tonsil.

> **Case 29.3** **Institutionalized Man with a Foreign Body Presenting as a Cough**
>
> An institutionalized man 39 years of age who lost his partial denture develops a cough. Several days later, his physician orders a chest radiograph, which unexpectedly identifies not only the source of the cough but the location of his "lost" denture (see Fig. 29.3A). Fiberoptic examination of the pharynx demonstrates that the foreign body is impacted in his pharynx (see Fig. 29.3B), with one prong of the denture impaling the epiglottis.
>
> Because endotracheal intubation is not feasible—and because removal under sedation is not believed to be feasible—a tracheotomy is performed, through which the patient is anesthetized and the foreign body is removed uneventfully. The tracheostomy tube is removed several days later, and the patient is discharged back to his institution.
>
> **Discussion**
>
> This case is unusual because the symptoms of this foreign body were minimal. If this had occurred in a cognitively intact individual, the pain would have resulted in immediate identification.

anesthesia and a McGill forceps or hemostat. If the object is sharp or irregular or if the patient uncooperative, he or she should be taken to the operating room where the object may be removed safely under controlled conditions.

Complications

Esophageal and pharyngeal foreign bodies have an increased rate of complications if the presentation or diagnosis is delayed. A foreign body, particularly a fish bone, in the posterior pharynx is the most common cause of retropharyngeal abscess formation in adults (13). Other complications of pharyngeal foreign bodies include perforation and cellulitis. Patients with these problems complain of increasing dysphagia, odynophagia, and fever. If severe enough, either retropharyngeal abscess or cellulitis may lead to swelling of the pharynx and airway compromise.

Foreign Bodies of the External Auditory Canal

Foreign bodies in the external auditory canal (EAC) can be inorganic objects, organic or vegetable matter, or insects. Removal not only relieves the symptoms of pain, pressure, and decreased hearing but also avoids infection, further hearing loss, and EAC stenosis.

The most common inorganic foreign body in the adult ear is a piece of a cotton-tipped applicator. This is commonly seen in institutionalized adults and should be sought in patients who complain of drainage or ear odor. Objects placed into the bowl of the ear for water protection also may become foreign bodies in the EAC.

History

Symptoms include pressure, discomfort or pain, hearing loss, itchiness, ear odor, and ear discharge. Insects in the EAC usually present with severe pain and complaints about the noise of the live insect. Button batteries in the EAC are considered an emergency and are removed as soon as possible to avoid canal burns.

A patient who presents with an EAC foreign body and is experiencing severe hearing loss, dizziness, vertigo, nausea, or vomiting may have an injury to the middle or inner ear (*see* Chapter 2). Urgent examination by an otologist is necessary.

Management

Peas, beans, and other vegetable material should be removed while dry and intact. Instrumentation and suction with visualization under an operating microscope is the best method. If irrigation is used or the objects become wet, they can swell and even germinate (*see* Fig. 2.9), causing obstruction, pain, and maceration of the EAC mucosa.

Only experienced personnel should use irrigation. Excessive water pressure can cause EAC laceration, tympanic membrane perforation, or middle ear damage. Furthermore water that is retained in the canal medial to a foreign body causes maceration and otitis externa. Dizziness, vertigo, bloody otorrhea, and complete hearing loss are contraindications to EAC irrigation.

Insect removal can be challenging. Occasionally, a flying insect will fly toward a bright light directed at the ear. Filling the EAC with body-temperature mineral oil or lidocaine drowns or paralyzes the insect; however, this method is contraindicated if the patient has a history of an unrepaired tympanic membrane perforation (mineral oil can irritate the middle ear mucosa). Once insect movement ceases, the patient is much more comfortable, and the insect can be removed with suction and a headlamp or an operating microscope. After removal, the remaining liquid is suctioned out and the canal is inspected for trauma. The integrity of the ear canal skin and tympanic membrane should be evaluated after removing any foreign body from the EAC. If hearing has not returned to baseline, assessment with an audiogram and further evaluation is recommended.

In uncomplicated cases, no further care is required; however, if the foreign body has been present for a few days, **maceration or even cellulitis** may occur. **Topical antibiotic and steroid drops** are used in these cases. The patient should be counseled to avoid getting any water in the ear for 7 to 10 days. If there is significant infection in the EAC or conchal bowl, systemic antibiotics that are effective against *Pseudomonas* and *Staphylococcus aureus* are used. If the canal has a laceration or is macerated extensively, one or two expandable wicks in the canal, followed by antibiotic and steroid drops, should be inserted for 2 to 3 days. Examination of the ear via an operating microscope after wick removal is recommended.

Unrecognized **lacerations** of the canal can produce infection, scarring, and eventual canal stenosis. Trauma to the tympanic membrane or ossicular chain can result in hearing loss, either from the foreign body itself or as a complication of the foreign body extraction.

Nasal Foreign Bodies

Foreign bodies of the nose are encountered commonly in children but are seen rarely in adults (e.g., institutionalized patients, patients who have undergone previous nasal procedures). Foreign bodies that are left in the nose after treatment of epistaxis can result in foul nasal drainage and sinusitis with fever, facial swelling, and, if untreated, chronic disease. Local infection that results in granulation tissue with bleeding and drainage is common. Rarely, concretions accumulate on the foreign body over the course of years, forming a rhinolith that may reach a size so large as to destroy bone and require surgical removal. Large crusts can be retained in the nose after the removal of indwelling tubes and often act like foreign bodies, causing foul odor, drainage, and bleeding. These crusts should be removed with suction after softening them with saline irrigation. Nasal foreign bodies, although rare, do occur and require a high index of suspicion for identification.

Summary

Treating foreign bodies of the head and neck is a challenge that requires a suspicious physician and a thorough investigation for a successful outcome. Interdisciplinary cooperation is often the key to prompt symptom resolution.

REFERENCES

1. **Limper AH, Prakash UBS.** Tracheobronchial foreign bodies in adults. *Ann Intern Med.* 1990;112.604–9.

2. **Healy GB.** Management of tracheobronchial foreign bodies in children: an update. *Ann Otol Rhino Laryngol.* 1990;99:889–91.
3. **Lan R-S.** Nonasphyxiating tracheobronchial foreign bodies in adults. *Eur Respr J.* 1994;7:510–4.
4. **McGuirt WF, Holmes KD, Feehs R, Browne JD.** Tracheobronchial foreign bodies. *Laryugoscope.* 1988;98:615–8.
5. **Webb WA.** Management of foreign bodies of the upper gastrointestinal tract update. *Gastrointest Endosc.* 1995;41:39–51.
6. **Taylor RB.** Esophageal foreign bodies. *Emerg Med Clin North Am.* 1987;5:301–11.
7. **Brady PG.** Esophageal foreign bodies. *Gastroenterol Clin North Am.* 1991;20:691–701.
8. **Ratcliff KM.** Esophageal foreign bodies. *Am Fam Phys.* 1991;44:824–31.
9. **Kost KM, Shapiro RS.** Button battery ingestion: a case report and review of the literature. *J Otolaryngol.* 1987;16:252–7.
10. **Papsin BC, Friedberg J.** Aerodigestive-tract foreign bodies in children: perils in management. *J Otolaryngol.* 1994;23:102–8.
11. **Towbin RB.** Removal of foreign bodies from the upper gastrointestinal tract of children. *Curr Op Radiol.* 1990;2:900–8.
12. **Stack LB, Munter DW.** Foreign bodies in the gastrointestinal tract. *Emerg Med Clin North Am.* 1996;14:493–521.
13. **Singh B, Kantu M, Har-El G, Lucente FE.** Complications associated with 3D foreign bodies of the pharynx, larynx, and esophagus. *Ann Oto Rhino Laryngol.* 1997;106:301–4.
14. **Sundgren PC; Burnett A, Maly PV.** Value of radiography in the management of possible fishbone ingestion. *Ann Otol Rhinol Laryngol.* 1994;103:628–31.

SUGGESTED READINGS

Kost KM, Shapiro RS. Button battery ingestion: a case report and review of the literature. *J Otolaryngol.* 1987;16:252–7.

This report details the dangers of button battery ingestion, and discusses strategies for preventing ingestion.

Limper AH, Prakash UBS. Tracheobronchial foreign bodies in adults. *Ann Intern Med.* 1990;112.604–9.

This article reviews 60 adults with foreign body aspiration, nearly half of whom had underlying impairment of the airway protection mechanism. Fourteen of 23 foreign bodies were successfully removed with flexible bronchoscopy and 43 of 44 with rigid bronchoscopy. Only three required thoracotomy for removal.

Taylor RB. Esophageal foreign bodies. *Emerg Med Clin North Am.* 1987;5:301–11.

This is an excellent and thorough review of the approaches to treating patients with esophageal foreign bodies.

30

Caustic Ingestion

Andrew J. Nemechek, MD
Ronald G. Amedee, MD

The upper aerodigestive tract is a conduit for inhaled and ingested materials, and its structures are at risk for significant injury when exposed to caustic substances. The word *caustic*—derived from the Greek root *kaustikos*, which means "burning"—applies to both acid- and alkali-containing substances. Successful treatment of caustic ingestion depends on the following factors: 1) prompt, early, emergent stabilization and resuscitation, 2) proper classification of the extent of mucosal injury, 3) judicious pharmacotherapy to limit further injury, and 4) prompt surgical management of complications and their sequelae.

This chapter addresses the history and epidemiology of caustic ingestion, reviews the pertinent anatomy, and describes the pathophysiology specific to caustic ingestion. The challenges of diagnosis and emergency management are addressed, and a current review of strategies for definitive management and treatment of complications is presented. Finally, current clinical strategies are presented to guide the decision-making process in treating these challenging patients.

Social History

As society rapidly became industrialized, potent cleaning agents became widely available to the general public. Early otolaryngologists such as Chevalier Jackson recognized the gravity of the increased incidence of caustic injuries and lobbied legislators aggressively to adapt laws mandating that containers holding these dangerous substances be labeled as poisonous. In 1927, Calvin Coolidge signed the Federal Caustic Act into law. Since then, other legislation has sought to further protect consumers against these hazardous materials. Both the Poison Prevention Packaging Act of 1970 and the Federal Hazardous Substance Act of 1972 have been executed by the United States Consumer Products Safety Commission. Antidote procedures and handling instructions are included on labels, and these regulations apply to materials that contain strong acids as well. Regulations also require that the substances be contained in child-resistant packaging.

Although these injuries still cause significant morbidity, the incidence of caustic ingestions in the United States has declined moderately over the past few decades. The National Safety Council reported 2600 deaths in 1981 secondary to poisonings, and there has been a decrease in incidents of caustic ingestion in children under 5 years of age. Many clinicians believe that these moderate improvements are a direct result of the legislative changes mentioned above.

Epidemiology

Early reports of caustic ingestion usually involve children playing with white crystalline substances that resemble sugar. The largest group of patients affected are those 3 years of age and younger. The U.S. Poison Control Center estimates that up to 26,000 caustic ingestions occur per year. In these instances, the patient may remain asymptomatic for a period of time. Cases of caustic ingestion exhibit a bimodal distribution, with the second peak occurring in patients having attempted suicide. Generally, these patients are older women. Alkali ingestion is responsible for 60% to 80% of the injuries, with the rest caused by acids.

Caustic alkaline substances commonly contain sodium or potassium hydroxide (e.g., lye, drain cleaners), sodium carbonate (e.g., washing soda), and sodium metasilicate (e.g., dishwashing detergent). The frequently ingested household bleach (sodium hypochlorite) has a near-neutral pH of 6 and has little affect on the mucosa of the upper aerodigestive tract. It is an irritant but does not cause tissue necrosis. Household cleaners that contain ammonia also contribute to caustic ingestion injuries. Acid corrosives include hydrochloric, sulfuric, nitric and phosphoric acids, which are contained in automobile batteries. Esophageal burns have been reported after ingesting Clinitest tablets, which are commonly used for testing urine. These tablets contain copper sulfate, citric acid, sodium hydroxide, and sodium carbonate. Ingestion of alkaline batteries that are small and disc-shaped (i.e., button batteries) also has been reported. Many batteries contain alkaline electrolyte solutions with a pH greater than 12. After button batteries are ingested, an electrochemical current develops across the battery seal, corroding it and causing its contents to leak. A severe local corrosive effect ensues.

Factors that seem relevant in cases of caustic ingestion include parental psychopathology, marital dissatisfaction, and mental illness. Studies conclude that accidental poisoning, whether or not there is a strong suspicion of purposefulness, should always be treated as a family emergency or as evidence of a family disturbance (Case 30.1). Psychiatric evaluation is necessary not just for the well-being of the patient but also to give emotional support to the surrounding family.

Case 30.1 Child with Caustic Ingestion of Battery Acid

A boy 5 years of age is brought into the emergency department by his parents, whose arguing you can hear before you enter the room. The boy is sitting up in no airway distress, but he is drooling and has sores around his lips and anterior oral cavity. A history of caustic ingestion is obtained from the parents, although there is much disagreement as to what the substance was and how much of it was consumed. After much questioning, it seems that the child drank battery acid.

The boy is stabilized with intravenous fluids, his electrolytes are normal, and a full otolaryngologic assessment is performed. The boy does not permit you to make a complete examination of the oral cavity, so you decide to take him to the operating room where a laryngoscopy is performed under inhalational anesthesia. Sores are noted around the patient's lips, tongue, and oral cavity, but they do not appear to be deep. Fortunately, the oropharynx, larynx, and hypopharynx are entirely normal. Esophagoscopy is also normal. The patient is awakened and taken to the recovery room.

An immediate consultation with the pediatric and childcare services is obtained, and the child is admitted to the hospital overnight until the family situation can be evaluated and the child safely placed.

Discussion

This case demonstrates the ability of a child to obtain acids that are stored carelessly. Fortunately, because of the bitter taste, the boy sustained injury only to the oral cavity. Lack of supervision was thought to contribute to the child's ability to obtain the acid. Fortunately, he recovered completely.

Relevant Anatomy and Physiology

The taste and burning sensation of an ingested corrosive may cause a person to spit it out immediately, limiting injury to the oral cavity and oropharynx. Even in these cases, however, the buccal mucosa, tongue, floor of mouth, and hard palate may be injured. The voluntary oral phase of swallowing is completed as the bolus of ingested material passes the anterior faucial (tonsillar) arches. Thereafter, swallowing is involuntary.

The oropharynx is the anatomic segment bounded superiorly by the soft palate, anteriorly by the anterior faucial arches, and posteriorly by the pharyngeal wall. It also includes tongue base structures and the vallecula. The oropharynx is a ring-like sphincter that opens and closes involuntarily with the second and third phases of swallowing. Ingested corrosives may bathe any or all of these areas during transit into the hypopharynx and proximal esophagus. With a competent velopharynx (i.e., soft palate), the reflux of ingested material into the nasopharynx is not common; however, evaluating the nasal cavity and nasopharynx does ensure a complete assessment of the patient's airway.

The larynx and associated structures are enveloped in the horseshoe-shaped hypopharynx, which is defined laterally by the pyriform sinuses and posteriorly by the posterior pharyngeal wall and the postcricoid region. Laryngeal involvement is more common in severe injuries. Aspiration is rare and may indicate an unnatural (i.e., purposeful) method of aspiration. A patient with an intact swallowing mechanism usually protects the supraglottic structures, which are at significant risk during ingestion; their involvement may compromise a patient's airway significantly.

Ingested caustic agents pause at the following specific areas along the upper alimentary tract: the cricopharyngeus, thoracic inlet, left hilar area (including the aorta, left main stem bronchus, and left atrium), gastroesophageal junction, and pylorus. The effect of the ingested material on these areas is directly related to pH, specific gravity, and viscosity—factors that combine to determine the site and the severity of injury. The evaluation of each segment of the aerodigestive tract defines appropriate treatment protocols.

Alkalis are bases that dissolve in water and have a positive radical and a hydroxyl group. Alkali burns occur most commonly in the esophageal regions that normally impede transit (Case 30.2). The extent of mucous membrane corrosion depends on the corrosive's type and concentration and the amount of time it came in contact with the mucosa. Alkalis produce liquefaction necrosis in which superficial tissue layers become separated by resultant edema. Consequently, the corrosive agent diffuses into deeper tissues, and the necrosis progresses.

> **Case 30.2 Male Psychiatric Patient Who Ingested Lye**
>
> You are called to the emergency department to evaluate a 27-year-old male patient who has a history of imbibing lye. Upon arrival, you see the patient in distress, unable to hold down his own secretions. He is writhing around on the bed because of abdominal discomfort and complaining of chest pain. A history is obtained while appropriate resuscitative measures are being undertaken. The gentleman has a past history of suicide attempts and is noted to have recently broken up with his girlfriend. His mother had brought him into the hospital with an empty bottle of lye, which she had found next to him as he was retching in the sink. A General Surgery consultation is obtained, and it is felt that he requires his abdomen to be explored, as well as stabilization of his upper airway in the operating room. He is taken to the operating room where severe burns of the oral cavity and oropharynx are visualized. The supraglottis is swollen and edematous, and he is intubated with difficulty. A severe burn of the esophagus at the postcricoid region is seen. Meanwhile, the general surgeons have performed a laparoscopic procedure and note that the stomach is grossly inflamed, red and partially necrotic superiorly.
>
> It is felt that this gentleman has suffered a severe necrotizing injury of his esophagus and part of his stomach. These areas are resected, requiring a total esophagectomy, partial gastrectomy, and reconstruction with a colon interposition flap.
>
> After a stormy postoperative course, the gentleman eventually returns home with multiple problems.
>
> **Discussion**
>
> This case demonstrates the ability of common household substances to induce tremendous injury to the upper aerodigestive and gastroesophageal tract. While most injuries are not as severe as the one suffered by this gentleman, other organ systems, including the esophagus and stomach, must be considered when evaluating patients with a history of lye ingestion.

The amount of a corrosive alkali that can cause significant injury is surprisingly small. It is reported that as little as 1 cm^3 of a highly concentrated lye solution may produce esophageal lesions. **Seemingly inconsequential amounts do not imply inconsequential lesions** and should not be treated with less vigilance than cases in which a massive ingestion is suspected.

Acids contain hydrogen atoms and one or more nonmetal compounds, are generally soluble in water, and often cause immediate pain on contact with mucous membranes. Injury may be limited to the oral cavity and oropharynx as the patient spits out the agent. Acid ingestion causes coagulation necrosis, with a thick eschar forming on injured tissue that prevents deeper penetration. Affected cells remain intact initially, but their protein becomes denatured. The resultant coagulum helps limit deeper penetration into muscular tissues. The esophagus normally has a slightly alkaline pH, and its squamous epithelium is somewhat resistant to acid burns; hence, esophageal burns from acids are relatively rare. The area most susceptible to burns caused by acidic agents is the gastric antrum, probably because of the pooling of material in the stomach secondary to reflex pyloric spasm.

The depth of mucosal burns is clinically relevant and is classified as follows: **first-degree burns** have hyperemia with superficial mucosal desquamation; **second-degree burns** have blistering and shallow transmural ulcers; and **third-degree burns** are full-thickness injuries, extending outside of the esophagus. First-degree burns generally do not progress to stricture; second degree burns may produce stricture in 15% to 30% of patients; and up to 90% of patients with third-degree burns develop clinically significant stricture.

Stabilization and Resuscitation

Acute care begins with **airway stabilization**. The most common cause of severe respiratory distress in patients with caustic ingestion is supraglottic swelling. The airway must be monitored continually, because mild stridor can progress rapidly to complete respiratory obstruction. However, the immediate loss of an airway is rare, as is the need for tracheostomy. Airway stabilization is achieved most optimally by endotracheal intubation with direct visualization by the oral route. Nasotracheal intubation is contraindicated because of its associated high risk of tracheal, pharyngeal, and esophageal perforation. When direct visualization of the airway is not possible, cricothyrotomy may be used. Cardiovascular compromise (e.g., hypotension, tachycardia) should be treated initially with large-bore intravenous access and crystalloid resuscitation. Attendant eye and other injuries should be sought. Identifying the type and quantity of ingested material and the situation surrounding the ingestion episode is helpful in planning treatment. If the episode is considered purposeful, appropriate psychiatric services should be alerted. **Neutralization is not recommended** because this may cause further injury or delay definitive treatment. Tissue damage after ingestion occurs rapidly; attempts to dilute or neutralize the ingested substance cannot prevent the damage that has already occurred. Emetics are not given because **vomiting may cause a worsening of the caustic injury by exposing mucosa to the offending substance**. **Vomiting also can cause aspiration**, exposing a previously noninjured airway to the substance. Activated charcoal does not absorb alkalis, and its administration may hamper the physician's ability to determine the extent of injury endoscopically.

Contrast radiography should be performed using a water-soluble agent if a perforation is suspected. This study can provide baseline results to which future study results can be compared. Symptoms of caustic ingestions include dyspnea, dysphagia, and thoracoabdominal pain; however, severe injury may be present in the absence of these symptoms. On initial examination, signs that suggest caustic injury include mucosal ulceration with discoloration, hypersalivation, and, less commonly, perioral lesions (including skin bleeding with ulceration). Hamman's sign (a precordial "crunch" on auscultation) may be present as "crackles" and "rubs" that indicate distal airway injury. Peritoneal signs that indicate perforation include rebound tenderness and guarding. There is a poor correlation between the symptoms and signs and the severity of distal injury after a caustic ingestion. The location of injuries may be divided into three zones: oropharyngeal (zone I), hypopharyngeal (zone II), and distal esophageal (zone III). Zone III lesions are rarely found without coexisting zone I or II injuries, and most zone III injuries are severe. If vomiting, drooling, or stridor is present, serious esophageal injury is likely. **Oropharyngeal burns do not predict esophageal injury** (e.g., second- or third-degree burns). Laboratory evaluation is not helpful in predicting distal aerodigestive injury.

Initial Evaluation

Endoscopy is performed after initial stabilization. Because there is a risk of perforation through an injured esophagus or stomach, some clinicians suggest using a **pediatric flexible esophagoscope** for this evaluation. Others conclude that esophagoscopy should be stopped just distal to the first burned segment encountered. Recent literature, however, reveals a low complication rate for endoscopy after caustic ingestion. The information gained from esophagoscopy more than offsets the relatively low risk of complications.

A common **grading system** based on endoscopic findings can be used. Grade I injuries are first-degree burns with mucosal hyperemia and edema and superficial mucosa desquamation. Grade II injuries are second-degree burns, with shallow ulcers limited to the mucosa. The ulcers may demonstrate a linear pattern. A psueodmembranous or fibrinous exudate may be present. Grade III injuries are third-degree burns with deep ulcerative lesions and obvious scarring and eschar formation.

Flexible esophagoscopy can be performed safely with sedation anesthesia, thereby avoiding possible vomiting after the general anesthesia that is required for rigid endoscopy. Endoscopy is best performed within 36 hours of injury unless medical instability contraindicates its use. Patients who have ingested ammonia bleach or mild laundry detergents may be observed without endoscopy. If drooling and stridor are present, endoscopy is required.

Treatment and Follow-Up

All patients with suspected caustic ingestion should be **admitted to the hospital** for observation and nursing support. Patients with grade I lesions should be observed, given a **slowly advancing diet**, and discharged to a confirmed "safe" environment with competent supervision. The incidence of esophageal or gastric sequelae in this group of patients is low. **Follow-up contrast radiography at 4 to 6 weeks** after the initial injury is recommended. If the ingestion is deemed accidental, ask the social services department to evaluate the home situation, which helps the physician provide adequate instruction about packaging and handling of corrosive agents. If the ingestion was purposeful, the patient and his or her family should receive aggressive psychiatric support while still in the hospital.

If a grade II lesion with transmucosal extension is identified on endoscopy, bacteria can potentially migrate through the defect (this is also true for grade III burns). **Prophylactic antibiotic treatment** (ampicillin for 7–14 days; gentamicin can be added to help eliminate oropharyngeal organisms more optimally) should be instituted in these patients. Nutritional support can be provided intravenously or enterally via nasogastric tube. **Blind (i.e., unguided) placement of a nasogastric tube in the emergency department should be avoided because of possible viscus perforation.** A nasogastric tube, placed under endoscopic guidance at the time of initial esophagogastroscopy, also decompresses the stomach and allows for gentle gastric lavage.

Most clinicians agree that systemic corticosteroids are not needed after superficial or grade I injuries. After grade II and III injuries, steroid therapy must be initiated within 48 hours unless perforation or stomach necrosis is suspected. Blockage of fibrin deposition and migration of cellular inflammatory elements are not seen if steroids are administered more than 48 hours after injury. Because of nonuniform lesion grading and steroid-dosage regimens, a comparison between studies is difficult; however, the general consensus is that **a tapering dosage of intravenous methylprednisolone** (0.5–1.0 mg/kg/d for over 2 weeks) is beneficial. The patient's diet should be slowly advanced, starting with clear liquids, while providing close monitoring for impending complications. Prednisone (0.5–1.0 mg/kg/d for 2–3 weeks and tapered thereafter) also may be used. **Adjunctive pharmacologic therapy** includes proton-pump inhibitors to decrease the amount of acid secreted into an injured stomach and to decrease acid reflux into an injured distal esophagus. N-acetylcysteine and penicillamine limit stricture formation. Because esophageal dysmotility is common after caustic ingestion, promotility agents used in combination with agents that alter the resting tone of the lower esophageal sphincter may prove effective; however, this regimen has not been studied.

Initial therapy is aimed at preventing stricture formation in the esophagus and lower alimentary tract. One method for preserving the esophagus lumen is placing a nasogastric tube as a stent at the time of the initial esophagogastroscopy. Silastic stenting that extends from the esophageal stricture through the gastroesophageal junction also can be used. Generally, stenting for at least 3 weeks is advocated. Gastrostomy puts the esophagus at rest and provides access for enteral feeding. As mentioned previously, steroids are advocated for grade II and III injuries, but their aggressive use is contraindicated after severe caustic injuries if perforation or stomach necrosis is suspected clinically and/or radiologically. Immediate evaluation by a general surgeon is required if the physical examination suggests viscus rupture or peritonitis or if radiographs reveal free air under the diaphragm, a widened mediastinum, or a pneumomediastinum. **Immediate exploration** is required if radiography shows extravasation of contrast material from the stomach or esophagus. Exploration also is indicated for severe back retrosternal pain or metabolic acidosis. Such patients are explored through the right abdomen, which permits the examination of all intra-abdominal organs and allows a resection of full-thickness viscus injuries. A cervical incision is added, if it is required for esophageal resection. If the upper esophagus is uninjured, cervical esophagostomy may be performed.

There is controversy about the timing of **alimentary tract reconstruction** if emergent resection is indicated. Some clinicians advocate deferring continuity restoration until the patient has recovered from the acute injury. All patients with grade II or III injuries on endoscopy should undergo **emergent exploratory laparotomy**; those with full-thickness lesions should undergo **esophagogastrectomy**. Other patients are treated by a silicon stent that is left in the esophagus for 3 weeks. No protocol effectively prevents stricture formation in every patient. Other types of stents may include a swallowed string, nasogastric tube, or formal silicone esophageal or gastric stent. Complications of esophageal stenting include esophagomegaly and chronic motility disorders. Early in the 20th century, prophylactic dilatation via bougienage was performed routinely to treat caustic esophageal burns. This treatment worked well but was based on 11 patients who normally would have had a low rate of stricture formation, and there was no endoscopic confirmation of injury. Later, delaying dilatation until 6 to 8 weeks after the injury (i.e., after reepithelialization of the injured segment had occurred) minimized the risk of esophageal perforation.

Prograde or retrograde methods can be used. Generally, the prograde method is used initially with subsequent dilatations that are performed with mercury-filled dilatators (e.g., the Maloney type). The patient should be counseled that the need for dilatation may be lifelong and that the timing of subsequent dilatation is based on a subjective increase in swallowing difficulty. Patients with more severe strictures are treated with retrograde dilatation using **Tucker bougienage**: A gastrostomy is required first, after which the instrument, made of soft rubber, is introduced into the stomach, passed in a retrograde fashion through the esophagus, and then pulled out through the mouth. A swallowed suture maintains the lumen between dilatations. The next time, the dilatator is again drawn through the gastrostomy, up through the strictured segment of esophagus where it can be left in place for 15 to 30 minutes. **Balloon-catheter dilatation** also can be used and is helpful in the management of very young children. Patients who fail repeated dilatation are candidates for **segmental reconstructive procedures**; the ileum and colon have been used for bowel interposition. Reestablishing continuity requires resection followed by interposition grafting rather than solely a bypass procedure. The colon has been used for interposition grafting, with a mortality of 5% to 10%.

Laryngeal complications can occur with caustic ingestion. Laryngeal stenosis occurs after severe injury to the supraglottic structures, and patients may be examined with high-resolution computed tomography scan. The carbon-dioxide laser is used in these patients under microlaryngoscopic control to recannulate the stenotic portion of supraglottic larynx. Stenting usually requires the placement of an inverted Montgomery tracheal T-tube stent. Speech pathologists play a major role in the rehabilitation of these patients.

Long-term sequelae include hiatal hernia, esophageal contraction that elevates the stomach into the chest, and achalasia from periesophageal fibrosis. The most serious long-term complication is carcinoma in the injured esophagus, which may present 10 to 20 years later. Carcinoma occurs more frequently after caustic ingestion—at least 1000 times more often than in the general population. Most of these esophageal carcinomas develop at the level of the carina (all are in squamous cells), and 5-year survival rates are low (10%). After caustic ingestion, late symptoms of progressive dysphagia, hoarseness, chest or abdominal pain, or hematemesis suggest a malignancy. Evaluation includes contrast radiography with water-soluble agents and endoscopy. The inability to dilate a chronic stricture that previously responded well to dilatation also suggests malignant degeneration. Biopsy of these lesions may be difficult because a lesion distal to the initial stricture can be missed with an esophagoscope, especially when the instrument cannot be advanced beyond the stricture. **Carcinomas that develop in strictures seem to behave less aggressively than do esophageal cancers that arise de novo**. The scar that envelops a caustic stricture may serve as a barrier to tumor extension. A high index of suspicion is required for the early detection and successful management of these patients, even though biopsy-proven carcinoma may be difficult to demonstrate.

Danger Signs

Any child or adult with a history of psychiatric illness who presents to the emergency department with burns around the oral cavity and a history of possible caustic ingestion should be evaluated immediately to rule out caustic ingestion. Profuse drooling and airway distress indicate a severe injury. Patients who have swallowed alkaline substances tend to have a greater severity of injury. Patients with a history of caustic ingestion who present with increasing dysphagia many years after the original esophageal insult require immediate assessment to rule out an esophageal carcinoma.

Summary

Physicians at the turn of the 20th century recognized that the best treatment for caustic ingestion is prevention. Grass-roots educational efforts and legislative changes during the past century have resulted in a better awareness of the risks of caustic ingestion. Nonetheless, the number of injuries remains disappointingly high. As our society and health care system have taken an aggressive stance on other health care issues, physicians must counsel patients on the proper storage, use, and disposal of these common household agents. Despite major advances in medical care, patients who are victims of caustic ingestion will continue to challenge primary care givers and subspecialists alike.

SUGGESTED READINGS

Anderson KD, Rouse TM, Randolph JG. A controlled trial of corticosteroids in children with corrosive injury of the esophagus. *N Engl J Med.* 1990;323:637.

This article presents a prospective randomized study performed over 18 years of children with corrosive esophageal injuries. The authors conclude that steroid administration does not affect later development of esophageal stricture and that the severity of mucosal injury is the only accurate predictor.

Andreoni B, Marini A, Gavinelli M, et al. Emergency management of caustic ingestion in adults. *Surg Today.* 1995;25:119.

This article reports the aggressive diagnostic and therapeutic protocols in use at the University of Milan. With early surgery for severe injuries, the university's acute mortality and long-term morbidity rates are excellent, suggesting that aggressive therapy is preferable for deep mucosal injuries.

Christesen HB. Prediction of complications following caustic ingestion in adults. *Clin Otolaryngol.* 1995;20:272–8.

This article reviews the course of 86 adults after caustic ingestion. Complications occurred only after ingesting lye or after deliberately ingesting ammonia or hydrochloric acid. More severe complications developed after the most severe mucosal injuries, such as circumferential esophageal burns or burns exposing the submucosa. Esophagoscopy is strongly recommended (for aggressive treatment) to identify the transmural injuries.

Crain EF, Gershel JC, Mezey AP. Caustic ingestions: symptoms as predictors of injury. *Am J Dis Child.* 1984;138:863.

This classic article reviews a pediatric population, but the findings are relevant to adult patients as well. The authors found that if patients had two or more of the three serious physical findings (i.e., vomiting, stridor, and drooling), then they had a 50% chance of having a serious esophageal injury. Patients with none of the serious findings had virtually no risk of having a serious esophageal injury. Oropharyngeal burns were not predictive of esophageal burns.

Ferguson MK, Migliore M, Staszak VM, et al. Early evaluation and therapy for caustic esophageal injury. *Am J Surg.* 1989;157:116.

This review of 43 patients with caustic ingestion found that esophagoscopy accurately predicted the risk of developing an esophageal stricture. Steroids did not influence the risk of stricture development.

Moore, William R. Caustic ingestion: pathophysiology diagnosis and treatment. *Clin Pediatr.* 1996;25:192.

This excellent article provides an overview of the current concepts of pathophysiology. Based on the pathophysiology, the authors suggest a diagnostic protocol and develop treatment plans based on the results of initial diagnostic evaluations.

31

Head and Neck Cancer: An Overview

Lyon L. Gleich, MD
David E. Eibling, MD

Approximately 5% of all malignancies in the United States each year arise in the head and neck. Approximately 12,000 new laryngeal cancers are diagnosed each year, whereas more than 150,000 cancers of the breast, lung, and colon are diagnosed. Primary care physicians are therefore unlikely to encounter, and may not suspect, the existence of an early head and neck cancer. This chapter covers squamous cell cancer of the upper aerodigestive tract. (Cancers of the skin, sinus, and thyroid are covered elsewhere in this text, and intracranial neoplasms have been omitted.)

Epidemiology

More than 90% of patients with squamous cell cancer of the oral cavity, hypopharynx, and larynx have smoked tobacco for years, and many of these patients have consumed substantial amounts of alcohol as well. However, some patients who develop squamous cell carcinoma of the head and neck have never used tobacco or alcohol. The disease usually appears in middle age (rarely in the young), with a peak incidence at 60 years of age.

Detection and Screening

More than half of head and neck cancers are in an advanced stage when treatment is begun. Two thirds of these patients have had symptoms or signs of cancer for some time, and half of these (one third of the total) knew there was something wrong but delayed visiting a doctor or dentist. The other half sought care promptly but their diagnosis was missed until symptoms were pronounced when the diagnosis was obvious. Symptoms of early head and neck cancer can masquerade as benign conditions, and examination of the affected region can be difficult. Table 31.1 is a list of symptoms and signs that suggest head and neck cancer that, if persistent, are indications for detailed investigation.

Oral cavity cancers are noted easily during routine oral cavity examination, typically during dental care. Although many edentulous patients do not visit a dentist, a good many do see their primary care physicians for chronic illnesses. In patients who are at risk for head and neck cancer, a routine examination of the oral cavity can be a life-saving evaluation. Examination of the larynx and hypopharynx requires specialized skills and instruments and is sel-

Table 31.1 Danger Signs or Symptoms That Suggest Head and Neck Cancer*

Presence of mucosal ulcerations that do not resolve within 10 days
Red or white patchy lesions within the upper aerodigestive tract
Appearance of a skin lesion that is new; has changed in size or color; or is associated with bleeding, pain, or numbness
Presence of hoarseness or change in the quality of voice that does not resolve after 2 weeks of observation or antibiotic therapy
Difficult or painful swallowing after a 10-day course of antibiotic therapy or after 2 weeks of observation
Aspiration or coughing while eating solids or liquids
Ear pain without evidence of ear abnormalities
Trismus (difficulty opening the mouth)
Presence of a neck mass that does not resolve after 7–10 days of antibiotic therapy or observation
Difficult or noisy breathing
New onset of nasal obstruction
Unilateral nasal polyps
Epistaxis or bloody secretions from the oral cavity, oropharynx, or larynx
Evidence of cranial neuropathies
Presence of masses within the parotid, thyroid, or parathyroid glands
A chronic draining ear that is refractory to topical or systemic antibiotic therapy
Hypercalcemia
Orbital masses or change in extraocular muscle function
Proptosis (with the other ocular symptoms)

* Early diagnosis and treatment of premalignant and malignant lesions of the head and neck dramatically improve the likelihood of disease control and survival.
Republished with permission from the Committee on Head and Neck Surgery, The American Academy of Otolaryngology–Head and Neck Surgery.

dom performed in a primary care setting. The head mirror ($37) and laryngeal mirror ($8) enable competent examination of the patient who has a persistently sore throat, especially if there is referred ear pain.

History

The patient may complain of localized pain, hoarseness, dyspnea, stridor, and dysphagia (perhaps also with weight loss). When these symptoms occur in a patient who uses tobacco, inspection of the pharynx, hypopharynx, and larynx is mandated. A neck mass in an adult suggests malignant tumor in a lymph node and prompts careful examination of the mouth, pharynx, and larynx. Complaints of sore throat or a "lump in the throat" that persists after a course of antibiotic therapy deserves further investigation. Pain referred to in the ear is a common symptom of hypopharyngeal cancer, and hoarseness can signal vocal cord cancer.

Physical Examination

The oral cavity and oropharynx are examined by both direct inspection and palpation. It is critical that all mucosal surfaces are examined, particularly the floor of the mouth and the ventral surface of the tongue. Patches of leukoplakia (hyperkeratosis) (Fig. 31.1) may be seen easily and are considered by some to be precancerous. The palpating index finger is invaluable in determining the size of an indurated, ulcerated, painful lesion. A useful rule is: any lesion that is not recognized easily as benign is considered to be malignant until proven otherwise (by biopsy if necessary).

Palpation of the neck is an integral part of the head and neck examination and includes tactile examination of the parotid glands, submandibular glands, larynx, and thyroid gland. The floor of the mouth is best examined using both hands, with one finger in the mouth pressing the sublingual and submandibular glands downward with the fingers of the other hand on the skin of the submandibular triangle. Grasping the tongue with one hand, and feeling first the mobile part of the tongue and then the base of the tongue has revealed many early malignant neoplasms that masqueraded as "chronic tonsillitis" (Case 31.1). Gagging is unavoidable but is diminished by topical anesthetic spray, and the patient retains a lasting impression of the examiner's thoroughness.

Hoarseness that persists for more than 2 weeks deserves examination of the larynx, either with a laryngeal mirror and head mirror (or headlamp), or with a flexible fiberoptic nasopharyngoscope. (These techniques are discussed

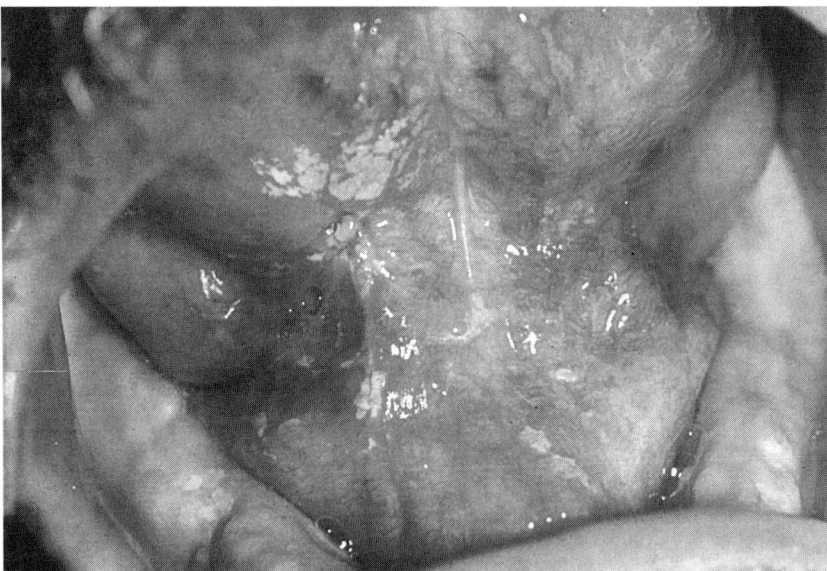

Figure 31.1 Leukoplakia of the ventral tongue. Leukoplakia is defined as a white lesion occurring on a mucosal surface. Although rarely representing cancer, it is a sign of abnormal mucosa and is often encountered in association with cancer (see Fig. 31.2).

in Chapter 1). Likewise, persistent dysphagia merits a thorough examination of the oropharynx, hypopharynx, and larynx. If the examination is normal yet difficulty swallowing persists, barium esophagography (of the entire esophagus) or cineradiographic esophagography can lead to the diagnosis or can give a basis for reassurance. Persistent symptoms with normal imaging generally deserve esophagoscopy by a gastroenterologist and, perhaps, esophageal manometric studies (*see* Chapter 15).

Otalgia without evidence of ear inflammation suggests pain referred from the tonsil, pyriform sinus, tongue base, or larynx. Examination of the nasopharynx (*see* Chapter 14) is important in cases of eustachian tube dysfunction, nasal obstruction, purulent drainage, and epistaxis (especially when accompanied by symptoms of cranial nerve I–VI dysfunction). Examination usually requires a rigid or flexible endoscope; however, using a nasopharyngeal or laryngeal mirror is entirely practical when the nose and throat are first sprayed with 4% lidocaine and when the soft palate is retracted. This is done with a soft, red, rubber catheter that is inserted into each nostril, brought out through the mouth, and then fastened with a pair of hemostats. Because adenoid tissue involutes during puberty, suspicious masses in the adult require biopsy.

> **Case 31.1** **Man with Tongue Cancer**
>
> An executive 55 years of age presents with a small ulcerative lesion on the lateral aspect of his tongue, which he had first noted approximately 3 weeks earlier (see Fig. 31.3). The lesion is only minimally tender, and he does not have a history of recurrent aphthous ulcerations. He has smoked approximately one pack per day for the past 40 years and uses alcohol socially. He has had no industrial exposures and sees his dentist regularly. His last examination was approximately 6 months ago.
>
> Digital examination reveals a 4 mm x 6 mm ulcerative lesion on the lateral margin of his tongue, with minimal surrounding induration. No other mucosal lesions are identified on examination of his oral cavity, oropharynx, larynx, and hypopharynx. Excisional biopsy of the ulcer reveals well-differentiated squamous cell carcinoma. Chest radiography and a barium esophagography are normal. The patient is determined to have stage I (T1,N0) cancer.
>
> One week later, the patient undergoes reexcision with 1-cm margins (similar to that noted in Fig. 31.5). An elective, unilateral, selective neck dissection is performed at the same time, removing nodes in zones I through III. No tracheostomy is required, and the excision site is closed primarily. Histologic examination of the resected specimens reveals no histologic evidence of residual tumor in the tongue specimen or in any of the 20 lymph nodes identified on the neck dissection specimen. The therapy is thought to have been curative, so adjuvant therapy is not recommended. The patient is reexamined monthly for 12 months and then followed at reduced intervals thereafter. His primary care physician initiates counseling and nicotine-replacement assistance for smoking cessation, and the patient has remained free of disease.
>
> **Discussion**
>
> This case demonstrates the value of early detection and treatment. This patient had minimal long-term sequelae of his tumor. Moreover, he undertook lifestyle changes (i.e., smoking cessation) to reduce his risk for the development of second primary tumors.

Radiographic Imaging

Radiographic imaging of the head and neck is commonly used for staging rather than for detecting head and neck cancer. Computed tomography (CT) is used most often and has real value in detecting metastases in the cervical nodes and in identifying masses within the sinonasal tract, nasopharynx, tongue, oropharynx, hypopharynx, and larynx. Unfortunately, CT is usually not helpful for detecting or evaluating early mucosal lesions. By the time a tumor is large enough to be apparent on CT, it has reached significant size and usually has associated symptoms. CT for evaluating vague head and neck symptoms should not be performed until after the mucosal surfaces have been examined.

Contrast imaging studies of the pharynx and esophagus are valuable for the detection of mucosal lesions below the esophageal inlet. Video fluoroscopic imaging permits frame-by-frame visualization and gives insight into function and anatomy (*see* Chapter 15). Magnetic resonance imaging (MRI) is useful for tumor mapping in the pharynx, sinuses, and neck. MRI is particularly valuable in defining intracranial extension and the invasion of nerves and bone marrow. However, for most purposes, CT is sufficient to suggest the diagnosis, whereas MRI is reserved for treatment planning.

Synchronous Second Primary Tumors

One out of every 20 patients diagnosed with head and neck cancer has a second undiagnosed primary cancer in the upper aerodigestive tract, esophagus, or lung. These so-called "synchronous primary cancers" often have a dramatic effect on prognosis and treatment planning; hence, the initial work-up of a patient with a head and neck malignancy routinely includes a search for these second primary tumors. We recommend chest radiography (posteroanterior and lateral views) and barium esophagography and/or esophagoscopy. Some centers use chest CT instead of plain radiography.

These patients need to be followed closely after treatment to detect recurrences and to discover metachronous primary tumors (i.e., second tumors that appear after and independently of the primary cancer) as early as possible. Certain chemopreventive agents may be effective in the prevention of metachronous head and neck cancers. There are no specific recommendations at present, but agents such as the retinoids have shown promise in investigational trials.

Biopsy and Staging

Biopsy and clinical staging of head and neck malignancies are accomplished before treatment. Staging has been standardized by the American Joint Council on Cancer and reflects tumor size, extension into surrounding structures, and impaired function. Each tumor is described with a combination of the symbols, T, N, and M. *T* indicates primary tumor characteristics, *N* indicates regional nodal status, and *M* indicates the presence of distant metastasis (Tables 31.2–31.5). Note that the presence of a single palpable cervical node immediately establishes the tumor as stage III, regardless of the extent of the primary tumor.

Table 31.2 Schema for T-Staging of Carcinoma of the Oral Cavity

T1	Tumor <2 cm in greatest dimension
T2	Tumor 2–4 cm in greatest dimension
T3	Tumor >4 cm in greatest dimension
T4	Tumor invading mandible, root of tongue, maxilla, or skin

Republished with permission from the American Joint Council on Cancer, 1988.

Table 31.3 Schema for T-Staging of Glottic Cancer

T1	Tumor involving one or both vocal cords
T2	Tumor existing above or below the level of the true vocal cords
T3	Tumor limited to the larynx, with vocal cord fixation
T4	Tumor invading the thyroid or cricoid cartilage or extending beyond larynx

Republished with permission from the American Joint Council on Cancer, 1988.

Table 31.4 Schema for N-Staging of Enlarged Regional Neck Nodes

N0	No palpable lymph node metastases
N1	Single ipsilateral node <3 cm
N2A	Single node 3–6 cm
N2B	Multiple nodes, all <6 cm
N2C	Bilateral or contralateral nodes <6 cm
N3	Metastases >6 cm

Republished with permission from the American Joint Council on Cancer, 1988.

Table 31.5 Relationship Between TNM Status and Tumor Stage*

	N0	N1	N2	N3	M+
T1	I	III	IV	IV	IV
T2	II	III	IV	IV	IV
T3	III	III	IV	IV	IV
T4	IV	IV	IV	IV	IV

* Notice that the presence of any palpable cervical node immediately establishes the tumor as stage III regardless of the extent of the primary tumor.
Republished with permission from the American Joint Council on Cancer, 1988.

Treatment

Treatment options for most squamous cell cancers of the head and neck are surgery, radiotherapy, or both, sometimes supplemented with (or preceded by) chemotherapy. Advanced tumors usually require combined therapy (surgery plus radiation), followed by chemotherapy. The range of therapeutic options reflects the variety of institutional experience with this disease, leading to ethical differences in therapeutic approaches. No one plan of treatment enjoys universal recommendation; however, there is justified optimism over the multi-institutional treatment protocols that are currently in use and under development.

Nasopharyngeal Cancer

Cancer of the nasopharynx is rare among whites but common in North American Inuit and in southeastern Chinese populations. The disease causes eustachian tube blockage and conductive hearing loss (from middle ear fluid accumulation). Later, nasal obstruction (often with blood-streaked nasal mucus) appears. Enlarged cervical lymph nodes are sometimes the first sign of the disease. Late in the disease, invasion of the foramina in the base of the skull leads to cranial nerve dysfunction (e.g., visual changes, facial pain).

Evaluating patients with suspected nasopharyngeal carcinoma includes directly examining the nasopharynx by flexible or rigid endoscopy or, in skilled hands, by nasopharyngeal mirror. Suspicious lesions deserve prompt biopsy. CT of the skull base and nasopharynx delineates the extent of tumor but cannot substitute for direct visualization. In patients who have metastatic cancer in a cervical node without evidence of a primary tumor (unknown primary), biopsy of the nasopharynx should be performed, even if nasopharyngeal examination is normal (*see* Chapter 20). An adult with recurrent or persistent unilateral middle ear effusion should be urged to undergo nasopharyngeal endoscopy and biopsy. Nasopharyngeal carcinoma may be the cause of the eustachian tube dysfunction.

The World Health Organization (WHO) has classified nasopharyngeal carcinoma, reflecting biological behavior and probable etiology. WHO type 3 (undifferentiated) nasopharyngeal carcinoma is most common, especially among Inuit and Chinese populations. In Hong Kong, this tumor type constitutes 18% of all malignancies and is associated with infection by the Epstein–Barr virus. The tumor metastasizes readily and is radiosensitive. Some Chinese treatment centers have adopted an alternative staging system for the disease because of its dramatic responsiveness to irradiation, which represents standard treatment. Concurrent chemotherapy seems to increase the cure rate. Epstein–Barr viral antibody levels can be used as a serologic tumor marker.

WHO types I and II (keratinizing and nonkeratinizing, respectively) are better differentiated and behave more like typical squamous cell cancer. Most of these tumors are treated by external-beam radiation. Surgical excision is offered in some centers, particularly for early lesions and in cases in which the tumor has recurred after radiation therapy.

Oral Cavity Cancer

Oral cavity cancer is the most common form of head and neck cancer. In the United States alone, approximately 30,000 new cases appear every year, and half of these patients present with advanced disease (Case 31.2). Most oral cavity cancers begin on the side of the tongue and the floor of the mouth, and in most instances arise in an area of preexisting mucosal change (Fig. 31.2). Leukoplakia ("white patches") rarely represents carcinoma, whereas erythroplakia ("red patches") is more likely to be invasive cancer.

Patients who have oral cavity cancer deserve careful palpation of the neck, searching for cervical lymph node metastases. Half of patients with early oral cavity cancers already have metastases in the regional lymph nodes that are often too small to be detected by the examiner. CT of the neck improves detection of metastases in cervical nodes, but still misses 10% to 15% of them. CT of the oral cavity cancer can identify extension to maxilla or mandible, and MRI shows depth and the extent of soft tissue invasion.

Treatment

Treatment of oral cavity cancer reflects tumor characteristics, institutional policies, and the patient's wishes. Surgical resection is the standard in most places, with radiation therapy as an acceptable alternative. Small tumors can be excised transorally, taking a margin of normal tissue around the tumor (Fig. 31.3). Microscopic examination (frozen section) of the resection margins is necessary to ensure complete removal.

Tumors adjacent to the mandible require resection of partial thickness of the mandible (marginal mandibulectomy). If the tumor invades bone, then a full-thickness piece of mandible must be removed (segmental mandibulectomy). Segmental resection of the mandible creates much more of a significant reconstructive challenge than does marginal mandibulectomy, in which the continuity of the mandible is preserved. The mandible may be divided to resect tumors in the back of the mouth. The mandible is then put back together using metallic plates or wires in a procedure called mandibulotomy, which is preceded by a lip-splitting incision and heals with an unobtrusive scar.

The incidence of cervical lymph node metastases is high in patients with oral cavity cancer, and selective neck dissection is standard therapy in most centers. An alternative for the clinically negative (N0) neck is radiation therapy.

Elective Neck Dissection

"Elective" neck dissection is performed in cases in which there are no palpable or enlarged cervical lymph nodes and when the likelihood of cervical lymph node metastasis exceeds 15% to 20%. This includes most head and neck cancers, with the exception of cancer of the sinuses and true vocal cords. Neck

Case 31.2 Man with Advanced Oral Cavity Cancer

A male Vietnam War veteran 46 years of age with posttraumatic stress disorder presents to the emergency room of a Veterans' Affairs hospital complaining of "sore mouth." The patient is not sure whether he had lost weight but notes that he has experienced increasing difficulty eating during the past several months. He is vaguely aware of an abnormality in his mouth but has not sought medical attention until now. His past medical history is significant for posttraumatic stress, including a service-connected disability. He has been followed infrequently at a Veterans' Affairs outpatient mental health center. He is unemployed, smokes approximately two packs of cigarettes per day, and is a heavy user of alcohol, admitting to drinking a six-pack of beer per day plus "a little whiskey."

Physical examination reveals a large tumor involving the floor of the mouth and the ventral tongue, with additional areas of abnormal mucosa in his oral cavity (similar to that pictured in Fig. 31.2). He has an enlarged ipsilateral submandibular mass and a palpable small jugulodigastric node. Many of his teeth are missing, and most of the remaining ones are carious. Chest radiography and barium esophagography are normal. Incisional biopsy at the margin of the tumor reveals invasive, poorly differentiated squamous cell cancer. CT of the neck with contrast reveals an enlarged ipsilateral submandibular gland with areas of necrosis (suggesting tumor infiltration), multiple ipsilateral cervical lymph nodes, and evidence of invasion of the mandibular bone along the anterior alveolus. No enlarged lymph nodes are identified on the contralateral neck. Medical consultation is obtained and reveals mild hepatic dysfunction and chronic obstructive pulmonary disease but no contraindications to surgical management. The patient is then presented to a multidisciplinary head and neck planning conference whose consensus is that combined therapy would provide him with the optimal chance of cure. The patient's family, who has not seen him for several years, is contacted and becomes involved in the planning process.

Primary tumor extirpation with mandibular reconstruction using vascularized bone with adjuvant postoperative radiation therapy is planned. Preoperative lower-extremity angiography is performed to document the status of the lower-extremity vessels to ensure that vascularized fibular bone could be used for reconstruction. Before surgical resection, the patient undergoes 1) direct laryngoscopy and esophagoscopy to rule out synchronous second primary tumors of the pharynx, larynx, and esophagus; 2) full-mouth dental extraction; and 3) a temporary tracheostomy. Then, in a 14-hour procedure, the patient undergoes excision of the tumor with segmental mandibular resection from the ipsilateral mandibular angle to the contralateral mental foramen. An ipsilateral modified neck dissection is attempted; however, because the tumor involvement near the spinal accessory nerve precludes its preservation, a radical neck dissection is performed. A contralateral selective neck dissection that removes nodes in levels I through III is performed.

After tumor extirpation, a separate surgical team performs reconstruction. Vascularized fibular bone is harvested as a free vascularized graft and is used for mandibular reconstruction. The donor vessels are anastomosed to the contralateral facial artery and internal jugular vein. The fibular bone is shaped by multiple osteotomies and is stabilized with a mandibular plate and screws.

Continued

> **Case 31.2 (continued)**   **Man with Advanced Oral Cavity Cancer**
>
> The patient has an uneventful initial postoperative course; however, on the second postoperative day, the patient becomes agitated and attempts to remove his nasogastric and tracheostomy tubes. Delirium tremens is diagnosed, and the patient is sedated initially with Midazolam, but he eventually requires propofol infusion and has to be placed back on the ventilator. During a period of 10 days, he is gradually weaned from sedation and from the ventilator and is able to begin ambulating with assistance shortly thereafter. His leg donor site heals well, but he remains in the intensive care unit for the next 14 days after his surgical procedure. During this time, he undergoes decannulation and begins attempting oral feedings. However, because he is unable to maintain adequate caloric intake because of persistent oral edema, he undergoes a percutaneous gastrostomy for prolonged feeding.
>
> Pathological examination of the surgical specimens reveals a tumor measuring 6 cm × 4 cm that involved the ventral surface of his tongue, floor of mouth, and mandible. There was tumor invasion into the bone of the mandibular alveolus, but it did not extend into the inferior alveolar canal. The submandibular mass is found to be squamous cell cancer. No nodal remnants are visualized, but the tumor had invaded the submandibular gland. Seven of the remaining 33 ipsilateral nodes reveal metastatic squamous cell carcinoma, with extracapsular extension of tumor in three of the nodes. Two involved nodes are identified in the contralateral neck, neither of which demonstrates extracapsular spread. Perineural invasion is seen on microscopic examination of the primary specimen. Despite the advanced nature of the disease, there is no histologic evidence of tumor involving the surgical margins.
>
> The patient is treated with planned adjuvant radiotherapy, which begins 3 weeks after surgery. He is enrolled in an investigational protocol using radiosensitizing doses of chemotherapeutic agents, which are administered weekly and concurrently with the radiotherapy. During this therapy, the patient develops severe mucositis that requires "break-in" treatment. He is able to begin swallowing adequately after finishing treatment, and the percutaneous endoscopic gastrostomy is removed. After completion of therapy, the patient is followed sporadically. He continues to use both tobacco and alcohol to excess.
>
> Three years after successful treatment of his lower mouth cancer, the patient presents again with increasing sore throat, otalgia, and weight loss. Physical examination reveals an ulcerated lesion of the pyriform sinus involving the larynx and displacing the true vocal cords toward the midline. Endoscopy and biopsies reveal moderately well-differentiated squamous cell cancer. Because the patient has previously received full-course radiotherapy as adjuvant therapy for his floor-of-mouth cancer, he is not a candidate for a laryngeal-preservation protocol. Therefore, he undergoes total laryngectomy and a complete neck dissection on his unoperated neck.

Case 31.2 (continued)   Man with Advanced Oral Cavity Cancer

Once again, he has a stormy postoperative course that is complicated not only by delirium tremens but also by significant edema of his head secondary to the sacrifice of his remaining dominant internal jugular vein. In addition, he develops a syndrome of inappropriate antidiuretic hormone (SIAH), with serum sodium levels dropping to 122 mg per 100 m^3 and urine osmolalities of greater than 600 mOsm. He is treated successfully with water restriction, and the condition resolves within 5 days. Thereafter the patient has a relatively uneventful course and is discharged after 3 weeks of hospitalization.

Discussion

Head and neck cancer is often part of a "lifestyle disease." This case illustrates the difficulties in managing a heavy alcohol and tobacco user who, despite relatively young age, presents with significant disease that requires heroic efforts to resect and rehabilitate. Unfortunately, for some of these patients, lifestyle changes are often extremely difficult because of contributing mental health problems (as in this case of a man with posttraumatic stress disorder that was incurred after his service in the Vietnam war). Therefore, they may be lost to follow-up, which precludes early identification of second primary tumors. It seems likely that this man remains at-risk for either recurrence of his hypopharyngeal tumor or for the development of additional primary cancers in his upper aerodigestive tract, esophagus, or lung.

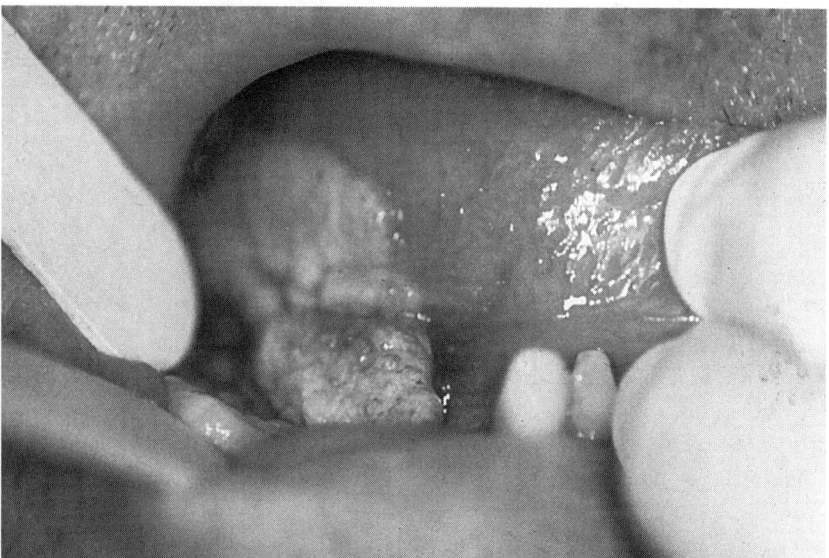

Figure 31.2 Tumor of the floor of the mouth arising in an area of leukoplakia. Here the tumor involves the right side of the tongue in a patient with heavy alcohol and tobacco use.

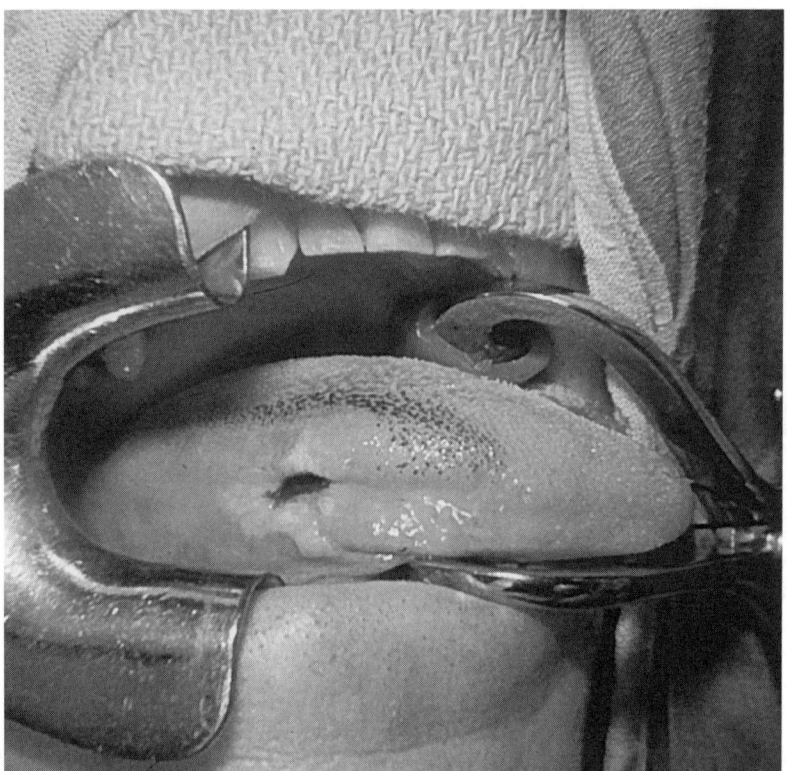

Figure 31.3 Small tumor of lateral tongue with surgical excision marked. Note the extent of normal tissue to be resected to assure an adequate margin.

dissection also facilitates biological staging of the tumor, often suggesting that additional therapy is required to optimize outcome. Traditional radical neck dissection has been the standard since it was described by Dr. Crile in 1906. In the past 25 years, however, modifications of this operation have been adopted. Neck dissections are now classified as radical, modified, or selective.

The radical neck dissection removes all of the lymphatics in the neck (sometimes called *comprehensive neck dissection*) except for the retropharyngeal nodes, the peritracheal nodes, and those that are deep to the trapezius muscle. The sternocleidomastoid muscle, internal jugular vein, and spinal accessory nerve are included in the en bloc resection. Shoulder stability is lost from partial denervation of the trapezius muscle (Fig. 31.4), leaving the patient with cosmetic and functional disabilities and discomfort. Physical therapy minimizes but does not eliminate these sequelae.

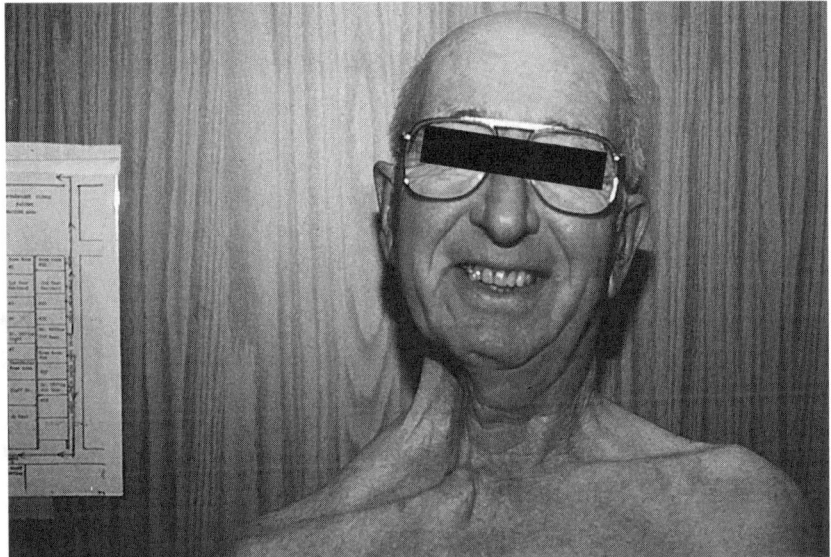

Figure 31.4 A patient who has undergone right radical neck dissection with sacrifice of the eleventh nerve. Note the drooping right shoulder and the obvious neck deformity.

The modified neck dissection removes all of the lymph nodes but preserves the spinal accessory nerve, internal jugular vein, and sternocleidomastoid muscle, avoiding shoulder disability and neck deformity.

Selective neck dissection removes only those lymph nodes that are at significant risk for metastasis from the primary lesion. The location of the primary tumor determines which nodes are resected. This procedure preserves as much of the neck anatomy as is consistent with good surgical principles, typically sparing the spinal accessory nerve, sternocleidomastoid muscle, internal jugular vein, and submandibular salivary gland. Oral cavity cancer characteristically spreads to submandibular nodes and the nodes along the internal jugular chain; hence, these are the only nodes that are typically removed.

Oral Cavity Reconstruction

Tumor site and extent and the patient's medical condition determine reconstructive options. Soft tissue reconstruction consists of epithelial resurfacing, adding bulk, or both. Small tumors of the lateral margin of the tongue can be resected with almost no loss of function (Figs. 31.3 and 31.5). Resecting tumors on the floor of the mouth limits tongue movement unless the operative site is covered with new epithelium immediately (Fig. 31.6). This can be done with a local mucosal flap, a split-thickness skin graft, a pedicled muscle flap

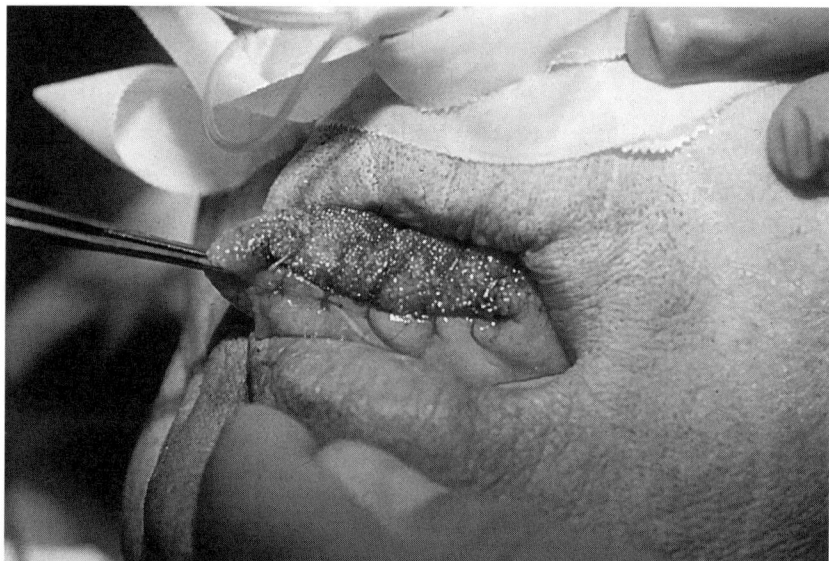

Figure 31.5 Primary closure of tongue after resection of tumor (similar to that pictured in Fig. 31.3). This type of closure will lead to very little impairment of tongue function, with expected normal speech and swallowing.

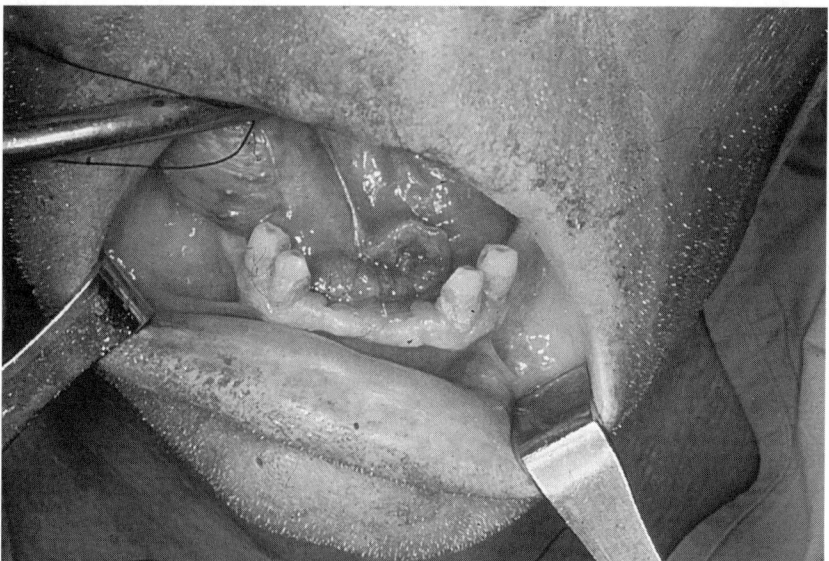

Figure 31.6 Ulcerated cancer of the floor of the mouth. Although this tumor can be easily resected surgically, a portion of the mandible must be removed to ensure an adequate resection. Replacing epithelial coverage is necessary to prevent tethering of the tongue with resultant severe disability of the oral cavity (see Fig. 31.7).

from the platysma, or a free microvascular flap (e.g., radial forearm flap). When bulk is needed, the pedicled pectoralis myocutaneous flap is the usual choice. Free vascularized flaps also can add bulk to the reconstruction. In most cases, epithelial reconstruction is sufficient and maximizes the mobility of the remaining structures (Fig. 31.7).

Reconstruction of the mandible is more difficult, especially when the anterior portion of the mandible has been removed. Without reconstruction, the defect causes an unsightly deformity and can rob the patient of intelligible speech (Fig. 31.8). Mandibular reconstruction is now used in nearly every head and neck cancer center. Reconstruction of lateral mandibular defects is also routine, although not as critical for function. Older techniques have been replaced by free flaps that contain vascularized bone in almost every center. The most popular donor site is the free vascularized fibula bone. Before harvesting this bone, patients undergo angiography of the lower extremities to make sure the vessels are healthy. Reconstruction by this technique is effective both cosmetically and functionally.

Swallowing Rehabilitation

Swallowing dysfunction is common after the resection of tumors of the oral cavity or pharynx. Prosthetic rehabilitation is effective for defects in the hard

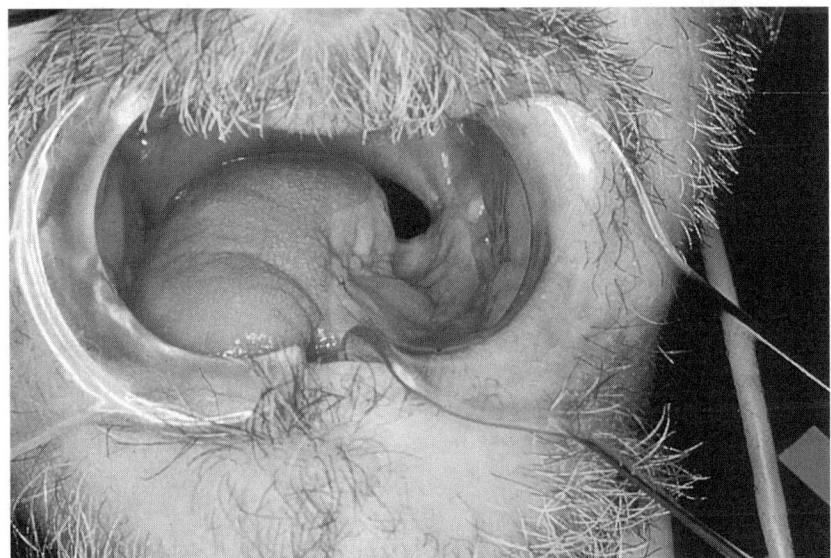

Figure 31.7 Split-thickness skin graft replacing the left side of the tongue and floor of the mouth. Replacing epithelial coverage after resection maximizes tongue mobility and reduces morbidity. Nevertheless, the extent of resection in this case resulted in permanent alteration in speech and swallowing function.

and soft palate (Fig. 31.9). Prostheses isolate the oral cavity from the nasal cavity, preventing "cleft palate" speech and nasal reflux during swallowing. The fashioning of prosthetic devices requires the services of a trained maxillofacial prosthodontist because it takes time to design, build, fit, and revise these prostheses and it costs money. Nevertheless, this is a critical step in rehabilitation and should be considered an essential part of the treatment plan. As of

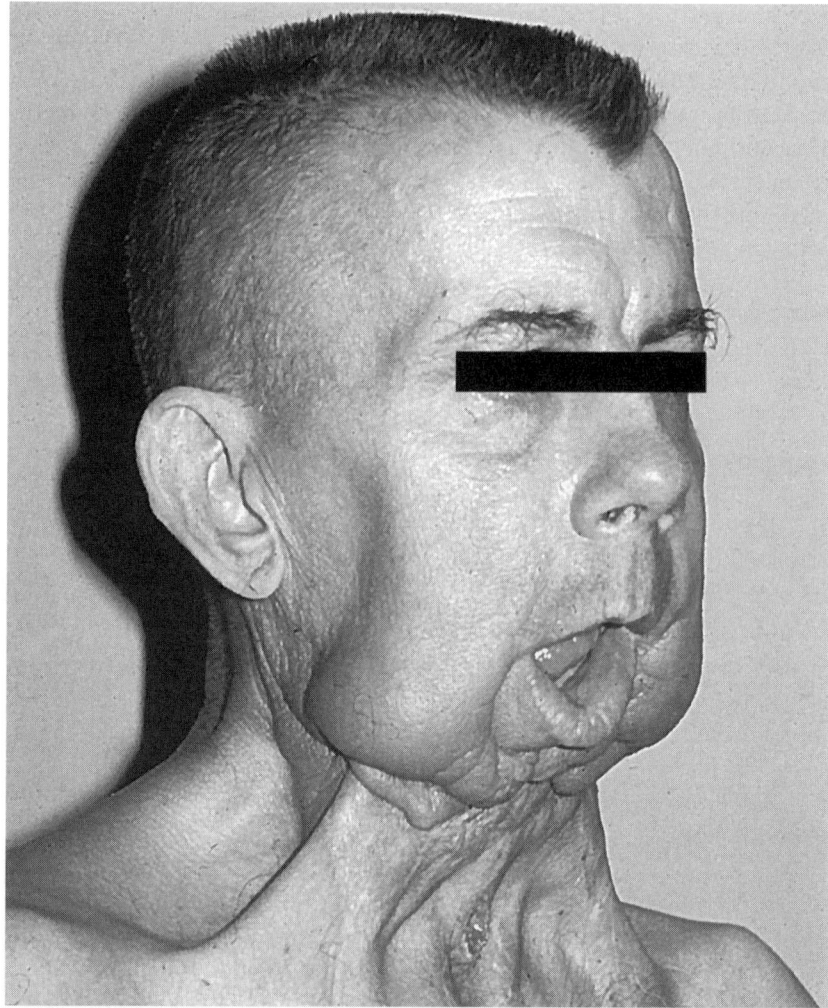

Figure 31.8 This patient underwent segmental resection of the anterior mandibular arch for advanced cancer with failure of reconstruction. The resultant defect created a severe functional and cosmetic deformity, often termed an "Andy Gump deformity." The patient later underwent repeat reconstruction with an alternate technique and was successfully rehabilitated.

Head and Neck Cancer: An Overview   621

2001, third-party payers have tended to disallow payments for prosthetic rehabilitation, and advocacy by the primary care physician is often necessary to educate the insurance carrier to its responsibility in cases of oral and oropharyngeal cancer.

Speech Therapy
Removing large cancers of the oral cavity can decrease tongue mobility, impairing swallowing and speech. The anterior tongue prepares the food bolus for swallowing, and the tongue base propels the food bolus toward the esophageal inlet and away from the upper airway. Aspiration of saliva and food can lead to recurrent episodes of pneumonia (*see* Chapter 19). This is a particular problem when tongue bulk or mobility has been reduced surgically. Myocutaneous flaps or vascularized free flaps used for surgical reconstruction lack normal sensation and mobility and place patients at risk for aspiration pneumonia. A temporary tracheostomy is essential for protecting the airway and pulmonary function. When healing has progressed so that the patient can begin to swallow again, the tracheostomy tube can be removed, and the patient should be instructed in swallowing techniques.

The services of a speech pathologist who is specially trained in swallowing rehabilitation are vital at this point. The speech therapist teaches the patient to form a food bolus with his remaining tongue and how to position the head to open the throat as much as possible during the pharyngeal phase of swallowing. The patient learns to expel any swallowed food remaining near the laryngeal inlet by coughing immediately after swallowing and before taking a breath. Because surgical treatment of oral cavity cancer affects speech as well,

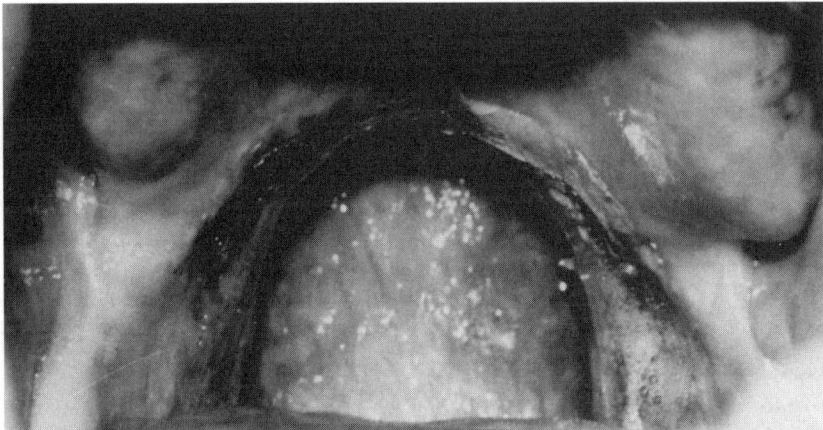

Figure 31.9 Palatal defect after resection of a soft palate cancer. A prosthesis is used after healing to enhance speech and swallowing.

the speech therapist can teach the patient to enunciate clearly by speaking slowly and by strengthening and mobilizing the remaining tongue muscle.

Radiation Therapy

Radiation therapy is also used as the primary treatment for oral cavity cancer, but treatment with this modality is not as benign as one might expect. Permanent loss of salivary function increases the risk of periodontitis, dental caries, and, in the worst case, osteoradionecrosis of the mandible. Once completed, radiation therapy is no longer an option for treatment of new tumors in the same region. The selection of therapy for an individual patient depends on specific tumor characteristics, institutional experience, and the patient's wishes.

Treatment is by external-beam to a dose of 6500 to 7000 cGy administered daily during a period of 5 or 6 weeks. Interruptions of treatment diminish its effectiveness, so these must be kept to a minimum (even if severe sore throat and mucositis occur). Supporting the patient with supplemental tube feedings and pain medication is preferable to discontinuing therapy for more than a day or two.

Implanted radiation sources (brachytherapy) are sometimes used as part of the treatment, particularly for large tumors or tumors of the tongue base. Brachytherapy requires hospitalization while the implants are in place, and a temporary tracheostomy is sometimes needed (Fig. 31.10).

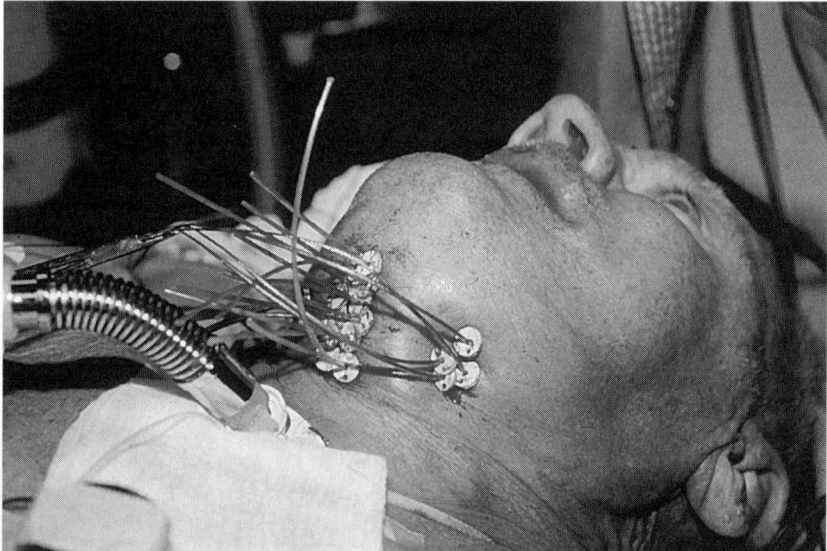

Figure 31.10 One technique used for administration of radiation to large tumors is brachytherapy. Catheters are placed through the tumor and then "after loaded" with high-dose radiation seeds. The seeds are left in place for 2 to 4 days, during which time patients must be isolated in a designated room because they represent a radiation hazard.

Adjuvant (assistive) radiotherapy is given after surgery for advanced-stage and biologically aggressive malignancies of the oral cavity. To be effective, it must begin within 6 weeks after surgery.

Acute radiation side effects include painful inflammation of the mucosa, severe dryness of the mouth, and burning of the throat. Radiation side effects also include the worsening of any dental or gum disease, so complete dental prophylaxis (and sometimes a full-mouth dental extraction) is required before beginning therapy. Radiation of an oral cavity in which bone is exposed because of a nonhealing surgical wound or from a recent dental extraction leads to osteoradionecrosis and chronic osteomyelitis. All dental extractions should be performed several weeks before starting radiation therapy. Regular dental prophylaxis and daily fluoride treatments will be needed for the rest of the patient's life to prevent radiation-induced caries. Oral pilocarpine 5 mg tid is often administered to augment salivary flow and to reduce the xerostomia due to radiation. Starting the prophylaxis regimen during radiotherapy reduces some of the annoying effects of radiation.

The swallowing difficulty that follows surgical excision typically worsens during radiation therapy. If swallowing difficulty is so severe that weight loss or aspiration pneumonia develops, a nasogastric tube or percutaneous feeding gastrostomy is indicated. Speech and swallowing therapy should be continued even during radiotherapy and until the patient recovers swallowing function. Occasionally, radiation therapy causes supraglottic swelling with partial obstruction of the patient's airway, necessitating tracheostomy. In most instances, this edema resolves in time, and the tracheostomy can be closed.

Although still investigational, adjuvant chemotherapy is sometimes used for head and neck cancer. There is some interest in induction chemotherapy as part of organ-sparing strategies, to be discussed later in this chapter.

Follow-Up

During the first two years after treatment of a primary tumor, the patient is at highest risk for recurrence; therefore, follow-up visits are scheduled every 1 to 3 months during this period. All patients remain at risk for second primary malignancies for the remainder of their lives. The risk of second primary tumor is 3% per year (higher if the patient continues to use tobacco and alcohol). Recent studies suggest that chemoprevention may be effective in this population.

Cancer of the Larynx

Cancer of the larynx occurs half as frequently as does oral cavity cancer, with 12,000 cases occurring in the United States each year. The cure rate is high, but some survivors eventually die of lung cancer. Cancer of the larynx occurs in two major types: cancer of the glottis (true vocal cords) and cancer of the supraglottis (epiglottis, false vocal cords, and aryepiglottic folds).

Glottic Cancer

Glottic cancer causes hoarseness and is usually diagnosed early. Staging is based on tumor extent and vocal cord mobility (*see* Table 31.3). Small (T1) glottic cancers are confined to the surface of the true vocal cords, which move normally (Fig. 31.11). Patients become aware of the problem when the tumor is only a few millimeters in size. At this stage, treatment is straightforward, and the cure rate is high. In fact, essentially all early glottic cancers can be cured if treated and followed appropriately, with preservation of the larynx in more than 90% of patients. However, early laryngoscopy for patients with hoarseness is critical to achieve these results (*see* Chapter 17). Tumor staging is based on tumor extent and vocal cord mobility. Cervical metastases are rare in glottic cancer, and CT of the neck is not required.

Large glottic cancers cause vocal cord fixation and may invade the thyroid and cricoid cartilages. Advanced tumors extend into the strap muscles and thyroid gland and are accompanied by airway distress and respiratory stridor. Occasionally, a patient with known lung disease has his unsuspected laryngeal

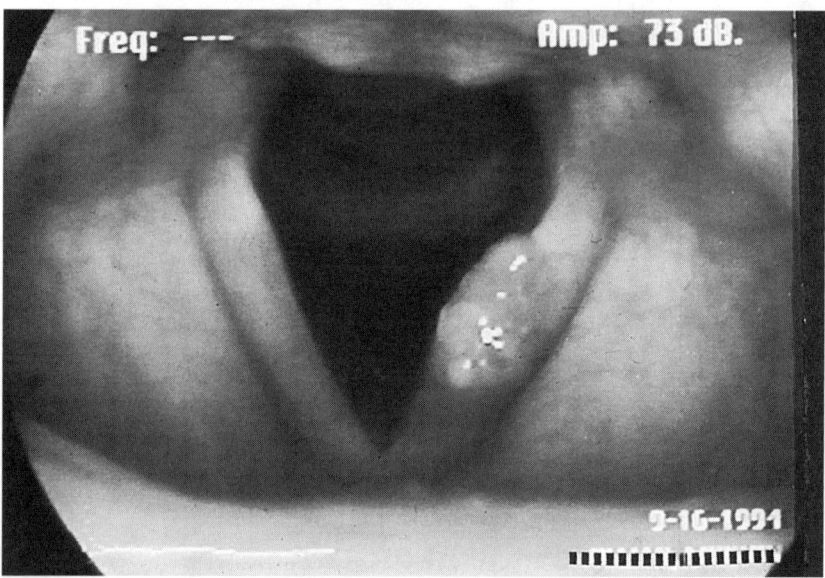

Figure 31.11 Small cancer arising on the left true vocal cord. This patient presented with hoarseness, and prompt evaluation identified tumor in early stage, permitting highly effective therapy with nearly no morbidity (see Case 31.3).

cancer misdiagnosed as asthma. CT is often required to assess the extent of the primary tumor and cervical lymph node metastases.

Treatment

Small glottic cancers (*see* Fig. 31.11) can be treated equally successfully by either surgery or radiation therapy (Case 31.3). Radiation therapy is popular in many centers, and external-beam treatment of 6500 to 7000 cGy cures 90% of T1 tumors. If a tumor persists or recurs, surgery is effective; however, the patient may require total laryngectomy if recurrence is not identified promptly. Very small glottic cancers can be treated by endoscopic excision (cordectomy), sometimes using a laser. Excision and histologic examination ensures complete excision and is preferred in many centers.

Surgical treatment of larger glottic tumors requires the removal of more of the vocal cord and typically is performed via hemilaryngectomy (an open surgical procedure). This and similar newer procedures remove one or even both vocal

---

Case 31.3   Man with Early Glottic Cancer

An automobile salesman 56 years of age develops hoarseness, which he attributes to postnasal drip. His primary care physician initially treats him with a combination of mucolytic and decongestant. When his symptoms persist, and he notices symptoms of gastroesophageal reflux, the patient is placed on a proton-pump inhibitor. Although he has significant improvement in his reflux symptoms, his hoarseness does not resolve and he is referred for laryngoscopy. Office laryngoscopy reveals a small lesion of his left true vocal cord (similar to that pictured in Fig. 31.11). Operative microlaryngoscopy and biopsy reveal squamous cell cancer.

The patient is very concerned about the quality of his voice and its association with his job and therefore refuses endoscopic laser cordectomy. He instead undergoes external-beam radiotherapy 5 days per week for 6 weeks (a total dose of 7000 cGy). He has only minimal sore throat and no significant difficulties with therapy. Empirical treatment with proton-pump inhibitors is continued throughout treatment. Follow-up after treatment reveals no evidence of recurrent tumor and he has successfully stopped using tobacco.

Discussion

This case demonstrates the confusion that often accompanies the development of glottic cancer. This patient's diagnosis changed during several weeks from postnasal drip to gastroesophageal reflux to squamous cell cancer of the larynx. Despite suspected benign diagnoses, voice abnormalities require a laryngeal examination if they do not resolve completely within 2 weeks. Early diagnosis facilitates a high probability of cure with any of a number of options. Treatment choices are made based on multiple factors; in this case, the patient's concern about potential hoarseness resulted in his refusal of offered laser excision.

cords. The voice is serviceable and often no more hoarse than when the tumor was present. In most instances, a permanent tracheostomy can be avoided.

Larger cancers require total laryngectomy, which removes the entire larynx and completely separates the air and food passages. The upper end of the trachea is sewn to the skin, producing a permanent tracheostoma (Fig. 31.12; *see also* Fig. 29.4B). Caring for the tracheostoma requires humidification and the removal of any crusts that may form. Tracheitis is a potential complication that occasionally requires hospitalization. Laryngectomy patients can take shower baths if they protect the stoma but cannot safely swim; however, some patients can wade or use a snorkel device in shallow water. Should it become necessary to do endotracheal intubation on a laryngectomy patient, the tube is inserted directly into the tracheostoma, not into the mouth or nose. Hence, in a respiratory emergency, it is a good idea to examine the patient's chest and neck for a tracheostoma. Many laryngectomy patients wear a Med-Alert bracelet that identifies them as a "neck breather."

Speech Rehabilitation After Laryngectomy

Despite the loss of the true vocal cords, it is possible to speak after having had a total laryngectomy. A voice can be produced by any of three different strategies: esophageal speech, electrically powered vibratory devices, and via a tracheopharyngeal fistula. Each of these techniques has specific advantages and disadvantages.

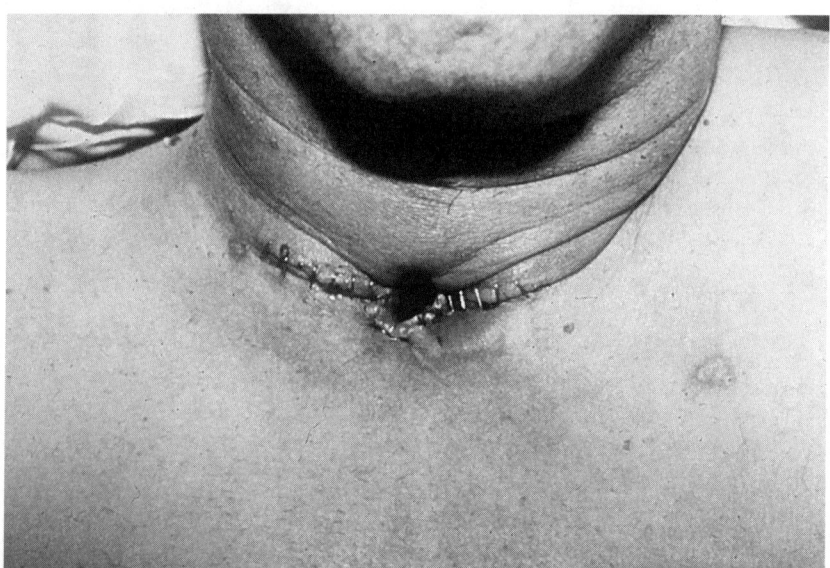

Figure 31.12 Laryngectomy stoma. Because there is no connection between the trachea and the pharynx, all air exchange must occur through this stoma (see Fig. 29.4B).

Esophageal speech arises from pharyngeal wall vibrations caused by regurgitation of previously inhaled air. The voice is deep, and sentences are short because of the limited quantity of air that can be stored in the esophagus. The technique requires no prosthesis but does require considerable practice. Only 25% of laryngectomy patients attain effective speech with this method.

Electrically powered prosthetic devices transmit vibrations through the skin of the neck or face or via a short tube placed in the open mouth. The voice is toneless and mechanical, but speech is easily learned.

A tracheo-esophageal puncture is a fistula created in the common wall shared by the posterior part of the trachea and the anterior part of the esophagus. The patient occludes the tracheostoma with his or her finger and then breathes out, diverting air through the fistula into the esophagus. This flow of air induces vibrations in the pharyngeal walls, enabling the patient to phonate. A small plastic valve called a tracheoesophageal prosthesis occludes the fistula and prevents aspiration of food and liquid during swallowing (Fig. 31.13). The fistula closes quickly if the prosthesis is dislodged, so replacing a lost prostheses within a few hours is necessary to prevent a return trip to the operating room for repuncture. In an emergency, the fistula can be stented with a 14 French catheter until the prosthesis can be replaced.

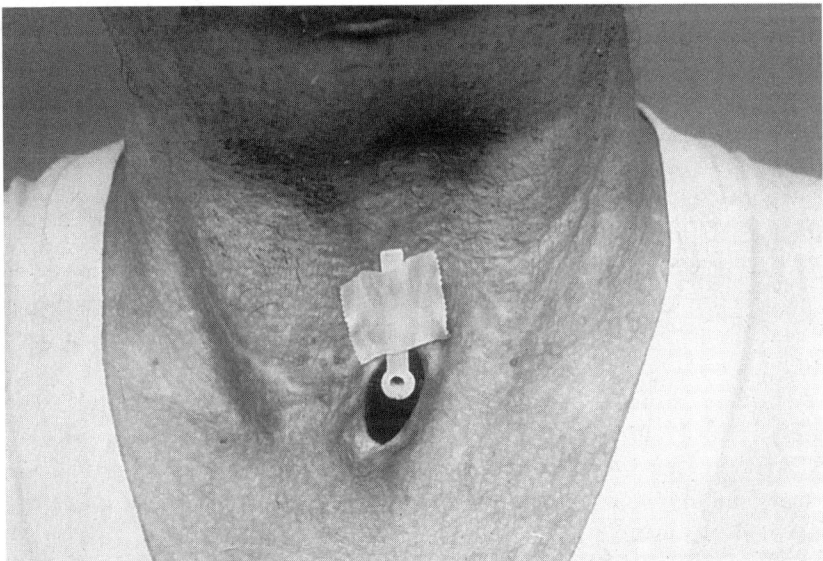

Figure 31.13 Tracheoesophageal speech prosthesis placed through the posterior tracheal wall. This prosthesis occludes the fistula during swallowing to prevent aspiration and is opened by air pressure generated by the occlusion of the stoma during exhalation. Vocalization is created by vibrations of the pharyngeal walls, not the prosthesis.

All of these speech rehabilitation techniques require that the patient be able to articulate to form useful speech from the vibrating air column. Other communication devices that are available for use by patients who have lost part or all of the tongue (or who have other defects that impair speech articulation) include signboards, magic slates, or simply pencil and paper; these are reliable and convenient for literate patients. However, now there are portable computerized speech synthesizers and software to adapt standard laptop computers for speech synthesis. These devices permit ordinary typing of messages, and they contain macros for uttering common phrases simply by striking one or two keys. They enable voice telephone communication and are indispensable for patients living alone. They cost approximately $3000 (for the dedicated synthesizer or laptop computer and the software). Unfortunately, health care organizations often require substantial documentation and physician advocacy (education) before agreeing to pay for these products. Furthermore, these techniques and devices require instruction provided by a specially trained speech pathologist, and health care organizations must be educated in the need to complete the treatment by ensuring maximal rehabilitation.

Supraglottic Cancer

Cancer of the larynx above the true vocal cords is called supraglottic cancer. These cancers constitute approximately one half of all laryngeal cancers, and their symptoms and biological behavior are different from glottic cancer. The supraglottic structures do not vibrate during phonation, and supraglottic cancer does not cause hoarseness. Symptoms of supraglottic cancer are ill defined, consisting of sore throat, irritation of the throat, varying degrees of dysphagia, and referred ear pain. Early diagnosis is unusual in supraglottic carcinoma, because general practitioners do not examine this area routinely. By the time the patient's symptoms have reached the point of serious concern, the tumor is usually very large. The supraglottis has a generous lymphatic drainage system, and metastasis to cervical lymph nodes occur early and bilaterally.

Airway obstruction can be the first symptom of supraglottic cancer because these tumors can grow to considerable size before they are diagnosed (Fig. 31.14). Hoarseness occurs only when the tumor spreads downward and involves the true vocal cords. It is common for patients to present to the otolaryngologist with a palpable cervical node metastasis and have it go undetected until laryngoscopy is performed. The evaluation of supraglottic cancer includes mapping the extent of the tumor and measuring pulmonary function. CT is useful for estimating the extent of the primary tumor and for identifying cervical lymph nodes metastases.

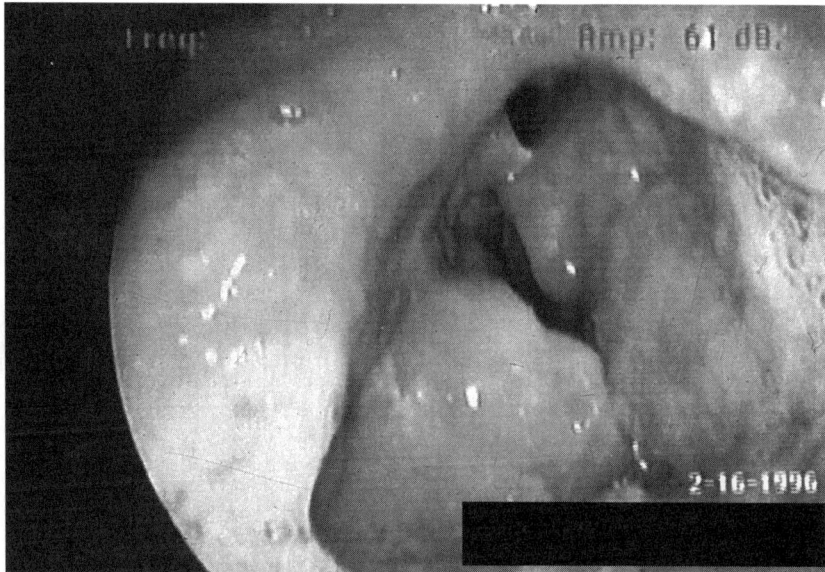

Figure 31.14 Large obstructing supraglottic cancer arising from the epiglottis and both false vocal cords (see Case 31.4). This patient presented with a sore throat and dysphagia. Despite the large size of this tumor, the voice was nearly normal because the tumor was situated superior to the true vocal cords and there was surprisingly little airway obstruction. Surgical management with supraglottic laryngectomy, preserving the vocal cords, is feasible; however, tumors of the supraglottis require that the neck nodes be addressed.

Treatment of supraglottic cancer uses radiation therapy, surgery, or both. Radiation cure rates are not as good as in glottic carcinoma because supraglottic tumors are more advanced at diagnosis. Furthermore, radiation therapy of the cervical lymph nodes affects a much larger tissue volume than in the treatment of glottic cancer; hence, the therapy's morbidity rate is greater.

Surgical treatment consists of either partial or total laryngectomy combined with bilateral dissection of the cervical lymph nodes because occult (i.e., not clinically detectable) metastatic cancer is frequently present in the cervical nodes. Total laryngectomy is effective but unnecessary in many cases. In these patients, a modification of the operation (called supraglottic laryngectomy) allows preservation of the true vocal cords but can, however, impair swallowing function and predispose the patient to aspiration pneumonitis. Therefore, the patient's pulmonary function must be documented before selecting this operation.

Supraglottic laryngectomy is the usual operation for small or medium-sized supraglottic cancers (Case 31.4). Tumors that begin on the supraglottis tend to remain above the level of the true vocal cords for a time and can grow very large while still amenable to resection without removing the vocal cords.

Case 31.4 — Man with Supraglottic Cancer

A man 51 years of age with a history of tobacco and alcohol use complains of unilateral sore throat, "throat mucus," and ear pain. He is not hoarse and does not have complaints of dysphagia. His primary care physician notes that his ear examination is normal and refers him for laryngoscopy. Office laryngoscopy reveals an ulcerative lesion involving the left false vocal cord and epiglottis, with extension onto the aryepiglottic fold (similar to but smaller than the tumor pictured in Fig. 31.14). Both vocal cords appear normal in both configuration and mobility. Palpation of the neck reveals a 2-cm, freely mobile lymph node in the jugulodigastric region. There are no other oral mucosal lesions. Chest radiography and barium swallow are normal. Direct laryngoscopy and biopsy confirm the office findings and reveal no evidence of other lesions. Biopsy of the tumor reveals moderately differentiated squamous cell cancer. CT reveals only a single ipsilateral node in the jugulodigastric region with a necrotic center that suggests metastatic cancer. The patient is determined to have stage III (T2,N1) cancer.

Because the patient is active and has excellent exercise tolerance, he is a candidate for a supraglottic laryngectomy. He is taken to the operating room where he undergoes 1) an uneventful supraglottic laryngectomy with a ipsilateral modified neck dissection, preserving the internal jugular vein and spinal accessory nerve; 2) a contralateral selective neck dissection, removing nodes in levels II through IV; and 3) a temporary tracheostomy.

The patient does well postoperatively, with the expected amount of postoperative aspiration, which is partially controlled with tracheostomy cuff inflation, early ambulation, and vigorous pulmonary toilet. Approximately 1 week after surgery, a trial deflation of the tracheostomy tube cuff is performed, which the patient does not tolerate. However, 2 days later, the deflation is successful. The patient has an adequate airway, with finger occlusion of the tracheostomy tube. Therefore, the tube is downsized and plugged, and the following day he is decannulated. Early attempts at oral feeding are unsuccessful, despite intensive efforts by speech therapy and swallow retraining. However, by the end of the second postoperative week, the patient was beginning to tolerate small amounts of applesauce—even so, because he had to concentrate on swallowing strategies with each swallow, it took over an hour to consume a 3-oz cup. By the end of the third week, the patient is tolerating a mechanical soft diet and aspirating only minimally on thin liquids. His feeding tube is removed, and he is discharged.

The final pathology report reveals moderately differentiated squamous cell carcinoma involving the false cord, epiglottis, and extending up to the aryepiglottic fold. All surgical margins are clear. Three ipsilateral nodes are positive for squamous cell carcinoma, and one has extracapsular spread. None of the 10 contralateral nodes contains deposits of metastatic cancer. Because of the presence of extracapsular spread and multiple ipsilateral nodes, the patient is at high risk for recurrence, and so postoperative radiotherapy is administered. At the end of his fourth week of radiotherapy, the patient has some difficulty with edema of his arytenoid mucosa. He is admitted for observation but responds to steroids and does not require tracheostomy replacement. He is placed on oral pilocarpine to reduce the effects of the radiation on salivation but still has significant difficulties with dry mouth and pharyngeal crusting.

> **Case 31.4 (continued)   Man with Supraglottic Cancer**
>
> Three months after surgery, his treatment is complete and he is tolerating an oral diet. He has regained nearly all of the 20 lb he lost throughout the course of his treatment. He has enrolled in a smoking-cessation course at his local clinic. After 3 years, he remains free of disease.
>
> **Discussion**
>
> This case illustrates the subtle symptoms associated with supraglottic cancer and the late-stage presentation (stage III) that is common in this disease process. Combined treatment with surgery and radiation was necessary to effect the highest chance of cure. The postoperative course after supraglottic laryngectomy is complex and entails orderly decannulation and intensive swallowing therapy that usually must be continued after discharge. The acute effects of radiotherapy resulted in prolonging the rehabilitation phase, but this patient was able to resume an essentially normal life after completion of his therapy. It is clear that his young age and excellent physical condition contributed to his satisfactory outcome.

Supraglottic laryngectomy patients require a tracheostomy for 2 or 3 weeks. Although the true cords are preserved, removing the epiglottis, false vocal cords, and aryepiglottic folds leaves them unprotected during swallowing. Incompletely swallowed material remains on the vocal cords and is aspirated into the trachea at the next breath unless the patient uses specific swallowing techniques. These techniques require that he or she have sufficient pulmonary reserve to clear the larynx by coughing; therefore, supraglottic laryngectomy is not selected for debilitated patients or for those with reduced pulmonary function. The services of a specially trained speech pathologist are invaluable in rehabilitating supraglottic laryngectomy patients.

Smaller cancers that are easily accessible can be treated by endoscopic laser excision. One benefit of endoscopic excision is that tracheostomy can be avoided. Even when the primary tumor is successfully resected endoscopically, treatment still must cover occult cervical lymph node metastases.

Laryngeal preservation protocols using chemotherapy and irradiation have received considerable attention in the lay press. As many as two thirds of patients who undergo these treatments can expect to keep their larynxes, and survival has not been affected adversely in randomized trials. These techniques are obviously an option for treating cancer of the larynx and hypopharynx, but they are not yet considered standard care. It must be noted that failure to identify recurrence early after induction therapy results in an increased risk of dying from a recurrent tumor. In many cases of advanced disease, larynx-preservation surgery leaves the patient with impaired laryngeal function and a permanent tracheostomy or feeding tube; however, this may be preferable to many patients.

Danger Signs

Tobacco and alcohol act synergistically to induce changes in the upper aerodigestive tract mucosa. Consequently, any patient who has a history of tobacco and/or alcohol abuse and complaints referable to the upper aerodigestive tract that have not resolved with conservative medical treatment within 2 or 3 weeks should be evaluated by an otolaryngologist. Symptoms that include hoarseness, dysphagia, mild discomfort, and severe pain may be presenting signs of an upper aerodigestive tract carcinoma.

Hoarseness without an underlying cause requires visualization of the larynx to rule out early laryngeal carcinoma. Dysphagia, odynophagia, or discomfort in the oral cavity or oropharynx requires evaluation of the oropharynx and hypopharynx to rule out an early carcinoma. Unfortunately, many of these tumors present late because of the propensity for them to remain asymptomatic until they become large enough to cause obstructive symptoms.

Summary

Cancer of the mucosal surfaces of the head and neck is usually squamous cell carcinoma. Epidemiologic studies confirm its association with excessive use of alcohol and tobacco. Cancer at most of these sites has a propensity to metastasize to the regional lymphatic system. Distant metastases are rare and treatment is effective if the tumor is diagnosed early. Unfortunately, one half of all head and neck cancers are diagnosed late, which increases treatment morbidity and reduces patient survival. Smaller tumors are treated with either surgery or radiation, whereas advanced tumors generally require a combination of both modalities. Chemotherapy can be used as adjuvant therapy, as a radiosensitizer, or as part of an organ-preservation therapy. Head and neck cancer patients remain at high risk for the development of a second primary malignant tumor (especially one of the upper aerodigestive tract, lung, and esophagus) and should be followed assiduously for the rest of their lives.

SUGGESTED READINGS

McQuarrie D, Adams G, Shons A, Browne G. *Head and Neck Cancer: Clinical Decisions and Management Principles.* Chicago: Year Book; 1986.

This text presents head and neck cancer through the Socratic method of posing questions and then discussing options and decisions.

Myers E (ed). *Operative Otolaryngology.* Philadelphia: WB Saunders; 1998.

This text deals primarily with surgical management of a variety of disease processes, including well-illustrated chapters on the treatment of head and neck cancer.

Myers E , Suen A. *Cancer of the Head and Neck,* 3rd ed. Philadelphia: WB Saunders; 1996.

Thawley S, Panje W, Batsakis J, Lindberg R. *Comprehensive Management of Head and Neck Tumors.* Philadelphia: WB Saunders; 1998.

These two texts are standard comprehensive reference materials for head and neck cancer.

32

Head and Neck Disorders in the Immunocompromised Patient

Thomas A. Tami, MD

Technological advances in medicine, improved drug therapy, and longer life expectancies have allowed more patients to develop immune dysfunction. Intrinsic (e.g., diabetes mellitus, immunoglobulin deficiencies), iatrogenic (e.g., neutropenia of chemotherapeutic agents), and infectious (e.g., AIDS) causes of immune dysfunction are encountered frequently in clinical practice.

Diabetes Mellitus

The most common cause of an immune deficiency–like state is diabetes mellitus. Chronic hyperglycemia is associated with neutrophil dysfunction, which facilitates head and neck infections. The metabolic changes in acute diabetic ketoacidosis also permit infections by opportunistic pathogens. The most commonly encountered condition is oropharyngeal candidiasis (thrush). Thrush can occur in normal infants, patients on broad-spectrum antibiotics, and patients with severe xerostomia caused by Sjögren's syndrome or previous head and neck radiation. Thrush also can occur with the use of inhaled steroids, so patients using these medications should be instructed to rinse their mouth after use. In the absence of these situations, oropharyngeal thrush suggests an underlying immune problem. Oral thrush is treated with topical nystatin (100,000 U/mL swish swallow) or clotrimazole lozenges (orally three times daily). Occasionally, a systemic agent, such as ketoconazole or fluconazole, is needed. Maintaining serum glucose near normal levels minimizes problems with thrush.

Necrotizing Otitis

Necrotizing otitis (malignant external otitis) occurs most commonly in diabetic patients, beginning as an external otitis that responds poorly to conservative medical therapy. Initially presenting as a soft tissue infection, it may progress to chondritis of the ear canal and then to osteitis in diabetes patients. Typically, granulation tissue develops on the floor of the external auditory canal at the bony–cartilaginous junction (Case 32.1). Radiographic imaging (computed tomography and/or magnetic resonance imaging) usually makes

---

Case 32.1 **Necrotizing Otitis in a Man with Diabetes Mellitus**

A man 58 years of age with insulin-dependent diabetes mellitus presents with right facial nerve paralysis. He developed a draining ear several weeks ago and, despite topical drops, had persistent drainage and developed severe pain. Several weeks before to the onset of his infection, he had attempted unsuccessfully to irrigate wax out of his ear.

Physical examination reveals pus and granulation tissue in his right ear canal, with total ipsilateral facial nerve paralysis. Laboratory studies reveal marked hyperglycemia and ketoacidosis. He is admitted to the hospital and his diabetic ketoacidosis is treated aggressively. His ear canal is cultured, and he is begun on intravenous gentamicin. Computed tomography reveals erosion of the inferior portion of the temporal bone.

After his hyperglycemia with ketosis and electrolyte disturbance are corrected, the patient undergoes surgical debridement with removal of necrotic tympanic bone and soft tissue inferior to his ear canal. The facial nerve is identified and decompressed by removing the necrotic bone. He is continued on antibiotics for 6 weeks, and his cavity heals uneventfully. He regains some facial nerve function at 3 months, with gradual improvement over the following year.

Discussion

This case represents an unusual and severe complication of necrotizing otitis externa. Once called *malignant otitis externa* due to the nearly universal fatal outcome, this disease can now be managed with antibiotics that are active against *Pseudomonas*, correction of diabetic ketoacidosis, and occasionally surgical debridement. Most early infections can be managed effectively with cleansing of the ear canal and oral ciprofloxacin and without surgical debridement.

the diagnosis. Bone scans may be helpful in defining the extent of the disease. If necrotizing otitis is not treated aggressively (i.e., with topical cleansings and debridement, long-term parenteral antibiotics, and occasionally hyperbaric oxygen therapy), it can progress to skull-base osteomyelitis (1). Because *Pseudomonas aeruginosa* is usually the implicated organism, ciprofloxacin or another antipseudomonal drug should be used. Water contamination of the external auditory canal predisposes to necrotizing otitis externa; thus, in patients with diabetes, irrigation to remove cerumen should be avoided. If irrigation is used, the canal must be dried meticulously. Diabetic ketoacidosis is often present and should be corrected.

Mucormycosis

A potentially lethal problem in diabetic or immunocompromised patients is mucormycosis, a deeply invasive and aggressive fungal infection of the nose and paranasal sinuses that is caused by multiple genera in the Mucoraceae family (*Rhizopus, Mucor,* and *Absidia*). Mucormycosis can occur in transplant patients and in patients with adrenal suppression, hematologic dyscrasias, and AIDS. Diabetes mellitus is the most common underlying condition.

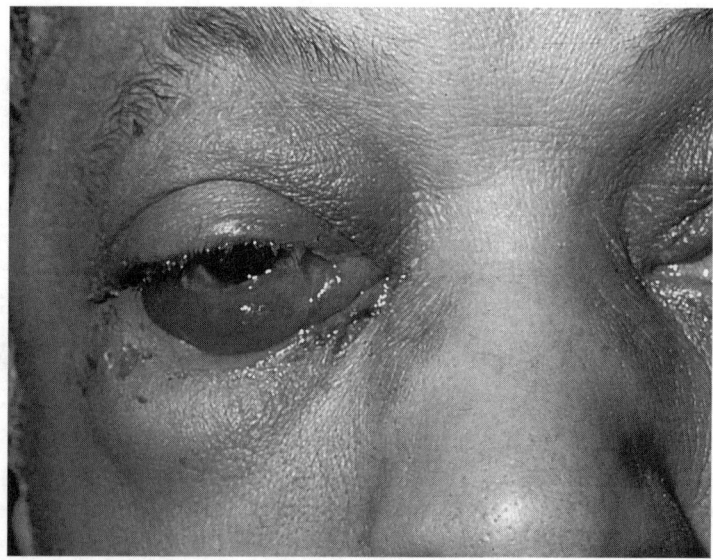

Figure 32.1 Right chemosis, proptosis, ophthalmoplegia, and apparent facial paralysis in a diabetic patient with orbital mucormycosis (see Case 32.2). (Republished with permission from Thatch LS, Kusne S, Eibling DE. Successful treatment of zygomycosis of the paranasal sinuses with surgical debridement and amphotericin-B colloidal dispersion. *Am J Otolaryngol.* 1993;14:249–53.)

Mucor fungi thrive in the glucose-rich acid environment of diabetic ketoacidosis. Blood vessel invasion with arterial and venous thrombosis leads to ischemic infarction and hemorrhagic necrosis. The clinical picture includes cranial nerve deficits, proptosis, chemosis, ophthalmoplegia, facial swelling, and palatal ulcers (Fig. 32.1). Intranasal examination often reveals dark areas on the nasal turbinates or septum that do not bleed when biopsied (Fig. 32.2). Histopathologic examination shows tissue necrosis and inflammatory cells. Nonseptate hyphae are diagnostic and are seen easily on silver methenamine stain (Fig. 32.3).

Early diagnosis of mucormycosis is essential for successful treatment; immediate, aggressive surgical debridement of all involved tissues, the administration of parenteral antifungal drugs, and the reversal of underlying condition are key. Correcting hyperglycemia and ketoacidosis can halt or slow disease progression. However, because conditions such as renal failure, posttransplant immunosuppression, and AIDS may not be reversible, the prognosis of mucormycosis is worse in these patients.

Radical surgical debridement removes devitalized and necrotic tissue that could serve as a reservoir of fungal elements. Thorough debridement often includes resection of facial skin, intranasal structures, the hard and soft palates, and sometimes even the orbit (Case 32.2). When infection spreads to the orbit, cavernous sinus, or cranium, survival rates decrease dramatically (<20%).

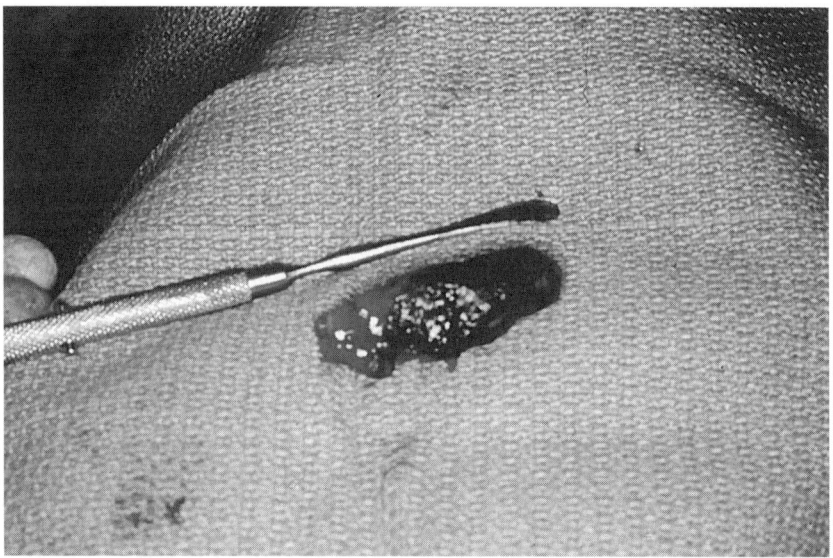

Figure 32.2 Necrotic inferior turbinate removed at time of surgical debridement in the patient shown in Figure 32.1. Necrosis results from intravascular invasion of fungal mycelia, which occlude blood flow.

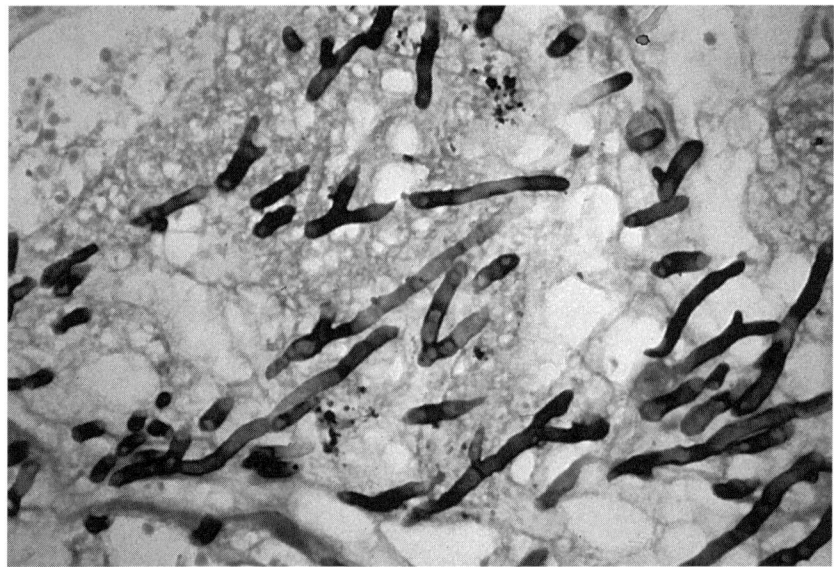

Figure 32.3 Typical nonseptate branching hyphae of *Mucor* invading tissue.

Amphotericin B is the drug of choice. Because it is fungistatic rather than fungicidal, long-term therapy is usually necessary. Prognosis is poor in patients with a low or decreasing neutrophil count. Cumulative doses of between 2000 and 4500 mg are common. When they become available, newer forms of the drug that are better tolerated and permit higher doses may save more patients.

Immunodeficiency with Neutropenia

Aspergillus Sinusitis

Neutropenia occurs in patients with blood dyscrasias, hematologic malignancies, chemotherapy-induced bone-marrow suppression, immunosuppression associated with organ transplantation, and chronic renal failure. Neutropenia provides an ideal setting for infection, and *Aspergillus* is the most common invasive fungal organism in the neutropenic patients without diabetes. Although invasive aspergillosis can present as a fulminant infection in severely neutropenic patients (e.g., those who have undergone a bone-marrow transplant), it is more often indolent and chronic, involving the paranasal sinuses.

Invasive *Aspergillus* sinusitis can be difficult to differentiate from nonfungal sinusitis. Imaging of the sinuses is useful: Computed tomography provides a

Case 32.2 Mucormycosis in a Man with Diabetes Mellitus

A man 78 years of age who has non–insulin-dependent diabetes mellitus presents with a 3-day history of swelling of his right eye with proptosis, ophthalmoplegia, and vision loss (see Fig. 32.1). He developed sinusitis 2 weeks ago and was treated with ceftriaxone but did not improve. He has no vision in his contralateral eye, and the vision in his involved eye is markedly decreased with an ophthalmoplegic globe. He has apparent ipsilateral facial nerve paralysis involving the lower division of the facial nerve.

Intranasal examination reveals a black right middle turbinate and a palatal ulcer over the maxillary tuberosity. Laboratory studies demonstrate ketoacidosis and hyperglycemia. Computed tomography without contrast reveals pansinusitis on the right, with soft tissue swelling over the maxilla.

The patient is taken to the operating room where he undergoes radical debridement of all necrotic tissue. The mucosa and bone of the maxillary and ethmoid sinuses are necrotic and are removed, along with the necrotic subcutaneous tissue of his cheek. The inferior turbinate is also necrotic (see Fig. 32.2). Necrotic orbital periosteum is debrided; however, because the patient is blind in his contralateral eye, preservation of his right eye is attempted. Pathologic examination of the resected tissue demonstrates nonseptate branching hyphae invading the soft tissues that is typical of mucormycosis (see Fig. 32.3).

Postoperatively, the patient is begun on intravenous amphotericin B and hyperbaric oxygen. He does not tolerate the drug, with elevation of his serum creatinine to 3.3 mg per 100 m^3, indicating renal failure. Compassionate use of an investigative colloidal form of amphotericin is obtained urgently, and the patient is treated with escalating doses. Additional debridement of necrotic tissue in his cavity is required on many occasions, but orbital exenteration is avoided. A total of 13.5 g of amphotericin (more than six times the usual maximum dose) is administered. His cavity eventually heals, the ophthalmoplegia resolves, and the vision in his right eye returns to normal.

Discussion

Although the presentation of *Mucor* in this patient was not uncommon, the treatment in this case was innovative because a condemned eye was preserved by the use of limited debridement and an investigative form of amphotericin. Early recognition, correction of ketoacidosis and hyperglycemia, surgical debridement, and antifungal therapy are the mainstays of successful management. Hyperbaric oxygen is probably helpful and was used in this case.

This case was reported previously in the *American Journal of Otolaryngology* (13).

view of the sinus bones, and magnetic resonance imaging can demonstrate extension of the disease into the soft tissues beyond the sinus cavities. Cultures establish the diagnosis. If neurological deficits, visual changes, or tissue necrosis occurs, aggressive surgical intervention and intensive medical therapy seldom produce a favorable outcome. The prognosis is grim if the underlying immune defect cannot be improved. If the neutropenia is reversible (e.g., secondary to immunosuppressive drugs) or if the production of neutrophils can be stimulated (with granulocyte colony–stimulating factor), the prognosis is better.

Bacterial Infections

Bacterial infections are common in patients with neutropenia. Seemingly minor infections can progress rapidly to life-threatening disease; hence, early diagnosis and therapy with appropriate drainage and/or antibiotics is critical (Case 32.3). Because typical signs of infection may be absent, a high index of suspicion is needed. Oncologists and infectious disease specialists are aware of the common upper airway infections (e.g., sinusitis) that occur in their patients with neutropenia, and early consultation for culture and drainage is usual. Nosocomial sinusitis is common and warrants early sinus puncture for culture and treatment in patients with neutropenia.

Case 32.3 **Life-Threatening Bacterial Infection in a Young Woman with Neutropenia**

A woman 26 years of age with juvenile rheumatoid arthritis who had been treated with colloidal gold developed *Listeria* meningitis that was treated successfully with intravenous ampicillin and gentamicin. After 14 days of therapy she presents with sudden painful swelling of her upper lip (resembling angioneurotic edema) and focal discoloration near the right side of her nose.

A complete blood count reveals total white blood cell count of 100 cells per 100 m^3, of which 71% were lymphocytes. Needle aspiration of the edema fluid reveals gram-negative rods and later grows *Pseudomonas* organisms.

The patient is admitted to the intensive care unit and is begun on high-dose, intravenous, broad-spectrum antibiotics. Over a 4-hour period after her initial presentation, she develops obvious necrosis of much of her face, including her upper lip and nose, and systemic sepsis with hypotension. Five days after being admitted, the patient dies of multiple-organ failure, despite appropriate antibiotic therapy and heroic measures.

Discussion

This disturbing case illustrates that overwhelming fatal sepsis can occur with very minimal clinical findings and can deteriorate rapidly toward patient demise in the setting of profound neutropenia. Treatment in such cases is often ineffective unless the neutropenia can be reversed.

This case was reported previously in the *American Journal of Medicine* (14).

Oral Ulcerations

Management of oral ulcerations is problematic in neutropenic patients. Viral infections such as herpes simplex can activate and result in painful ulcerations over the tongue, gingiva, lips, and buccal mucosa. Leukemic ulcers, mucositis, and oral ulcerations are common in patients who receive chemotherapy and defy effective management. Topical therapy with a variety of compounds may provide symptomatic relief, but resolution does not occur until the disease process is controlled and the neutrophil function returns. Oral feeding during therapy may be nearly impossible because of pain. Narcotics and alternative feeding routes often are required.

Serum-Immunoglobulin Deficiencies

Head and neck infections often occur in patients with serum-immunoglobulin (Ig) deficiency syndromes. Chronic sinusitis and otitis media that are refractory to medical treatment sometimes prompt the search for these disorders.

X-linked (Bruton's) agammaglobulinemia is an unusual inherited condition that affects male children. At approximately 9 months of age, these children begin developing frequent pyogenic infections, including sinusitis and otitis media. Serum concentrations of IgG, IgA, and IgM are below normal. The tonsils, adenoids, and peripheral lymph nodes are hypoplastic.

The most common congenital Ig deficiency is **selective IgA deficiency**, occurring as often as in three of every 1000 patients. These patients are otherwise healthy but often experience recurrent respiratory infections. Concentrations of other serum Ig types are usually normal, although there may be a relative deficiency of IgG2.

Common variable immunodeficiency (acquired hypogammaglobulinemia) is similar to X-linked agammaglobulinemia except for having a later age of onset. The infections are milder, and there is an equal sex distribution. These patients usually have normal levels of circulating B lymphocytes, but the cells are unable to differentiate into mature Ig-producing cells. Cultures obtained from the maxillary antrum by puncture or endoscopic culture of the sinus ostium can be helpful in determining recurrent sinus infections, because unusual and resistant organisms are common.

IgG-subclass deficiencies can be associated with multiple or chronic infections; however, completely asymptomatic individuals have been described who have a complete lack of IgG1, IgG2, and IgG4. An IgG2-subclass deficiency occasionally occurs with a selective IgA deficiency, causing susceptibility to upper respiratory tract infections. It is generally recommended that intravenous Ig therapy not be given to patients who are IgG-subclass deficient unless a deficiency of antibodies to a broad array of antigens can be demonstrated.

Mycobacterial Infections

As immunocompromised patients survive longer, once-rare mycobacterial infections are being seen with increasing frequency (2). **Tuberculosis** (from *Mycobacterium tuberculosis*) usually begins with a pulmonary infection (3). The most common head and neck manifestation of tuberculosis is infected cervical lymph nodes (scrofula) (4). Clinical suspicion, skin testing, cultures, and computed tomography of the neck usually make the diagnosis; however, excisional biopsy is sometimes required. Other head and neck sites of presentation include the larynx, middle ear and mastoid, oral cavity, pharynx, nasal cavity, and salivary glands (5). Long-term multiple drug therapy is required for eradication. Longer therapy is required in AIDS patients.

Atypical mycobacterial infections are more common in the head and neck than are typical mycobacterial tuberculosis infections. Infections of the cervical lymph nodes and the middle ear and, occasionally, skin involvement are seen most often. Diagnosis is approached as with tuberculosis; however, excisional biopsy of neck nodes for diagnosis is required more frequently than with tuberculosis. Pharmacotherapy is the mainstay of treatment. Surgical treatment is reserved for persistent neck masses and tympanic membrane perforations.

In AIDS patients, disseminated mycobacterial infections occur more frequently, involvement of the skin (plaques or ulcerations) and joints is not uncommon (6), and long-term pharmacotherapy is the key to control and resolution.

AIDS

Otologic Manifestations

The most common otologic problem in AIDS patients is **acute otitis media**. Ear infections are frequent because of the underlying immune deficiency and the generalized adenoidal lymphoid hypertrophy many patients develop. When the CD4 count (T-helper lymphocyte level) is greater than 500 cells/mm^3, otitis media usually responds to standard antibiotics. As immune function deteriorates (i.e., low CD4 cell count), antibiotic therapy becomes less effective. Myringotomy with or without ventilating tubes can be useful in preventing recurrent infections and in relieving the associated conductive hearing loss.

Sensorineural hearing loss is common in AIDS patients (20%–50% of HIV-positive patients experience it) and probably originates from a central demyelinating process (7).

Chronic external otitis can be frustrating in AIDS patients. The high incidence of generalized dermatitis suggests an underlying predisposition to cutaneous disorders. Although standard otic antibiotic preparations (e.g., neomycin plus polymyxin plus corticosteroid) are occasionally effective, they often do not resolve the inflammatory process adequately. Frequent cleaning and debridement using adequate illumination and magnification can help control the problem. Culture-directed antibiotic therapy is useful for persistent infections, because some of these may be fungal rather than bacterial.

Occasionally, **otitis externa** spreads out of the external auditory canal onto the conchal bowl and pinna. When this occurs, viral cultures should be obtained, because herpes simplex or zoster also can have this appearance. Acyclovir therapy is usually effective.

When **necrotizing otitis (malignant external otitis or skull-base osteomyelitis)** occurs in AIDS patients, the hallmark granulation tissue may be absent, and *Pseudomonas* is not always the responsible organism. The approach to diagnosis and treatment is the same as in other patients, but the prognosis is worse than the usual necrotizing otitis in diabetes patients (8).

Nasal and Sinus Manifestations

Chronic sinusitis occurs in up to 65% of AIDS patients. Nasal congestion with postnasal drainage and abnormal mucus production is often a nagging problem. During the early stages of HIV disease, the treatment of sinusitis is the same as in the general population. As the CD4 cell count decreases, the incidence of IgE-related atopic disease increases. When paired with the progressive underlying systemic humoral and cellular immune dysfunction, acute infections become recalcitrant to standard treatment. The acute infections develop into a chronic sinusitis, the treatment of which is challenging.

Chronic sinusitis in AIDS patients usually is caused by *Staphylococcus* (40%) or *Pseudomonas* (20%) species; anaerobic bacteria are less common causes. Because many infections are polymicrobial, either ciprofloxacin with clindamycin or levofloxacin with metronidazole is a good empirical choice. Early culture is recommended so that organism-specific therapy can be instituted and fungal pathogens can be excluded.

Steroid nasal sprays, systemic nasal decongestants (e.g., pseudoephedrine) and mucolytics (e.g., guiafenesin 2400 mg/d) are also helpful. When troublesome symptoms persist despite full medical therapy, endoscopic surgical drainage of the sinuses may produce clinical improvement.

Nasal vestibular infections are common and are usually staphylococcal infections of the hair follicles (vibrissae) in the nasal vestibule. Because retrograde venous spread of infection from the nose can cause intracranial spread and meningitis, every infection near the nose should be treated aggressively.

Systemic antistaphylococcal antibiotics and topical mupirocin are usually effective. As with infections of the ear canal, when the infection begins to spread out of the nasal vestibule and onto the adjacent facial skin, the possibility of a herpes simplex infection must be considered.

Oral Cavity, Laryngeal, and Pharyngeal Manifestations

Oral disease develops in almost all patients with AIDS. **Oral thrush** is common and may be one of the earliest presenting signs of HIV infection. Involved mucosa has a patchy, pseudomembranous, "cottage cheese" appearance; it also can appear flat with erythematous atrophic mucosal patches. Topical nystatin or clotrimazole is usually effective. If the infection recurs immediately after treatment, systemic therapy with fluconazole or ketoconazole is helpful, and long-term prophylaxis with these agents is sometimes necessary. If severe sore throat, hoarseness, or odynophagia accompanies oral thrush, then pharyngeal, laryngeal, and esophageal candidiasis should be considered. These more serious conditions usually respond to intravenous amphotericin-B therapy.

Another common oral condition in AIDS patients is asymptomatic **hairy leukoplakia of the tongue,** which appears as a whitish, vertically corrugated area on the lateral edges of the tongue and is probably caused by a viral infection. Although it is of no clinical significance, hairy leukoplakia can be confused with malignant conditions and oral thrush, occasionally requiring a biopsy for differentiation.

Periodontal disease is common. HIV gingivitis produces a band of marked erythema along the gingival margin that bleeds easily (7). Gingival inflammation and atrophy can be controlled by good oral hygiene and frequent dentist visits. Occasionally, despite these preventive measures, acute fulminant necrotizing gingivitis and periodontitis caused by anaerobic oral bacteria are encountered. These diseases produce severe inflammation of the gingiva and the underlying alveolar bone, which in turn loosen the teeth. Even aggressive local care and intravenous antibiotic administration may not halt their progression.

Recurrent **aphthous stomatitis** is often seen throughout the oral cavity but has a particular affinity for the cheeks, oropharynx, and tonsillar fossae. Lesions can coalesce to form giant aphthous lesions that measure more than 2 cm. Severe odynophagia and dysphagia can cause significant weight loss due to decreased oral intake. Topical anesthetics and steroids are occasionally effective. The combination of systemic steroids and an antibiotic (e.g., clindamycin) can help when there is secondary infection. Recent experimental studies have shown dramatic clinical responses after thalidomide therapy for giant aphthous ulcers.

The oral cavity is a common site for **Kaposi's sarcoma (KS).** Interestingly, men who becomes HIV positive from a transfusion or intravenous drug use have only an approximate 20% chance of developing KS, whereas men who become HIV positive from engaging in homosexual sex have a 15% to 30% chance of developing KS (9) (Case 32.4) (Fig. 32.4). This violaceous neoplasm has a predilection for the palate and gingiva but can occur throughout the upper aerodigestive tract. Generally, treatment is not required for asymptomatic KS. If lesions become ulcerated, painful, and infected, or if they interfere with function (e.g., eating, swallowing, breathing), then surgical excision, laser ablation, radiation therapy, and intralesional vinblastine can be offered. Other less-common conditions that occur in the oral cavity of AIDS patients include oral histoplasmosis, herpes simplex and zoster, cytomegalovirus infections, non-Hodgkin's lymphoma, and squamous cell carcinoma (10).

Neck Manifestations

Neck masses are seen almost universally in patients with HIV infection. The most common mass is **generalized lymphadenopathy**, a symmetric enlarge-

Case 32.4   Kaposi's Sarcoma in a Young Man with HIV

A man 26 years of age presents with a severely sore throat and a "hot potato" voice.

Physical examination reveals an erythematous, swollen epiglottis and an adequate airway. He is admitted to the intensive care unit and is placed on intravenous antibiotics. Tracheostomy or other airway interventions are not required. Blood cultures are positive for *Haemophilus influenzae*, and his infection responded within 72 hours.

Routine reexamination reveals a violaceous area on his palate (similar to that pictured in Fig. 32.4). On further questioning, the patient confirmed that he is homosexual and has a history of multiple partners. HIV testing is positive, and his T4 count is 450 cells per 100 cm^3. The palate lesion is diagnosed clinically as Kaposi's sarcoma and is not biopsied.

Discussion

The occurrence of an unusual infection such as adult epiglottitis should have prompted further questioning by the admitting physician to determine whether some predisposing factor (e.g., AIDS) was present. In fact, the diagnosis was not considered until the palate lesion was noted. This patient had avoided being tested for HIV, despite a lifestyle that placed him at high risk for infection. Biopsy confirmation of Kaposi's is not necessary, because no therapy is warranted unless the lesions become symptomatic. This case is also an object lesson in reinforcing the value of universal precautions. Because the diagnosis of HIV seropositivity had not been made or considered at his initial presentation, examination without eye protection or gloves would have placed the examining physician at risk.

ment of cervical lymph nodes caused by lymphoid follicular hypertrophy. **Tuberculosis and atypical mycobacterial infections** are becoming more common in AIDS patients and often present as neck masses, as do toxoplasmosis, histoplasmosis, and other fungal infections. Therapy is directed at the particular organism. Metastatic KS or squamous cell carcinoma is a rare cause of a neck masses.

AIDS-related lymphoma is always a concern, because it is the most common neoplasm to present as a neck mass in AIDS patients (11). Medium- or high-grade B-cell lymphoma is the most common type. AIDS-related lymphoma is also rapidly increasing, and it has a poor prognosis. Unfortunately, the chemotherapy used to treat the lymphoma also worsens the patient's immunosuppression, and radiation therapy is poorly tolerated (12).

Frequently, the diagnosis of a neck mass can be made by fine-needle–aspiration biopsy. Open biopsy is required when lymphoma is suspected, so that the nodal architecture is available. Other indications for open neck-mass biopsy include 1) marked constitutional symptoms with an otherwise normal clinical evaluation, 2) localized enlarging lymphadenopathy, 3) a single disproportionately large node with persistent generalized lymphadenopathy, and 4) the need for reassurance about an ambiguous cytologic diagnosis after fine-needle–aspiration biopsy.

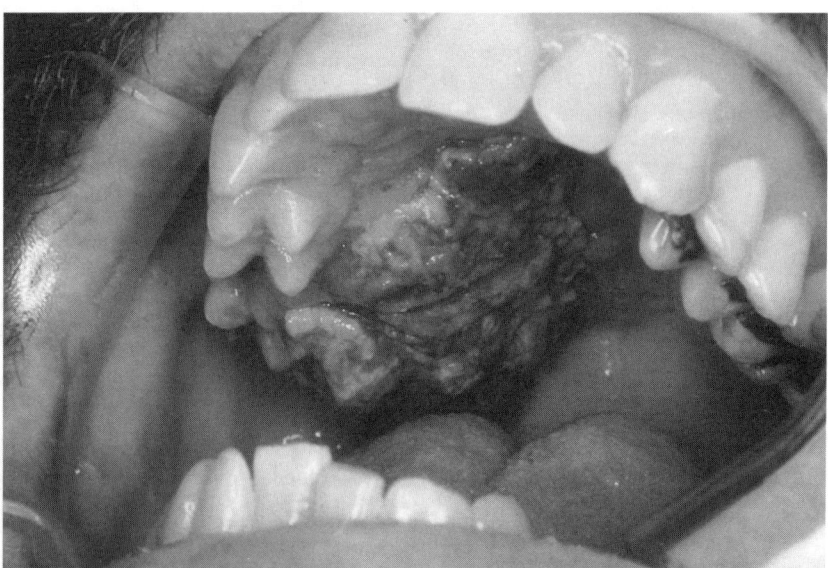

Figure 32.4 Kaposi's sarcoma of the hard palate in a patient with AIDS. (Republished with permission from Tami TA, Lee KC. *AIDS and the Otolaryngologist SIPac*. Alexandria, VA: American Academy of Otolaryngology–Head and Neck Surgery Foundation; 1993.)

Head and Neck Disorders in the Immunocompromised Patient   647

Salivary Gland Manifestations

A common complaint in HIV-infected patients is dry mouth (**xerostomia**). Histopathologic evaluation of the salivary glands reveals chronic inflammatory infiltrates similar to Sjögren's syndrome. **Generalized parotid gland enlargement** caused by chronic inflammatory cell infiltration is common, especially in HIV-infected children. In adults, **benign lymphoepithelial cysts of the parotid gland** often are encountered and can become massive (Fig. 32.5). These parotid masses are diagnosed by needle aspiration or imaging studies. Treatment, if required, consists of multiple needle aspirations to decompress the cyst. A recent paper describes **sclerosis** occurring after needle aspiration and tetracycline injection. Open surgical parotidectomy is reserved for cases in which 1) the diagnosis is in question, 2) recurrent infections have occurred, or 3) severe cosmetic deformity is present.

Summary

Patients with compromised function of their immune system are vulnerable to infections that would be less serious or would not occur at all in patients with

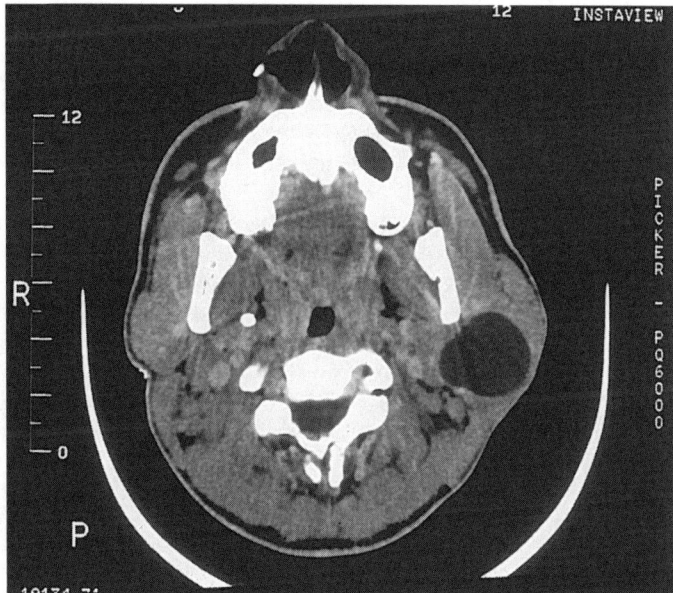

Figure 32.5 Computed tomography scan of massive parotid cysts in a patient with AIDS. Needle aspiration can provide temporary symptomatic relief.

normally functioning immune systems. Physicians who treat such patients should be vigilant to detect these often-unusual infections and to initiate aggressive therapy early in the disease process, for this offers the best possible chance for successful treatment.

REFERENCES

1. **Slattery WH, Brackmann DE.** Skull-base osteomyelitis: malignant external otitis. *Otolaryngol Clin North Am.* 1996;29:795–806.
2. **Williams RG, Douglas-Jones T.** Mycobacterium marches back. *J Laryngol Otol.* 1995;109:5–13
3. **Preheim LC, Smith TL.** Mycobacterial infections: new threats from old disease. *Compr Ther.* 1997;23:310–8.
4. **Fliss DM, Barki Y, Leiberman A, Hertzanu Y.** Mycobacterial cervical adenitis. *Ann Otol Rhinol Laryngol.* 1995;104:409–12.
5. **Cleary KR, Batsakis JG.** Mycobacterial disease of the head and neck: current perspective. *Ann Otol Rhinol Laryngol.* 1995;104:830–3.
6. **Zanelli G, Webster GF.** Mycocutaneous atypical mycobacterial infections in acquired immunodeficiency syndrome. *Clin Dermatol.* 1995;13:281–8.
7. **Moazzez AH, Alvi A.** Head and neck manifestations of AIDS in adults. *Am Fam Phys.* 1998;57:1813–22.
8. **Ress BD, Luntz M, Telischi FF, et al.** Necrotizing external otitis in patients with AIDS. *Laryngoscope.* 1997;107:456–60.
9. **Conant MA.** Management of human immunodeficiency virus–associated malignancies. *Recent Results Cancer Res.* 1995;139:423–32.
10. **Langford A, Langer R, Lobeck H, et al.** Human immunodeficiency virus–associated squamous cell carcinoma of the head and neck presenting as oral and primary intraosseous squamous cell carcinomas. *Quintessence Int.* 1995;26:635–54.
11. **Denton AS, Brook MG, Miller RF, Spittle MF.** AIDS-related lymphoma: an emerging epidemic. *Br J Hosp Med.* 1996;55:282–8.
12. **Carbone A, Vaccher E, Barzan L, et al.** Head and neck lymphomas associated with human immunodeficiency virus infection. *Arch Otolaryngol Head Neck Surg.* 1995;121:210–8.
13. **Thatch LS, Kusne S, Eibling DE.** Successful treatment of zygomycosis of the paranasal sinuses with surgical debridement and amphotericin B colloidal dispersion. *Am J Otolaryngol.* 1993;14:249–53.
14. **Kusne S, Eibling DE, Yu VL, et al.** Gangrenous cellulitis associated with gram-negative bacilli in pancytopenic patients: dilemma with respect to effective therapy. *Am J Med.* 1988;85:490–4.

SUGGESTED READINGS

Blitzer A, Lawson W. Fungal infections of the head and neck. *Otolaryngol Clin North Am.* 1993;26:1007–68.
  This article reviews the various head and neck presentations of fungal infections, many of which occur in immunocompromised patients.

Tami TA. The management of sinusitis in patients infected with the human immunodeficiency virus (HIV). *Ear Nose Throat J.* 1995;74:360–3.

This article reviews the pathophysiology of sinusitis in this immunocompromised patient population and describes approaches to treatment.

Tami TA, Lee KC. *AIDS and the Otolaryngologist SiPac.* Alexandria, VA: American Academy of Otolaryngology–Head and Neck Surgery; 1993.

This self-instructional monograph discusses the varied head and neck manifestations of AIDS infection and their diagnosis and management.

33

Smell and Taste Disorders

Thomas Hummel, MD
Michael Knecht, MD

Problems with smell and taste can have an enormous effect on our lives. These senses contribute substantially to the enjoyment of what we eat and drink and may even contribute to the selection of a spouse. When the sense of smell is lost, it becomes a difficult task to differentiate between cardboard and a hamburger. We also lose the sense that alerts us to dangers from fire or rotten food.

Disturbances of the chemical senses occur frequently. It is estimated that a complete loss of the sense of smell is found in at least 1% of the U.S. population. In addition, hundreds of thousands of patients complain to their physicians about disturbances of smell or taste each year. However, compared with the other senses, relatively little is known about the origins of smell and taste disorders and their treatment.

The perception of a certain flavor results from the interplay between three sensory systems: 1) the olfactory nerve, which mediates olfactory sensations (e.g., the pleasant odor of vanilla or the rotten smell of hydrogen sulfide); 2) the gustatory system, which mediates the basic tastes (i.e., sweet, salty, sour, and bitter); and 3) the trigeminal nerve, which mediates, for example, the burning and stinging of chili peppers and the cooling of menthol. The vagal and glossopharyngeal nerve–innervating areas in the back of the throat–also may contribute to these sensations. The physiologic significance of other systems (e.g., the vomeronasal organ located at the bottom of the anterior third

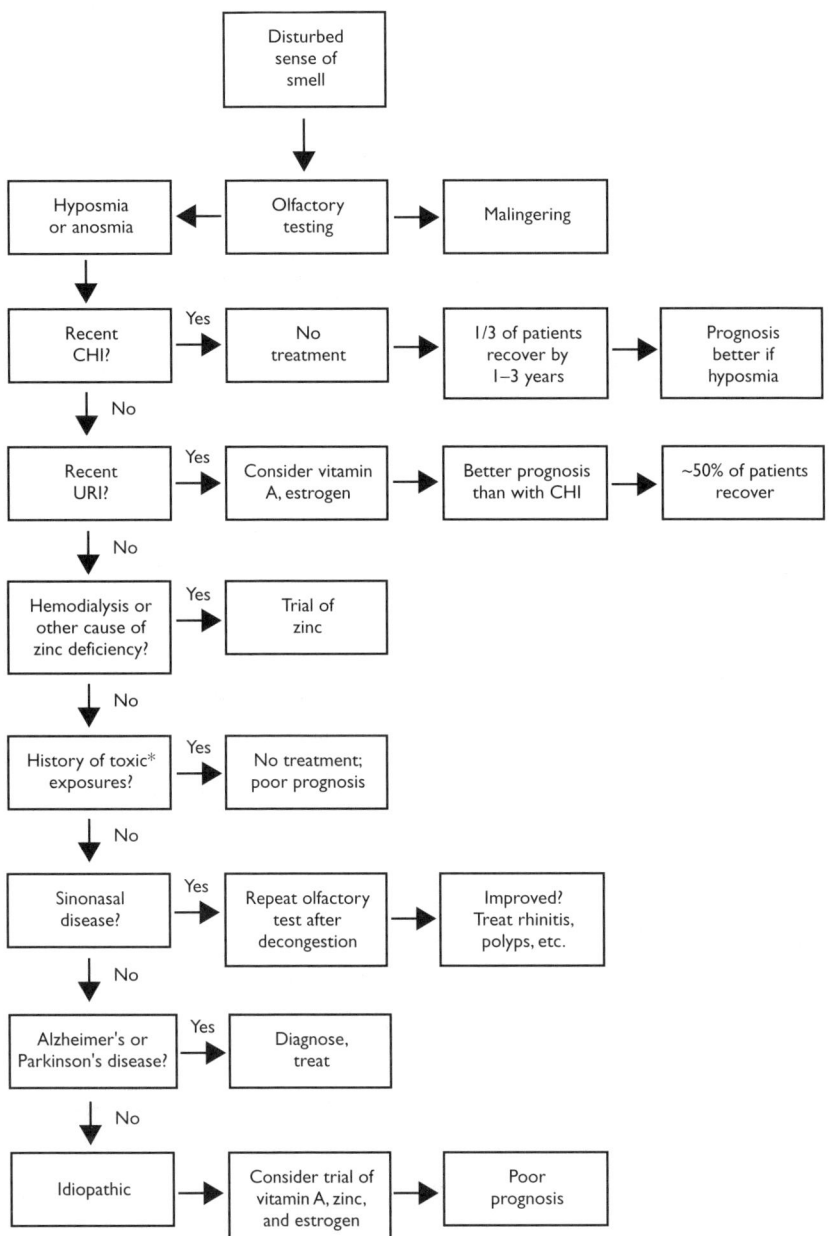

*Including benzene, acetone, hydrazine, paint solvents, trichloroethylene, cadmium, nickel, carbon disulfide, and ammonia.

Algorithm A Management of olfactory disorders. CHI = closed head injury; URI = upper respiratory infection.

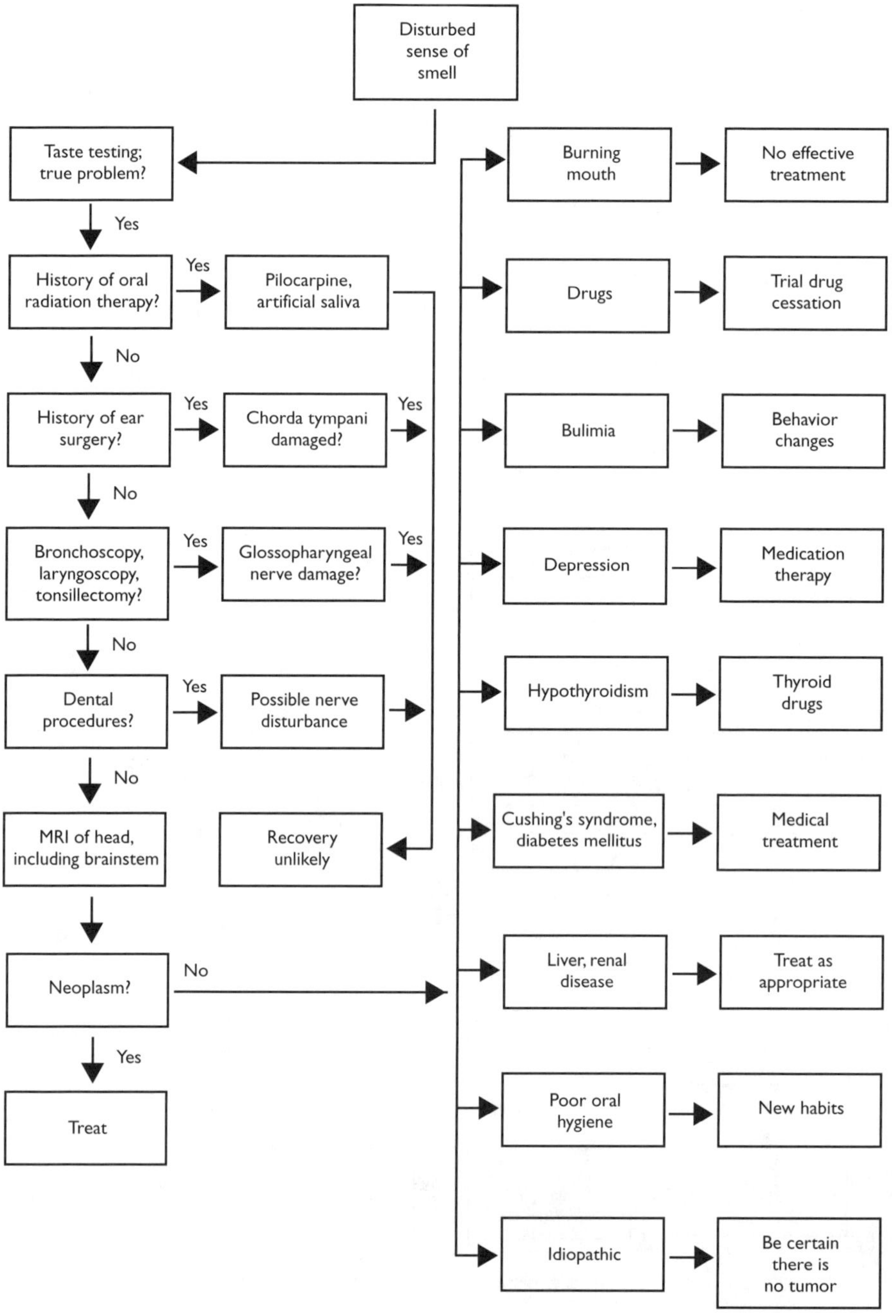

Algorithm B Management of gustatory disorders. MRI = magnetic resonance imaging.

of the nasal septum, 1–2 cm dorsal to the columella) is under investigation. Owing to this diversity, disturbances of the chemosensory perception may have a large variety of causes; however, the most frequent causes are disturbances related to the olfactory and gustatory systems.

Olfactory Disorders

Physiology

The olfactory neuroepithelium is found in the roof of the nasal cavity, mostly out of the direct path of respiratory air flow where it is accessible to odors that are presented either retropharyngeally (i.e., during eating and drinking) or in front of the nostrils. At this location, the local concentration of odorants is partially controlled by respiration.

The perception of odorants is believed to be due to the interaction between the odorants and the olfactory receptors located on the cilia of the bipolar olfactory receptor neurons (ORNs). Before this contact can be established, odorants must diffuse through a mucus layer. This transport may be facilitated by the olfactory binding protein, which also may play a role in removing odorants from the receptor site. A unique feature of primary ORNs is that they are regularly replaced throughout life.

Approximately 600 to 1000 different olfactory receptors are encoded in the human genome, and different ORNs respond to different spectrums of odors. Transduction is G-protein mediated and involves the cyclic adenosine monophosphate (cAMP) system and possibly the inositol-1,4,5-triphosphate (IP_3) system. The activation of cation channels (Na^+, K^+) results in the depolarization of the ORNs. This information is then transmitted via the olfactory nerve (fila olfactoria) through the cribriform plate to the mitral cells in the olfactory bulb. Unlike with vision, audition, and the somatosensory system, a large portion of the incoming olfactory information is processed ipsilaterally to the side of odor presentation.

Olfactory sensitivity is determined by gender and age, and it is well known that women have a higher olfactory sensitivity. The exact reason for this remains unclear, but social, hormonal, or genetic factors are thought to be involved. Using different measures, studies have shown a decrease of olfactory sensitivity after 60 years of age. In terms of odor identification, more than 50% of people 80 years of age exhibit olfactory disturbances. Another determinant of olfactory sensitivity is smoking, which leads to a mild but significant decrease of olfactory function that is related to the number of cigarettes smoked. Fortunately, it can be reversed if cigarette smoking is stopped.

Definition

Anosmia describes a complete loss of smell; the term *specific anosmia* refers to someone's inability to perceive a certain odor. **Hyposmia** describes a diminished olfactory sensitivity. **Hyperosmia** is an enhanced odor sensitivity (as in epilepsy and mucoviscidosis). **Dysosmia** is defined as a distorted olfactory perception that may occur intermittent or continually. Among dysosmia disorders, **parosmia** occurs in the presence of an odor, whereas **phantosmia** refers to an olfactory perception when no odor source is present (i.e., olfactory hallucination). Parosmia is typically associated with reduced olfactory sensitivity, particularly when virally induced. In sinus disease, parosmia may be associated with odors that emanate from infected cavities. Interestingly, less than 10% of individuals with parosmia report the perception of pleasant odors; most find these odors unpleasant. Signs of depression have been reported in approximately one third of patients who have dysosmia or dysgeusia.

Approximately two thirds of patients with olfactory disorders complain not only of a decreased olfactory function but also of taste loss. Approximately 10% of patients with olfactory disorders complain of a gustatory loss only. However, decreased gustatory function is present only in less than 5% of patients with chemosensory disorders.

Etiology

The three major causes of olfactory disorders are **head injury** (20%), **infections of the upper respiratory tract** (20%), and **nasal and sinus diseases** (20%). The major determinants of these three causes are summarized in Table 33.1.

Other frequent causes include **congenital anosmia** (5%) and **exposure to toxic substances** (5%). A wide variety of other causes include psychiatric disorders (e.g., schizophrenia, depression), epilepsy, Parkinson's disease, Alzheimer's disease, sarcoidosis, lupus erythematosus, multiple chemical sensitivities, pregnancy, diabetes, hypothyroidism, renal failure, liver disease, olfactory meningiomas, and brain neoplasms. In both Alzheimer's and Parkinson's diseases, the loss of olfactory sensitivity is thought to be among the earliest signs. Finally, iatrogenic causes of olfactory disorders include rhinoplasty, neurosurgery, and radiation and drug therapies (Table 33.2). In an additional 20% of patients, a cause for the chemosensory disturbance cannot be identified (**idiopathic**) (Case 33.1).

Diagnostic Evaluation

The first step in patient evaluation is to take a thorough **history**, including demographics; eating, drinking, and smoking habits; past major illnesses and in-

Table 33.1 Olfactory Dysfunction in Relation to the Three Major Causes

	Head Trauma	Upper Respiratory Infection	Nasal and Sinus Disease
Probable cause	Shearing of olfactory filaments at the cribriform plate	Viral destruction of olfactory epithelium	Polyps; secondary edema due to local inflammatory processes
Epithelial findings	Degeneration	Metaplasia; defective development of ORNs	Mostly normal
Occurrence of olfactory disturbances	≤5 %	≤1 %	Frequent
Approximate age	20–50 years	>60 years	20–60 years
Rapid onset of olfactory dysfunction	*	*	†
Degree of olfactory loss	*	‡	‡
Frequent occurrence of parosmia	‡	*	†

ORNs = olfactory receptor neurons.
* Patients are responsive to surgical therapy or treatment with corticosteroids.
† Improvement occurs mostly in hyposmic patients and mostly within the first year.
‡ Improvement is possible, even over a period of several years.

Table 33.2 Drugs Considered To Be Possible Causes of Olfactory Disturbances

Antibiotics (e.g., streptomycin)
Antirheumatics (e.g., D-penicillamine)
Antihypertensives (e.g., diltiazem, nifedipine)
Antidepressants (e.g., amitriptyline)
Chemotherapy drugs (e.g., methotrexate)
Local anesthetics (e.g., tetracaine, cocaine)
Opioids (e.g., codeine, morphine)
Psychopharmaceuticals (e.g., amphetamine, alcohol)
Sympathomimetics (e.g., chronic use of local vasoconstrictors)
Others (e.g., strychnine, acetylcholinergic drugs)

juries; medications taken in relation to symptom onset; history of present illness; endocrine information, including questions about menstrual status or thyroid function; general nasal health information, including obstruction, rhinorrhea, and postnasal drip; and any changes in the sense of smell.

> **Case 33.1 Woman with Anosmia Occurring After an Upper Respiratory Infection**
>
> A woman 63 years of age presents with an inability to smell that began rather abruptly last fall after an episode of influenza. Now, 6 months later, she is still unable to smell.
>
> A complete history and physical examination fails to reveal any other pertinent data, and olfactory testing demonstrates complete dysfunction of cranial nerve I.
>
> Over the next several months, she is empirically tried on oral vitamin A, estrogen, and zinc, with no improvement. Three years later, she still has a complete lack of the sense of smell.

The **physical examination** typically includes an evaluation of the patient's head and neck, with the remainder of the investigation directed by the patient's history. Frequently, a detailed neurological examination may be necessary. Specific nasal examination should include **nasal endoscopy**.

Radiologic evaluation may be helpful to rule out the presence of olfactory meningiomas, pituitary tumors, frontal lobe gliomas, large aneurysms, and other cerebral tumors. Computed tomography also may be useful in identifying the olfactory loss as conductive. **Additional diagnostic tests** may include the search for other underlying causes of the olfactory disorders (e.g., diabetes; hypothyroidism; lupus; deficiency of zinc, vitamin A, and vitamin B_{12}). Finally, **biopsies** of the olfactory epithelium may be helpful in the diagnosis of olfactory disorders.

Olfactory Testing

During the past decade, standardized tests of olfactory dysfunction have been developed, including the following:
- **University of Pennsylvania Smell Identification Test (UPSIT):** a "scratch and sniff" odor-identification test (Sensonics, Inc; Haddon Heights, New Jersey; phone: 856-428-1161; fax: 856-547-5665; Web site: http://www.smelltest.com)
- **"Sniffin' sticks":** pen-like odor-dispensing devices that include tests for odor identification, discrimination, and thresholds (Kobal; Erlangen, Germany; phone: 011-49-9131-807111; fax: 011-49-9131-807131; e-mail: kobal@t-online.de)
- **Connecticut Chemosensory Clinical Research Center (CCCRC) test:** a combined odor-identification and odor-threshold test (*see* list of centers below for contact information)

Testing of olfactory sensitivity typically includes the testing of **detection thresholds** for odors such as phenyl ethyl alcohol and butanol. Odors are either presented several times in ascending concentrations (ascending method of limits) or in a single staircase (different odor concentrations are presented in both ascending and descending orders around the level of the "threshold"). In addition, all tests involve **odor-identification** tasks. The most widely used olfactory test in the United States—the self-administered UPSIT—is based solely on this task. Various versions of the UPSIT have been established, including tests used for rapid screening (3 items) and the thorough chemosensory investigation (40 items). Odor identification is typically performed using multiple-choice lists of verbal descriptors, with the number of items correctly identified being the test measure. Other tests of olfactory function include **odor memory**, **odor discrimination**, **intensity scaling**, and **differential thresholds**.

Specialized testing may include electroencephalography-derived measures such as the recording of **olfactory brain potentials**. These responses seem to be especially helpful in cases in which anosmia needs to be definitively verified. In the United States, these recordings are available in only a few specialized centers, including the Smell and Taste Center at the University of Pennsylvania (*see* list of centers at the end of this chapter for contact information) and San Diego State University's Department of Psychology (San Diego, California; 619-594-4559).

Treatment

Therapeutic possibilities in olfactory disorders are limited. Therapy has been proven to be effective only for olfactory dysfunction due to nasal and sinus diseases (Case 33.2). Specifically, both **surgery** (e.g., antrostomy, polypectomy, sinusotomy, ethmoidectomy) and topical or systemic **corticosteroids**

Case 33.2 **Man with Hyposmia Caused by Nasal Polyps**

A man 54 years of age is distressed with his lack of ability to smell any but the strongest odors, a condition that has worsened gradually over the past 5 years. He also has noted increasing nasal obstruction and an increasing number of episodes of acute sinusitis that have required antibiotic therapy for resolution.

Fiberoptic rhinoscopy reveals multiple nasal polyps, filling both nasal cavities.

After pretreatment with a short course of oral steroids, the patient undergoes nasal polypectomy and endoscopic sinus surgery. After an uneventful recovery from the surgery, he regains his sense of smell.

may be helpful. In both steroid-dependent hyposmia and anosmia, high doses of steroids restore sense of smell. A trial of high-dose steroids may serve as a diagnostic test; if the sense of smell returns, then low-dose, long-term steroid therapy can be used to maintain olfactory sensitivity. A different approach to the treatment of olfactory disorders is the **detection and treatment of underlying causes**, which may also involve the **discontinuation and replacement of drugs** that are suspected to affect the sense of smell (*see* Table 33.2).

Studies with **zinc** have produced controversial results; however, zinc may be of therapeutic value in patients with zinc deficiency (e.g., hemodialysis patients). Studies have suggested that **estrogens** may provide some protection against olfactory disturbances. Consequently, despite the lack of adequate studies, estrogens may be tried in appropriate cases. The therapeutic use of orally administered **vitamin A** also may be tried on a similar basis.

The management of olfactory disorders is outlined in Algorithm A.

Gustatory Disorders

Physiology

Gustatory receptor cells are located within the taste buds of the visible papillae (~250 buds per circumvallate papilla). Taste cells are known to have regenerative capabilities, with an approximate life span of 10 to 20 days. Afferent nerves make contact with the receptor cells at the base of the taste bud. A single taste bud may be innervated by several afferents, and a single fiber may innervate several taste buds. Fungiform papillae are found on the anterior portion of the tongue, whereas circumvallate and foliate papillae are located on the posterior portion of the tongue.

Transduction of sour stimuli (H^+) may be produced by the block of K^+-channels in the membrane of taste receptors. Voltage independent Na^+-channels are involved in the transduction of salty stimuli. The transduction of sweet and bitter stimuli seems to involve specific membrane receptors that are linked to second messenger systems (e.g., cAMP, IP_3).

Gustatory sensations are mediated via three different pathways: 1) sensory branches of cranial nerve (CN) VII, which innervate the taste buds of the anterior part of the tongue (chorda tympani) and the palate (greater superficial petrosal nerves); 2) CN IX (lingual tonsillar branch), which innervates taste buds of the posterior tongue; and 3) CN X (superior laryngeal nerve), which innervates taste buds in the oropharynx and on the pharyngeal part of the epiglottis. In addition, the trigeminal nerve contributes to taste-mediating sensations such as texture, spiciness, and warmth. This diverse innervation may explain why loss of the sense of taste is much less frequent than is the loss of the sense of smell.

Taste sensitivity has been shown to decrease with age, but these findings are less robust compared with those of olfaction. As with the sense of smell, there are gender-related differences in the sense of taste, with women being more sensitive than men.

Definition

Ageusia describes a complete loss of taste. **Hypogeusia** is a diminished sense of taste. **Hypergeusia** refers to an enhanced gustatory sensitivity. **Dysgeusia** relates to a distorted taste perception, which is by far the most common complaint in self-identified patients with gustatory disorders. In patients with dysgeusia, gustatory stimuli are reported to be different from what they had been previously (i.e., they are often perceived to be bitter or metallic). **Taste hallucinations** have been reported in both epilepsy and schizophrenia.

Etiology

Overall, gustatory dysfunction is rare, occurring in less than 5% of all patients who present to specialized clinics with complaints of altered or lost taste or smell. Although the majority of the patients report taste loss, most of them suffer from loss of olfactory sensitivity. It is the olfactory loss that contributes to the loss of the perception of flavor (*see* above). Major causes of gustatory sensitivity are **head trauma, infections of the upper respiratory tract, exposure to toxic substances, iatrogenic causes** (e.g., dental procedures or radiation), **drugs**, and **burning-mouth syndrome**.

Head trauma is thought to produce lesions that involve the processing of gustatory sensations (i.e., in the thalamus, brainstem, or ventral forebrain). Fractures of the mandibular and temporal bones may lead to CN VII damage, whereas CN IX and X are relatively well protected in the depth of the neck. Recovery is possible. For example, in cases where the chorda tympani is sectioned bilaterally, complete restitution of gustatory function has been reported after several months in approximately 20% of the patients. The chorda tympani is a sensory branch of the facial nerve (CN VII) that carries taste sensation from the anterior two thirds of the tongue. For part of its route back to the brain, it is suspended within the middle ear space, making it susceptible to surgical trauma, blunt head trauma, and infections.

Infections may involve the taste buds, the nerves innervating the taste buds, or the central structures of the brain. CN VII is especially vulnerable to infections (e.g., herpes zoster [Ramsey–Hunt syndrome]) where it travels through the middle ear. A large number of drugs have been implicated in the etiology of taste disorders (Table 33.3); however, little is known about the mechanisms that underlie these changes. For some drugs, interference with gustatory sensations seems obvious—there are those that decrease salivation (e.g., drugs with

Table 33.3 Drugs Considered To Be Possible Causes of Gustatory Disturbances

Amebicides, antihelmintics (e.g., metronidazole)
Antibiotics, antimycotic drugs (e.g., amphotericin B, griseofulvine, ampicillin, cefamandol, tetracycline, bleomycin, lincomycin, ethambutol)
Antiepileptics (e.g., carbamazepine, phenytoin)
Antigout drugs (e.g., allopurinol, colchicine)
Antihistamine (e.g., chlorpheniramine, trifluoperazine)
Antiproliferatives, immunosuppressives (e.g., doxorubicin, methotrexate, azathioprine, vincristine)
Antirheumatics (e.g., gold, D-penicillamine, phenylbutazone)
Antiseptics (e.g., hexetidine)
Antithyroid drugs (e.g., thiouracil, methimazole, carbimazole, thiouracil)
Corticosteroids (e.g., dexamethasone, hydrocortisone)
Dental hygiene agents (e.g., sodium lauryl sulfate, chlorhexidine)
Diuretics, antihypertensive agents (e.g., acetazolamide, amiloride, captopril, diazoxid, diltiazem, enalapril, ethacrynic acid, nifedipine)
Hyperlipoproteinemia drugs (e.g., clofibrate)
Antidiabetics (e.g., glipizide, phenformin)
Local anesthetics (e.g., tetracaine, benzocaine, lidocaine)
Muscle relaxants, antiparkinson drugs (e.g., baclofen, chlormezanone, levodopa)
Psychopharmaceuticals (e.g., amphetamine, psilocybin)
Vasodilators (e.g., dipyridamole, nitroglycerin)
Others (e.g., etidronate, iron, phenindione, lithium)

anticholinergic effects such as tricyclic antidepressants) and those that damage the intraoral mucosa (e.g., antiproliferative drugs such as vincristine). Recent studies indicate that the function of gustatory Na^+-channels may be modulated by hormones, growth factors, and cytokines, which might help explain the gustatory changes in several diseases of internal medicine.

Burning-mouth syndrome is an intraoral pain disorder that is frequently associated with dysgeusia and often described as the persistent presence of a metallic or bitter taste. Other symptoms include dry mouth and thirst. Frequently, burning increases throughout the day. It is most prevalent in postmenopausal women. Partial spontaneous remission may occur in approximately half of these patients within 6 years of onset. Possible causes include psychological (e.g., anxiety, depression), hormonal (e.g., estrogen-related changes), and nutritional (e.g., deficiency of zinc and vitamins B_1, B_2, B_6).

Other causes of taste dysfunction may include **neoplasms, depression, bulimia** (Case 33.3), **hypothyroidism, Cushing's syndrome** (with an apparent inverse relation between the plasma level of glucocorticosteroids and taste sensitivity), **diabetes mellitus, liver disease,** and **renal disease. Poor oral hygiene** may be another factor.

> **Case 33.3** **Young Woman with Bulimia Presents with Dysgeusia**
>
> A woman 24 years of age presents with complaints of a chronic bad taste in her mouth. She has been treated recently for presumed sinusitis, with no change in her sense of taste.
>
> Physical examination reveals mild bilateral parotid swelling. The patient also has had multiple recent restorations of dental caries. These findings prompt you to ask her about diet and eating habits. She eventually tells you that she has been in the habit of intermittently eating large meals and then forcing herself to vomit as a means of weight control. At the end of your lengthy discussion, she agrees to a referral to a dietitian and a therapist.
>
> At follow-up, 6 months later, the patient reports that she no longer engages in bulimic behavior, and the bad taste in her mouth is gradually resolving.

Diagnostic Evaluation

Evaluation of the patient with a taste disorder should be performed similarly to the evaluation of patients with a smell disorder mentioned above. A special focus on the oral cavity and the ear canal is necessary because the lesions of the chorda tympani may be present. The **history** should focus on dentures, dental procedures, salivary status, and, of course, the sense of taste. It has been reported that, in a patient who answers the question "Do you have trouble tasting salt, sweet, sour, bitter?" with a "No," there is a 94% chance he or she has no measurable taste deficit for the four basic tastes. The history also should include questions related to salivation, swallowing, chewing, oral pain, previous ear infections (possibly indicated by hearing or balance problems), oral hygiene, and stomach problems. **Radiologic evaluation** should be directed toward possible central nervous lesions in the brainstem, thalamus, or pons. **Cultures** are indicated when fungal or bacterial infections are suspected.

Additional diagnostic tests should include the search for other underlying causes of the taste disorder (e.g., diabetes, hypothyroidism). **Olfactory assessment** (as described earlier in this chapter) is needed to complete the patient's evaluation.

Gustatory Testing

Gustatory testing is performed as either a whole-mouth or a regional procedure, and both natural and electrical stimuli are used. Regional tests give the most precise source of information about gustatory function. Frequently,

20 to 50 μL of liquid stimuli are presented to the anterior and posterior part of the tongue. Other methods are based on taste stimuli presented to the tongue by either soaked filter-paper disks or cotton swabs. In contrast, whole-mouth testing is a way to quantify "real world" taste function. Small quantities (2–10 mL) of tastant solution are kept in the oral cavity for a few seconds and then spat out (i.e., the "sip and spit" method); the solution should not be swallowed.

Tests for the natural-stimuli threshold are typically performed with sucrose (sweet), citric acid (sour), sodium chloride (salty), and quinine or caffeine (bitter). Among the methods used is the two-alternative, forced-choice, detection-threshold procedure in which solutions are sampled from two cups (one containing the tastant, the other water), with the mouth rinsed out between trials. The patient is forced to identify the cup with the tastant. As with the assessment of olfactory thresholds using the previously described single-staircase procedure, it is possible to track and, finally, to determine the threshold with this method.

One of the most frequently used techniques is the **"three-drop test."** In this test, three drops of liquid (one of them the taste stimulus, the other two pure water) of less than 0.1 mL are presented to the subject. The threshold is defined as the concentration at which the patient correctly identifies the tastant three times consecutively.

Electrogustometry is based on the induction of gustatory sensations by means of an anodal direct current (DC) of electricity. For example, in patients with a sectioned chorda tympani, detection thresholds have been reported to be significantly higher than in controls. Electrogustometry is widely used; however, recent investigations indicated a poor correlation between electrically and chemically induced sensations, which may limit the clinical applications of this test (especially with respect to the diagnosis of dysgeusia).

Suprathreshold tests are used to assess a patient's ability to discriminate different intensities and to estimate the magnitude of suprathreshold loss. Estimates of pleasantness are of value in the diagnosis of dysgeusia. Although many of the tests are based on ratings by means of visual analogue scales, some of these methods use magnitude-matching procedures in which patients estimate the intensity of a series of weights and compare them with a concentration series of sucrose, sodium chloride, citric acid, and caffeine. Other tests include the identification or discrimination of common taste substances.

Topical anesthesia has been reported to be helpful in the diagnosis of dysgeusia. Because the sensorial function of a certain area of the oral cavity can be anesthetized, the disappearance of a dysgeusic sensation indicates the particular gustatory pathways involved in the generation of the taste distortion. Additionally, in cases of peripheral origin, a drastic reduction of dysgeusia has been observed after topical antibiotic use.

Treatment

As with olfactory disturbances, there are few therapeutic options. Treatment with zinc is frequently tried despite the equivocal results of clinical studies. Similarly, both systemic **corticoids** and **vitamin A** have been used to treat taste disorders despite the lack of convincing clinical studies. **The main focus of gustatory disorder therapy is the search for and therapy of possible underlying diseases**, which includes a thorough revision of any drugs taken by the patient (*see* Table 33.3).

In **burning-mouth syndrome**, the use of low-dose tricyclic antidepressants (e.g., imipramine, amitriptyline) has been found to relieve dysgeusia. Other therapeutic approaches include the use of clonazepam. The management of specific gustatory disorders is shown in Algorithm B.

Danger Signs

Patients who present with an acute loss of smell should have a comprehensive history taken to evaluate concomitant symptoms. The presence of other sinonasal symptoms (e.g., unilaterality of symptoms, discharge, bleeding, optical problems) should prompt immediate referral to rule out a neoplastic process. Anosmia with nasal obstruction requires a thorough evaluation of the nasal cavities.

Summary

Disturbances of the chemical senses occur frequently and can affect our lives severely. Appropriate testing is needed to determine the nature of a patient's complaints. Because many chemosensory disorders are secondary to a wide variety of diseases (e.g., Parkinson's disease), olfactory and/or gustatory complaints may help in the development of certain differential diagnoses. In turn, treating the underlying disease may restore chemosensory function in these patients.

More research is needed because therapeutic options for chemosensory disorders are limited. In this context, the unique regenerative capabilities of the olfactory epithelium are thought to be of special significance. Future developments also seem to be possible with the use of the standardized tools that have been developed over the past decade for assessing chemosensory dysfunction.

Centers That Specialize in the Evaluation of Smell and Taste

Smell and Taste Center. University of Pennsylvania; Philadelphia, Pennsylvania; 215-662-6580.

Connecticut Chemosensory Clinical Research Center. University of Connecticut; Farmington, Connecticut; 860-679-2459.

SUNY Upstate Clinical Smell Research Center. Syracuse, New York; 315-473-5591.

Monell Chemical Senses Center. Philadelphia, Pennsylvania; 215-898-6666.

Rocky Mountain Taste and Smell Center. University of Colorado; Denver, Colorado; 303-315-5650.

SUGGESTED READING

Beauchamp GK, Bartoshuk LM. *Handbook of Perception and Cognition: Tasting and Smelling.* San Diego: Academic Press; 1997.

An excellent overview of the physiology and pathophysiology of taste and smell.

Doty RL. *Handbook of Olfaction and Gustation.* New York: Marcel Dekker; 1995.

Another detailed resource for physiology and abnormal mechanisms of taste and smell disorders.

Getchell TV, Doty RL, Bartoshuk LM, Snow JB Jr. *Smell and Taste in Health and Disease.* New York: Raven Press; 1991.

Seiden AM. *Taste and Smell Disorders.* New York: Thieme; 1997.

These two references discuss the clinical occurrences of taste and smell disorders, their evaluation, and possible treatments.

Index

Note: *f* following page number indicates figure; *t* indicates table.

A-beta fibers, 481
A-delta fibers, 479
Abductor muscle paralysis, 350
Abscess, CNS, 126
Acetylsalicylic acid, 405
Achalasia, 292
  balloon dilatation of, 301-302
  with caustic ingestion, 601
Acid corrosives, 593
Acid ingestion, 596-597
Acidosis, upper airway obstruction, 344
Acoustic nerve, malfunction of, 59-60
Acoustic neuroma, 122-123
  computed tomographic scan of, 62*f*
  in hearing loss, 61
Acoustic-reflex testing, 61
Acquired immunodeficiency syndrome (AIDS)
  Kaposi's sarcoma in, 263
  laryngeal, and pharyngeal manifestations of, 644-645
  mycobacterial infections in, 642
  nasal and sinus manifestations of, 643-644
  nasopharyngeal fungal infections with, 272-273
  neck manifestations of, 645-646
  necrotizing otitis externa in, 40
  oral cavity lesions of, 234, 250, 644-645
  otologic manifestations of, 642-643
  salivary gland manifestations of, 647
Actinic keratosis
  diagnosis and management of, 507-509
  treatment options for, 510*t*
Actinomyces infection
  in granulomatous lymphadenopathy, 404
  in inflammatory neck masses, 421
Actinomycosis
  in granulomatous lymphadenopathy, 404
  salivary involvement in, 440-441
Acupuncture, for hiccups, 565
Acyclovir
  for Behçet's syndrome, 241
  for chemical peel infection, 544-545
  for facial paralysis, 496

for herpes zoster oticus, 493
Addison's disease, vertigo with, 124
Adenoid cystic carcinoma, 277, 442
  epistaxis with, 210
  external auditory canal, 100*f*
  of minor salivary gland, 262*f*
  parotid, 443*f*
  salivary, 417
Adenoid pad, 266
Adenoid tissue, 272*f*
Adenoidectomy, 274
  for obstructive sleep apnea, 318
Adenoids, 274
Adenoma, thyroid gland, 411
Adenopathy, mediastinal, 334
Adnexal lesions, 516
Adrenocortical insufficiency, 124
Aerodigestive tract, foreign bodies in, 567-590
Afrin, 212, 214
Agammaglobulinemia, X-linked, 641
Ageusia, 659
Aging
  dizziness with, 128
  in sensorineural hearing loss, 68
AIDS-associated salivary gland cysts, 444
Air-conduction hearing, 63
  audiogram of, 65*f*, 66*f*
Airway
  after laryngectomy, 576*f*
  foreign bodies in
    asymptomatic phase of, 569
    complications of, 577, 578*t*
    delayed diagnosis of, 567-569
    diagnostic evaluation for, 570
    differential diagnosis of, 570*t*
    impairment from, 567
    management of, 570-576
    physical examination for, 569-570
    symptoms of, 569*t*
  normal anatomy of, 576*f*
  obstruction of
    with goiter, 462-463
    subglottic, 347-350
    with supraglottic cancer, 628
  protection against esophageal foreign body, 583

Airway—*continued*
　stabilization of with caustic burn injury, 597-598
　support of for upper airway obstruction, 346-347
　tracheostomy tube in, 576*f*
Airway-protective mechanisms, 577
Alcohol abuse
　in aerodigestive tract squamous cell carcinoma, 260
　in dysphagia, 288
　in head and neck cancer, 632
Alimentary tract reconstruction, 600
Alkali burns, 595
Alkali ingestion, 596
Alkaline batteries, ingestion of, 593-594
Alkaline substances, 593-594
Allergen-specific IgE, 165
Allergic disorders
　in differential diagnosis of dizziness, 114*t*
　immunotherapy for, 175-176
　in itchy ears, 86
　of nose and sinuses, 169-174
　of oral cavity, 240-246
　vertigo with, 124
Allergic fungal sinusitis, 172-173
　computed tomography of, 174*f*
　thick inspissated pus of, 175*f*
Allergic rhinitis, 169-172, 195
　eustachian tube dysfunction with, 128
　management algorithm for, 162*f*
　pale nasal mucosa with, 20
　topical cromolyn sodium for, 196
Allergic rhinosinusitis, 93
　in aural itching, 88
　management of, 87*f*
Allergy
　diagnosis of, 161-165
　impaired sinus drainage with, 183-184
　inhalant, 271-272
　in throat, 174-175
　triggers of, 163-164
　　in nasal obstruction, 150
Allergy dipstick test, 165
Alligator forceps, 42
Alpha-hydroxy acids, 541
　before chemical peeling, 542
Alzheimer's disease, 654
Amalgam tattoo, 263*f*
Aminoglycosides
　dizziness and, 127, 129
　for necrotizing otitis externa, 40
　in tinnitus, 134
　transtympanic, for Meniere's disease, 115
Amitriptyline
　for atypical odontalgia, 487
　for burning-mouth syndrome, 663
　for hiccups, 564*t*, 565
Amoxicillin
　for acute otitis media, 45
　for acute sinusitis, 182
　for furunculosis, 42
　for rhinosinusitis, 193-194
Amoxicillin/clavulanate (Augmentin), 45
Amphotericin, 194
Amphotericin B
　for AIDS-related oral candidiasis, 250
　for *Histoplasma capsulatum*, 252
　for histoplasmosis, 405, 424
　for mucormycosis, 638
　　with diabetes, 639
　for oral thrush, 644
Ampicillin, 45
Ampulla, 102-104
Amyloidomas, nasopharyngeal, 276
Amyloidosis, 361
Anaplastic thyroid carcinoma, 420
Anemia, pernicious, 289
Anesthesia, topical, 662
Angiocath, large-gauge, 570-572
Angioedema
　angiotensin-converting enzyme inhibitor-associated, 358-360
　hereditary, 360
　in supraglottic obstruction, 358
　in upper airway obstruction, 344
Angiofibroma
　juvenile nasal, with epistaxis, 211
　juvenile nasopharyngeal, 210
　of nasal vault, 209*f*
Angiography
　for hemangiomas, 401
　for tinnitus, 137
Angioneurotic edema, medication-induced, 255
Angiotensin-converting enzyme inhibitors
　in angioedema, 358-360
　in angioneurotic edema, 255
　for upper airway obstruction, 345
Angular vein thrombophlebitis, 18
Animal bites, facial, 538
Ankyloglossia, 238
Anosmia, 538, 654

after upper respiratory infection, 656
congenital, 654
in nasal obstruction, 151, 159, 663
in nasopharyngeal disorders, 267
steroid-dependent, 658
Anterior compartment lymph nodes, 388
anatomical areas drained by, 388*t*
Antibiotics
after cerumen curettage and suction, 85
for chronic otitis media, 46
for diffuse bacterial external otitis, 38-39
for necrotizing otitis externa, 40
ointment for epistaxis, 213, 214
prophylactic for caustic ingestion, 599
for rhinosinusitis, 193-194
for upper airway obstruction, 347
Anticholinergics
for dizziness, 128-129
in dysphagia, 295
Anticonvulsants, 565
Antidepressants, 295
tricyclic, 481, 486, 487, 663
Antidote procedures, 593
Antiemetics, 128-129
Antifungals
for rhinosinusitis, 194, 196
for seborrheic dermatitis of ear, 99
Antihistamines
for allergic rhinitis, 169, 170, 171
for allergic rhinosinusitis, 93
in dysphagia, 295
laryngeal dryness with, 337
in nasal spray, 195
for rhinosinusitis, 179, 195-196
Antihypertensives, 295
Antimalarial drugs, 134
Antimetabolite agents, 241
Antimicrobials
broad-spectrum, for rhinosinusitis, 194
for necrotizing otitis externa, 40
resistance to, 192-193
for rhinosinusitis, 179
Antireflux medications, 301
Antrochoanal polyps, 274
Aphthous stomatitis, AIDS-related, 250, 644
Aphthous ulcers
in AIDS patients, 234
in Crohn's disease, 244, 246*f*
multiple, 245*f*
recurrent, 240-241
stress-associated, 245
Aplastic thyroid carcinoma, 467

Aristotle, 11
Arnold-Chiari malformation
in dysphagia, 286
in vocal cord paralysis, 352-353
Arnold's nerve, 50-51
Arrhythmia
dizziness with, 126
with sleep apnea, 308
Arteriography, 153
Arteriovenous malformation, 138
Aryepiglottic folds, 17*f*
Arytenoid adduction, 377
Arytenoid cartilage, 4
Arytenoids, 17*f*
Aspergillosis, labyrinth, 118
Aspergillus
flavus otomycosis, 40-41
fumigatus, 40-41
niger, 40-41
sinusitis with neutropenia, 638-640
Aspiration, 378-379
after stroke, 367
causes and complications of, 365-371
of caustics, 595
chronic, 364
signs of, 365*t*
classic presentation of, 363
diagnostic evaluation of, 371-373
in dysphagia, 298-299
with head and neck cancer, 367
management algorithm for, 364*f*
management of, 302, 373-378
massive, 363-364
signs of, 365*t*
modified barium swallow demonstrating, 298*f*
in pharyngeal and oral disorders, 284
stroke and neurological diseases in, 365, 366*t*
with tracheostomy, 369-371
with vocal cord paralysis, 368-369
Aspiration pneumonia, 366
Aspirin
in dizziness, 127
in epistaxis, 215
in tinnitus, 134
Assisted-listening devices, 69-70, 73*f*
Atherosclerosis
dizziness with, 125-126
epistaxis with, 210
Atomizers, 6
Atopic dermatitis, 97

Audiograms, 63-64
  for sensorineural hearing loss, 68
  showing air- and bone-conduction lines, 65*f*, 66*f*
Audiologic testing
  for facial paralysis, 494-495
  for tinnitus, 137
Audiologic testing booth, 67*f*
Audiometric testing, 110-111
Auditory brainstem response test, 61, 67*f*
  for dizziness, 103*f*, 111
  for hearing loss, 65-66
  for tinnitus, 141
Auditory canal
  anatomic relationships of, 55*f*
  external
    adenoid cystic carcinoma of, 100*f*
    anatomy of, 55-56, 75, 86
    beefy or ulcerative lesion of, 99
    cellulitis of, 590
    curettage and suction of, 78-80
    disorders of, 40-43
    epithelial migration in, 77
    foreign bodies in, 588-589
      management of, 589-590
    inflammatory polyp of, 48*f*
    irrigating device in, 82*f*
    lacerations of, 590
    mycelial elements in, 42*f*
    otoscopic evaluation of, 31
    physiology of, 86
    pruritus of, 86
    skin dryness of, 86
    traumatized with cerumen removal, 84
    ulcerating squamous cell carcinoma of, 96*f*
Auditory meatus, external, 54
Auditory rehabilitation, 68
Auditory system
  central, 53
  peripheral, 53
Aural discharge, 70-71
Aural itching, 100-101
  causes of, 86
  danger signs in, 99-100
  diagnosis of
    local causes, 88-96
    systemic dermatologic disease in, 97-99
  history of, 88
  management algorithm for, 87*f*
  physical examination for, 88
Aural polyps, 100
Aural syringing, 40
Auralgen, 43
Auricle
  anatomy of, 54
  deformity of, 37*f*
  disorders of, 35-39
    treatment of, 36*t*
  trauma to, 35
    hematoma with, 37*f*
    treatment of, 36*t*
Auricular chondritis, 38*f*
Auriculitis, 36
Auscultation, 136
Auspitz's sign, 98
Autoimmune disease
  in dysphagia, 281*t*, 288-289
  of inner ear, 124
  oral, 240-246
  subglottic stenosis with, 347-348
  in sudden hearing loss, 69
Autoimmune hyperthyroidism, 465
Autoimmune interstitial keratitis, 124
Autoimmune stomatitis, 234
Autolaryngoscope, 4
Avatene, 212
Azelastine (Astelin), 170

B-cell lymphomas, non-Hodgkin's, 420
Bacitracin, 213, 214
Baclofen, 564*t*, 565
Bacteremia, 258
Bacterial external otitis, diffuse, 36-39
Bacterial infections
  life-threatening with neutropenia, 640
  in neck masses, 423-424
  oral cavity, 234
Bacterial lymphadenopathy, 402
Bactroban, 213, 214
Balance impairment, age-related, 128
Ball valve foreign body, 571*f*
Balloon-catheter dilatation
  of achalasia, 301-302
  for caustic ingestion, 601
  for esophageal foreign body, 584-585
Barium esophagography
  for advanced oral cavity cancer, 613
  for dysphagia, 297
Barium swallow
  for esophageal foreign body, 583
  modified
    for aspiration, 371-372
    for dysphagia, 297-299

in swallowing evaluation, 284-285
Barotrauma, otitic, 47-49
Barrett's esophagus, 292
  diagnosis of, 294
  esophagoscopy for, 300*f*
Bartonella (Rochalimaea) henselae, 403
Basal cell carcinoma
  differential diagnosis of, 508
  of face or scalp, 512-515
  in H zone, 514
  of head, 506
  versus keratoacanthoma, 510*t*
  over cheek, 514*f*
  sclerosing or morpheic type, 513
  stages of reconstruction in, 519*f*
Basilar artery aneurysm, 126
Battery acid ingestion, 594
Bayonet forceps, 207
Beclomethasone, 194
Behçet's syndrome, 241
Bell's palsy
  diagnosis of, 495
  facial nerve injury in, 491
  family history of, 494
  features of, 492-493
  herpes simplex virus I in, 496
  treatment of, 492, 496-497
Benadryl, 241
Benign familial hypocalciuric hypercalcemia, 471
Benign lymphoepithelial lesions, 438
Benign paroxysmal positional vertigo, 119
  canalith repositioning procedure for, 121*f*
  case history of, 120
Benign tumors
  oral, 258-260
  upper airway, 348*t*
Benzodiazepam
  for cholesteatoma, 123
  for vestibular neuronitis, 117
Bernoulli effect, 349*f*
Bernstein test, 291
Bimanual examination
  for salivary gland disorders, 432-433
  for suppurative sialadenitis, 436
Bimaxillary advancement, 317-318
Biofeedback, 140-141
Biopsy. *See also* Fine-needle-aspiration biopsy
  for advanced oral cavity cancer, 613
  for facial and scalp skin malignancy, 507
  for head and neck cancers, 609
  for mucosal lesions, 261
  for nasal obstruction, 157-158
  for olfactory disorders, 656
Bipolaris, 173
Birch shampoo, 167*f*
Black hairy tongue, 238
  treatment of, 242-244
Blastomycosis, labyrinth, 118
Bleaching compounds, prophylactic, 546
Blepharoplasty
  before and after, 552*f*
  lower-eyelid, 549-550, 551*f*
  upper-eyelid, 549
Blistering, chemical peel infection, 544-545
Blood-clotting abnormalities, 210-212
Blood oxygenation, 344
Blow out fracture, zygomatic, 529, 530*f*
Bone-conducting hearing aid, 72*f*
Bone-conduction hearing, 63
  audiogram of, 65*f*, 66*f*
Bone-mineral density, 460
Bony-cartilaginous spur, 198
Bony exostoses, 89, 90*f*
Bony labyrinth, structures of, 104*f*
Bony reduction, nasal fracture, 225
Botulinum toxin
  for facial rejuvenation, 548-549
  for functional inspiratory adduction, 355
Bozzini, Phillip, 4
Brachytherapy, 622*f*
Bradycardia, 308
Brain
  aspiration after injury to, 373
  auditory areas of, 53
  catarrhal secretions from, 2-3
  in hearing, 56
Brain breathing, 1-2
Brainstem, 56
Brainstem auditory evoked response, 65-66
Brainstem evoked response, 65-66
Branchial abnormalities
  first, 397
  second, 397, 398*f*
  third, 397-398
Branchial cleft
  cysts of, 396-398
  fistula of, 396-398
  sinuses, 396-398
Branhamella catarrhalis tonsillitis, 249
Breath of Life (Caitlin), 3-4
Breslow's staging, 517*t*
Bronchorrhea, 369
Bronchoscope, rigid, 573-575
Bronchoscopy, 583-584

Bronchus, dental appliance in, 572*f*
Bruits, 136
Buccal linea alba, 257
Buccal mucosa, 231
Buccogingival sulcus, 231
Budesonide (Rhinocort)
  for allergic rhinitis, 170, 172
  for rhinosinusitis, 194
Bulimia, in gustatory dysfunction, 660, 661
Bullous myringitis, 43
  blebs of, 44*f*
Bullous pemphigoid, oral, 244
Burkitt's lymphoma, 413*f*
Burning-mouth syndrome, 483
  differential diagnosis of, 485-486
  in gustatory dysfunction, 659, 660
  treatment of, 663
Burns, depth of, 597
Burow's aluminum solution (Domeboro), 93
Burton's agammaglobulinemia, 641
Button batteries
  in external auditory canal, 589
  ingestion of, 593-594

C1-esterase inhibitors, 360
C fibers, 479, 481
Caitlin, George, 3-4
Calcipotriene, 98
Calcitonin
  serum levels with medullary thyroid carcinoma, 420
  in thyroid disorders, 454
Calcium-channel blockers, 255
Calcium levels, 454
Caldwell-Luc procedure, 199
Caloric testing
  for dizziness, 109-110
  results of, 110*t*
Canalicular apparatus, injuries to, 537
Canalith repositioning, 119
  for benign paroxysmal positional vertigo, 121*f*
Canalithiasis, trauma-related, 119
Cancer
  esophageal, dysphagia with, 293-294
  glottic, 337
  head and neck, 604-632
    aspiration with, 367
  laryngeal, 293, 336
  nasopharyngeal, 392*f*
  obstructing supraglottic, 355-356, 357*f*
  oral cavity, 260-261
  danger signs suggesting, 234*t*
  oropharyngeal, 260-261
  of pharynx, 293
  staging of, 609-610
  thyroid, 466-468
  of tongue, 608
  of vocal folds, 333-335
Candida
  albicans
    oral, 251
    in otomycosis, 40-41
    with chemical peel, 544
Candidiasis
  AIDS-related oropharyngeal and esophageal, 250
  in dysphagia, 289
  esophageal, 302
  of labyrinth, 118
  oral, 252*f*
    diabetes-associated, 244
Canker sores, 240-241
Carbamazepine, 140
Carbenicillin, 210
Carbogen, 129
Carbon dioxide laser, 545-546
Carcinoma
  with caustic ingestion, 601
  in esophageal foreign bodies, 578
  ex-pleomorphic adenoma, salivary, 417-418
  in itchy ear, 96
Cardano, Gerolamo, 2
Cardiac arrhythmia
  dizziness with, 126
  with sleep apnea, 308
Cardiovascular disease
  in differential diagnosis of dizziness, 114*t*
  in dysphagia, 281*t*
  risk of with hyperparathyroidism, 472-473
  vertigo with, 124-126
Carotid angiography, 137
Carotid arteries, 202
  in nasal mucosa, 204*f*
Carotid bruits, 107
Carotid endarterectomy, 352
Carotid massage, 564
Carotid paraganglioma, 408-409
Carotidynia, 482-483
  diagnosis of, 484
Cartilaginous folds, external ear, 18*f*
Cat-scratch disease, 403
  skin test for, 422

Catarrh, 2-3
Cauliflower ears, 35
Caustic burns, grading system of, 598
Caustic ingestion, 592
 danger signs for, 601-602
 epidemiology of, 593-594
 initial evaluation for, 598
 oral burns from, 257, 258f
 relevant anatomy and physiology of, 595-597
 social history of, 592-593
 stabilization and resuscitation for, 597-598
 treatment and follow-up for, 599-601
Cautery, nasal, 212-213
Cavernous lymphangioma, 399-400
Cavernous sinus thrombophlebitis, 18
Cefaclor (Ceclor), 45
Cefpodoxime proxetil, 193
Cefprozil, 193
Ceftazidime, 40, 194
Cefuroxime axetil, 193
Cefuroxime (Ceftin), 45
Cellulitis, pharyngeal, 588
Central nervous system diseases
 in differential diagnosis of dizziness, 114t
 dizziness with, 126-127
Cephalexin, 544
Cephalgia, 189
Cerebellar disorders, 127
Cerebellar function, 108
Cerebellopontile angle, 491
 acoustic neuroma in, 62f
 masses of
  diagnosis and management of, 122-123
  in dizziness, 112
Cerebral cortex, 56
Cerebral secretions, 2
Cerebral ventricles, 2
Cerebrospinal fluid leakage
 with facial trauma, 537-538
 with nasal fractures, 220, 226
Cerebrovascular accident, aspiration after, 373
Cerumen, 56, 86
 composition of, 75-77
 in dizziness, 128
 impacted, 134
 impaction of, 40
  danger signs of, 84
  direct removal of, 78-80
  etiology of, 77

 history and physical examination in, 77
 incidence of, 75
 irrigation of, 81-83
 management algorithm for, 76f
 management and follow-up for, 78-84
 prevention of, 84
 relevant anatomy and physiology of, 75-77
 removal of, 58
 topical antibiotic drops after curettage and suction for, 85
 types of, 76-77
Cerumen curettes, 78, 80f
Cerumenolytics, 83-84
Cervical artery, lymph nodes along, 387
Cervical arthritis, 479
Cervical lymph nodes, 387, 391
Cervical lymphadenopathy, 252
 examination for, 454
 viral, 401-402
Cervical metastasis, 413-416
 in glottic cancer, 624
 non-squamous, 412
Cervical osteophytes, 260
Cervical plexus, benign tumors of, 406-407
Cervical spine
 disease of, 292-293
 injury to, 523-524
Cervicofacial actinomycosis, 251
Cetirizine, 195-196
Charcot-Leyden crystals, 173
Cheeks
 basal cell carcinoma over, 514f
 rejuvenation surgery for, 550
 squamous cell carcinoma of, 515f
 swelling of in nasal obstruction, 159
Chemical cauterization, 485
Chemical peeling, 541-543
 complications of, 543-545
 depth of, 542-543
 inadequate depth of, 543-544
 uneven, 543
Chemodectomas, 407
Chemoradiation, 467
Chemotherapy
 in dizziness, 127
 for head and neck squamous cell cancer, 610-611
 for malignant melanoma of head and neck, 517
 for nasopharyngeal carcinoma, 611
 oral lesions with, 234

Chemotherapy-induced mucositis, 252, 254
Chemotherapy-induced stomatitis, 253*f*
Chest physical therapy, 576
Chest radiography
　for advanced oral cavity cancer, 613
　for airway foreign bodies, 570
　for esophageal foreign body, 580-582
　for goiter, 463
　for hiccups, 562
　for malignant neck masses, 422
Chevers, Norman, 11
Chlorambucil, 241
Chloramphenicol, 210
Chlorpheniramine (Chlortrimeton), 170
Chlorpromazine (Thorazine), 564-565
Choanal atresia, 275
　CT scan showing, 158*f*
Cholesteatoma, 66, 100
　in facial paralysis, 498
　vertigo with, 123
Cholesterol granuloma, 62*f*
Cholinergic drugs, 302
Chondritis
　auricular, 36, 38*f*
　early signs of, 100
Ciprofloxacin
　for AIDS-related sinusitis, 643
　for furunculosis, 42
　for necrotizing otitis, 635
　for necrotizing otitis externa, 40
　for *Pseudomonas aeruginosa* ear infection, 96
　for rhinosinusitis, 194
Circummandibular wiring, 528
Circumvallate papillae, 16, 658
Clark staging, 517*t*
Clavulanate, 42
Clear cell squamous cell carcinoma, 515
Cleft lip, 232
Cleft palate, 232
Clindamycin
　for AIDS-related sinusitis, 643
　for bacterial lymphadenopathy, 402
Clinitest tablets, 593
Clonazepam, 663
Clotrimazole lozenges, 634
Coagulation necrosis, 596
Coagulopathy, epistaxis with, 210
Coal tar shampoo, 99
Cocaine, 207
Cochlea, 53, 56
　hair cells in, 57*f*
　inflammation of, 68-69

　malfunction of, 59-60
Cochlear implants, 70
　basic system of, 73*f*
Cochlear nerve, acoustic neuroma of, 122
Cochleovestibular cerebrovascular accident, 122
Cogan's syndrome, 124
Colchicine, 241
Collagen injection, 553-554
Collagenesis, 553
Colloid adenomas, 411
Coly-Mycin
　in contact dermatitis, 93
　for diffuse bacterial external otitis, 38
Complete blood count, 61
Computed tomography
　for advanced oral cavity cancer, 613
　of allergic fungal sinusitis, 174*f*
　for *Aspergillus* sinusitis, 638-639
　for benign salivary neoplasms, 410, 411
　of choanal atresia, 158*f*
　for deviated septum, 155*f*
　for dizziness, 112
　for facial trauma, 526
　for fibrous dysplasia, 500
　for goiter, 463
　for head and neck cancer, 608-609
　for hearing loss, 61, 62*f*
　for hiccups, 562-563
　for lymphangiomas, 400
　for malignant external otitis, 41*f*
　for mandible fractures, 526-528
　for nasal fractures, 224-225, 535
　for nasal obstruction, 156-157
　in nasopharyngeal examination, 271
　for neck masses, 422-423
　for necrotizing otitis externa, 40
　for neurofibromas, 407
　for olfactory disorders, 656
　for oral cavity cancer, 612
　for oral cavity lesions, 236
　for rhinosinusitis, 179, 190-191
　for salivary gland disorders, 435
　for thyroglossal duct cysts, 396
　for tinnitus, 137
Concha, 54
　bullosa, 184*f*
Concussion, labyrinthine, 122
Conductive hearing loss, 53
　audiograms for, 63-64
　with cerumen impaction, 77
　differential diagnosis of, 59-60
　management of, 66, 68-70

para-auditory tinnitus with, 134
  testing for, 59
Congenital disorders, nasopharyngeal, 275
Congenital neck masses, 423
Congenital torticollis, 399
Connecticut Chemosensory Clinical
  Research Center (CCCRC) test, 656
Connective tissue disorders, 281*t*
Consciousness, loss of, 524
Contact dermatitis, 93
  in aural itching, 88
  of external ear, 165-166
  of hand, 167*f*
  on neck, 167*f*
Continuous positive airway pressure
    (CPAP)
  mask for, 3
  model of, 315*f*
  nasal mask for, 316*f*
  for obstructive sleep apnea, 306*f*, 313-314
Contrast imaging
  for caustic ingestion, 597-598, 599
  for dysphagia, 297-299
  for head and neck cancer, 609
Corneal injury, 221
Coronal lift, 548
Coronary artery disease, 212
Corti, organ of, 56
Corticosteroids
  for airway foreign body complications, 577
  for allergic fungal sinusitis, 172-173
  for allergic rhinitis, 169-170, 172
  for caustic ingestion, 599
  for Eagle's syndrome, 484
  for gustatory disorders, 663
  for olfactory disorders, 657-658
  for rhinosinusitis, 194
  for seborrheic dermatitis of ear, 99
Cortisporin
  in contact dermatitis, 93
  for diffuse bacterial external otitis, 38
Coryza, 2
Cotton impaction, 94
Cotton swab use, 89
Coumadin, 210
Cranial nerve VIII, 53, 56
Cranial nerves
  benign tumors of, 406-407
  examination of
    for lesions, 23
    for rhinosinusitis, 186

in pain perception, 479
in referred otalgia, 49-50
sensory branches of, 658
testing of for dizziness, 107
in vestibulo-ocular system, 105
Cranial neuropathy, 159
Cranialization, 536
Craniofacial disjunction, 533*f*
Craniofacial structure, 309-310
Cresylate, 41, 91
Cricoarytenoid joint
  fixation of, 350
  diagnosis and management of, 351
  injury of, 353
Cricopharyngeal achalasia
  in dysphagia, 289
  esophageal manometry for, 300-301
Cricopharyngeal joint, long-standing dysfunction of, 289-290
Cricopharyngeal myotomy, 289
  for aspiration, 376
  for Zenker's diverticulum, 291
Cricopharyngeus muscle
  caustics in, 595
  in swallowing, 283-284
Cricothyroid cartilage, 16
Cricothyrotomy
  for airway foreign bodies, 573
  for upper airway obstruction, 342, 347
Crista, 102-104
Crohn's disease
  aphthous ulcers in, 246*f*
  oral manifestations of, 244
Cromolyn sodium, 196
Croup, 349*f*
Cryosurgery, 508-509
Cryptococcosis, labyrinth, 118
Cultures
  for *Aspergillus* sinusitis, 639
  for gustatory dysfunction, 661
  for inflammatory neck masses, 421
  for rhinosinusitis, 191-192
Cupula, 104
Cupulolithiasis, trauma-related, 119
Curettage
  for keratoacanthoma, 510
  for malignant melanoma of head and neck, 517
Curettage and suction
  for cerumen impaction, 40, 78-80, 85
  topical antibiotic drops after, 85
Cushing's syndrome, 660
Cutter, Ephraim, 4-6

Cyclophosphamide, 241
Cyclosporine
  for Behçet's syndrome, 241
  xerostomia with, 255
Cylindromas, 277
Cystic hygromas, 259, 399-400
Cysts, salivary gland, 434t, 446-447
Cytomegalovirus
  AIDS-related, 645
  in viral lymphadenopathy, 401
Czermak, Johann, 4

Deafferentation pain, 481
Debridement
  for mucormycosis, 637
    with diabetes, 639
  for necrotizing otitis externa, 40
Decannulation, 374-376
Decongestant spray, 19, 20-21
Decongestants
  for AIDS-related sinusitis, 643
  for allergic rhinitis, 170, 171
  for nasal fractures, 225
  for rhinosinusitis, 179, 195
Deep lobe parotid gland tumors, 443-444
Deglutition, 282-283
Dental amalgam implantation, 263f
Dental caries, 22
Dental examination, 188
Dental infections
  in bacterial lymphadenopathy, 402
  facial pain in, 479
Dental loss, 159
Dental radiographs, 236
Dentition, 282
Depression
  in gustatory dysfunction, 660
  sinus-type symptoms with, 188t
  tinnitus and, 135, 140
Dermabrasion, 546-548
Dermatitis
  atopic, 97
  contact, 88, 93, 165-166, 167f
  nonspecific, 91-92
  seborrheic, 98-99
Dermatophytid reaction
  of external ear, 166
  from fungal infection at distant site, 168
Dermoid cysts, 396
Dexamethasone, 347
Diabetes
  in dysphagia, 288
  mellitus

  in gustatory dysfunction, 660
  head and neck disorders in, 634-635
  mucormycosis in, 636-638, 639
  necrotizing otitis in, 635-636
  oral candidiasis with, 244
  vertigo with, 124
Diagnostic tests
  for aspiration, 371-373
  for atypical facial pain, 484-486
  for dizziness, 110-114
  for dysphagia, 297-302
  for epistaxis, 208
  for esophageal foreign body, 580-583
  for facial paralysis, 494-496
  for fibrous dysplasia, 500
  for gustatory dysfunction, 661
  for hearing loss, 59-66
  for hiccups, 561-563
  for hyperparathyroidism, 471-472
  for nasal fractures, 222-225
  for neck masses, 393-394
  for olfactory disorders, 654-656
  for oral cavity lesions, 236
  for salivary gland disorders, 433-435
Diaphragm
  irritation of with lung cancer, 563
  unintentional contraction of. *See* Hiccups
Dickens, Charles, 3
Dicloxacillin, 42
Dieffenbach, Ernst, 10
Diffuse esophageal spasm, 290, 301
Dilutional intradermal testing, 163-164
Dioxybenzones, 541
Diphenhydramine (Benadryl)
  for allergic rhinitis, 170
  for burning-mouth syndrome, 486
Diphenylhydantoin, 564t, 565
Dipyridamole, 210
Diplopia
  in rhinosinusitis, 185
  with zygomatic trauma, 531
Disequilibrium, 117
Diuretics
  in dizziness, 127
  loop, 134
  for Meniere's disease, 115, 116
Dix-Hallpike maneuver, 109, 110f
Dix-Hallpike test
  for benign paroxysmal positional vertigo, 119, 120
  for dizziness, 103f
Dizziness, 102
  anatomy of, 102-104

cardiovascular disorders causing, 114t
  dangers signs in, 129-130
  diagnostic evaluation of, 110-112
  differential diagnosis of, 113-115
  history of, 105-107
  idiopathic disorders causing, 114t
  key points of history for, 115t
  management algorithm for, 103f
  physical examination for, 107-110
  physiology of, 104-105
  precipitating events of, 107
  with short-lived neurological symptoms, 130
  in specific disorders, 115-129
Docusate sodium, 83-84
Dorsal spinal cerebellar tract, 106f
Droperidol, 128
Drug-related allergy, external ear, 166
Dry eyes, 242-244
Dugas, Louis, 3
Duplex carotid ultrasound, 137
Dynamic posturography, 112
Dysgeusia, 659
  bulimia in, 661
  diagnosis of, 662
  treatment of, 663
Dysosmia, 654
Dysphagia, 279
  aspiration and, 363, 367
  with caustic ingestion, 601
  danger signs in, 302-303
  diagnostic evaluation for, 296-301
  differential diagnosis of, 284-294
  with esophageal foreign body, 580
  in head and neck cancer, 607, 632
  history of, 294-295
  hypersalivation and, 447
  local problems causing, 281t
    diagnosis of, 289-294
  management of, 301-302
    algorithm for, 280f
  physical examination for, 295-296
  relevant anatomy and physiology of, 279-284
  systemic causes of, 281t
    diagnosis of, 285-289
Dysphonia. See Hoarseness

Eagle's syndrome, 482
  diagnosis of, 484
  elongated styloid process with, 485f
  physical examination for, 483
  treatment of, 486

Ear canal, 17
Ear candles, 84
Ear pain
  danger signs of, 51
  history and physical examination for, 31-34
  referred, 49-51
Ear wax phenotype, 77
Ear-wick, 42
Ears. See also Auditory canal; Auricle; Pinna
  allergic conditions of, 161-165, 168-169, 175-177
  anatomic relationships of, 55f
  anatomy and physiology of, 53-56
  external, otolaryngic allergy manifestations of, 165-166
  foreign objects in, 11
  inner
    allergic conditions of, 169
    anatomic relationships of, 55f
    irrigation of, for foreign bodies, 589
    itchy, 86-101
  middle
    allergic conditions of, 168-169
    anatomic relationships of, 55f
    bony cavity of, 56
    disorders of, 45-49
    structures of, 53
  squamous cell carcinoma of, 516f
  surgery of for dizziness, 107
  topographic anatomy of, 16-18
Ectropion, 553
Eczema, external ear, 166
Edison, Thomas, 6
Electrical testing, facial nerve, 495
Electrocautery, nasal, 213f
Electrodesiccation
  for acinic keratosis, 508-509
  of pyogenic granulomas, 260
Electrogustometry, 662
Electromyography, 138
Electroneurography, 495-496
Electronystagmography
  for dizziness, 111
  for tinnitus, 137
Electrophysiologic tests, 137-138
Embolization, 153
Embryonal adenomas, 411
Endocrine diseases, salivary gland, 434t
Endocrine/metabolic disorders, 114t
Endolymph, 56, 102
Endolymphatic fluid pressure, 134
Endolymphatic sac decompression, 129

Endoscope
  fiberoptic, passed through nose, 270f
  nasal, in office settings, 156f
  in nasopharyngeal examination, 21-22
Endoscopic examination of swallowing, 372-373
Endoscopic photography
  of nasopharynx, 268f
  of posterior nasal cavity, 267f
Endoscopic sinus surgery, 197
Endoscopy
  for airway foreign bodies, 573
  for caustic ingestion, 598
  for dysphagia, 299
  for esophageal foreign body, 583-584
  in facial rejuvenation surgery, 548
  flexible, for gastric aspiration, 364
  for gastric aspiration, 364
  for hiccups, 563
  for juvenile nasopharyngeal angiofibroma, 153
  meatus, 192f
  nasal
    for chronic sinusitis, 198
    for rhinosinusitis, 179, 191
    in nasopharyngeal examination, 21-22
    for olfactory disorders, 656
Endotracheal intubation
  for bacterial lymphadenopathy, 402
  for facial trauma, 524
  for upper airway obstruction, 345, 346-347
  in vocal cord fixation, 353
  in vocal cord paralysis, 353
ENG. *See* Electronystagmography
Enophthalmos, 531-532
Enucleation, 409
Enzymatic digestion, 585
Enzyme-linked immunosorbent (ELISA) test, 164-165
Epidermophyton, external ear, 166
Epiglottis, 16, 357
  dentures caught on, 574-575f
  laryngoscopic view of, 17f
Epilepsy, 126-127
Epinephrine
  for ACE-inhibitor induced angioneurotic edema, 360
  for airway foreign body complications, 577
  for epistaxis, 214
Episodic laryngospasm, 354
Epistaxis, 202

  in acute rhinosinusitis, 185
  with adenoidal enlargement, 274
  anatomy and physiology of, 202-205
  danger signs for, 216
  diagnostic evaluation of, 208
  differential diagnosis of, 209-212
  history of, 205
  local causes of, 209-210
  management algorithm for, 203f
  management and follow-up for, 212-216
  with nasal fracture, 219
  in nasal obstruction, 152, 159
  physical examination for, 205-207
  systemic causes of, 210-212
Epstein-Barr virus
  with nasopharyngeal carcinoma, 611
  in viral lymphadenopathy, 401
Epulis, pregnancy-associated, 244
Epworth Sleepiness Scale, 309, 310t
Erbium:yttrium-aluminum-garnet laser, 546
Erosive lichen planus, 246
Erythrocyte sedimentation rate, 61
Erythroplakia, 256-257
  in oral cavity cancer, 612
Eryximachus, 11-12
Esophageal sphincters, 579-580
Esophagectomy, trans-hiatal, 294
Esophagitis, 578
Esophagogastrectomy, 600
Esophagogastroduodenoscopy
  with balloon dilatation, 581
  for Barrett's esophagus, 292, 294
Esophagoscopy
  for caustic ingestion, 598
  for dysphagia, 299-300
  for esophageal foreign body, 583
  for impacted foreign body, 581
Esophagus
  cancer of with dysphagia, 293-294
  candidiasis of, 250
  caustic burns of, 593-594, 598
  contraction with, 601
  coin in, 582f
  diffuse spasm of, 290, 301
  disorders of
    in dysphagia, 281t
    with obstructive-type symptoms, 284
  examination of for dysphagia, 297
  foreign bodies in, 577-580
    causes of, 579t
    complications of, 586
    diagnostic evaluation for, 580-583
    history of, 580

management of, 583-586
physical examination for, 580
symptoms of, 581*t*
manometry of, 300-301
perforation of, 586
physiologic narrowing of, 579-580
strictures of
with caustic ingestion, 600
in esophageal foreign bodies, 578
in swallowing, 283-284, 285*f*
tack lodged in, 579*f*
Estrogens
nasal congestion and, 150
for olfactory disorders, 658
Ethmoid arteries, anterior, 204-205
Ethmoid bone, 2, 218
Ethmoid sinuses, 183*f*
Ethmoid sinusitis, subperiosteal abscess in, 186*f*
Ethmoidal neoplasm, 151
Ethmoidectomy, 198
Ethmoid arteries, ligation of, 206*f*
Eustachian tubes
allergic conditions of, 168-169
dysfunction of, 607
dizziness with, 128
in equalizing ear pressure, 47-48
function of, 56
orifices of, 15, 265
patency of, 31
patulous, 267, 274
Eutectic mixture of local anesthetics (EMLA), 78
Examination, head and neck, 13-26
Excisional biopsy
for facial and scalp skin malignancy, 507
for malignant melanoma of head and neck, 517
for malignant neck masses, 415-416
for nevus, 511
for tongue cancer, 608
Exostoses, benign, 239-240
Expiratory speaking valve, 375
Exposure keratitis, 496
External ear. *See* Auricle
Extraocular motility, nasal, 221
Extraocular muscle mobility, 524
Eyebrows, 548-549
Eyelids
injuries of, 537
lower, 551*f*
Eyes
closing of, 494

examination of for nasal fractures, 221
opening of, 494
painful movement of in rhinosinusitis, 185
rejuvenation surgery for, 549-550

Face
anatomy and physiology of, 504-506
examination of for rhinosinusitis, 185-186
injuries of, 257-258
Facelift, 550
Facial asymmetry
differential diagnosis of, 489
facial paralysis in, 489-499
fibrous dysplasia in, 499-500
management algorithm for, 490*f*
progressive hemifacial atrophy in, 500-501
tumors and infection in, 501-502
Facial fractures, 526-536
Facial lesions, 520-521
danger signs for, 520
diagnosis and management of, 507-520
history of, 506
physical examination for, 506-507
Facial lines, 506
Facial nerve, 506
anatomy of, 491
damage to, 536-537
electrical testing of, 495
function of in salivary gland disorders, 433
Facial pain
atypical
danger signs for, 487
diagnosis of, 479
differential diagnosis of, 484*t*
history of, 481-483
management algorithm for, 480*f*
management of, 484-487
physical examination for, 483-484
relevant anatomy and physiology of, 479-481
infectious causes of, 481-482
in rhinosinusitis, 184-185, 200
Facial paralysis
after closed head injury, 498
anatomy and physiology of, 491
danger signs of, 499
diagnostic evaluation of, 494-496
differential diagnosis of, 492*t*
in facial asymmetry, 489-499

Facial paralysis—*continued*
  grade 6/6, 495*f*
  in herpes zoster oticus, 129
  herpes zoster oticus in, 493
  history of, 491-493
  House-Brackman scale of, 492, 493-494
  management and follow-up for, 496-499
  with orbital mucormycosis, 636*f*
  with parotidectomy, 444-445
  physical examination for, 493-494
  temporal bone fracture with, 129
  traumatic, 448, 497
  zygomaticomaxillary fracture with, 535
Facial reconstruction, 9-10
Facial rejuvenation, 539
  collagen injection in, 553-554
  implants in, 553-554
  skin damage and, 539-541
  with skin resurfacing, 541-548
  surgery for, 548-553
    around eyes, 549-550
    for cheeks and jowls, 550
    complications of, 552-553
    for forehead and eyebrows, 548-549
    for neck, 550-552
Facial trauma, 523
  diagnosis and management of conditions in, 526-538
  differential diagnosis for, 525
  history of, 523-524
  physical examination for, 524-525
  radiographic studies for, 525-526
  sinus-type symptoms with, 188*t*
  soft tissue injuries with, 536-538
Fallopian canal, 491
Fallopio, Gabriele, 2
Federal Caustic Act, 593
Federal Hazardous Substance Act, 593
FEES. *See* Flexible endoscopic examination of swallowing
Fexofenadine (Allegra)
  for allergic rhinitis, 170
  for rhinosinusitis, 195-196
Fiber optics, 6
Fiberoptic esophagoscopy, 299-300
Fiberoptic laryngoscopy, 310
Fiberoptic pharyngoscopy, 587
Fibromas, submucosal, 260
Fibromatosis colli, 399
Fibrous dysplasia, 499
  danger signs for, 500
  history of, 499
  management and follow-up for, 500
  physical examination for, 500
Filiform papillae, 232
Fine-needle-aspiration biopsy
  for AIDS-related lymphoma, 646
  for bacterial lymphadenopathy, 402
  for benign salivary neoplasms, 410, 411
  for benign thyroid gland neoplasms, 411
  for branchial abnormalities, 398
  for congenital torticollis, 399
  of dominant thyroid nodule, 454
  for enlarged jugulodigastric lymph nodes, 414
  for granulomatous lymphadenopathy, 403
  for granulomatous neck masses, 424
  for head and neck masses, 422
  for inflammatory neck masses, 423-424
  for malignant thyroid neoplasms, 419
  for mucoepidermoid carcinoma of parotid, 417
  for neck masses, 415, 427
  for neoplastic neck masses, 425, 426
  for oral cavity lesions, 236
  for salivary gland disorders, 433-435
  for thyroglossal duct cysts, 395-396
  for thyroid gland disease, 457-459
  with thyroid suppressive therapy, 460
  for tuberculosis, 404
Fingernail fungal infection, 168
Fissured tongue, 238, 242*f*
Fitzpatrick scale, 512
Fitzpatrick sun-reactive skin types, 513*t*, 544
Flare, 163
Flavors, perception of, 650
Fletcher, Horace, 7
Fletcherization, 7
Flexible endoscopic examination of swallowing, 299
  for aspiration after stroke, 367
Flocculonodular lobe, 106*f*
  vestibular input to, 105
Fluconazole (Diflucan)
  for AIDS-related oral candidiasis, 250
  for oral thrush, 634-635, 644
Flunisolide (Aerobid), 170
Fluorescent treponemal antibody absorbed (FTA-Abs) test, 60-61, 118
Fluoroscopy, 373
5-Fluorouracil
  for acinic keratosis, 508-509
  for keratoacanthoma, 511
Fluticasone
  for allergic rhinitis, 172

for rhinosinusitis, 194
Folic acid deficiency, 240
Follicular adenomas, 411
    fine-needle-aspiration biopsy for, 459
Follicular carcinoma, thyroid, 419, 466
Follicular neoplasms, 425-426
Food
    allergies to, 168-169
    oral preparation of, 282
Food bolus, 282
    impacted, 578-580
    premature loss of, 373
    propulsion of, 283
Food filter, invisible, 7
Foramen cecum, 232
Fordyce's spots, 239, 243f
Forehead, facial rejuvenation surgery for, 548-549
Foreign bodies, 11
    airway, 567-577
    in aural itch, 93-94
    in dizziness, 128
    in dysphagia, 289
    esophageal, 577-586
    in external auditory canal, 42, 43f, 588-590
    incidence of, 567
    ingestion of, 578-579
    inhaled, 577
    in itchy ear, 95
    laryngeal, 569
    management algorithm for, 568f
    nasal, 590
    pharyngeal, 586-588
Fractures
    facial, 526-536
    nasal, 218-226
Fragrance, contact dermatitis, 93
Frazier-tip suction, 81f, 207
Free-tissue transfer, 518t
Frenzel lenses, 108
    in positioning test, 109
    with video camera, 109f
        rotation chair testing with, 112f
Frey's syndrome, 444-445
Frontal mucocele, 187f
Frontal sinus disease, chronic, 199
Frontal sinus fracture, 535
    treatment of, 535-536
Frontal sinus wall fracture, 530
Frostbite
    in aural itching, 88
    in itchy ear, 96

FTA-Abs testing, 60-61, 118
Functional dysphonia, 338t
Functional inspiratory adduction, 355
Fundoscopic examination, 136
Fungal infections
    of labyrinth, 118, 129
    nasopharyngeal, 272-273
    oral, 251-252
Fungal otitis externa, 92
Fungal sinusitis, 172-173
    allergic
        computed tomography of, 174f
        thick inspissated pus of, 175f
Fungiform papillae, 232
Furunculosis, 41-42

G-proteins, 653
Gadolinium imaging, 495
Gait, 108
Galen, 1-2
Garcia, Manuel, 4
Gastric contents, 363
Gastric distention hiccups, 559
    postoperative, 561
Gastroesophageal junction, caustics in, 595
Gastroesophageal reflux disease, 290-291
    in burning-mouth syndrome, 486
    dysphagia representing, 292
    episodic laryngospasm and, 354
    esophageal obstruction with, 581
    hoarseness with, 326f, 328, 329-331
    management of dysphagia with, 301
    posterior laryngeal erythema of, 26
    in upper airway obstruction, 348
Gastroscope, flexible fiberoptic nasal, 300f
Gastrostomy feeding
    for aspiration, 374, 379
    for caustic ingestion, 600-601
    for lymphangiomas, 400
Gatifloxacin, 193
Gelatin sponge, 213
Gelfoam, 377
Genesis, 1
Genioglossal advancement, 317-318
Geniohyoid muscle, 232
Genioplasty, advancement, 319f
Gentian Violet
    for fungal otitis externa, 92
    for otomycosis, 41, 91
Geographic tongue, 238, 240f
GERD. *See* Gastroesophageal reflux disease
Giant cell epulis, 244

Gingiva, 231
  hypertrophy of, 244
Gingivitis, 244
Glasgow Coma Scale, 498
Globus, 292
Globus hystericus, 291-292
Glogau classification system, 540
Glomus tumors, 407
Glossectomy, 317-318
Glossitis
  median rhomboid, 238, 239f
  migratory, 238, 240f
Glossopharyngeal nerve, 650
Glottic airway configuration, 343f
Glottic cancer, 624-625
  early treatment of, 625
  hoarseness with, 337
  speech rehabilitation after, 626-628
  T-staging for, 610t
  treatment of, 625-626
Glottic closure
  hiccups and, 557
  procedures to enhance, 376-377
  short latency of, 558-559
Glottic obstruction
  diagnosis of conditions causing, 350-356
  with removal of airway foreign body, 573
Glottic stenosis, 350
Glottis
  too open, 376-377
  tracheal rings below, 16
Glucagon, 585-586
Goiter, 461-462
  evaluation for, 462-463
  management of, 463-465
  multinodular, 463
  physical examination for, 454
  substernal, 464
  surgical therapy for, 450
  in upper airway obstruction, 344
Gout, parotitis with, 446
Grafting, 518t
Granular cell myoblastoma, 260
Granulation polyps, postintubation, 338
Granulation tissue, tracheostomy stomal, 349-350
Granulomatous disease
  in neck masses, 390
  salivary involvement in, 440
Granulomatous lymphadenopathy, 402-405
Granulomatous neck masses, 424
Graves' disease, 450
  fine-needle-aspiration biopsy for, 458
  goiter and, 465
  in hyperthyroidism, 465
Guiafenesin
  for acute sinusitis, 182
  for AIDS-related sinusitis, 643
  for patulous eustachian tubes, 274
  for rhinosinusitis, 196
Gustatory disorders, 650
  danger signs in, 663
  definition of, 659
  diagnostic evaluation of, 661
  etiology of, 659-661
  gustatory testing in, 661-662
  management algorithm for, 652f
  physiology of, 658-659
  treatment of, 663
Gustatory receptor cells, 658
Gustatory sensation pathways, 658
Gustatory system, 650
Gustatory testing, 661-662

H_2 blockers
  for episodic laryngospasm, 354
  for GERD, 292
  for reflux laryngitis, 329-331
Habituation, 141
Haemophilus influenza
  in acute otitis media, 45
  in acute tonsillitis, 249
  in Kaposi's sarcoma, 645
  in rhinosinusitis, 193
  in supraglottitis, 357-358
  vaccine, 357
Hair cells, 56, 57f, 102-104
  hyperactivity of in sensorineural tinnitus, 134
Hair dye ingredient, 93
Hairy leukoplakia of tongue, AIDS-related, 250, 644
Hamman's sign, 598
Hammer nose. *See* Rhinophyma
Hard palate, 232
  punctate red spots on, 22-23
Hashimoto's thyroiditis, 458
Head
  cancer of, 367
  injury of
    anosmia after, 538
    in facial nerve paralysis, 497-498
    in olfactory disorders, 654
  trauma to
    in gustatory dysfunction, 659

intractable hiccups with, 562
in olfactory disorders, 655t
with unsteadiness, 129
with vertigo, 119-122, 129
Head and neck
disorders of in immunocompromised patient, 634-648
examination of
pearls and pitfalls of, 18-26
topographic anatomy of, 13-18
lymphatic drainage of, 504-506
malignancies of
biopsy and staging of, 609-610
danger signs in, 605t, 632
detection and screening of, 604-606
epidemiology of, 604
glottic cancer, 624-628
history of, 606
incidence of, 604
laryngeal cancer, 623-624
nasopharyngeal cancer, 611
oral cavity cancer, 612-623
physical examination for, 606-607
radiographic imaging for, 608-609
supraglottic cancer, 628-632
synchronous second primary tumors, 609
treatment of, 610-611
Head mirror/light, 22f
Headlight, 23f
with indirect laryngoscopy, 24
Hearing
anatomy of, 53-57
asymmetry of, 141
Hearing aids, 69-70
behind-the-ear, 70f
body, 72f
bone-conducting, 72f
components of, 70f
implantable, 70
in-the-canal, 71f
in-the-ear, 71f
for sensorineural hearing loss, 68
for tinnitus, 140
Hearing-conservation programs, 68
for noise-hazardous environments, 139
Hearing loss
asymmetrical with sudden vertigo, 129
with bullous myringitis, 43
causes of, 53
with cerumen impaction, 77
conductive
with nasopharyngeal masses, 267

para-auditory tinnitus with, 134
danger signs for, 70-71
diagnostic evaluation for, 60-66
differential diagnosis of, 59-60
history of, 57-58
low-frequency sensorineural, 115
management algorithm for, 54f
management and follow-up of, 66-70
noise-induced in tinnitus, 139
physical examination for, 58-59
relevant anatomy and physiology in, 53-56
sensorineural
AIDS-related, 642
tinnitus with, 134
in serous labyrinthitis, 118-119
sudden, 68-69
with cerumen impaction, 78-80
Hearing threshold level, 63
Heerfordt's disease, 441
Heimlich maneuver, 570
Helium-oxygen mixture, 347
Hemangiomas, 400-401
diagnosis and management of, 423
epistaxis with, 210
oral, 259
Hematoma
auricular, 35, 37f
with facial rejuvenation surgery, 552-553
Hemithyroidectomy, 466
Hemotympanum, with barotrauma, 49
Hennebert's sign, 118
Heparin, 210
Hereditary hemorrhagic telangiectasia, 210
Herpes simplex infection
AIDS-related, 645
in nasal vestibular infection, 644
oral manifestations of, 246-247
vesicular eruption of, 248f
Herpes simplex neuritis, 491
Herpes simplex virus, 496
Herpes zoster, 248f
AIDS-related, 645
oral, 247
Herpes zoster oticus
in chronic otitis externa, 90f
diagnosis of, 495
with dizziness, 118
facial nerve injury in, 491
with facial nerve paralysis, 129
in facial paralysis, 498
presenting symptoms of, 491-492
treatment of, 493

Herpetic recrudescence, 544-545
Hiatal hernia, 601
Hiccups, 557
  after head trauma, 562
  central causes of, 560t
  classification of by duration, 559t
  diagnostic evaluation of, 561-563
  etiology of, 559-561
  history of, 11-12
  management algorithm for, 558f
  peripheral causes of, 560t
  physiology of, 557-559
  treatment of, 563-566
Hippocrates, 1
Histamine
  for dizziness, 129
  in impaired sinus drainage, 183-184
Histoplasma capsulatum
  in granulomatous lymphadenopathy, 405
  oral ulcerations in, 252
Histoplasmosis
  AIDS-related, 234, 645
  in granulomatous lymphadenopathy, 405
  treatment of, 424
Hoarseness, 325
  characteristics of, 328t
  chronic, 340
  common causes of, 327t
  danger signs for, 340
  defining, 327t
  diagnosis and management of, 329-336
  differential diagnosis of, 331t
  with glottic cancer, 624
  in head and neck cancer, 606-607, 632
  history of, 326-328
  with laryngoceles, 399
  management algorithm for, 326f
  physical examination for, 328-329
  prevention of, 336-337
  therapy for, 337-339
Hodgkin's lymphoma, 277, 412
  incidence of, 416
House-Brackman Scale
  of facial paralysis, 493-494
  grading system of, 494t
  for salivary gland disorders, 433
Human bites, facial, 538
Human immune deficiency virus (HIV) infection
  Kaposi's sarcoma in, 645

  in viral lymphadenopathy, 401-402
  xerostomia and, 441
Hürthle cell adenoma, 459
Hürthle cell carcinoma, 459
Hürthle cell neoplasm, 419
Hydralazine, 129
Hydrocephalus, 352-353
Hydrochlorothiazide, 115
Hydrocortisone
  for burning-mouth syndrome, 486
  for nonspecific dermatitis of external ear, 92
Hyoid advancement, 317-318
Hyoid bone, greater cornu of, 16
Hyoid cartilage, 16
Hyoid suspension
  anatomical changes with, 319f
  for obstructive sleep apnea, 318
Hyoid syndrome, 482
  diagnosis of, 484
  physical examination for, 483
Hyperbaric oxygen
  for mucormycosis with diabetes, 639
  for necrotizing otitis externa, 40
Hypercalcemia
  causes of, 469t
  chronic, 471t
  with thyroid disease, 473
Hypercapnia, 342, 344
Hypercarbia, 308
Hypergeusia, 659
Hyperglycemia, chronic, 634
Hyperosmia, 654
Hyperparathyroidism, 468-470
  evaluation for, 471-472
  giant cell epulis and, 244
  primary, 469-470
  secondary, 470
  surgical therapy for, 472-473
  tertiary, 470
Hyperpigmentation
  with chemical peel, 544
  with laser resurfacing, 546
Hypersalivation, 434t, 447
Hypertension
  dizziness with, 125-126
  long-standing, epistaxis with, 208
  with profuse epistaxis, 211
Hyperthyroidism, 452, 465
  autoimmune, 465
  with goiter, 463
Hyperviscosity syndrome, 126

Hyphema, nasal fracture, 221
Hypnosis, 565
Hypogeusia, 659
Hypoglossal nerve lesion, 23
Hypopharyngeal cancer, 606
Hypopharyngeal disorders, 281*t*
Hypopharyngeal dysfunction, 295
Hypopharynx
  corrosives in, 595
  laryngoscopic view of, 17*f*
  topographic anatomy of, 16
  tumor of, 353*f*
Hypopigmentation, 544
Hyposmia, 654
  nasal polyps in, 657
  steroid-dependent, 658
Hypotension, orthostatic, 107
Hypothyroidism, 452
  in dysphagia, 286
  in gustatory dysfunction, 660
  nasal congestion and, 150
  vertigo with, 124
Hypoxemia, 342
Hypoxia
  dizziness with, 126
  with sleep apnea, 308

Ibuprofen, 486
ICD-9 diagnosis code, 279
Ice-cold gauze pads, 225
IgG antibody, 175
Image-analysis cytometry, 103*f*
Imaging studies, ear, 61, 62*f*
Imepenam, 194
Imipramine, 663
Immune compromise, 647-648
  abnormal nasal mucosa in, 188
  head and neck disorders in, 634-648
Immunodeficiency
  common variable, 641
  diabetes mellitus in, 634-636
  mucosal, 184
  with neutropenia, 638-641
Immunoglobulin A deficiency, selective, 641
Immunoglobulin E, allergen-specific, 161, 165
Immunoglobulin G-subclass deficiencies, 641
Immunologic disease
  in differential diagnosis of dizziness, 114*t*
  vertigo with, 124
Immunosuppression, mucosal, 189

Immunotherapy
  for allergic conditions, 175-176
  for inner ear allergy, 169
  for malignant melanoma of head and neck, 517
Impedance audiometry, 137
Implants, facial rejuvenation, 553-554
Incisional biopsy, facial and scalp, 507
Incus, 57*f*
Infections
  with chemical peel, 544-545
  dizziness with, 115-118
  in gustatory dysfunction, 659-660
  in itchy ears, 86
  in upper airway obstruction, 348*t*
Infectious disorders
  in differential diagnosis of dizziness, 114*t*
  differential diagnosis of sinus-type symptoms of, 188*t*
  in facial asymmetry, 501-502
  of oral cavity, 246-252
Inflammation, nasopharyngeal, 271
Inflammatory bowel disease, 240
Inflammatory diseases
  differential diagnosis of sinus-type symptoms of, 188*t*
  in nasal obstruction, 152*t*
  of salivary glands, 434*t*
    acute, 436-438
    chronic, 438-441
  vertigo with, 123
Inflammatory neck masses, 389
  management and follow-up for, 423-424
  work-up for, 421
Inflammatory processes
  of diaphragm, 559-561
  in upper airway obstruction, 348*t*
Inhalant allergies
  of middle ear and Eustachian tube, 168-169
  nasopharyngeal effects of, 271-272
Insects
  in external auditory canal, 42, 589
  in itchy ears, 93-94
  in nose and throat, 11
Inspiratory stridor, 342-343
Instruments, development of, 4-8
Intermaxillary fixation, 528
  for mandibular fractures, 528*f*
Intoxication, inhaled foreign body during, 577
Intracranial hypertension, 134

Intracranial injuries, 524
Intradermal allergy testing, 163-164
Intraoral examination, 433
Intubation
   granulation polyps after, 338
   for upper airway obstruction, 346-347
   in vocal cord fixation, 353
   in vocal cord paralysis, 353
In vitro allergy testing, 164-165
Iodine deficiency, 462f
Iodine scanning, 455
Irrigation systems, ear, 81-83
Isopropyl alcohol, 93-94
Isotretinoin (Accutane), 255
Itard, Jean, 4

Jackson, Chevalier, 592-593
Jod-Basedow phenomenon, 463
Jowls, rejuvenation surgery for, 550
Jugular lymph nodes
   anatomical areas drained by, 388t
   lower, 387
   middle, 387
   upper, 386-387
Jugulo-omohyoid lymph nodes, 387
Jugulodigastric lymph nodes
   benign neoplasms of, 410
   enlarged and tender, 391, 414

Kaposi's sarcoma
   AIDS-defining, 250, 263
   of hard palate, 646f
   oral manifestations of, 234, 644-645
   salivary gland masses from, 441
   ulcerated, 262f
Kawasaki disease, 249
   in lymphadenopathy, 405
Kellogg, Dr. J. H., 7
Keratitis, exposure, 496
Keratoacanthoma
   diagnosis and management of, 510-511
   of head, 506
Keratoconjunctivitis sicca, 438
Keratolytics, 99
Ketoacidosis, diabetic
   with mucormycosis, 639
   in necrotizing otitis, 635, 636
Ketoconazole
   for *Histoplasma capsulatum*, 252
   for oral thrush, 634-635, 644
Kiesselbach's plexus, 204
Kyphoscoliosis, 351

Labial artery, superior, 202-205
Labiogingival sulcus, 231
Laboratory tests
   for dizziness, 112
   for hearing loss, 60-61
   for hyperparathyroidism, 468-469
   for sleep apnea, 311-312
Labyrinth, 102
   bony, 104f
   caloric testing of, 109-110
   fungal infection of, 118, 129
   membranous, 56
Labyrinthectomy, 129
Labyrinthine apoplexy, 126
Labyrinthine concussion, 122
Labyrinthitis
   in dizziness, 129
   luetic, 118
   in mumps, 437-438
   serous, 118-119
   suppurative, 118
Lacrimal system injuries, 537
Lagophthalmos, 553
Laminar flow, 147
Lamm, Heinrich, 6
Laparotomy, emergent exploratory, 600
Laryngeal cartilages, 16
Laryngeal granuloma, postintubation, 26
Laryngeal mirror, 25, 235
   for head and neck cancer diagnosis, 607
Laryngeal muscle tension
   hoarseness with, 335
   inappropriate, 333
Laryngeal nerve
   paralysis of with thyroid cancer surgery, 468
   paresis of, 26
   recurrent, 451
      injury to, 332
      path of, 368f
      superior, 658
Laryngectomy
   for advanced oral cavity cancer, 614
   airway after, 576f
   for airway foreign bodies, 573
   for glottic cancer, 625-626
   speech rehabilitation after, 626-628
   stoma, 626f
   for supraglottic cancer, 629-632
Laryngitis, reflux, 332
   treatment of, 329-331

Laryngoceles, 398-399
Laryngopharyngeal abnormalities, 371
Laryngoplasty, medialization, 332
  custom-designed implant with, 335f
Laryngoscope, flexible fiberoptic, 21-22
  for aspiration, 371
Laryngoscopy, 4
  indirect, 24-26
  for lymphangiomas, 400
  for sleep apnea, 310
  for supraglottic cancer, 630
  telescopic indirect, 329
Laryngospasm
  episodic, 354
  functional, 354-355
Laryngostroboscopy, video
  for hoarseness, 329
  typical setup for, 332f
Laryngotracheal separation
  after stroke, 379
  for aspiration, 377-378
Larynx
  cancer of, 333-335
    above true vocal cords, 628-632
    dysphagia with, 293
    hoarseness with, 336
    incidence of, 623-624
  corrosives in, 595
  endoscopic examination of, 299
  erythema of, 26
  examination of, 24-26
    for neck masses, 390-391
  foreign bodies in, 569t
  laryngoscopic view of, 17f
  malignancy of with tobacco use, 333-335
  neoplasms of, 355-356
  papilloma of, 338t
  stenosis of with caustic ingestion, 601
  topographic anatomy of, 16
  visualization of, 328-329
Larynx-preservation surgery, 631-632
Laser ablation, 348-349
Laser-assisted uvulopalatoplasty, 317
Laser cordotomy, 351
Laser excision, supraglottic cancer, 631
Laser skin resurfacing, 545-546
Laser vaporization, 260
Lee, Edward W., 11
Leech, 6
Leser-Trélat sign, 509
Leukemia, AIDS-related, 250

Leukocytosis
  in infectious mononucleosis, 249
  in suppurative sialadenitis, 436
Leukoplakia, 256-257
  in oral cavity cancer, 612, 615f
  snuff-dipper's, 233f
  of ventral tongue, 607f
Levator muscles, 494
Levofloxacin
  for AIDS-related sinusitis, 643
  for rhinosinusitis, 193
Lichen planus, 246, 247f
Lidocaine
  for aphthous ulcers, 245
  for foreign bodies in external auditory
    canal, 42
  for insect removal from ear, 93-94, 589
  for tinnitus, 140
Lifestyle change
  after oral cavity cancer, 615
  for dizziness, 129
  for tinnitus, 140
Light sources, 6
Lightheadedness
  with abnormal blood glucose, 130
  with cardiovascular disease, 124-125
  with hypo- or hyperglycemia, 124
Lingual frenulum, 232
  short, 238
Lingual thyroid, 238
Lingual tonsil, 232
Lingual tonsillar nerve, 658
Lip pits, 238
Lipomas, 409
Liposarcomas, 409
Lips, 231
  angioneurotic edema of, 255
  cystic mucoceles on, 259
  lacerations of, 257
Liquefaction necrosis, alkali-induced, 595
Liquid nitrogen cryosurgery, 508-509
Liver disease, 660
Local pain, 481
Loop diuretics, 134
Loratadine (Claritin)
  for allergic rhinitis, 170
  for rhinosinusitis, 195-196
Lothrop procedure, 199
Lotrimin
  for fungal otitis externa, 92
  for otomycosis, 41, 91

Ludwig's angina, 344
  angioedema in, 360f
  features of, 345
  of floor of mouth, 360f, 361
Lungs
  cancer of, 563
  hyperinflation of, 571f
Lupus erythematosus, 99
Lye ingestion, 596
Lymph nodes
  anterior compartment, 388
  collections of in neck, 385f
  drainage routes of, 387f
  lower jugular, 387
  malignancies of, 413-416
    Hodgkin's and non-Hodgkin's, 412
  management of in malignant melanoma, 517
  middle jugular, 387
  posterior triangle, 387
  primary groups of in head, 388t
  submandibular, 384, 385-386
  submental, 384, 385-386
  upper jugular, 386-387
Lymphadenopathy
  AIDS-related, 645-646
  bacterial, 402
  granulomatous, 402-405
  miscellaneous causes of, 405
  supraclavicular, 414
  viral, 401-402
Lymphangioma, 399-400
  diagnosis and management of, 423
  simplex, 399-400
  tongue, 259
Lymphatic drainage, head and neck, 504-506
Lymphoepithelial cysts
  parotid gland, 411
    AIDS-related, 647
  salivary gland masses from, 441
Lymphoma
  AIDS-related, 645, 646
  Burkitt's, 413f
  Hodgkin's and non-Hodgkin's, 416
  nasopharyngeal, 277
  non-Hodgkin's, 412
  oral, AIDS-related, 250
  salivary gland masses from, 441
  thyroid, 420
Lymphosarcomas, 416

Macroglobulinemia, 126
Macrolides, 193-194
Macula, 104
Magnetic resonance angiography, 137
Magnetic resonance imaging
  for benign salivary neoplasms, 410, 411
  for carotid paragangliomas, 408
  for dizziness, 103f, 112
  for facial paralysis, 495
  for head and neck cancer, 609
  for hearing loss, 61, 62f
  for hiccups, 562-563
  for lymphangiomas, 400
  for nasal obstruction, 157
  for nasopharyngeal carcinoma, 392f
  in nasopharyngeal examination, 271
  for neck masses, 423
  for neurofibromas, 407
  for oral cavity lesions, 236
  for rhinosinusitis, 190-191
  for salivary gland disorders, 435
  for tinnitus, 141
Mal de debarquement syndrome, 128
Malabsorption syndromes, 240
Malar eminence, 528-532
Malar fat pad, 550
  elevation of, 551f
Malassezia furfur infection, 99
Malignancy. *See also specific types*
  in ear pain, 51
  nasopharyngeal, 276-278
  oral, 260-263
  skin biopsy for, 507
  of thyroid gland, 454
  upper airway, 348t
Malignant neck masses
  neoplastic, 412-420
  work-up for, 422
Malignant neoplasms
  of salivary glands, 434t, 441
  of submandibular gland, 446
Malignant otitis externa, 635
  AIDS-related, 643
Malignant thyroid nodules, 460
Malleus bone, 56, 57f
Malocclusion
  with mid-face injuries, 532-533
  with nasal fractures, 220
Mandible
  fractures of
    diagnosis and management of, 526-528

Index 687

distribution of, 527*f*
fixation plate for, 529*f*
segmental resection of, 612
Mandibular arch, 620*f*
Mandibular fixation plate, 529*f*
Mandibular reconstruction, 613
Mandibulotomy, 612
Manometry, 300-301
Masking, tinnitus, 140
Mastoid, 56
Mastoiditis, 56
  acute, 49*f*
  chronic, 49*f*
  in facial paralysis, 498
  suppurative, with chronic otitis media, 46-47
Maxilla
  fractures of, 532
  nasal process of, 218
Maxillary crest, 218
Maxillary rhinosinusitis, 185
Maxillary sinus
  mucosal drainage pattern of, 182
  normal, 183*f*
  squamous cell carcinoma eroding floor of, 157*f*
  surgical procedures for disease of, 199
  tap of, 198-199
Maxillomandibular wiring, 528*f*
McCune-Albright syndrome, 499
McGill forceps, 588
Meat impaction, 577
  enzymatic digestion of, 585
  treatment of, 581
Meclizine, 128
Medialization laryngoplasty
  custom-designed implant with, 335*f*
  for hoarseness, 332
Medialization thyroplasty, 377
Mediastinal adenopathy, 334
Medication-induced disorders
  olfactory, 654
    drugs involved in, 655*t*
  oral, 252-255
Medications
  in dysphagia, 281*t*
  in gustatory dysfunction, 659, 660*t*
Medicine, history of, 1-12
Medullary thyroid carcinoma, 418, 419-420
  calcitonin as marker for, 454-455
  management of, 466-467
  thyroid, 466

Melolabial fold basal cell carcinoma, 513*f*
Melanoma
  epistaxis with, 210
  malignant
    diagnosis of, 516-517
    of head, 506
    of head and neck, 516-517
    staging of, 517*t*
    treatment of, 517
  mucosal, 263
Melkersson-Rosenthal syndrome, 244
  family history of, 494
Melkersson's syndrome, 238
Membranous tonsillitis, 234
Meniere's disease, 169
  diagnosis and management of, 115
  management of, 68
  natural history and treatment of, 116
Meningismus, 130
Meningitis, 126
Meningoencephalitis, 118
Messerklinger approach, 197
Metabolic diseases of salivary glands, 434*t*
Metastasis, nasopharyngeal, 277-278
Methotrexate, 511
Methylcellulose nasal tampons, 214
Methylmethacrylate, 93
Methylprednisolone, 599
Metoclopramide, 564*t*, 565
Metronidazole
  for AIDS-related sinusitis, 643
  for fungal otitis externa, 92
Microaspiration, 363
  with presbylarynx, 372
Microdebrider surgical instruments, 197
Microfibrillar collagen, 213
Microfollicular adenomas, 411
Microvascular decompression, 565
Microvascular disease, 553
Mid-face bones, 532*f*
Mid-face fractures, 532-533
  repairing, 533
Migraine, 185
Mikulicz's syndrome, 438
Mineral oil, 42, 589
MMS, 520
Mohs' defect, 519*f*
Mohs' micrographic surgery
  for basal cell carcinoma, 514
  for keratoacanthoma, 510

Mononucleosis
  with massive tonsillar swelling, 362
  oral manifestations of, 234, 249
  shaggy exudate of, 361*f*
  in viral lymphadenopathy, 401
Mononucleosis tonsillitis, 249
Moraxella
  in acute otitis media, 45
  catarrhalis, 193
Motility disorders, 301-302
Motion sickness, 128
Motor neuron disorders, lower, 286
Mouth. *See also* Oral cavity
  floor of, 232
  ulcerated cancer of floor of, 618*f*
Mouth breathing, 3-4
Moxifloxacin, 193
Mucoceles
  on lips, 259
  obliterating frontal sinus, 187*f*
Mucoepidermoid carcinoma, 442
  parotid, 417
Mucolytics
  for AIDS-related sinusitis, 643
  for rhinosinusitis, 196
Mucor
  branching hyphae of, 638*f*
  nasopharyngeal, 273
Mucormycosis
  with diabetes mellitus, 639
  in immunocompromised patient, 636-638
  of labyrinth, 118
Mucosal burns, depth of, 597
Mucosal challenge testing, 163
Mucosal immunosuppression, 189
Mucosal melanoma, 263
Mucosal stasis, 182-183
Mucosal-transport disorders, 189
Mucositis, 234
  chemotherapy-induced, 252, 254
  radiation-induced, 252, 253*f*
Müller maneuver, 21
Multiple sclerosis
  dizziness with, 127
  in dysphagia, 286
Multiple sleep latency test, 312
Mumps, 437-438
Mupirocin, 644
Muscle relaxation, 339
Muscular disease, 286
Muscular dystrophy
  in dysphagia, 286

  family history of, 295
Muscular tension dysphonia, 333
Musculoaponeurotic system, superficial, 550
Musculoskeletal disorders, 281*t*
Myasthenia gravis, 286-287
Mycobacterial infections, 642
  atypical, 642
  neck masses with
    AIDS-related, 646
  skin tests for, 421-422
  salivary involvement in, 440-441
Mycobacterium
  atypical, in granulomatous lymphadenopathy, 402-403
  nasopharyngeal, 272-273
  tuberculosis
    in granulomatous lymphadenopathy, 403
    in inflammatory neck masses, 421
Mycoplasma pneumoniae, 43
Mycostatin, 486
Mycotic infections, oral, 251-252
Myelomeningocele, 352-353
Mylohyoid muscle, 232
Myofascial pain syndrome, 482, 483
  physical examination for, 483-484
  treatment of, 486
Myxedema, classic, 468*f*

N-acetylcysteine, 599
N-staging, enlarged regional neck node, 610*t*
Narcolepsy, 312
Nasal airflow, 146
  measurement of, 148
  obstruction of, 146-147
Nasal angiofibroma, juvenile
  diagnosis of, 158
  epistaxis with, 211
Nasal blood supply, 202-204
Nasal bones, 218
Nasal cavity
  anatomy and physiology of, 202-205
  before decongestion, 14*f*
  endoscopic view of, 267*f*
  tumors of, 210
  visualization of for nasal fractures, 222
Nasal channels, 2
Nasal congestion, 185
Nasal corticosteroids, 169-170
Nasal cycle, 147
  in nasal obstruction, 151

Nasal dilator adhesive strips, 316*f*
Nasal discharge, 185
Nasal disease, 654, 655*t*
Nasal endoscopy
 for nasal obstruction, 156-157
 for olfactory disorders, 656
Nasal examination
 for facial trauma, 525
 for nasal fracture, 221
Nasal fractures, 218, 534-536
 anatomy and physiology of, 218
 complex, 223*f*
 danger signs in, 225-226
 diagnostic evaluation for, 222-225
 displaced, 226
 frontal and base views of, 220*f*
 history for, 219-220
 management algorithm for, 219*f*
 management and follow-up for, 225
 physical examination for, 221-222
Nasal mask, CPAP, 316*f*
Nasal mucosa
 dryness of, 202
 erythematous, cobblestoned, 188
Nasal obstruction
 in anosmia, 663
 bilateral, 151
 causes of, 145, 152*t*
 danger signs in, 159
 diagnostic evaluation for, 155-158
 epistaxis with, 209-210
 history of, 150-153
 management algorithm for, 146*f*
 management and follow-up for, 158-159
 with minor nasal trauma, 224*f*
 in nasopharyngeal disorders, 266-267
 physical examination for, 153-155
 self-treated, 145
 treatment of in obstructive sleep apnea, 314
Nasal packing, 216f
 for epistaxis, 214*f*, 215
 for nasal fracture, 219
 for nasal hematoma or abscess, 226
Nasal passages, 145-150
Nasal polypectomy, 156
Nasal polyposis, bilateral, 157-158
Nasal saline irrigations, 196
Nasal septum, 13, 218
 abscess of, 226
 with nasal fractures, 220

 blood supply of, 205*f*
 deviated, 13-14
  coronal CT showing, 155*f*
  examination for, 19-21
  nasal obstruction and, 147
 hematoma of, 224*f*
  indications of, 225
  treatment of, 226
 hematomas of, 222
 in nasal airflow, 148
 parts of, 150*f*
 trauma to, untreated, 224*f*
Nasal speculum, 19-20, 207
Nasal sprays
 for allergic rhinitis, 170-171, 195
 for rhinosinusitis, 196
Nasal turbinates, 13, 15*f*
 concha bullosa in, 184*f*
 engorgement of, 147-148
 in nasal obstruction, 154
 hypertrophy of, 149
 middle, 14
 turgidity of, 149-150
 visualization of, 268
Nasal valve, 146-147
Nasal vault angiofibroma, 209*f*
Nasal vestibule, 13
 AIDS-related infections of, 643-644
 furunculosis of, 18
Nasal wall, lateral, 151*f*, 218
Naso-orbital-ethmoid complex fracture, 535
Nasogastric intubation
 for aspiration, 373-374
 for caustic ingestion, 599
 for hiccups, 563-564
Nasolacrimal apparatus, 148-149, 535
Nasopharyngeal angiofibroma, juvenile, 274-275
 in nasal obstruction, 153
Nasopharyngeal carcinoma
 epistaxis with, 210
 MRI showing, 392*f*
 neck metastases from, 276*f*
Nasopharyngeal mirror, 269*f*, 607
Nasopharyngitis, acute, 273
Nasopharyngoscope, 268
 inserting into nose, 25*f*
Nasopharyngoscopy
 flexible fiberoptic, 329
 mirror, 191
 technique of, 24*f*

Nasopharynx
  anatomic structures surrounding, 269f
  anatomy and physiology of, 265-266
  cancer of
    evaluation of, 611
    incidence of, 611
    WHO classification of, 611
  disorders of, 265-278
    congenital, 275
    danger signs in, 278
    diagnosis and management of, 271-278
    differential diagnosis of, 273t
    history in, 266-267
    local, 274-275
    management algorithm for, 266f
    physical examination for, 267-271
  endoscopic view of, 268f
  examination of, 21-22
    for neck masses, 390-391
    optimal positioning for, 270f
  lateral radiography of, 272f
  masses in, 267
  packing of, 215f
  polyps in, 274
  rare tumors of, 277-278
  topographic anatomy of, 14-15
  tumors of
    benign, 276
    malignant, 276-278
  visualization of, 267-268
Nasopharyngeal lymphoepitheliomas, 277
Nasotracheal intubation, 524
Neck. See also Head and neck; Neck masses
  anatomic triangles of, 384f
  anatomical triangles of, 383
  anatomy of, 383-388
  anterior triangle of, 383-384
  aspiration with cancer of, 367
  carotid triangle of, 384-385
  contact dermatitis on, 167f
  levels of, 386f
  muscular triangle of, 385
  nasopharyngeal carcinoma metastasis to, 276f
  palpation of for cancer, 606
  posterior triangle of, 383
  rejuvenation surgery for, 550-552
  submandibular triangle of, 384
  submental triangle of, 384
  topographic anatomy of, 16
Neck dissection
  comprehensive, 616
  neck deformity after, 616, 617f
  for oral cavity cancer, 612-617
  for thyroid cancer, 467-468
  for tongue cancer, 608
Neck lifts, 550-552
Neck masses, 426-427
  age and location of, 389
  AIDS-related, 645-646
  benign neoplastic
    diagnosis and management of, 406-412
  classification of, 389t
  congenital, 389
    diagnosis and management of, 394-401
    differential diagnosis of, 393t
    location of, 390t, 391f
    type and location of, 394t
  diagnosis of, 383
  diagnostic categories of, 394t
  differential diagnosis of, 393-394
  examination for, 390-391
  history and physical examination for, 389-393
  inflammatory, 389
    diagnosis and management of, 401-406
    differential diagnosis of, 393t
    type and location of, 394t
  location, size, color, and consistency of, 391
  management and follow-up for, 423-426
  in nasal obstruction, 159
  neoplastic, 389
    differential diagnosis of, 393t
    malignant, 412-420
    type and location of, 394t
  painful, 390
  in upper airway obstruction, 344
  work-up for, 420-423
Necrosis, facial, 553
Necrotizing otitis
  AIDS-related, 643
  in immunocompromised patient, 635-636
Necrotizing otitis externa, 40
Necrotizing sialometaplasia, 246
Neomycin
  in contact dermatitis, 93
  for diffuse bacterial external otitis, 38
  topical sensitivity to in ear drops, 39f
Neoplasms
  adnexal, 516

benign oral, 258-260
differential diagnosis of sinus-type symptoms of, 188*t*
in facial asymmetry, 501-502
in gustatory dysfunction, 660
laryngeal, 355-356
malignant oral, 260-263
in nasal obstruction, 151, 152*t*, 154, 159
pharyngeal, 51
in referred otalgia, 50-51
with rhinosinusitis, 200
of salivary glands, 434*t*, 441-445
sinonasal, 189
in vocal cord paralysis, 352
Neoplastic neck masses, 389
benign, 406-412
management of, 425
Neurofibromas, 407
Neurogenic neck masses, 406-407
Neurological disorders
aspiration associated with, 365, 366*t*
in dysphagia, 281*t*
in vocal cord paralysis, 352-353
Neurological examination, 136
Neuroma, acoustic, 61
computed tomographic scan of, 62*f*
Neuropathic disorders, 188*t*
Neurosurgery, 654
Neutropenia
Aspergillus sinusitis and, 638-640
bacterial infections and, 640
oral ulcerations and, 641
Nevus, face or scalp, 511
Niacin, 129
Nickel contact dermatitis, 93
Nociception
categories of, 481
cranial nerves in, 479
Nodular leukoplakia, 256
Noise exposure, 68
Nonsteroidal anti-inflammatory drugs (NSAIDs)
epistaxis with, 210, 215
for furunculosis, 42
Nose
abnormal anatomy of, 184*f*
AIDS-related infections of, 643-644
allergic conditions of, 161, 162*f*, 169-174
anatomy of, 145-147
artificial, 8-10
biopsy for masses in, 157-158
cross-sectional area of, 147
early reconstructive surgery for, 8

examination of, 18-21
foreign bodies in, 11, 590
functions of, 145
injury of, 8
large, 7-8
medical history of, 7-10
physiology of, 146-150
polyps in, 173-174
in hyposmia, 657
in nasal obstruction, 154, 156
in sinus disease, 20-21
posterior choanae of, 265-266
in respiration, 2
rhinoplasty for, 8-10
squamous cell carcinoma of, 515*f*
topographic anatomy of, 13-14
trauma to, 534-536
dislocated septum in, 19
Nosocomial sinusitis, 640
NPO, 373-374
Nystagmus, 105
in dizziness, 107, 108
left-beating, 105
with suppurative labyrinthitis, 118
Nystatin, 634

Obesity-related sleep apnea, 307
Observationes Anatomicae (Fallopio), 2
Obstructive sleep apnea syndrome, 304, 320
complications of, 304
danger signs for, 319
diagnostic tests for, 311-312
differential diagnosis of, 310-311
history for, 309
management of, 312-318
algorithm for, 306*f*
medical consequences of, 305*f*
physical examination for, 309-310
presenting symptoms of, 305-307
relevant anatomy and physiology of, 307-309
therapy for, 304
Occupational Health and Safety Act, noise hazards, 139
Ocular disorders, 127
Ocular emergency treatment, 525
Oculopharyngeal dysphagia, 295
Oculopharyngeal syndrome, 286
Odontalgia, atypical, 483
treatment of, 487
Odontogenic infections
in bacterial lymphadenopathy, 402
of neck, 424

Odor detection thresholds, 657
Odor discrimination, 657
Odor-identification test, 656, 657
Odor memory, 657
Odorants, perception of, 653
Odynophagia, 279
 with esophageal foreign body, 580
 in head and neck cancer, 632
Oidiomycetes, 166
Olfactory assessment, 656-657, 661
Olfactory brain potentials, 657
Olfactory disorders, 650
 danger signs in, 663
 definition of, 654
 diagnostic evaluation of, 654-656
 etiology of, 654
 major causes of, 655*t*
 management algorithm for, 651*f*
 olfactory testing for, 656-657
 physiology of, 653
 treatment of, 657-658
Olfactory nerve, 650
Olfactory neuroepithelium, 653
Olfactory receptor neurons, 653
Olfactory sensitivity testing, 653, 657
Omohyoid muscle, 385
Oncocytomas, 411
Ondansetron (Zofran), 128
Open reduction, frontal sinus fracture, 535-536
Ophthalmic artery, 204
Optical forceps, 578*f*
Orabase, 241
Oral cavity
 acquired conditions of, 237*t*
 allergic disorders of, 237*t*
 anatomic aberrations and inherited conditions of, 237*t*
 diagnosis and management of, 238-240
 anatomy and physiology of, 231-233
 autoimmune and allergic conditions of, 237*t*, 240-246
 benign neoplasms of, 237*t*
 cancer of, 260-261, 605-606
  advanced, 613-615
  danger signs suggesting, 234*t*
  examination for, 606
  follow-up for, 623
  incidence of, 612
  as lifestyle disease, 615
  speech therapy after, 621-622

 swallowing rehabilitation after, 619-621
 T-staging for, 610*t*
 treatment of, 612-623
 examination of, 22-23, 188, 606
 functions of, 231
 hemangiomas of, 259
 infections of, 361-362
 infectious lesions of, 237*t*
 malignancies of, 22, 237*t*
 medication-induced conditions of, 237*t*
 mucosal lesions of, 231
  diagnosis and management of, 236, 238-264
  differential diagnosis of, 236-238
  history of, 233-234
  physical examination for, 234-236
 reconstruction of, 617-619
 systemic disorders of, 237*t*, 240-246
 trauma to, 237*t*, 257-258
Oral contraceptives, 244
Oral devices, 317*f*
Oral hygiene, 660
Oral jet irrigator, 81-83
Oral lichen planus, AIDS-related, 250
Oral thrush
 AIDS-related, 644
 in diabetes mellitus, 634-635
Oral ulcerations, 641
Orbicularis oris muscle, 257-258
Oropharyngeal dysphagia, 302
Oropharynx
 anatomy and physiology of, 232-233
 burns of, 598
 cancer of, 260-261
 candidiasis of, 250
 caustic burn of, 595
 disorders of, 281*t*
 examination of, 22-23
 for cancer, 606
 functions of, 231
 lesions of, 236
 mucosal lesions of, 231
 squamous papillomas of, 250
 topographic anatomy of, 15-16
 tuberculosis of, 251
Orotracheal intubation, 523-524
OSAS. *See* Obstructive sleep apnea syndrome
Osler-Weber-Rendu disease, 210
Ossicles, 56
Osteoarthritic spurs, cervical, 293

Osteomeatal complex, 182
    inflammation and obstruction of, 190f
Osteomyelitis, 49f
Otalgia, 607
    differential diagnosis of, 34t
    evaluation of, 32
    head and neck examination for, 31-32
    in hearing loss, 70-71
    history in, 32-34
    management of, 32f
    referred, 31, 49-51
        causes of, 33f
        neural pathways of, 33f
Otitic barotrauma, 47-49
Otitis, necrotizing, 635-636
Otitis externa
    AIDS-related, 643
    with cerumen removal, 84
    chronic
        AIDS-related, 643
        diagnosis and management of, 89-91
    diffuse bacterial, 36-39
    eczematoid, 92
    evaluation for, 31
    fungal, 92
    malignant, 41f, 51
    necrotizing, 40
    nonspecific dermatitis preceding, 91
Otitis media, 56
    acute, 45-46
        AIDS-related, 642
    chronic, 46-47, 118
        with tympanic membrane perforation, 48
    evaluation for, 31
    in facial paralysis, 498
    intracranial spread of, 50f
    serous, with nasopharyngeal masses, 267
    with tympanic membrane perforation, 44
Otoconia, 104
Otolaryngic allergy, 165-168
Otolaryngology
    development of instruments for, 4-8
    history of, 1-12
Otolith-repositioning procedure, 120
Otologic disease, 498
Otomycosis, 40-41, 91
    mycelial elements in, 42f
Otorrhea, 100
    cerebrospinal fluid, 538
    differential diagnosis of, 34t

    in dizziness, 107
Otosclerosis, 128
Otoscope, 4, 6f, 35f
    pneumatic and surgical, 79f
Otoscopy
    for cerumen impaction, 77
    for facial paralysis, 494
    of otalgia, 31
    for tinnitus, 136
Ototoxicity, 68
Oxidized cellulose packing, 213
Oxybenzones, 541
Oxycel, 213
Oxygen therapy, 347
Oxymetazoline
    for epistaxis, 207, 214
    plus lidocaine, 207
    for rhinosinusitis, 195

Paget, Sir James, 11
Pain perception, 479
Palatal advancement, 317
Palatal myoclonus, 133-134
Palate. *See also* Hard palate; Soft palate
    defect of after soft palate cancer resection, 621f
    distortion of in nasal obstruction, 159
    ulcers of with mucormycosis, 639
Palatine tonsils, 16
Palpitation, with dizziness, 130
Panendoscopy, 414
Papain, 585
Papillary cystadenoma lymphomatosum, 410-411
Papillary thyroid carcinoma, 419, 466
Papilledema, 107
Papilloma
    epistaxis with, 210
    of head, 506
Para-auditory noises, 132-134
Para-aminobenzoic acid, 541
Paradoxical vocal fold motion, 354-355
Paragangliomas, 407-408
    carotid, 408-409
    management of, 425
    nonchromaffin, 407-408
    vagal, 408
Paranasal sinuses, 148-149
Paranasal tumors, 153
Parapharyngeal masses, 260
Parapharyngeal nodes, 387
Parapharyngeal parotid tumors, 443-444
Paraphenylenediamine, 93

Parasympathetic efferent fibers, 491
Parasympathetic tone, 149-150
Parasymphyseal mandible fracture, 527f
Parathormone
   intraoperative assay of, 473
   production of, 469
   serum levels of in hyperparathyroidism, 471
Parathyroid adenoma
   location of, 471-472
   sestamibi scan of, 472f
Parathyroid glands
   anatomy of, 450-451
   carcinoma of, 470
   function of, 469
   location of, 470f
Paré, Ambrose, 2, 8-10
Parkinson's disease
   in dysphagia, 286, 287
   managing dysphagia of, 302
   in olfactory disorders, 654
Parosmia, 654
Parotid duct injuries, 537
Parotid glands, 429
   adenoid cystic carcinoma of, 443f
   AIDS-related massive cysts of, 647f
   congenital masses of, 400-401
   deep lobe and parapharyngeal tumors of, 443-444
   drainage of, 430
   enlarged, AIDS-related, 647
   examination of, 235
   injury to, 448
   lymphoepithelial cysts in, 441
   mass in, 431f
   neoplasms of, 416-417
   palpation of in facial paralysis, 494
   pleomorphic adenoma of, 442f
   sarcoidosis involving, 441
   swelling of, 439
      in Sjögren's disease, 440f
Parotidectomy
   for parotid gland masses, 442-443
   sequelae and complications of, 444-445
   for sialadenitis, 437
Parotitis, 446
   acute, 436-437
Parry-Romberg syndrome, 500-501
Passy-Muir valve, 375
Pediatric disorders, 114t
Pemburton's sign, 454, 461-462
Pemphigus, oral, 244
Penicillamine, 599

Penicillins
   for necrotizing otitis externa, 40
   for rhinosinusitis, 193
Pentagastrin infusion, 454
Peptic strictures, 580
Peptostreptococcus, 193
Percutaneous gastrostomy, 614
Peri-auricular edema, 100
Perichondritis
   early signs of, 100
   edema and erythema in, 95f
   in itchy ears, 94-96
Perilymph, 102
   fistula of, 122
Periodic movement syndromes, 311
Periodontal disease, AIDS-related, 644
Periodontitis, 22
Periorbital examination, 524-525
Periparotid lymph node actinomycosis, 440-441
Peritonsillar abscesses, 362
Pernicious anemia
   with aphthous ulcers, 240
   in dysphagia, 289
Petroleum-jelly strip gauze, 214
Petrous bone, cholesterol granuloma of, 62f
Phantosmia, 654
Pharyngeal abscess, bleeding of, 6
Pharyngeal bands, lateral, 239
Pharyngeal paresis, 368f, 369
Pharyngeal reflux, 354
Pharyngeal stimulation, 565-566
Pharyngitis, granular, 239
Pharyngoscope, flexible fiberoptic nasal, 300f
Pharyngoscopy, 400
Pharynx
   aspiration in disorders of, 284
   cancer of, 293
   dentures impacted in, 588
   endoscopic examination of, 299
   fish and chicken bones in, 586-587
   foreign bodies in, 586
      complications of, 588
      history of, 586-587
      management of, 587-588
      physical examination for, 587
   hemangiomas of, 259
   neoplasms of in referred otalgia, 51
   in swallowing, 282-283
Phenol peel, 543
   hypopigmentation with, 544
Phenothiazines, 295, 296

Phenytoin
  in Stevens-Johnson syndrome, 254
  xerostomia with, 255
Pheochromocytoma urine studies, 454-455
Phlebotomy, 6
Phonation, 330f
Photodamage
  protection against, 541
  skin, 539-540
Photodynamic therapy, 520
Phrenic nerve
  in hiccups, 559
  inflammation of, 561
  section of for hiccups, 565
Physical examination
  for advanced oral cavity cancer, 613
  for airway foreign bodies, 569-570
  for allergic conditions, 161
  for atypical facial pain, 483-484
  for aural itching, 88
  for cerumen impaction, 77
  for cervical metastasis and lymph node malignancies, 413-415
  for dizziness, 107-110
  for dysphagia, 295-296
  for epistaxis, 205-207
  for esophageal foreign body, 580
  for face and scalp lesions, 506-507
  for facial paralysis, 493-494
  for facial trauma, 524-525
  for fibrous dysplasia, 500
  for goiter, 463
  for head and neck cancer, 606-607
  for hearing loss, 58-59
  for hiccups, 562
  for hoarseness, 328-329
  for nasal fractures, 221-222
  for nasal obstruction, 153-155
  for nasopharyngeal disorders, 267-271
  for neck masses, 389-393
  for obstructive sleep apnea, 309-310
  for olfactory disorders, 656
  for oral cavity lesions, 234-236
  for pharyngeal foreign bodies, 587
  for rhinosinusitis, 185-188
  for salivary gland disorders, 432-433
  of thyroid gland, 453-454
  for tinnitus, 135-136
  for upper airway obstruction, 344-345
Pickwick Papers (Dickens), Joe the Fat Boy in, 3, 305
Pickwickian syndrome, 305
  true, 307

Pilocarpine, 448
Pinna, 53, 56
  atopic dermatitis of, 97
  with cartilaginous folds, 18f
  congenital malformations of, 58
  convoluted cartilage of, 55f
  unusually shaped, 16-17
Pipe-smoker's stomatitis, 22-23
Plain radiography
  for nasal fractures, 223-225
  Waters-view, 190
Plato, 11-12
Pleomorphic adenoma, 410, 442
  complications of parotidectomy for, 445
  nasopharyngeal, 276
Plummer-Vinson syndrome, 289, 485
  family history of, 295
Pneumatic massage, 136
Pneumatic splinting, 313f
Pneumococcus otitis media, 45
Pneumocystis infection, nasopharyngeal, 272-273
Pneumonia, aspiration, 366
Poiseuille's law, 147
Poison Prevention Packaging Act, 593
Poisoning, caustic, 592-602
Politzer, Adam, 4
Polycythemia, 126
Polymyxin, 38
Polypectomy
  for hyposmia, 657
  for rhinosinusitis, 197-198
Polypoid corditis, 26
Polyposis, 198
Polyps, nasal, 173-174
Polysomnography, 311
Polytetrafluoroethylene implant, 554
Positioning test, 109
Postintubation granulation polyp, 338
Postpolio syndrome, 286
Posturography
  six positions in, 113f
  for tinnitus, 137
PPD skin testing
  for granulomatous lympadenopathy, 403
  for inflammatory neck masses, 421
  for tuberculosis, 404
Prednisone
  for allergic fungal sinusitis, 173
  for Bell's palsy, 492
  for facial paralysis, 496
  for herpes zoster oticus, 493

Pregnancy, oral lesions associated with, 244
Presbycusis, 68
Presbylarynx, 372
Pressure-equalizing tube, 119
Prick allergy testing, 163
Processed acellular cadaveric skin (AlloDerm), 553
Progressive hemifacial atrophy, 500
 history and physical examination for, 501
 management and follow-up for, 501
Proprioceptive disorders, 127
 dizziness with, 127
Proprioceptive system, 105
Proptosis, 159
Prosthetic rehabilitation, oral cavity, 619-621
Proteus external otitis, 36
Proton-pump inhibitors
 for caustic ingestion, 599
 for episodic laryngospasm, 354
 for reflux laryngitis, 329-331
Pruritus, external auditory canal, 86
Pseudocysts, salivary gland, 446
Pseudoephedrine
 for acute sinusitis, 182
 for AIDS-related sinusitis, 643
 for rhinosinusitis, 195
Pseudoepitheliomatous hyperplasia, 510
Pseudomonas aeruginosa
 in diffuse bacterial external otitis, 36
 in itchy ear, 96
 in necrotizing otitis, 40, 635-636
 in rhinosinusitis, 193, 194
 in AIDS-related sinusitis, 643
 with chemical peel, 544
Pseudoxanthoma elasticum, 539-540
Psoriasis, ear, 97-98
Psychiatric evaluation, 594, 596
Psychic pneuma, 2
Psychoactive agents, 255
Psychogenic pain, facial, 481
Psychogenic vertigo, 128
Psychotherapy, 565
Ptotic submandibular glands, 16
Puberty, oral lesions associated with, 244
Pulmonary complications, aspiration-related, 363, 366
Pulmonary function tests, 346
Pulse irregularity, 107
Punch biopsy
 for facial and scalp skin malignancy, 507

 technique of, 508f
Pupillary light response, 524
Pupillary reaction, 107
Pure-tone audiometry, 137
Pylorus, caustics in, 595
Pynchon, Thomas, 10
Pyogenic granulomas, 260
Pyriform sinuses, 16
 ulceration of, 614
Pyrimethamine, 405, 424

Quincke's disease, 238
Quinine, 127

Radiation-induced mucositis, 252, 253f
Radiation-induced xerostomia, 434t
Radiation therapy
 adjuvant, 623
 for advanced oral cavity cancer, 614
 for basal cell carcinoma, 514-515
 for glottic cancer, 625
 for head and neck squamous cell cancer, 610-611
 for hemangiomas, 401
 for laryngeal cancer of vocal folds, 334-335
 for malignant melanoma of head and neck, 517
 for nasopharyngeal carcinoma, 611
 for neoplastic neck masses, 425
 in olfactory disorders, 654
 for oral cavity cancer, 622-623
 oral lesions with, 234
 for paragangliomas, 408
 side effects of, 623
 for skin cancer, 520
 for supraglottic cancer, 629
 xerostomia with, 448
Radioactive iodine ablation, 465
Radioallergosorbent test (RAST), 164, 165
 immunotherapy and, 176
Radiofrequency fibrosis, 317
Radiography
 for caustic ingestion, 597-598, 599
 for epistaxis, 208
 for esophageal foreign body, 580-582, 584
 for facial trauma, 525-526
 for head and neck cancer, 608-609
 for hiccups, 560-561, 562-563
 for mandible fractures, 526-528
 for nasal fractures, 222-225
 for rhinosinusitis, 190

for salivary gland disorders, 435
Radiology
　for airway foreign bodies, 570
　for dysphagia, 297-299
　for gustatory dysfunction, 661
　for olfactory disorders, 656
　for upper airway obstruction, 346
Radiolucent foreign bodies, 583
Ragweed pollen, 171
Ramsey-Hunt syndrome. *See also* Herpes zoster oticus
　in chronic otitis externa, 90f
　with dizziness, 118
Ranula, 260, 446-447
Rapid-sequence induction, 364
Rathke's pouch, 266, 275
RDI. *See* Respiratory disturbance index
Reactive airway disease, 363
Reconstructive surgery
　for advanced oral cavity cancer, 613
　for facial or scalp malignancy, 507
　options for skin cancer, 518-520
　for oral cavity cancer, 617-619
Reduction, nasal fracture, 225, 226
Reepithelialization, 546
Referred pain, 481
　trigger area of, 483
Reflux laryngitis
　case of, 332
　treatment of, 329-331
Regional skin flaps, 518t
Rehabilitation
　after oral cavity cancer surgery, 619-621
　after supraglottic laryngectomy, 630
Rehabilitative vestibular exercises, 117
Reinke's edema, 355
　cause and treatment of, 338t
Relaxation therapy
　for functional inspiratory adduction, 355
　for tinnitus, 140-141
REM sleep, monitoring of, 308-309
Renal disease, 660
Resection
　for hemangiomas, 401
　for oral cavity cancer, 612
Respiration
　Galen's description of, 1-2
　upper airway in, 1
Respiratory alkalosis, 557
Respiratory distress, 399
Respiratory disturbance index, 317
　for sleep apnea, 306f, 311
Respiratory failure, 346

Respiratory papillomatosis, recurrent, 355
Respiratory support, 339
Resuscitation, 597-598
ret oncogene analysis, 455
Reticular system, 105
Retin-A, 541
Retinal disease, 107
Retinoids, 511
Retroglossal airway
　enlargement of, 319f
　oral devices to open, 317f
Retromastoid craniotomy, 116
Retropharyngeal abscesses, 361
　with pharyngeal foreign bodies, 588
Retropharyngeal nodes, 387
Rhabdomyosarcoma, 420
　nasopharyngeal, 277
Rheum, 2
Rhinitis, allergic, 169-172
Rhinitis medicamentosa, 148
　in nasal obstruction, 150
Rhinolalia, 232
Rhinolith, 11
Rhinomanometry, 148
　mask for, 149f
　for nasal obstruction, 154-155
Rhinophyma, 8, 9f
Rhinoplasty
　descriptions of, 10
　history of, 8-10
　in olfactory disorders, 654
Rhinorrhea
　allergic, 195
　cerebrospinal fluid, 537-538
　with nasal fractures, 220, 226
　watery, 226
Rhinoscopy, 4
　anterior, for rhinosinusitis, 186-188
　in foreign object removal, 11
　for nasal obstruction, 154
Rhinosinusitis, 172
　acute, 193
　allergic, 93
　anatomy and physiology of, 182-184
　chronic, 181
　　management of, 193
　danger signs of, 199-200
　diagnostic evaluation for, 20, 190-192
　differential diagnosis of, 188-189
　factors associated with, 181t
　history of, 184-185
　incidence and costs of, 179
　indications of, 179-181

Rhinosinusitis—*continued*
  infectious, 188
  management algorithm for, 180*f*
  management and follow-up for, 192-199
  physical examination for, 185-188
  recurrent acute, 181-182
  subacute, 181
  treatment of, 179
Rhinosporidium, nasopharyngeal, 272-273
Rhytidectomy, 540*t*
Rinne test, 59, 60*f*
Rosenmüller's fossa, 15, 265
  visualization of, 268
Rotation chair testing, 112*f*
Rotational studies, 137
Rush, Benjamin, 6

Saccule, 102, 104, 398
Saddle-nose deformity, 224*f*, 534
Sagittal mandibular osteotomy, inferior, 318
Saliva
  in food preparation, 282
  hypersecretion of, 447
  reduced flow of in dysphagia, 295
  uric acid crystals in, 446
Salivary ducts
  obstruction of, 260
  strictures of, 441
Salivary glands
  AIDS-associated cysts of, 444
  AIDS-related infection of, 647
  anatomy and physiology of, 429-432
  benign neoplasms of, 409-411
  disorders of, 429
    danger signs for, 449
    diagnostic tests for, 433-435
    differential diagnosis of, 433, 434*t*
    history of, 432
    management algorithm for, 430*f*
    management of, 436-448
    physical examination for, 432-433
  dysfunction of with Sjögren's syndrome, 242-244
  in gustatory dysfunction, 661
  malignant neoplasms of, 416-418
  minor, 232, 429
    adenocystic carcinoma of, 262*f*
    malignancies of, 261-263
  secretomotor innervation of, 430-432
  swelling of, 429
Salivary pooling, 372
Salivary stone, 235*f*

Salivation
  enhancement of, 301
  reticular system in, 105
Salogen, 448
Salt-restricted diet, 115
Sarcoidosis
  diagnosis of, 421
  in granulomatous lymphadenopathy, 404-405
  management of, 424
  parotid enlargement with, 441
  in supraglottic obstruction, 360-361
Scalp
  anatomy and physiology of, 504-506
  layers of, 504
  lesions of, 520-521
    danger signs for, 520
    diagnosis and management of, 507-520
    physical examination for, 506-507
    squamous papilloma of, 512*f*
SCALP mnemonic, 504
Scarring
  with chemical peel, 545
  with dermabrasion, 548
Schatzki's ring, 580
Schirmer's test, 405
Schwannomas, neck, 407
Sclerosis, salivary gland, 647
Scratch testing, 163
Screening, head and neck cancer, 604-606
Scrotal tongue. *See* Fissured tongue
Sebaceous glands, benign ectopic, 243*f*
Seborrheic dermatitis, 98-99
Seborrheic keratosis, 508
  diagnosis and management of, 509
Secretomotor nerves, 430-432
Segmental reconstructive procedures, 601
Selenium sulfide shampoo, 99
Semicircular canal, 102
Sensitivity studies, 421
Sensorineural auditory noises, 133, 134
Sensorineural hearing loss, 53
  with acoustic neuroma, 122
  AIDS-related, 642
  audiograms for, 63-64
  differential diagnosis of, 59-60
  with labyrinthine concussion, 122
  low-frequency, 115
  management of, 68-70
  sudden, 69
  with suppurative labyrinthitis, 118

with temporal bone fracture, 119, 120-122
testing for, 59
Sensory system, 650-653
Sentinel-node mapping, 517
Septoplasty
  for nasal fractures, 225
  for rhinosinusitis, 197
Sequential intradermal tests, 163
Serial end point titration testing, 164f
Serologic studies, 421
Serous labyrinthitis, 118-119
Serous otitis, 159
Serous otitis media, 267
Serum-immunoglobulin deficiencies, 641
Sestamibi scanning
  for hyperparathyroidism, 471
  showing parathyroid adenoma, 472f
Sharpened Romberg test, 108
Shave biopsy
  for malignant melanoma of head and neck, 517
  for nevus, 511f
Shunting, 129
Sialadenitis, 235
  acute suppurative, 405-406, 436
  chronic, 406, 441
  chronic punctate, 438
  diagnosis of, 424
  in lymphadenopathy, 401
  parotid gland, 242
Sialography, contrast, 435
Sialolithiasis, 406
  chronic, 438, 439
Sicca complex, 438
Sickle cell anemia, 126
Siegle pneumatic otoscope, 4, 6f
Signet-ring cell squamous cell carcinoma, 515
Silicone gels, 545
Silicone hearing aids, 93
Sinclair, Upton, 7
Singultus, 557. See also Hiccups
Sinonasal neoplasms
  epistaxis with, 210
  with nasal obstruction, 151
  versus rhinosinusitis, 189
Sinus culture, 191-192
Sinuses
  allergic conditions of, 169-174
  innervation of, 188-189
  normal, 183f

obstructed drainage of, 189
in olfactory disorders, 654, 655t
Sinusitis, 172. See also Rhinosinusitis
  allergic fungal, 172-173
  computed tomography of, 174f
  thick inspissated pus of, 175f
  Aspergillus, 638-640
  bony-cartilaginous spur with, 198
  chronic, AIDS-related, 643
  nosocomial, 640
Sinusoidal harmonic acceleration, 111-112
Sjögren's disease
  conditions associated with, 439-440
  in dysphagia, 288-289
  parotid swelling in, 440f
Sjögren's syndrome, 242-244
  diagnosis of, 421
  in granulomatous lymphadenopathy, 405
  salivary gland inflammation in, 438-439
  thickened mucosal secretions in, 271
  treatment of, 448
Skin
  cancer of, reconstructive options for, 518-520
  damage to, 539-541
  eradicating malignancies of, 507
  hemangiomas of, 400
  lesions of, management algorithm for, 505f
  resurfacing of
    chemical peeling for, 541-545
    dermabrasion, 546-548
    laser, 545-546
    topical therapy for, 541
Skin flaps, 518t
Skin grafts, tongue and mouth floor, 619f
Skin testing
  allergy, 163
  for neck masses, 421-422
Skull-base neoplasm, 151
Skull-base osteomyelitis, AIDS-related, 643
Sleep apnea, 3
  laryngoscopic evaluation of, 21-22
  obstructive, 304-320
  physiologic consequences of, 308
Sleep deprivation, 310-311
Sleep monitoring, 308-309
Smell
  centers specializing in, 664
  disorders of, 650. See also Olfactory disorders
    management algorithm for, 651f

Smoking
    in aerodigestive tract squamous cell carcinoma, 260
    in ear pain, 32
    enlarged jugulodigastric lymph nodes with, 414
    facial rejuvenation surgery complications with, 553
    glottic cancer with, 337
    in head and neck cancer, 632
    hoarseness with, 333-335
    in leukoplakia, 256
    oral disease and, 22-23
    upper aerodigestive trace carcinoma with, 293
Sneezing, 11
Snellen chart test, 221
SNHL. *See* Sensorineural hearing loss
Sniffin' sticks, 656
Snore ball, 314-315
Snoring
    harmful effects of, 3
    new-onset, 267
    treatment of in obstructive sleep apnea, 314-315
    weight loss for, 307
Snoring caps, 3
Snuff-dipper's leukoplakia, 233*f*
Soft palate, 16, 232
    defects in, 232
Soft tissue injuries, facial, 536-538
Soft tissue scarring, 350
Sound, 56
    air conduction of, 63
    bone conduction of, 63
Sour stimuli, 658
Spasmodic dysphonia, 338*t*
Speech
    esophageal, 627
    hypernasal, 232
Speech audiometry, 137
Speech discrimination, 69
Speech-reception threshold, 68, 69
Speech rehabilitation, 626-628
Speech therapy
    after supraglottic laryngectomy, 630
    for oral cavity cancer, 621-622
    with vagal lesion, 370
Sphenoid rhinosinusitis, 185
Sphenopalatine artery, 204-205
Sphenopalatine ganglion, 485
Sphenopalatine neuralgia, 482
    diagnosis of, 484

    physical examination for, 483
    treatment of, 485
Spider, in ear, 95
Spinal accessory lymph nodes, 387, 388*t*
Spinal accessory nerve, 387
Splinting, mandibular fracture, 528
Squamous cell carcinoma
    aerodigestive tract, 260
    in airway obstruction, 356
    diagnosis of, 426
    differential diagnosis of, 508
    dysphagia with in alcoholic man, 288
    of ear, 516*f*
    epistaxis with, 210
    of face and scalp, 515
    of glottis, 337
    of head and neck, 506
        treatment options for, 610-611
    in itchy ears, 86
    versus keratoacanthoma, 510*t*
    laryngeal, 26, 355-356
    lymphatic spread of, 260
    metastatic, 425
        to neck, 415
    in nasal obstruction, 157*f*
    nasopharyngeal, 276-277
    oral, AIDS-related, 645
    in referred otalgia, 51
    supraglottic, 630
    of tongue, 261*f*
    ulcerating external auditory canal, 96*f*
    upper neck, 412*f*
Squamous epithelium, migration of, 77
Squamous papillomas, 512
    oropharyngeal, 250
SS-A antibodies, 439
SS-A autoantibodies, 421
SS-A autoantibody tests, 405
SS-B antibodies, 439
SS-B autoantibodies, 421
SS-B autoantibody tests, 405
Stapes, 57*f*
    disruption from oval window, 44-45
Staphylococcus
    in acute otitis media, 45
    in AIDS-related sinusitis, 643
    aureus
        in bacterial lymphadenopathy, 402
        coagulase-positive in suppurative sialadenitis, 405-406
        in diffuse bacterial external otitis, 36
        in epistaxis, 214
        of external ear, 97

in rhinosinusitis, 193, 194
in supraglottitis, 357
with chemical peel, 544
in furunculosis, 41-42
in rhinosinusitis, 194
in suppurative sialadenitis, 436
Stensen's duct
injury to, 537
traumatic injury to, 448
Sternocleidomastoid muscle, 16, 383
Sternotomy, 463
Steroid nasal sprays
for AIDS-related sinusitis, 643
for allergic rhinitis, 170-171
Steroids
for aphthous stomatitis, 644
for aphthous ulcers, 241
for chemical peel scarring, 545
for chronic otitis media, 46
for congenital neck masses, 423
for contact dermatitis, 93
for facial paralysis, 496
for hemangiomas, 401
for nasal polyps, 156
for psoriasis of auricle, 98
for upper airway obstruction, 347
Stevens-Johnson syndrome, 234, 252-254
Stomatitis, 234
chemotherapy-induced, 253f
recurring aphthous, 241
Streptococcus
in bacterial lymphadenopathy, 402
with chemical peel, 544
in diffuse bacterial external otitis, 36
group A, in inflammatory neck masses, 421
pneumoniae
rhinosinusitis in, 193
in supraglottitis, 357
pyogenes, 36
in rhinosinusitis, 194
in suppurative sialadenitis, 436
viridans, 357
Stress-related aphthous ulcers, 245
Stroke
aspiration after, 365, 366t, 367
in dysphagia, 285
laryngotracheal separation after, 379
Styloid process, elongated, 239
Subclavian steal, 126
Subcutaneous hemangiomas, 400-401
Subglottic airway obstruction
diagnosis and management of, 347-349

tracheostomy stomal granulation tissue in, 349-350
Subglottic secretions, continuous suction of, 374
Subglottic stenosis, 347-348
Sublingual glands, 233, 429
masses in, 431
secretomotor innervation of, 431-432
Submandibular duct stone, 437f
Submandibular glands, 232-233, 429
masses in, 431
neoplasms of, 416-417
malignant, 446
physical examination of, 236
secretomotor innervation of, 431-432
Submandibular lymph nodes, 385-386
anatomical areas drained by, 388t
Submaxillary glands, masses in, 431
Submental lymph nodes, 384, 385-386
anatomical areas drained by, 388t
Submucosal carcinoma, 23
Subperiosteal abscess, 186f
Subphrenic abscess, 560
Sulfonamides
oral lesions with, 234
in Stevens-Johnson syndrome, 254
Sun exposure, 506, 539-540
Sunscreens, 541
Suppressive thyroid therapy, 459-461
Suppurative labyrinthitis, 118
Supraclavicular lymph nodes, 387
Supraglottic cancer, 628
from epiglottis, 629f
late-stage presentation of, 630-631
obstructing, 357f
treatment of, 629-632
Supraglottic obstruction, 357-361
Supraglottic tumors, 356
Supraglottitis, infectious, 357-358
Suprathreshold tests, 662
Surgery
for advanced oral cavity cancer, 613-614
for allergic fungal sinusitis, 172
for *Aspergillus* sinusitis, 639-640
for aspiration, 376-377
aspiration after, 367
for basal cell carcinoma, 514
for branchial abnormalities, 398
for chronic otitis media, 46
for dizziness, 129
for epistaxis, 216
facial rejuvenation, 548-553
for glottic cancer, 625-626

Surgery—*continued*
  for goiter, 463
  for head and neck squamous cell cancer, 610-611
  for hyperparathyroidism, 472-473
  for keratoacanthoma, 510
  for laryngeal cancer of vocal folds, 334-335
  for Meniere's disease, 116
  for neoplastic neck masses, 425
  for obstructive sleep apnea, 312*t*, 315-318
  for olfactory disorders, 657-658
  for rhinosinusitis, 196-199
  for supraglottic cancer, 629-632
  for thyroid cancer, 450, 466-468
  for tinnitus, 141
Surgical debridement
  for mucormycosis, 637
  for mucormycosis with diabetes, 639
Surgical excision
  of lymphangiomas, 400
  for squamous papilloma, 512
  of thyroglossal duct cysts, 396
  of Warthin's tumor, 411
Surgical instruments, 5*f*
Surgical resection, basal cell carcinoma, 513
Surgicel, 213
Susruta, 8
Swallow scintigraphy, 371-372
Swallowing, 265
  after oral cavity radiation therapy, 623
  anatomy and physiology of, 279-284
  difficulty in. *See* Dysphagia
  endoscopic examination of, 372-373
  esophageal phase of, 283-284, 285*f*
  evaluation of, 284-285
  flexible endoscopic examination of, 299
  oral phase of, 282, 283*f*
  oral preparation phase of, 282
  painful. *See* Odynophagia
  pharyngeal phase of, 282-283, 284*f*
  therapy for in aspiration, 376
Swallowing rehabilitation
  after supraglottic laryngectomy, 630
  for oral cavity cancer, 619-621
Swimmer's ear, 36
Swimming, 88
Synchronous primary cancers, 609
Syncope, 125
Syndrome of inappropriate antidiuretic hormone, 615

Syphilis
  dizziness with, 118
  oral chancre of, 251*f*
  oral lesions of, 234, 250
Systemic disease
  dermatologic, 97-99
  nasopharyngeal effects of, 271-274
Systemic lupus erythematosus
  itchy ears with, 99
  management of aural itching in, 87*f*

T-staging
  of glottic cancer, 610*t*
  of oral cavity carcinoma, 610*t*
T_4 suppression, 459-461
Tachycardia, 107
Tagliocotti, Gasparo, 9-10
  patient of, 10*f*
Tandem walk, 108
Taste
  centers for, 664
  sensitivity of, 659
Taste buds, giant, 16
Taste cells, 658
Taste disorders, 650. *See also* Gustatory disorders
  management algorithm for, 651*f*
Taste hallucinations, 659
Taste stimuli thresholds, 662
Tear ducts, drainage of, 148-149
Technetium-99-labeled scintigraphy, 455
  for aspiration, 371-372
  for salivary gland disorders, 435
Teflon injection, 376-377
Telecanthus
  increased intercanthal distance in, 222*f*
  in nasal fracture, 221
Temporal bone
  computed tomographic scan of, 62*f*
  fractures of
    with facial nerve paralysis, 129
    in facial paralysis, 497
    longitudinal, 120-122
    vertigo with, 119-122
Temporomandibular joint
  disease of, 481
  facial pain in, 479
  in ear pain, 32-34
  pain, 185
  in referred otalgia, 51
Temporomandibular joint syndrome, 189
Teratomas, 396

Index   703

Terminal sulcus, 232
Tetracaine, 207
Tetracycline, 486
Thalidomide
　for aphthous stomatitis, 644
　for Behçet's syndrome, 241
Thermal injury, ear, 96
Thoracic esophageal disorders, 281t
Thoracic inlet, 595
Thoracic sympathetic nerve inflammation, 561
Thoracotomy, 463
Thorazine, 564-565
Three-drop tests, 662
Throat
　allergic conditions of, 161, 174-175
　foreign objects in, 11
Thrombophlebitis, with otitis media, 50f
Thrush
　oral, 251, 252f, 634-635
　treatment of, 242-244
Thymic cysts, 399
Thyroglossal duct, 451
　cysts of, 451
　　diagnosis and management of, 395-396
　　removal of, 395f
Thyroid artery, superior, 451
Thyroid-binding globulin, 451-452
Thyroid cartilage, 16
Thyroid function tests, 451-452
　for goiter, 463
Thyroid glands
　anatomy of, 450-451
　cancer of, 466
　　incidence of, 450
　　management of, 466-468
　　occurrence, survival, and characteristics of, 467t
　carcinoma of
　　aplastic, 467
　　risk of, 452
　cysts of, 458f
　disorders of, 473
　masses in, 453f
　　with airway obstruction, 350f
　　tracheal deviation with, 456f, 457f
　neoplasms of
　　benign, 411-412
　　malignant, 418-420
　palpable, 16
　vascular supply to, 450-451

Thyroid hormone
　production and secretion of, 451
　suppression of, 464-465
Thyroid isthmus, 450
Thyroid lobes, 450
Thyroid lymphomas, 420
Thyroid nodules
　carcinoma of, 455t
　differential diagnosis of, 460t
　disease of
　　fine-needle-aspiration biopsy for, 457-459
　　history of, 452
　　physical examination for, 453-454
　　with substernal goiter, 464
　　suppressive therapy for, 459-461
　　work-up for, 454-455
　fine-needle-aspiration biopsy of, 457-459
Thyroid-stimulating hormone
　assessment of, 454
　levels of, 451-452
　suppression of, 459-461
Thyroid ultrasound, 455
Thyroxine (T_4), 451-452
　suppression of, 459-461
TIE reaction, 166
Tinnitus, 132
　anatomy and physiology of, 132-134
　causes of, 137t
　danger signs in, 141
　depression and, 135
　diagnostic evaluation of, 137-138
　differential diagnosis for, 136
　history for, 134-135
　incidence of, 132
　management algorithm for, 133f
　management and follow-up for, 138-141
　with noise-induced hearing loss, 139
　objective, 136, 137t
　　arteriovenous malformation in, 138
　physical examination for, 135-136
　pulsatile, 136
　with sensorineural hearing loss, 68
　subjective, 136, 137t
Titanium dioxide, 541
TNM staging, 610t
Tobacco
　in aerodigestive tract squamous cell carcinoma, 260
　in head and neck cancer, 632
　in hoarseness, 333-335
　in leukoplakia, 256

Toenail, fungal infection of, 168
Tongue
  anatomy of, 232
  angioneurotic edema of, 358*f*
  base of, 16
  cancer of, 608
  decreased mobility of after oral cavity cancer, 621
  fissured, 242*f*
  functions of, 231
  hairy leukoplakia of, 644
  leukoplakia of, 607*f*
  lymphangioma of, 259
  mucosal lesions of, 231
  primary closure of, 618*f*
  small lateral tumor of, 616*f*
  squamous cell carcinoma of, 261*f*
  in swallowing, 282, 283
  trauma to, 258
  wandering rash of, 238
Tongue depressor, 4, 207
Tongue devices, 315
Tongue muscle, neoplasm of, 23
Tonsillar enlargement, 361*f*
Tonsillar pillars, 282
Tonsillectomy
  to cure snoring, 3
  for infectious mononucleosis, 362
  for obstructive sleep apnea, 318
Tonsillitis
  acute bacterial, 249
  acute follicular, 250*f*
Tonsils, fish bone embedded in, 587*f*
Topographic anatomy, head and neck, 13-26
Tornwaldt's bursa, 266
Tornwaldt's cysts, 275
Torticollis, congenital, 399
Torus mandibularis, 239-240, 243*f*
Torus palatinus, 240, 244*f*
Torus tubarius, 15*f*, 265
  visualization of, 268
Touch-perception fibers, 481
Toxic shock syndrome, 214
Toxic thyroid nodules, 450, 465
Toxins, 127
  in gustatory dysfunction, 659
Toxoplasma gondii, 405
Toxoplasmosis
  in granulomatous lymphadenopathy, 405
  treatment of, 424
Toynbee maneuver, 31-32

Toynbee otoscope, 4
Trabecular adenomas, 411
Tracheal mucosal injury, 349
Tracheal rings, 16
Tracheitis, 626
Tracheobronchial foreign body, 573-575
Tracheoesophageal puncture, 627
Tracheoesophageal speech prosthesis, 627-628
Tracheostoma, 626
Tracheostomy
  aspiration with, 369-371
  for bacterial lymphadenopathy, 402
  permanent, 576*f*
  for squamous cell carcinoma, 356
  for upper airway obstruction, 342, 345, 347
Tracheostomy stomal granulation tissue, 349-350
Tracheostomy tube
  for aspirated secretions, 370-371
  for aspiration, 374
  placement of, 576*f*
  removal of for aspiration, 374-376
Tragus, 54
  skin tag on, 58*f*
Transient ischemic attacks, 126
Trapezius muscle, 383
Trauma
  auricular, 35
    hematoma with, 37*f*
    treatment of, 36*t*
  in differential diagnosis of dizziness, 114*t*
  facial, 523-538
  in facial asymmetry, 501-502
  in facial paralysis, 497
  multisystem, 523
  nasal, 209
  in nasal obstruction, 152*t*
  to oral cavity, 257-258
  oral manifestations of, 256-258
  salivary gland, 434*t*, 448
  sinus-type symptoms with, 188*t*
  vertigo with, 119-122
Trench mouth, 249-250
Tretinoin (Retin-A), 541
  before chemical peeling, 542
Triamcinolone
  for aphthous ulcers, 245
  for rhinosinusitis, 194
Triamcinolone acetonide (Nasacort), 170
Trichloroacetic acid, 542-543
Trichophyton, 166

Tricyclic antidepressants
  for atypical odontalgia, 487
  for burning-mouth syndrome, 663
  for deafferentation pain, 481
  for myofascial pain, 486
Trigeminal nerve, 650
  innervating sinuses, 188-189
  in taste-mediating sensations, 658
Triiodothyronine (T_3), 451-452
Trimalar fracture, 529
  displaced, 531f
Trimethoprim-sulfamethoxazole, 45
Tripod fracture, 529
Trismus, 153, 159
Trisulfapyrimidines, 405, 424
TSH. *See* Thyroid-stimulating hormone
Tuberculin test, 404
Tuberculosis
  AIDS-related, 646
  diagnosed as carcinoma, 404
  diagnosis and management of, 424
  in immunocompromised patient, 642
  nasopharyngeal lesions in, 273-274
  oropharyngeal, 251
Tucker bougienage, 600-601
Tullio's phenomenon, 118
Tumarkin, crisis of, 115
Tumors
  CNS, 126
  extirpation of for oral cancer, 613
  of hypopharynx, 353f
  nasopharyngeal, 276-278
  neurogenic neck, 406-407
  resection of
    oral cavity, 617-619
      primary closure of tongue after, 618f
    thyroid, 350f
    upper airway, 348t
Tuning fork tests, 59
  for tinnitus, 136
Turkey gobbler deformity, 550
Tympanic canal, 11
Tympanic membrane, 17-18, 56, 57f
  in acute otitis media, 46f
  cerumen impaction obscuring, 75
  disorders of, 43-45
  in ear pain, 31
  examination of, 58-59
  granulation tissue near, 91f
  movement of, 31-32
  normal, 19f
  paper patching of, 44
  perforation of, 100

  in chronic otitis media, 46, 47f, 48
  in hearing loss, 70-71
  irrigation and, 81-83
  traumatic, 43-45
  testing mobility of, 4
  translucency of, 59
  trauma to, 590
  with cerumen removal, 79
Tympanometry, 137

UltraPulse 5000 laser, 546
Ultrasonography
  for bacterial lymphadenopathy, 402
  for malignant thyroid gland neoplasms, 418-419
  for neck masses, 422
  for oral cavity lesions, 236
  for thyroid gland diseases, 459
Ultraviolet A light, 539-540
Ultraviolet B light, 539
  in basal cell carcinoma, 512
University of Pennsylvania Smell Identification Test (UPSIT), 656, 657
Upper airway
  foreign bodies in, 11
  obstruction of, 342
    history of, 345-346
    locations of, 308f
    major causes of, 348t
    management of, 346-347
    physical examination for, 344-345
    pulmonary function tests for, 346
    radiologic studies of, 346
    signs of, 342-343
    specific pathologic processes associated with, 347-362
Upper respiratory infections
  in anosmia, 656
  in gustatory dysfunction, 659-660
  hoarseness from, 325
  in nasal obstruction, 150
  in olfactory disorders, 654, 655t
U.S. Consumer Products Safety Commission, 593
U.S. Poison Control Center, 593
Utricle, 102, 104
Uveoparotid fever, 441
Uvula, unusual configurations of, 238
Uvulopalatopharyngoplasty
  anatomical changes during, 318f
  for obstructive sleep apnea, 314, 317
Uvulotomy, 3

Vagal interruption, 369
Vagal nerve, 650
Vagal paraganglioma, 408
　aspiration with, 370
Vagal stimulation, 564
Vagus nerve
　in hiccups, 559
　inflammation of, 561
　path of, 368f
　vestibular nucleus and, 105
Vallecula, 26
Valproic acid, 564t, 565
Valsalva maneuver, 4
van Helmont, Jan Baptista, 2
Vancomycin, 194
Vapocoolant sprays, 564
Varicella virus, 247
Vascular cephalgia, 188t
Vascular disorders, 114t
Vascular headaches, 189
Vascular loop, 126
Vascular malformations, 133-134
Vascular neoplasms, 133-134
Vascular studies, 137
Vasoconstrictors
　for epistaxis, 207
　rebound from, 148
Vasodilators, 129
Vasomotor rhinitis, 149-150
　in nasal obstruction, 150
VDRL testing, 118
Velopharynx, 595
Venography, 137
Vermis, 105
Verrucous carcinoma, 515
Vertebral artery, 565
Vertigo
　benign paroxysmal positional, 119, 120
　　canalith repositioning procedure for, 121f
　cholesteatoma causing, 123
　psychogenic, 128
　in serous labyrinthitis, 118-119
　with temporal bone fracture, 119-122
Vesalius, Andreas, 2
Vestibular autorotation testing, 111-112
Vestibular exercises, 129
Vestibular labyrinth, 102
Vestibular nerve section, 129
Vestibular neuronitis
　case history of, 117
　diagnosis and management of, 115-117
Vestibular rehabilitation, 123

Vestibular spinal tract
　lateral, 106f
　medial, 106f
Vestibular suppressants
　for dizziness, 128-129
　for Meniere's disease, 115
　for vestibular neuronitis, 117
Vestibular system
　dysfunction of, 102
　pathways of, 105, 106f
　peripheral, 53
　physiology of, 104-105
Vestibular testing
　for dizziness, 108
　for tinnitus, 137
Vestibulo-ocular reflex, 105, 106f
Vestibulospinal reflex, 105, 106f
Video laryngostroboscopy
　for hoarseness, 329
　typical setup for, 332f
Videostroboscopy
　for aspiration, 373
　for presbylarynx, 372
Vincent's angina, 249-250
Viral infections
　in neck masses, 423-424
　of oral cavity, 246-250
Viral lymphadenopathy, 401-402
Viral warts, head, 506
Visual acuity assessment, 524
Visual changes, 185
Vitamin A
　for gustatory disorders, 663
　for olfactory disorders, 658
Vitamin D, 98
Vocal abuse, 339t
Vocal cord medialization, 370
Vocal cords
　cancer arising on, 624f
　cysts of, 338t
　fixation of, 353-354
　granuloma of, 335
　　cause and treatment of, 338t
　immobility of, 370
　laryngoscopic view of, 17f
　in midline position during phonation, 330f
　paralysis of, 16, 330f
　　aspiration due to, 368-369
　　causes of, 352-353
　　in dysphagia, 283
　　examination for, 454
　　in glottic obstruction, 351-352

with thyroid cancer surgery, 468
treatment of, 332
polyps of, 338*t*
visualization of, 4
Vocal folds
assessing motion of, 329
benign polyps of, 355
false, 16
immobility of, 350
unilateral, 352
irregular mucosa of, 26
laryngeal cancer of, 333-335, 336
lesions of, 348*t*
mobility disorders of, 348*t*
nodules of, 331
hoarseness with, 333
paradoxical motion of, 354-355
paralysis of, 350
with mediastinal adenopathy, 334
unilateral, 331
in upper airway obstruction, 348*t*
true, 16
Vocal hygiene, 336, 338
Vocal mechanism education, 339
Vocal personality type, 327-328
Vocal production, 339
Voice disorders, 325
danger signs for, 340
diagnosis and management of, 329-336
history of, 326-328
physical examination for, 328-329
prevention of, 336-337
therapy of, 337-339
Voice production, 325
Voice quality, 328*t*
Voice therapy
for hoarseness, 337-339
for laryngeal muscle tension, 335
Vomer, 218
visualization of, 268
Vomiting, reticular system in, 105
von Recklinghausen's disease, 407
Vosol
for diffuse bacterial external otitis, 38
for furunculosis, 42

Wallenberg's syndrome, 126
Warthin-Starry silver stain, 403
Warthin's tumor, 410-411, 442
Weber-Rendu-Osler syndrome, 259
Weber tuning fork test
for acoustic neuroma, 61
for hearing loss, 59

Wedders, Tomas, 7-8
Wegener's granulomatosis, 347-348
Weight loss
for obstructive sleep apnea, 312-313
for snoring, 307
Weisman, August, 11
Welch Allyn LumiView, 23*f*
Wepfer, Johann Jakob, 2-3
Wharton's duct, 232-233
impacted salivary stone of, 235*f*
inflammatory obstruction of, 436*f*, 437
Wheal, 163
Wicking, 38-39
Wigand procedure, 197
Wilde, Sir William, 4
Willis, Thomas, 3
Woodruff's plexus, 205
World Health Organization, nasopharyngeal carcinoma classification of, 611
Wrinkling, causes of, 539-540

X-linked agammaglobulinemia, 641
Xerostomia
AIDS-related, 647
in diabetes mellitus, 634
with glandular lymphocytic infiltration, 438
in HIV infection, 441
psychoactive agent-induced, 255
radiation-induced, 434*t*, 448
in salivary gland disorder, 439
with Sjögren's syndrome, 242-244
Xylocaine, 95

Yankauer suction, 207
Yawning, 265
chronic, 11

Zenker's diverticulum
in dysphagia, 289-290
in elderly man, 291
management of, 301
Zerbi, 2
Ziehl-Neelsen staining, 403
Zinc, 658
Zinc oxide, 541
Zinc pyrithione shampoo, 99
Zygoma, 528-529
fractured with resultant trismus, 531*f*
Zygomatic arch fractures, 531-532
Zygomatic complex fracture, 529-531
Zygomatic trauma, 528-532
Zygomaticomaxillary fracture, 535